SECOND EDITION

ADVANCED PRACTICE NURSING

Evolving Roles for the Transformation of the Profession

Edited by

SUSAN M. DENISCO, CNL
Associate Professor of Nursing
Sacred Heart University
Fairfield, Connecticut

ANNE M. BARKER, EDD, RN
Professor of Nursing
Sacred Heart University
Fairfield, Connecticut

JONES & BARTLETT
LEARNING

World Headquarters
Jones & Bartlett Learning
5 Wall Street
Burlington, MA 01803
978-443-5000
info@jblearning.com
www.jblearning.com

Jones & Bartlett Learning books and products are available through most bookstores and online booksellers. To contact Jones & Bartlett Learning directly, call 800-832-0034, fax 978-443-8000, or visit our website, www.jblearning.com.

The authors, editor, and publisher have made every effort to provide accurate information. However, they are not responsible for errors, omissions, or for any outcomes related to the use of the contents of this book and take no responsibility for the use of the products and procedures described. Treatments and side effects described in this book may not be applicable to all people; likewise, some people may require a dose or experience a side effect that is not described herein. Drugs and medical devices are discussed that may have limited availability controlled by the Food and Drug Administration (FDA) for use only in a research study or clinical trial. Research, clinical practice, and government regulations often change the accepted standard in this field. When consideration is being given to use of any drug in the clinical setting, the health care provider or reader is responsible for determining FDA status of the drug, reading the package insert, and reviewing prescribing information for the most up-to-date recommendations on dose, precautions, and contraindications, and determining the appropriate usage for the product. This is especially important in the case of drugs that are new or seldom used.

Production Credits

Publisher: Kevin Sullivan
Acquisitions Editor: Amanda Harvey
Editorial Assistant: Sara Bempkins
Associate Production Editor: Cindie Bryan
Marketing Manager: Elena McAnespie
Associate Marketing Manager: Katie Hennessy
V.P., Manufacturing and Inventory Control:
  Therese Connell
Composition: Arlene Apone
Permissions: Danny Meldung, Photo Affairs, Inc.
Cover Design: Kristin E. Parker
Cover Image: © Creatas/ShutterStock, Inc.
Printing and Binding: Malloy, Inc.
Cover Printing: Malloy, Inc.

Some images in this book feature models. These models do not necessarily endorse, represent, or participate in the activities represented in the images.

Library of Congress Cataloging-in-Publication Data
Advanced practice nursing : evolving roles for the transformation of the profession / [edited by] Susan DeNisco, Anne M. Barker. -- 2nd ed.
   p. ; cm.
Includes bibliographical references and index.
ISBN 978-1-4496-6506-7 (pbk.) -- ISBN 1-4496-6506-3 (pbk.)
I. DeNisco, Susan. II. Barker, Anne M.
[DNLM: 1. Advanced Practice Nursing--trends. 2. Nurse's Role. WY 128]
   610.73--dc23
                    2011042012

6048

Printed in the United States of America
16 15 14 13 12   10 9 8 7 6 5 4 3 2 1

Contents

Contributors

Anne M. Barker, EdD, RN
Professor of Nursing
Sacred Heart University
Fairfield, Connecticut

Emily Barey, MSN, RN
Director of Nursing Informatics
Epic Systems Corporation
Madison, Wisconsin

Audrey Beauvais, DNP, MSN, MBA, RN-C, CNL
Assistant Professor of Nursing
Sacred Heart University

Michael Carter, DNSc, APRN, BC, FAAN
Dean Emeritus
College of Nursing
The University of Tennessee, Memphis
Memphis, Tennessee

Lisa Astalos Chism, DNP, GNP, BC, NCMP, FAANP
Nurse Practitioner
Alexander J. Walt Comprehensive Breast Center
High Risk Breast Clinic
Karmanos Cancer Institute
Detroit, Michigan

Anita Finkelman, MSN, RN
Visiting Faculty, School of Nursing, Bouvé College of Health Sciences
Northeastern University
Boston, Massachusetts

Michelle Godin, RN, EdD, BC, CNA
Saint Mary's Hospital
Waterbury, Connecticut

Susan R. Gortner, MN, PhD, FAAN
Professor Emeritus
University of California, San Francisco
San Francisco, California

Janet Houser, PhD, RN
Academic Dean, Rueckert-Hartman College for Health Professions
Regis University
Denver, Colorado

Janet W. Kenney, RN, PhD

Jacqueline M. Loversidge, PhD(c), MS, RN, C
Assistant Professor
Ohio State University
Columbia, Ohio

Jeri A. Milstead, PhD, RN, FAAN
Professor and Dean
College of Nursing
The University of Toledo
Toledo, Ohio

George D. Pozgar, MBA, CHE
Consultant and Hospital Surveyor
Gp Health Care Consulting, International
Annapolis, Maryland
Surveyor
The Joint Commission
Oakbrook Terrace, Illinois

Joyce Pulcini, PhD, RNCS, PNP, FAAN
Associate Professor
School of Nursing
Boston College
Chestnut Hill, Massachusetts

Leiyu Shi, DrPH, MBA, MPA
Professor
Johns Hopkins School of Public Health
Co-Director
Johns Hopkins Primary Care Policy Center for
    the Underserved
Johns Hopkins University
Baltimore, Maryland

Douglas A. Singh, PhD, MBA
Associate Professor
School of Public Health and
    Environmental Affairs
Indiana University, South Bend
South Bend, Indiana

Patricia St. Hill, PhD, RN, MPH
Associate Professor
Hunter-Bellevue School of Nursing
Hunter College of the City University of
    New York
New York, New York

Dori Taylor Sullivan, PhD, RN, CAN, CPHQ
Associate Dean and Professor
School of Nursing
Duke University
Durham, North Carolina

Harry A. Sultz, DDS, MPH
Professor Emeritus
School of Preventive Medicine
School of Medicine and Biomedical Sciences
Dean Emeritus
School of Health Related Professions
State University of New York at Buffalo
Buffalo, New York

John G. Twomey, PhD, RN
Associate Professor
MGH Institute of Health Professions
Boston, Massachusetts

**Catherine Tymkow, DNP, APN,
    WHNP-BC, CNE**
Associate Professor
College of Health and Human Services
Governors State University
University Park, Illinois

Deborah Washington, RN, MSN
Director
Diversity, Patient Care Service
Massachusetts General Hospital
Boston, Massachusetts

Jill White, RN, RM, MEd, PhD
Dean
Faculty of Nursing
Midwifery and Health
University of Technology
Sydney, Australia

Karen A. Wolf, PhD, APRN, BC
Clinical Associate Professor and Chair of
    Generalist Level Nursing
Graduate Program in Nursing
MGH Institute of Health Professions
Boston, Massachusetts

**Mary E. Zaccagnini, DNP, RN,
    ACNS-BC, AOCN**
Clinical Associate Professor
University of Minnesota, School
    of Nursing
Minneapolis, Minnesota

Introduction

Advanced practice nursing education has been rapidly evolving over the past decade, with much attention given to the unique differences between "advance practice nursing" and the four traditional advanced practice roles—that is, certified registered nurse anesthetists (CRNAs), certified nurse–midwives (CNMs), clinical specialists (CNSs), and nurse practitioners (NPs)—as direct care providers. The second edition of this book was conceived in response to several new national initiatives including the evolution of the doctor of nursing practice (DNP) degree and the American Association of Colleges of Nursing's (AACN) recently revised *Essentials of Master's Education for Advanced Practice Nursing* (2011). These initiatives, which were developed in response to healthcare reform legislation and the focus on patient safety and quality care, have provided curricular guidance to master's programs transitioning to the doctoral level for advanced practice. The content of this book was then cross-referenced with *The Essentials of Doctoral Education for Advanced Nursing Practice* (AACN, 2006). The task force that developed the *Doctoral Essentials* built their work on the former *Master's Essentials*. **Table I-1** displays the new essential core curriculum content for both the master's and doctoral programs. The last column lists the chapters in this book that address this content.

The publisher, Jones & Bartlett Learning, under the guidance of editor Susan M. DeNisco, embarked on a quest to produce a new book that would compile selected chapters from existing books in the Jones & Bartlett Learning collection. The strength of this approach is that experts in each of the content areas author each chapter in the book.

The revision of this textbook comprehensively addresses the core curriculum content requirements of the MSN and DNP *Essentials,* recognizing that broad content areas and role competencies cannot be covered in separate courses due to credit limitations. In addition, this book addresses an audience of nurses in a variety of advanced practice nurse roles, including nurse executives, nurse educators, and entrepreneurs—not just those nurses who provide direct clinical care.

This book is divided into six parts that are meant to be read in sequence:

1. Professional Roles for the Advanced Practice Nurse
2. Healthcare Delivery Systems and Health Policy for Advanced Practice: Core Knowledge
3. Quality, Safety, and Information Systems for Advanced Practice
4. Theoretical Foundations, Research, and Evidence-Based Practice
5. The Role of Race, Culture, Ethics, and Advocacy in Advanced Nursing Practice
6. Leadership and Role Transition for the Advanced Practice Nurse

The goal of the book is to provide core knowledge that all nurses in advanced practice roles require, regardless of their specialty or functional focus. This knowledge can then be built

TABLE I-1 Comparison of *Master's Essentials, Doctoral Essentials,* and Book Content

Master's Essentials 2011	Doctoral Essentials	Book
I. Scientific and Humanistic Background for Practice	I. Scientific Underpinnings for Practice	Chapters 17 and 18
II. Organizational and Systems Leadership	II. Organizational and Systems Leadership for Quality Improvement and Systems Thinking	Chapters 8–12
III. Quality Improvement and Safety	II. Organizational and Systems Leadership for Quality Improvement and Systems Thinking; IV. Information Systems/Technology and Patient Care Technology for the Improvement and Transformation of Health Care	Chapter 13
IV. Translating and Integrating Scholarship into Practice	III. Clinical Scholarship and Analytical Methods for Evidence-Based Practice	Chapters 19–21
V. Informatics and Healthcare Technologies	IV. Information Systems/Technology and Patient Care Technology for the Improvement and Transformation of Health Care	Chapters 14–16
VI. Health Policy and Advocacy	V. Health Care Policy for Advocacy in Health Care	Chapters 6–11, 25, and 26
VII. Interprofessional Collaboration for Improving Patient and Population Health Outcomes	VI. Interprofessional Collaboration for Improving Patient and Population Health Outcomes	Chapters 24 and 30
VIII. Clinical Prevention and Population Health for Improving Health	VII. Clinical Prevention and Population Health for Improving the Nation's Health	Chapters 6, 7, and 22–24
IX. Master's-Level Nursing Practice	VIII. Advanced Nursing Practice	Chapters 1–5 and 27–29

upon as graduate students precede into their specialty foci.

New to this edition are the following topic and content areas:

- Focus on both direct and indirect provider roles
- Role of the clinical doctorate in advanced practice nursing
- Reimbursement and credentialing issues for nurse practitioners
- Federal and state regulation of advanced practice nursing
- Budgeting and finances for advanced practice
- Electronic health records and clinical informatics
- Evidence-based practice and clinical scholarship
- Special populations and healthcare disparities
- Role transition and professional development

The content of this book has been carefully selected based on the editor's 26 years' experience as a primary care provider, educator, and administrator. This content is essential to all levels of graduate nursing preparation. With the recent revision and sophistication of the *Master's Essentials,* there is closer application in each content area to the *Doctoral Essentials.* Thus the book can be used in both master's-level and post-baccalaureate doctoral programs in the beginning core courses to lay a foundation for advanced nursing practice. As with any textbook, additional scholarly readings, especially research- and evidence-based articles, will enhance the content.

As previously mentioned, some confusion exists regarding the terminology "advanced nursing practice" versus "advanced practice nursing." Over time, the terms "advanced practice nursing" and "advanced practice nurses" have become commonly used to indicate master's-prepared nurses who provide direct clinical care and include the roles of clinical nurse specialist, nurse practitioner, certified nurse–midwife, and certified registered nurse anesthetist, with the last three roles requiring a license beyond the basic RN license to practice. This book has adopted a broader, more inclusive definition (AACN, 2004), which reflects the current thinking about advanced practice. Advanced practice nursing is defined as follows:

> Any form of nursing intervention that influences health care outcomes for individuals or populations, including direct care of individual patients, management of care for individuals and populations, administration of nursing and health care organizations, and the development and implementation of health policy. (p. 2)

In this book, nurses in advanced practice are defined as any nurse who holds a master's degree or higher in nursing and whose role is consistent with this definition. "Advanced practice nursing," "advanced practice nurses," and "advanced nursing practice" are used interchangeably throughout the book.

Currently, several major professional forces are influencing graduate education in nursing and promise to have dramatic effects on nursing education both today and into at least the next decade:

- The 2010 Affordable Care Act represents the broadest healthcare overhaul legislation passed since the 1965 creation of the Medicare and Medicaid programs.
- The Institute of Medicine report *The Future of Nursing: Leading Change, Advancing Health* (2010) positions nurse regulators to provide leadership on the critically important challenge of assigning accountability for quality and patient safety at the state and local levels.
- The clinical doctorate, designated as a doctor of nursing practice (DNP), has been mandated as the entry to advanced nursing practice (see the introduction to Part 1 for more details).
- A consensus model for advanced practice nurse regulations has been developed through work by the Advanced Practice

Registered Nurse Consensus group (2008) and the National Council of the State Boards of Nursing (NCSBN).

■ A new role in nursing, the clinical nurse leader (CNL), has been introduced. This role is designed to address many of the problems currently evident in health care, including the nursing shortage, patient safety and medical errors, and fragmentation of the healthcare system. The AACN (2007) provides this definition of the CNL:

The CNL functions within a microsystem and assumes accountability for healthcare outcomes for a specific group of clients within a unit or setting through the assimilation and application of research-based information to design, implement, and evaluate client plans of care. The CNL is a provider and a manager of care at the point of care to individuals and cohorts. The CNL designs, implements, and evaluates client care by coordinating, delegating, and supervising the care provided by the health care team, including licensed nurses, technicians, and other health professionals. (p. 6)

■ CNLs are considered generalists who will be prepared at the master's level and require the same core curriculum knowledge as do other master's-prepared nurses.

In both the *Master's Essentials* and *Doctoral Essentials* documents, the AACN lays out the foundation for core knowledge needed by all graduate nursing students. This book provides in one manuscript a foundation for this core knowledge. It does not address any of the specific content needed by the specialties. Moreover, this foundational content should be further integrated and applied throughout the rest of the curriculum.

Professional Roles for the Advanced Practice Nurse

In Part 1 of this book, we will consider the role of the advanced practice nurse from historical, present-day, and future perspectives. This content is intended to serve as a general introduction to select issues in professional role development for the advanced practice of nursing. As students progress in the educational process and develop greater knowledge and expertise, role issues and role transition should be integrated throughout the entire program.

In Chapter 1, Wolf presents a brief history of nursing and its progress toward professional practice. Although not specific to the role of the advanced practice nurse, the information presented in this chapter will assist the advanced practice nurse to gain a broader perspective on nursing and healthcare organizations and their future. This discussion lays the foundation for a deeper understanding of the historical development, current practice, and future opportunities for advanced practice in nursing.

In Chapter 2, Pulcini defines advanced practice nursing from a traditional perspective and traces the history of the roles. Traditionally, and as discussed by Pulcini, advanced practice has been limited to clinical roles and includes the clinical nurse specialist, nurse practitioner, certified nurse–midwife, and certified registered nurse anesthetist; the last three roles require a license beyond the basic RN license to practice. This book, however, uses an expanded definition of the advanced practice nursing that reflects current thinking. As you read this chapter, keep in mind this expanded definition and at the same time appreciate the development of the advanced clinical roles for nursing practice.

Since Pulcini's work in 2004, much has transpired related to the role and education of nurses for advanced practice. Most revolutionary is the mandate to have the clinical doctorate as the requirement for advanced clinical practice nursing by 2015 (American Association of Colleges of

Nursing, 2007). With this change, many master's programs for advanced practice nurses will transition to the doctoral level. The rationale for this position by the American Association of Colleges of Nursing (AACN) was based on several factors:

- The reality that current master's degree programs often require credit loads equivalent to doctoral degrees in other healthcare professions
- The changing complexity of the healthcare environment
- The need for the highest level of scientific knowledge and practice expertise to assure high-quality patient outcomes

In an effort to clarify the standards, titling, and outcomes of clinical doctorates, the Commission on Collegiate Nursing Education (CCNE)—the accreditation arm of AACN—has decided that only practice doctoral degrees awarding a doctorate of nursing practice (DNP) will be eligible for accreditation. In addition, the AACN has published *The Essentials of Doctoral Education for Advanced Nursing Practice,* which sets forth the standards for the development, implementation and program outcomes for DNP programs.

Needless to say, this recommendation has not been fully supported by the entire profession. For instance, the American Organization of Nurse Executives (AONE, 2007) does not support requiring a doctorate for managerial or executive practice based on expense, time commitment, and the cost benefit of the degree. It also suggests nurses may migrate toward a master's degree in business, social sciences, and public health in lieu of nursing. Further, AONE suggests there is a lack of evidence to support the need for doctoral education across all aspects of the care continuum. In contrast, doctoral and master's education for nurse managers and executives is encouraged.

For other advanced practice roles, including those of the clinical nurse leader, nurse educator,

and nurse researcher, a different set of educational requirements exists. The clinical nurse leader as a generalist will remain as a master's program. For nurse educators, the position of AACN, although not universally accepted within the profession (as demonstrated by the existence of master's programs in nursing education), is that didactic knowledge and practical experience in pedagogy is additive to advanced clinical knowledge. Nurse researchers will continue to be prepared in PhD programs. Thus there will only be two doctoral programs in nursing, the DNP and the PhD. It will be important for readers to keep abreast of this movement as the profession further develops and debates this issue for implications for their own practice and professional development and within their own specialty. The best resource for this is the AACN website and the websites of specialty organizations.

The last three chapters of Part 1 discuss the future of advanced practice nursing and the evolution of doctoral education—in particular, the practice doctorate. Within today's rapidly changing and complex healthcare environment, members of the nursing profession are challenging themselves to expand the role of advanced practice nursing to include highly skilled practitioners, leaders, educators, researchers, and policymakers.

In Chapter 3, Carter reviews the historical development of doctoral programs, which provides important background information regarding how the profession has arrived at the aforementioned decisions. Of particular note is his discussion of the controversy surrounding the development of the clinical doctoral programs. Carter traces the roots of the PhD for research and clinical doctorate for practice. As doctorates in nursing developed in the latter part of the last century, the emerging diversity in titling and role expectations called for clarity and direction for the profession.

In Chapter 4, Chism defines the DNP degree and compares and contrasts the research doctorate and the practice doctorate. The focus of the DNP degree is expertise in clinical practice. Additional foci include the *Essentials of Doctoral Education for Advanced Nursing Practice* as outlined by the AACN (2007), which include leadership, health policy and advocacy, and information technology. Role transitions for advanced practice nurses prepared at the doctoral level will call for an integration of roles focused on the provision of high-quality, patient-centered care.

Lastly, in Chapter 5, the authors discuss emerging roles of DNP graduates as nurse educators, nurse executives, and nurse entrepreneurs, along with advanced practice nurses' increased involvement in public health programming and integrative and complementary health modalities.

REFERENCES

American Association of Colleges of Nursing. (2007). Doctor of Nursing Practice. Retrieved from http://www.aacn.nche.edu/DNP/DNPPosition Statement.htm

American Organization of Nurse Executives. (2007). Consideration of the Doctorate of Nursing Practice. Retrieved from http://www.aone.org /aone/docs/PositionStatement060607.doc

CHAPTER 1

The Slow March to Professional Practice

Karen A. Wolf

CHAPTER OBJECTIVES

1. Define professionalism.
2. Discuss the development of nursing as a profession over the last century.
3. Consider future trends in nursing that have the potential to positively affect the profession of nursing.

INTRODUCTION

Nursing's quest for professionalism has shaped nursing education and practice, past and present, in the United States and abroad. The emergence of professional practice models over the past quarter century represents the latest in professionalizing trends. This effort by nurses and healthcare managers to restructure the workplace and nursing work highlights the evolution of nursing from a simple matter of tasks to the complexity of knowledge-based practice in rapidly changing healthcare organizations. The current healthcare environment is faced with a wide range of regulatory and financial pressures. These include demands to justify healthcare service outcomes, the drive to maintain biomedical and technological currency, and a recurrent nursing shortage. Looking back through nursing history, one can see that crises in the healthcare system create opportunities for nursing. Too often, nursing's responses to crises have not created outcomes that serve both the interests of the profession and the public. Today, as nurses once again find themselves in the midst of a crisis, there is an opportunity to renegotiate the organizational realities of health care and to advance the contribution of professional nursing to healthcare outcomes.

NURSING AS A PROFESSION: KEY IDEAS FOR INTEGRATION

What makes work professional work? Nursing has struggled with this question throughout its history. For most of the 20th century, nursing was considered a semiprofession or a profession in progress by sociologists (Bucher & Strauss, 1961; Etzioni, 1969). The attention that nursing leaders have given to professional development is manifest in the push for control over educational standards, efforts to develop a theory base for nursing practice, the growth of professional organizations and journals, and, more recently, the reorganization of nursing work within professional nursing practice models. The nature of professional nursing work differs today from what it did for the sacred three professions of medicine, law, and the clergy in 1900. The autonomous solo professional serving the public with expert knowledge and skill is now a rare phenomenon. Few occupations can claim pure professional autonomy, because the reach of corporate and institutional control now dominates most sectors of the economy.

Autonomy, a hallmark of professionalism, can be differentiated into autonomy of decision making relative to the client and/or patient care and autonomy from the employing institution (Manthey, 1991). Autonomous practitioners are those who have direct lines of access to clients, who are responsible for their own practice decisions, and who are accountable to clients, peers, and professional organizations, as well as to the courts, for their conduct (Marram, Schlegel, & Bevis, 1974). The nursing profession has struggled with the idea of autonomy because most nurses are employed and subordinated to the authority of organizations such as hospitals (Ashley, 1976; Reverby, 1987; Wolf, 1993). The claim to autonomy with regard to the freedom to make decisions about patient care has advanced over the past few decades, fueled by the development of primary nursing models (Hegyvary, 1982). More recently, health services research studies have integrated the concept of nursing autonomy. For example, a recent study by Aiken, Clarke, Sloane, Sochalski, and Silber (2002) suggested that increasing nursing autonomy and control over the practice setting was associated with improved patient care outcomes.

Nursing can no longer be viewed as a subsidiary function of medicine that is proscribed by doctors' orders; nursing care now reflects a patient-centered approach based on nursing theory and shaped by a nursing process of reasoning. Current legal and professional regulations legitimate this nurse-driven process of practice. The body of statutory and case law that governs nursing practice holds nurses accountable to a definition of practice that recognizes and codifies practice in accordance with current nursing knowledge and clinical practice standards. Accountability is inherent to autonomy. By definition, accountability calls for professionals to accept responsibility or to account for their actions (*Merriam-Webster's Collegiate Dictionary*, 2006). The demand for professional accountability has been spurred on by the health-outcomes movement and patient safety concerns.

Professionalism should and does benefit the public. However, professionalism also arises out of self-interest and provides a means by which occupational groups exert influence to advance their own interests in society. The interest may reflect a desire for greater societal power and/or an increase of rewards or benefits for the group. As such, the quest for professional status by nursing reflects an attempt to access and achieve mobility. Professionalism, by reflecting the underlying meritocratic values of our society, offers a rational system for distributing status and rewards.

Professionalization provides access to social mobility. According to Hughes (1971), there are two types of mobility. The first is the rise of the individual by entering an occupation of high prestige or by achieving special success in his or her profession. The second is the collective effort of an organized occupation to improve its place and increase its power in relation to other occupational groups. In the case of nursing, mobility has traditionally been measured against or referenced to other groups, such as physicians.

Since the 1970s, interest in professionalizing nursing work has emerged in healthcare organizations as a means to provide a substitute motivation for workers with blocked access to structures of mobility. The ideological draw of professionalism is that it offers the promise of higher status and control. A crucial issue that arises out of the trend to professionalize work is the struggle of workers, including nurses, to exercise control over the context (environment) and content of their work. The ability to exercise control, however tentative, appears to mediate individual and collective tensions that arise from the heightened expectations of a more educated nursing workforce. By professionalizing the workplace, management seeks to counter more traditional collective action, such as unionism. Educated to be professionals in colleges and universities, nurses now expect to exercise their knowledge and skills without organizational or bureaucratic constraint. The heightened expectations of nurses represent a double-edged sword, offering a challenge to traditional hierarchical controls and opportunity for institutional enhancement.

As hospitals and other healthcare institutions confront the increasing complexity in health care, the application of professional knowledge and skills becomes essential to institutional functioning. That professional knowledge and skills serve institutional goals to solve institutional problems is now embraced by healthcare administrators as an asset, rather than a threat to traditional authority. Perrow (1972) observed in his classic treatise on bureaucracy that professionals, far from antithetical to institutional bureaucracy, are in fact readily harnessed to serve the needs and problems of organizations. Nurses have historically highlighted this phenomenon. More recently, other traditional professions (physicians, lawyers) have become organizational professions. Yet, despite nurses' central role in healthcare services, they have struggled to develop, assert, and be recognized for their professional expertise. Imbued with managerialism, nursing work in hospitals has evidenced a professional paradox (Fourcher & Howard, 1981). The application of nursing knowledge and skill in managing patient care in hospitals has a long history of being subjugated to nursing and hospital administration. Nursing expertise has more often than not been invisible and undervalued, and autonomy of practice has been absent.

ROOTS OF NURSING CONTRADICTIONS

The concept and actual practice of nursing work has evolved dramatically over the past 100 years. But like many evolutionary paths, old or outdated conceptions of nursing persist. As a result, both popular and professional conceptions of nursing are riddled with contradictory views. Prior to Florence Nightingale's reforms in England, nursing was largely women's work. Nursing was viewed as an extension of motherhood, midwifery, or religious duty. By the late 19th century, women working as nurses began to fill a role in the administration of poverty. Because health care and nursing care of the sick were intertwined with poverty, caring for the sick was largely caring for the poor. Nursing was commonly carried out by impoverished women who worked as nurses in almshouses caring for the poor, the sick, and the destitute. These untrained, able-bodied paupers worked for room and board. The harsh reality was that these nurses were viewed as part of the chaotic environments in which they worked. The Dickinsonian image of Sairey Gamp, a low-class drunkard and disheveled woman, was reflective of the persistent stigma that Nightingale sought to escape with the formal education of a higher class of women (Dean & Bolton, 1980; Williams, 1980).

Although some few nurses saw their work as a religious service, the role of religious values waned with the disintegration of church-based nursing orders with the rise of Protestantism in England. Hospitals, lacking the support of religious nursing orders, struggled to provide nursing care that was haphazard at best. Nurses lacked a systematic set of skills, a knowledge base, or training. Nightingale sought to modernize nursing by developing a trained nursing labor force composed of a higher class of women.

Nightingale also sought to link nursing education with the more formalized development of hospitals. Influenced by her experiences in the Crimea, Nightingale recognized that nursing care was the major determinant of hospital outcomes. A brilliant and politically astute woman, she took on nursing reformation with a passion born of her religious beliefs and desire to reform social expectations for women. Nightingale advanced her case for training nurses based on data. Nightingale contributed some of the earliest biostatistical data of hospital conditions and outcomes, drawing connections between the environments of care and the contribution of nurses (Dossey, 1999).

Despite Nightingale's innovative ideas to systematize the education of nurses, the origins of modern nursing were seeded with social constraints. Nightingale (1866) wrote to a friend that "the whole reform in nursing both at home and abroad has consisted of this: to take all power over the nursing out of the hands of men and put into the hands of one female trained head and making her responsible for everything. . ." (p. 25). Nightingale and her contemporaries purposely overlooked the traditions of men in nursing, such as the work of the Knights Templar (Bullough & Bullough, 1984). The concept of nursing discipline projected by Nightingale, as well as by nursing leaders in the

20th century, held nursing to conventional standards of female subservience within a hierarchy of a moral female authority. Nursing was embraced as a feminine endeavor that was to be the singular focus of the nurse's life. Imbued with inherent religious values, nursing was viewed as a selfless act, and the reward for nursing work was deemed intrinsic to the work itself. Nightingale, although a feminist and supporter of women's suffrage, struggled with contradictions of class and gender as she advanced her campaigns for nursing and health. Despite Nightingale's political opinions, modern nursing was reconceptualized as a woman's calling, and hence doubly subordinated to the paternalism of society.

NURSING TAKES ROOT IN THE UNITED STATES

The universal traditions and nursing functions of caring for the sick have existed for centuries. The power of Nightingale's reforms to formalize and reshape nursing has been evident in their global reach. In the United States, as in many other countries, the importation of the Nightingale schools of nursing legitimated nursing work as an occupation for women. Hospital-based schools of nursing offered women access to education and the potential for employment, creating an option for a sustainable livelihood. Employment as a head nurse or private duty nurse was a welcome alternative to agrarian domesticity or mill work.

The demand for nursing grew in response to hospital growth. As industrialization spurred the growth of larger communities, hospitals proliferated and became a central feature of community life (Rosenberg, 1989). Social reformism was a major force because it spurred the development of both public health and hospital-based services to provide health care to the growing industrial labor force (Rosenberg, 1989; Starr, 1982). From 1875 to 1924, the number of hospitals grew from just over 170 to more than 7,000 (Rosner, 1989). However, as noted by Stevens (1989), the central role that health care would take in American society was being shaped by the growing power of medicine. A benevolent paternalism pervaded the structure of healthcare services and harnessed the potential of nursing to support the role of medicine and hospitals (Ashley, 1976). By the early 1900s, the growth of hospitals in the United States generated an unprecedented demand for nurses. The growth of technology from basic advances such as X-rays and anesthesia fueled excitement in hospital investment. Physicians invested their money and technology into hospitals, securing power in their communities as well. Hospitals became a focal point of community life, and hospitals became both a symbol of the prosperity of a community and a focus for social reformism.

The thirst for a cheap and rapidly produced labor supply overshadowed concerns over standards of quality education. From 1900 to 1920, the nursing profession grew "from one in which there were more than 10 times as many physicians as nurses, to one in which there was less than one physician for every nurse" (Burgess, 1928, p. 43). As hospitals grew, schools of nursing were created to provide a labor force for the hospitals, often at the expense of adequate education (Ashley, 1976). As Dock and Stewart (1938) noted in their history of nursing, "the excess of poor schools and poorly prepared nurses was attributed in large measure to the apprenticeship system that prevailed, with its overemphasis on practice service at the expense of education" (p. 183). Formal studies of nursing education, such as the Goldmark report (1923) and the grading committee report of the National League for Nursing Education (1926), addressed the issue of raising standards for nursing education. Dock and Stewart (1938) suggested that despite the many recommendations for reform, "the system was too deeply rooted and the funds for putting nursing schools on a sound economic and education basis were sim-

ply not generally available" (p. 183). Despite forward movement with the establishment of university schools of nursing at Columbia, Yale, and Western Reserve, the push to establish college entrance as a requirement for practice was eclipsed by the hospital training schools. The fundamental professional goal to control the entry into the profession was overridden by hospitals' needs for a cheap labor supply.

The rapid expansion of a nursing labor force occurred with little regard for educational quality. Hospital administrators recognized the economic benefit of using student labor, and physicians began to appreciate the good nursing care offered by graduates of such training. But by the 1930s, concerns about overproduction of nurses emerged and were underscored by the Great Depression. A third of all hospital schools of nursing closed between 1929 and 1939. Nurses, no longer able to secure private duty work, sought employment in hospital wards for hourly or group nursing work. But as Reverby (1979) noted, hospitals were slow to hire graduates as staff nurses, despite admonishments by the nursing leaders and the American Nurses Association. Modified grouped private duty nursing efforts served as a transition to the development to staff nursing. The dire economic conditions of the Depression reshaped nursing work and healthcare services. Nursing shifted away from private freelance work to organized nursing services in hospitals and public health. As nursing became embedded in hospitals, the primacy of the nurse–patient relationship—a characteristic of private duty nursing—eroded, and the nurse became subordinated to the paternalism of the hospital (Ashley, 1976; Dock & Stewart, 1938).

THE CHANGING ORGANIZATION OF WORK

The organizational culture of hospitals, characterized by strong gender-based roles and a hierarchical authority structure, was fertile ground for the application of industrial management methods. The ideas of scientific management made an easy leap from factory floor to hospitals in the first half of the 20th century. Frederick Taylor, the architect of many scientific management ideas, was of a new breed of industrial engineers. His primary concerns were enhancing worker productivity and limiting the threats of unions so as to increase the profits from capitalism. Scientific methods were intended to extract labor from workers at the shop-floor level by dividing work into discrete tasks to be done by individual workers. "Taylorism" spread to hospitals and was embraced by nursing leaders, and the quest for efficiency in hospital operations mirrored the factory push toward mechanistic functioning. The application of Taylor's scientific management methods to hospitals included division of labor, the task orientation of functional nursing, and standardized and proscriptive procedure manuals. Hospitals were in a unique position to maximize the control and the execution of nursing work, because they were often both the diploma schools for training nurses and the employer. The hospital culture was able to secure the loyalty of nurses through both school ties and training (Wolf, 1993).

Management in hospitals emerged largely at the ward level. Mobility in nursing became tied to the management structure. Nursing leadership embraced managerialism, because it offered the potential for mobility and status recognition for women. Subordinated to physicians, nurses were unable to gain control over access to patients, use of technology, or application of knowledge. Nursing leader Isabel Stewart attempted to advance scientific nursing, which she thought could be employed in conjunction with industrial methods for standardization and efficiency of hospital care to wrest control from hospitals. However, her academic approach to building a scientific basis for practice was viewed skeptically by nurses and never gained sufficient financial support (Reverby, 1987). Nurses continued to follow or-

ders under a system where work conception was clearly separate from execution.

That the adage "a nurse is a nurse is a nurse" was born in this period reflects the view that nurses were considered an interchangeable part of the hospital machine. Although many nurses preferred to work as private duty nurses, the changing economics of the Great Depression made this an unstable option by the 1930s (Reverby, 1999). As a result of application of scientific management methods to nursing, patient care became fragmented, task oriented, and management focused. Case-based nursing, rooted in the tradition of private duty nursing, fell victim to what was viewed as progress. New models of care, such as group nursing and functional nursing, reflected the pooling of scarce nursing labor resources to meet the needs of the organization, not the patient.

Following World War II, team nursing became the common model of nursing care organization. The team nursing concept was influenced by wartime experiences and the emerging human relations school of management. The goal was to create a team of nursing care providers led by a professional nurse. Emphasis was placed on effective communication and delegation to enhance team functioning. However, nursing shortages often resulted in team leaders struggling to provide care with inadequately trained staff. The result of the team approach was more a functional approach to care, with emphasis on task completion rather than patient care (Hegyvary, 1982). Because of tradition and nursing shortages, remnants of mechanistic task performance continued to permeate the work culture of hospitals and counter professionalization attempts.

Nursing leader Lydia Hall, a fierce opponent of team nursing, challenged nursing to put its rhetoric of professionalism to the test of practice. In 1963, she instituted a system of professional nursing practice at the Loeb Center, Montefiore Medical Center, in New York City. The Loeb model of care emphasized nursing autonomy and accountability, giving the nurse responsibility for providing care and making care decisions for his or her patients during the full duration of their hospital stay (Hall, 1969). Her visionary efforts planted ideas for change; however, few hospitals adopted her model.

INSTABILITY IN THE NURSING LABOR FORCE

Despite the emphasis on efficiency and rationality in hospital management, the nursing labor force continued to be wracked by instability. Recurrent nursing shortages during the 1940s and 1960s led to the policies that increased the production of more nurses—short-training nurses in particular. These nursing shortages set the pattern for subsequent policy initiatives dominated by hospital interests (Grando, 1998). Hospital administrators and nursing leaders first encouraged licensed practical nurses and then associate degree nurses. In the midst of the shortages, attempts to fill nursing positions were like filling a leaking bucket. Nurses were clearly unhappy with work conditions and compensation. Shortages of nurses left team nurse leaders working alone as captains of understaffed nursing teams. While hospital nursing administrators struggled with the outflow of nurses, nursing educators struggled with the quest to professionalize nursing. The development of nursing knowledge and skills took on renewed urgency at mid-century. Nursing scholars such as Virginia Henderson (1966) sought to reclaim the primacy of the nurse–patient relationship and expand the focus of nursing care beyond efficiency to a process-oriented effectiveness.

The post–World War II period led to increased federal funding for nursing and health care. Along with the funding came a new closer scrutiny of hospital costs. As the federal government became more involved with funding hospital care, the drive to disentangle educational costs from nursing care costs took force.

By the late 1960s, funding of nursing education began to move away from the hospital training schools to colleges and universities. Early doctoral programs developed as hybrid degrees, between nursing and fields such as education, sociology, psychology, and biology. These graduate programs had as their primary focus the development of a pool of nursing educators. But within a few years, collegiate nursing education institutions expanded programs in nursing administration and clinical specialization. Graduate education became the primary incubator for nursing theory and the growth of professional knowledge and values.

By the 1970s, a culture of professionalism emerged in nursing, fueled by the growth of nursing scholarship. This resulted in a gap between nurses' expectations and the experiential reality of nursing work. This gap, or reality shock (Kramer, 1974), was evidenced by the rapid turnover in staff nursing and nurses' growing discontent. Despite the move to a more efficient hospital functioning, the nursing labor force continued to be wracked by instability. Once again, nursing shortages led to the increased production of nurses, in particular short-training nurses. Hospital administrators and nursing leaders encouraged the addition of associate degree nurse production as a solution.

Nursing education, long tied to hospitals through the tradition of hospital diploma schools, began to break free in the 1960s. The federal government took up more of the financial burden for nursing education. But as nursing education moved into colleges, the trade-off was the loss of nurses' loyalty to hospitals, a central characteristic of hospital-diploma-school nurses. While hospital administrators struggled with the outflow of nurses, the growth of college-based programs at the baccalaureate and associate degree levels infused nursing with a new drive for professional status. As the development of nursing knowledge and skills took on more status and legitimacy, the predominance of nursing management as the primary means of career mobility came to an end (Wolf, 1993).

MILITANCY ROCKS THE HOSPITAL BOAT

Discontent with the reality of nursing work reflected the changing values and expectations of nurses. With rising expectations of professionalism, nurses' desires for control over their work were influenced by the new social realities of women's employment. Nursing was no longer viewed as a transient occupation for women to keep them busy until they married. The growing careerism sharpened nurses' lenses to workplace realities. Turnover rates in hospitals reflected the discontent with working conditions and benefits. Nurses, college educated and empowered by the emerging women's movement, were no longer willing to bow to the paternalism of hospital administrators.

At various points in nursing history, nurses had discussed or attempted the use of collective action or unionism. The rate of nurses organizing for collective bargaining began to increase in the 1960s, but it was not until 1974, with the addition of amendments to the federal Taft-Hartley Act, that the potential impact of collective bargaining was realized (Foley, 1993). These amendments provided federal protection to nurses and other healthcare employees of nonprofit healthcare institutions with regard to the right to organize. The operational structure of the amendments emphasized that nurses were to be a separate and distinct bargaining unit.

The potential of the nursing labor force to be a catalyst for the unionization of the entire hospital labor force was clearly recognized by hospital administrators and union busting consultants. This, in turn, resulted in the idea of requiring hospital employees to organize into separate bargaining groups. Nurses were courted initially by professional nursing organizations, such as the ANA-affiliated state nursing organizations. Within a few years, more traditional industrial and trade unions, such as the United Auto Workers (UAW) and the American Federation of Teachers (AFT) joined efforts to organize nurses and other healthcare workers. The ANA-associated state nursing organizations were viewed as the lesser of two evils because the professionalism inherent in the nursing leadership tempered the militancy.

Hospital administrators explored a variety of means to fight the spread of hospital unionism (Kohles, 1994). Treating various types of hospital workers as contract workers was common, but this approach was neither cost- nor outcome-effective for nursing. Another approach was to create a new work culture and structure that would divide nurses from other hospital employees. This served a double purpose. First, it helped to insulate other hospital workers from nursing collective action. Second, it held the potential to curb the militancy. To effectively bridge the reality gap that had led to nurse militancy, nursing and hospital administrators needed to realistically grapple with the roots of nurses' frustration. The long-standing paternalism was no longer an effective means of controlling nurses.

NURSING IS NOT ALONE: THE NATIONAL CRISIS IN THE QUALITY OF WORK LIFE

By the late 1970s, professionalism, long viewed as an unnecessary extravagance, was to become a mantra for nursing management. The growing belief that creating a more professional work climate could mitigate the potential for workplace militancy shaped efforts to restructure nursing work in hospitals. As hospital administrators and nursing grappled with what was perceived to be an issue of militancy versus professionalization, the issue was reflected in broader discussions of an emerging national crisis in workplace relations. Nationally, as concerns over decreases in worker productivity grew, labor experts debated the origins and solutions to worker discontent across a wide range of occupations and professions. The U.S. Department of Health, Education, and Welfare (1973) funded a study—"Work in America"—that asked the question, "What do workers want?" The study yielded the following answers: interesting work, enough help and equipment to get the job done, enough information to get the job done, enough authority to get the job done, good pay, opportunities to develop special abilities, job security, and the ability to see the results of one's work. National labor and management experts debated innovations such as worker control programs and work restructuring. However, the long-standing dominance of industrial labor skewed the perspective of labor experts who were slow to recognize the power and problems of the emerging service sector, and specifically the healthcare labor force.

By the mid-1970s, the nursing profession was in the midst of a collective feminist consciousness raising (Wolf, 1993). Nursing's perspective on nurses' discontent with their work held that the conditions nurses faced were unique and were often viewed within the context of gender and professionalism. Jo Ann Ashley (1996), a feminist nursing historian, offered the most vocal of the feminist perspectives. She described nurses' perceived powerlessness to change their situations as a consequence of their unique socialization as a female-gendered occupation and a result of the cultural barriers to the exercise of the power of nursing within paternalistic institutions.

Caught in a rapid current of cultural change, nursing and hospital administrators were pushed by nurses and pulled by larger social, economic, and political currents to face change in healthcare organizations. Collegiate nursing education, which had begun to embrace the notion of nurses as change agents, contributed to a new professional consciousness. The power to change nursing realities was slowly unleashed.

The unfreezing of hospital nursing to change was rapidly catalyzed as the potential threat of collective bargaining became evident to nursing and hospital industry management. Nurses, like workers in other industries and service sectors, wanted control over their work

and a more equitable and open system of resource allocation and rewards. Control involved complex problems of achieving and sustaining authority and ensuring accountability for nursing practice. The potential scope of control ranged from specific day-to-day patient care decision making to participation in organizational governance, such as goal setting and finance (Siriani, 1984; Witte, 1972). Hospital decision making is typically viewed as hierarchical, with organizational control at the top and bedside or patient-care issues at the bottom. But in reality, the arenas of decision making are overlapping and interconnected within hospital organizations.

PATIENT-CENTERED CARE AND THE EMERGENCE OF PRIMARY NURSING

As the workplace reforms movement moved forward in the 1970s, the desire for control over patient care took precedence in most organizations. This reflected the growing necessity for greater nursing decision making given the rapidly increasing complexity of the patient care. The most influential development was primary nursing. According to Marram, Schlegel, and Bevis (1974), primary nursing was a developmental step in professional practice development that supported "the distribution of nursing so that the total care of an individual patient is the responsibility of one nurse, not many nurses" (p. 1). Many of the ideas inherent in primary nursing were previously noted by Lydia Hall (1969) at the Loeb Center. Influenced by the wave of quality in work life ideas in the contemporary management literature, primary nursing was invented as an approach to job redesign. This job-redesign approach had been applied successfully in industrial management in Europe and Japan. The primary nursing model offered hospital management a way to counter worker complaints about deskilling. The work of nursing was restructured and enlarged to make nurses accountable for the whole of patient care rather than just for specific tasks.

Primary nursing was also ideologically imbued with professionalism.

The association between primary nursing and enhanced professional orientation was noted in many studies beginning in the 1970s (Marram, Schlegel, & Bevis, 1974). Manthey (1980), an early proponent of primary nursing, noted that primary nursing reflected a philosophical commitment to decision making at the level of action. Primary nursing, drawing on professionalism, sought increased accountability by the nurse for patient care, a rational system of care provided by the nurse who is most knowledgeable about the patient, individualized and personalized patient care, and increased equality among nursing staff (Marram, Schlegel, & Bevis, 1974). To support the initiation of primary nursing, registered nurses had to be reskilled, and hospitals sought to increase the staffing levels of registered nurses while decreasing the employment and roles of licensed practical nurses and nursing assistants. In most instances, this necessitated increased funding or significant reallocation of funds, made possible in the late 1970s by government and private support to hospitals.

Primary nursing provided a process by which patient-centered care could be individualized yet applied within a standardized nursing process. However unique each patient-care situation might be, the process of nursing judgment and discretion became predictable. The application of the nursing process as a method of solving nursing care problems became central to nursing education and practice in the 1970s. The development of professional nursing standards for care by the ANA further codified this process orientation. However, the growing complexity of patient care and the increasing body of nursing theory would soon shift nursing's emphasis to critical thinking.

Despite the shift in control over nursing education from hospitals to academic institutions, the reality was that most nursing graduates were going to be employed by hospitals. Nursing educators faced pressure to produce a product nurse that met the hospital labor market needs in terms of skill as well as price.

As legal and regulatory pressures for greater accountability mounted, new demands for documentation shaped the day of hospital nurses. Nurses expressed a sense of being pushed into documentation at the expense of being pulled away from patient care. As one primary nurse noted, "Make sure your patient care is your priority, but don't forget your paperwork" (Wolf, 1993, p. 115). The strain of competing demands between the work of nursing and the documentation of the work emerged as a recurring theme underlying alienation and nurse dissatisfaction. As nurses grappled with the potential of primary nursing to provide rewards, the reality of the system's constraints and the contextual issues of organizational control became more apparent.

THE MISSING LINKS: SHARED GOVERNANCE AND RECOGNITION

The initiation of shared governance in healthcare institutions in the 1980s highlighted an attempt to ease the tensions between administrative controls and professional work. Primary nursing, while restructuring nursing work, was quickly found to be limited in its scope. The work of nurses was embedded in the organizational context and was shaped by decisions that were often removed from their sphere of action. From staffing to equipment choice, these decisions often impacted patient care, leaving nurses frustrated, which compounded problems of turnover and militancy. Just as American industry struggled with the push to expand worker control without sacrificing managerial prerogatives, the push for workplace participation in decision making grew. Genuine participation was made difficult by the complex hospital authority structure, which kept nurses trapped between the dual hierarchies of medicine and the hospital administration.

The climb by nurses out from between these two systems of control generated both a threat and an opportunity for the reallocation of power in hospitals. Nursing leaders such as Manthey (1991) cautioned that for the reallocation of power to occur, a major change was required in the structure and operation of nursing departments. Change would require a major dismantling of the hospital hierarchy, beginning with the nursing departments. As Porter-O'Grady (2001) noted, "Implementing an empowered format such as shared governance means that the relationships, decisions, structures, and processes will be forever changed at every level of the system and that all the players in the organization will be different and behave differently as a result" (p. 5). The changes in patterns of communication and behaviors extended across relationships, not only nurse–nurse or nurse–patient, but also nurse–physician. Many physicians were initially ambivalent and threatened by shared governance (Wolf, 1993).

In the 1980s and 1990s, many hospitals moved toward flatter management structures in an effort to move toward shared governance. Work, previously viewed as a management prerogative, was typically distributed across the flattened structure to involve staff nurses as well as administrators in decision-making processes at the committee level. Nurse participation was concentrated at the committee level. A study by Jenkins (1988) observed that the expanded committee structure resulted in more time spent in meetings and an overall drop in hours per full-time employee. For example, Massachusetts General Hospital provides a wide range of committees in its governance structure, including such foci as patient-care quality, diversity, and staff recruitment (Erickson, 1996). Participation is based on an application; it is a selective process that draws from a pool of dedicated full- and part-time nursing staff who give generously of their time and expertise.

A parallel concern to expanded decision making has been the need to recognize nurses for their efforts (McCoy, 1999). Hospital nursing is complex and difficult work. Keeping experienced nurses at the bedside improves the quality of patient care and reduces recruitment and orientation costs. The challenge has been to find a way to reward nurses for a career in direct care rather than management. Career ladders typify the development of new reward systems. Career ladders provide a hierarchical system of rewarding professional behaviors, such as advanced education; scholarship; and contributions to the institution, such as committee work or clinical projects. This system provides the semblance of mobility by recognizing those nurses who choose to stay at the bedside. Given the recurrent stresses of nursing shortages, career ladders have provided another mechanism to attract and retain clinically expert nurses. The career ladder system has codified the job enlargement of the professional nurse, while stimulating nurse productivity in a variety of areas, such as quality assurance, practice policy development, hospital public relations, and nurse recruitment (Wolf, 1993).

However, the linking of remuneration with career-ladder progression historically has been problematic for many hospitals. The hospital budget process and pressures to control nurse salaries has thwarted career-ladder development efforts in some hospitals. Many senior nurses find themselves hitting the glass ceiling with new hires rapidly gaining more compensation. Healthcare organizations have also adopted nonmonetary systems of nurse recognition, such as the professional nurse of the month awards. These symbolic rewards, while recognizing clinical excellence, divert attention away from the concrete contextual realities of practice.

THE ATTRACTION OF MAGNET HOSPITALS

In the early 1980s, the American Academy of Nursing launched an effort to recognize hospitals for their ability to attract and retain nursing staff (Upenickes, 2003). The Magnet

Hospital program was launched based on a study that identified hospitals having low staff turnover, high nurse job satisfaction, and low staff nurse vacancy rates. The initial recognition went to some 41 hospitals. The results of the early magnet hospital studies highlighted the importance of organizational factors, such as participatory structures and processes, perceived autonomy of nurses, and empowering leadership (Scott, Sochalski, & Aiken, 1999). The characteristics of these hospitals paralleled many of the recommended changes of the quality of work life advocates. Policy reports by the Institute of Medicine (1981) and the National Commission on Nursing (1981) report by the American Hospital Association gave added legitimacy to the move to restructure hospitals to better attract and retain nursing staff. Some 20 years after the initial magnet studies, a body of research has been collected to justify continuing support for the restructuring of systems of care. Current efforts focus on validating outcomes of care in magnet hospital systems, but a better understanding of the relationship between outcomes and nurses' autonomy is needed (Havens & Aiken, 1999; Ritter-Teital, 2002; Scott et al., 1999).

PROFESSIONAL NURSING AND NURSE STAFFING: CHICKEN OR EGG?

How well hospitals are able to sustain professional models is dependent on the political and economic climate of the healthcare market. Past nursing shortages generated greater leverage for nursing stakeholders. Yet as tensions in labor ease or are overcome by greater organizational pressure to contain or depress labor costs, the potential for backpedaling on professional nursing gains increases. Nursing has a greater potential to enhance quality outcomes by maximizing the use of professional expertise. As has been noted in recent studies, sustaining adequate nurse staffing may be one of the most important key factors in patient care outcomes (Aiken et al., 2002; Cho, Ketefian, Barkauskas,

& Smith, 2003). Such research further underscores the importance of continuing professional models of development as they support the recruitment and retention of staff. For too long the value of nursing has been hidden in health care by data collection and information systems that give primacy to medicine. Ideally, emerging advances in nursing informatics will add to nursing's visibility and support continued vitality. A firm investment in professional models will also call for healthcare organizations to effectively match nursing education and talents with the complexity of the work. The corporatization of hospitals provides a relative opportunity for nursing to gain power in the healthcare organization. It is time for nursing to cease its dependence on the good will of institutions and to demand full participation in institutional policy making.

CONCLUSION

Throughout the history of nursing, professionalization has been a driving force for change. From the earliest innovations of Nightingale to the most recent nursing shortage, the work culture of nursing has been reshaped to meet the needs of society or managerial interests, often in the midst of crises. The slow march toward professional practice continues as models of nursing practice offer a powerful ideological hold. Nursing has been influenced by ideas drawn from sociology, management, and industry, resulting in workplace reforms reframed within a professional lens. The power of professionalization has contributed significantly to the success of this reform, offering benefits to both healthcare institutions and nurses. However, nursing shortages remain. Challenging questions for the future include the following: To what extent are professional models of practice sustainable in the face of economic uncertainty? Can institutional control truly be ceded to nurses without a fundamental revolution in the overall restructuring of healthcare financing and service structure?

DISCUSSION QUESTIONS ─────────

1. In this chapter, the author argues that nursing's role in hospitals is imbued with managerialism, causing a paradox (Fourcher & Howard, 1981). The application of nursing knowledge and skill in managing patient care in hospitals has a long history of being subjugated to nursing and hospital administration. Nursing expertise has more often than not been invisible and undervalued, and autonomy of practice has been absent. Reflecting on this statement, do you agree or disagree?

2. How has societal and healthcare policy affected the development of nursing?

3. What are the pros and cons of unionization in nursing?

4. How will the Magnet Hospital program, shared governance, and mandated staffing ratios affect nursing in the future?

REFERENCES ─────────

Aiken, L. H., Clarke, S. P., Sloane, D. M., Sochalski, J., & Silber, J. H. (2002). Hospital nurse staffing and patient mortality, nurse burnout, and job satisfaction. *Journal of the American Medical Association, 288,* 1987–1993.

American Association of Colleges of Nursing. (2007). Doctor of Nursing Practice. Retrieved July 14, 2007, from http://www.aacn.nche.edu/DNP/DNPPositionStatement.htm

Ashley, J. (1976). *Hospitals, paternalism, and the role of the nurse.* New York: Columbia University Press.

Ashley, J. (1996). This I believe about power in nursing. In K. Wolf (Ed.), *Selected readings of Jo Ann Ashley* (pp. 23–34). New York: NLN Press/Jones and Bartlett.

Bucher, R., & Strauss, A. (1961). Professions in progress. *American Journal of Sociology, 66*(4), 325–334.

Bullough, V., & Bullough, B. (1984). *The history, trends, and politics of nursing.* Norwalk, CT: Appleton Century Crofts.

Burgess, M. (1928). *Nurses, patients, and pocketbooks.* New York: Committee on the Grading of Nursing Schools.

Cho, S. H., Ketefian, S., Barkauskas, V. H., & Smith, D. G. (2003). The effects of nurse staffing on adverse events, morbidity, mortality, and medical costs. *Nursing Research, 52,* 71–79.

Dean, M., & Bolton, J. (1980). The administration of poverty and the development of nursing practice in nineteenth-century England. In C. Davies (Ed.), *Rewriting nursing history* (pp. 76–101). London: Croom Helm.

Dock, L., & Stewart, I. (1938). *A short history of nursing.* New York: G. P. Putnam's Sons.

Dossey, B. (1999). *Florence Nightingale: Mystic, visionary, healer.* Springhouse, PA: Springhouse Corporation.

Erickson, J. I. (1996). Our professional practice model. *MGH Patient Care Services, Caring Headlines, 2*(23).

Etzioni, A. (1969). *The semi-professions and their organization.* New York: Free Press.

Foley, M. (1993). The politics of collective bargaining. In D. Mason, S. Talbot, & J. Leavitt (Eds.), *Policy and politics for nurses* (2nd ed., pp. 282–302). Philadelphia: W. B. Saunders.

Fourcher, L., & Howard, M. (1981). Nursing and the managerial demiurge: Social science and medicine, Part A. *Medical Sociology, 15*(Pt. 3), 299–306.

Goldmark, J. (1923). *Nursing and nursing education in the U.S. Report of the Committee for the Study of Nursing Education.* New York: Macmillan.

Grando, V. T. (1998). Making do with fewer nurses in the United States, 1945–1965. *Image: Journal of Nursing Scholarship, 30*(2), 147–149.

Hall, L. E. (1969). The Loeb Center for Nursing and Rehabilitation, Montefiore Medical Center, Bronx, New York. *International Journal of Nursing Studies, 16,* 215–230.

Havens, D., & Aiken, L. (1999). Shaping systems to promote desired outcomes: The magnet hospitals model. *Journal of Nursing Administration, 29*(2), 14–20.

Hegyvary, S. T. (1982). *The change to primary nursing.* St. Louis, MO: C. V. Mosby.

Henderson, V. (1966). *The nature of nursing.* New York: MacMillan.

Hughes, C. E. (1971). *The sociological eye.* Chicago: Aldine.

Institute of Medicine. (1981). *The study of nursing and nursing education.* Washington, DC: National Academy of Science Press.

Jenkins, J. (1988). A nursing governance and practice model: What are the costs? *Nursing Economics,* 302–311.

Kohles, M. K. (1994). Commentary on union election activity in the health care industry. *Health Management Review, 19*(1), 18–27.

Kramer, M. (1974). *Reality shock: Why nurses leaving.* St. Louis, MO: C. V. Mosby.

Manthey, M. (1980). *The practice of primary nursing.* Boston: Blackwell Scientific Publications.

Manthey, M. (1991). Delivery systems and practice models: A dynamic balance. *Nursing Management, 22*(1), 28–30.

Marram, G., Schlegel, M., & Bevis, E. O. (1974). *Primary nursing: A model for individualized care.* St. Louis, MO: C. V. Mosby.

McCoy, J. M. (1999). Recognize, reward, retain. *Nursing Management, 30*(2), 41–43.

Merriam-Webster's Collegiate Dictionary, 4th ed. (2006). p. 8.

National Commission on Nursing. (1981). *Summary of public hearings.* Chicago, IL: The Hospital Research and Educational Trust.

National League for Nursing Education. (1926). *The grading committee report of the National League for Nursing Education.* New York: NLNE.

Nightingale, F. (1866). Letter to Mary Jones. Cited on p. 25 in B. Abel-Smith, *A history of the nursing profession* (1960). London: Heinmann.

Perrow, C. (1972). *Complex organizations: A critical essay.* Glenview, IL: Scott Foresman.

Porter-O'Grady, T. (2001). Is shared governance still relevant? *Journal of Nursing Administration, 31*(10), 467–473.

Reverby, S. (1979). The search for the hospital yardstick. In S. Reverby & D. Rosner (Eds.), *Health care in America* (pp. 206–225). Philadelphia: Temple University Press.

Reverby, S. (1987). *Ordered to care, the dilemma of American nursing, 1850–1945.* Cambridge, England: Cambridge University Press.

Reverby, S. (1999). Neither for the drawing room nor for the kitchen: Private duty nursing in Boston, 1873–1914. In J. Waltzer Leavitt (Ed.), *Women and health in America* (pp. 460–474). Madison: University of Wisconsin Press.

Ritter-Teital, J. (2002). The impact of restructuring on professional nursing practice. *Journal of Nursing Administration, 32*(1), 31–41.

Rosenberg, C. (1989). Community and communities: The evolution of the American hospital. In D. Long & J. Golden (Eds.), *The American general hospital* (pp. 3–17). Ithaca, NY: Cornell University Press.

Rosner, D. (1989). Doing well or doing good: The ambivalent focus of hospital administration. In D. Long & J. Golden (Eds.), *The American general hospital* (pp. 157–169). Ithaca, NY: Cornell University Press.

Scott, J. G., Sochalski, J., & Aiken, L. (1999). Review of magnet hospital research: Findings and implications for professional nursing practice. *Journal of Nursing Administration, 29*(1), 9–19.

Siriani, C. (1984). Participation, opportunity, and equality: Towards a pluralist organization model. In F. Ficher & C. Siriani (Eds.), *Critical studies in organization and bureaucracy* (pp. 482–503). Philadelphia: Temple University Press.

Starr, P. (1982). *The social transformation of American medicine.* New York: Basic Books.

Stevens, R. (1989). *In hospitals and in wealth: American hospitals in the twentieth century.* New York: Basic Books.

Upenickes, V. (2003). Recruitment and retention strategies: A magnet hospital prevention model. *Nursing Economics, 21*(1), 7–13, 23.

U.S. Department of Health, Education & Welfare. (1973). *Work in America, HEW report.* Cambridge, MA: MIT Press.

Williams, K. (1980). From Sarah Gamp to Florence Nightingale: A critical study of hospital nursing systems from 1840 to 1897. In C. Davies (Ed.), *Rewriting nursing history* (pp. 41–75). London: Croom Helm.

Witte, J. (1972). *Democracy, authority and alienation in work.* Chicago: University of Chicago Press.

Wolf, K. A. (1993). *The professionalization of nursing work: The case of nursing at Mill City Medical Center.* Dissertation microfilms PUZ9322364. Ann Arbor: University of Michigan.

CHAPTER 2

Advanced Practice Nursing: Moving Beyond the Basics

Joyce Pulcini

CHAPTER OBJECTIVES

1. Define advanced practice nursing and explain how the term is currently expanding and evolving.

2. Articulate the history, similarities, and differences of each of the traditional roles categorized as advanced practice nursing.

3. Consider how the roles of entry-level nurses through advanced practice nurses should be conceptualized for the future.

INTRODUCTION

According to the *American Heritage Dictionary* (1980), the term *advanced* means "ahead of contemporary thought or practice or at the highest level of difficulty." *Practice* is defined as "the exercise of an occupation or profession." *Nursing* has been defined as "The diagnosis and treatment of human responses to actual and potential health problems" (American Nurses Association [ANA], 1995).

In the last century, nursing has undergone many changes that have reshaped and expanded what is considered to be basic nursing. As nursing's role has evolved, so has its scope of practice. Many of today's nursing functions were originally within the realm of medicine or other disciplines. This metamorphosis has been part of the profession's gradual evolution and maturity over time.

Advanced practice nursing is defined by Hamric, Spross, and Hanson (2005) as "the application of an expanded range of practical, theoretical, and research-based competencies to phenomena experienced by patients within a specialized clinical area of the larger discipline of nursing" (p. 89).

This term was coined to encompass four major roles within nursing: clinical nurse specialist (CNS), nurse practitioner (NP), certified nurse–midwife (CNM), and certified registered nurse anesthetist (CRNA). It distinguishes these nurses with advanced skills from those who practice as more traditional staff nurses and allows for a distinction between the nurse functioning at a more specialized level than the registered nurse. These roles also have been considered to be equally complex or at the same level of advanced practice. A common characteristic of these roles is the application of a greater breadth of knowledge and complexity of decision making to the problems of nursing care. Although each of these roles is distinct with regard to the specific areas of knowledge and skills that it draws on, all of them require high levels of critical thinking, independence, and decision making.

Finally, use of the term "advanced practice" has allowed for legislative changes to proceed with a minimum of confusion over how advanced practice and staff nurses differed. This distinction has created opportunities for advanced practice nurses (APNs), but also established a new class of nurses who seemed to some to be more privileged than their peers.

Each of these roles evolved a bit differently. The CNM evolved from the historical role of the midwife, who even today can be a non-nurse. The CRNA role evolved from the experiences of nurses in the Civil War, who provided pain relief for soldiers (Hamric, Spross, & Hanson, 2005).

The CNS began to flourish in the 1950s and 1960s due to interest in promoting the highest level of nursing practice that coincided with the strong evolution of nursing theories and frameworks. This early CNS role had its roots in psychiatric nursing in the late 19th century and in specialist nursing roles in the early 1900s (Hamric, Spross, & Hanson, 2005). Initially, the CNS tended to work in hospitals or chronic care facilities caring for ill patients with specific health conditions. A major focus was the performance of indirect roles in nursing, such as consultation, research, staff education, and patient/family education. Much of the practice—though certainly not all of it—was also directed toward care coordination or institutional management of care. This specialty practice often dealt with symptom management or diagnosis of responses to illness rather than health promotion, and it focused on a unique set of problems emanating from illness. CNSs are highly competent nurses with a specialty focus who effectively meet the needs of patients in an increasingly complex healthcare system.

However, as cost-containment concerns became paramount and hospitals had to begin to cut costs in the 1980s, many of these CNS positions were eliminated even as staff nurses began to deal with sicker patients who had shorter stays in hospitals. In contrast, an increasing demand for nursing care in the community and long-term settings led to new opportunities for CNSs in home health care or specialized care for persons with HIV/AIDS or other chronic illnesses. At that time, CNSs began to function in community and long-term care settings as shortened hospital stays led to the "quicker and sicker" discharge of patients from hospitals or tertiary care facilities. In the past 10 years, the CNS has reemerged as an important component of patient care. The renewed interest in the CNS role has been fueled by regulatory and professional concerns. Pressures to demonstrate outcomes of care and to reduce risks such as patient injury or financial loss have generated a demand for the advanced practice knowledge and skills offered by the CNS (Heitkemper & Bond, 2004).

The NP role evolved from a shortage of primary care medical providers in underserved areas in the 1960s. Efforts to train NPs were spurred by progressive legislation of the Great Society era. As the federal government expanded financial access to care funded by Medicare, Medicaid, and community health center legislation, the need for more primary care providers became acute. The efforts to expand nursing practice were viewed by some in both medicine and nursing as a way for doctors to extend their care for patients using this new care provider.

This early concept of the NP role led many nurse educators to reject the idea of an advanced practice nurse and to close many avenues to university education. Thus, in the beginning years of NP role preparation, the majority of NP educational programs evolved outside of traditional nursing education in continuing education programs rather than in traditional master's degree programs. These early programs reflected the collaborative intent of nurses and more progressive doctors to create a new role for primary care practice. Through the NP role, the nurse's scope of practice expanded into realms that were previously only within the scope of medical practice, such as health assessment, medical diagnosis, and treatment of common and chronic illnesses. Most NPs functioned within the realm of primary care or generalist care, adding a strong health-promotion focus, while substituting for physicians who were not numerous enough to meet client needs. As the role has evolved, NPs have assumed greater responsibility in the management of more complex and chronic illnesses, and some have branched into specialty areas such as oncology, cardiology, or emergency care. When the NP role emerged, health promotion and disease prevention were being emphasized as an important component of primary care in all sectors of the healthcare system. As a result, NPs have a very strong foundation in direct patient care rather than in indirect nursing roles (Hamric & Hanson, 2003).

By the 1980s, the original community or public health focus of advanced practice was diluted as medical care became more individually focused and health financing failed to address public health needs. In this period, containment of healthcare costs was paramount in the minds of health policy makers, and the country was on the brink of replacing a public health focus with a system dominated by managed care. One exception was the community health

CNS who continued to work in community settings such as Visiting Nurse Associations or home care agencies.

As more patients were discharged from the hospital due to shortened stays and prospective payment methodologies, the need for home care skyrocketed, and an entirely new sector of the healthcare system emerged. Cost-containment efforts of the 1980s were also a major force in the realignment of nursing roles. Diagnosis-related groups (DRGs) and cost-containment efforts led the public, insurers, and policy makers to demand more cost-efficient care. This changed the face of hospital nursing forever. Demands on nurses in inpatient settings increased exponentially. These developments led to nursing shortages and to periodic staffing crises, as were seen in 1989 and 2001.

Several occurrences led to fundamental changes in the mix of roles and the level of independence in nursing and to increasing difficulties in differentiating the various roles for nursing. An overarching factor was the women's movement, which reached its peak in the 1960s and 1970s, because it influenced the increased desire by nurses to have autonomy from other providers, such as physicians. This had a major effect on the nursing profession.

In the 1980s and 1990s, the NP role was viewed as a potentially cost-effective option to fill the growing need for healthcare services. It also received an enormous amount of attention in the public and professional press. Another important change was the increased movement of NPs into acute care and medical specialties from primary care settings. As NP education began to be housed in universities, the distinction between the NP and the CNS was blurred.

In the 1980s, the CNS role was seen as too costly by hospital administrations because of reduced reimbursements from Medicare and shrinking hospital budgets. Thus many CNS positions were lost across the country as hospitals eliminated any position viewed as providing indirect care. Education for the CNS specialty suffered from a lack of consistency across programs and confusion over the definition of terms. Educational programs reflected this confusion by using the designations NP and CNS interchangeably or by creating blended roles. The blended role was intended to combine the best of both roles, but it also confused those credentialing or hiring these advanced practice nurses (Hamric & Hanson, 2003; Hamric, Spross, & Hanson, 2005). Currently, the predominant view is that the CNS and the NP roles are distinct from each other and should have separate educational programs (Hamric & Hanson, 2003; NACNS, 2004).

Since the inception of advanced practice nursing, health policy and regulatory advances enabling practice have moved forward with unprecedented swiftness and congruity. These advanced practice roles seem to have captured the imagination and interests of nurses who want more independent decision making and relief from what has been an increasingly stressful hospital environment. Barriers to practice for advanced practice nurses have decreased greatly over the past 20 years as legislative reforms have swept the nation. Third-party reimbursement for services and legislation for prescriptive privileges are now almost universal for NPs, CNMs, and CRNAs. These regulatory reforms have been far-reaching and now have been adopted by virtually every state (Pearson, 2004; Towers, 2004).

The role of advanced practice nurses has expanded well beyond initial expectations, and demands on practice continue to increase. For example, prescription writing now is almost universal, and the types and breadth of prescribing have increased across all categories of NPs (Pulcini & Vampola, 2002; Pulcini, Vampola, & Levine, 2005). Moreover, practice barriers may be lowest in rural areas or other areas where there is a greater need for healthcare services.

EDUCATIONAL STANDARDS

Educational standards have evolved in different ways for each specialty. CNMs and CRNAs took the lead in establishing national standards for certification and program accreditation. The American Association of Nurse Anesthetists (AANA) established its own separate certification process in 1945 and an accreditation process in 1952 (AANA, 2004). The American College of Nurse Midwives (ACNM) established its certification process in 1971 and its own separate accreditation process in 1982 (ACNM, 2004). These efforts enabled these specialties to evolve with a consistency not seen in either NP or CNS educational programs, which expanded with less consistency and homogeneity.

Yet regulatory changes and reimbursement efforts for CNSs have lagged behind and are surrounded by controversy, such as whether prescribing should be part of the role (Lyons, 2004). Recently, CNSs have organized under the National Association of Clinical Nurse Specialists (NACNS) and have begun to standardize their education, regulations, and practice, publishing the NACNS's landmark document, *Statement on Clinical Nurse Specialist Practice and Education* (2004).

Master's degree education preparation for NPs became the norm by the mid-1980s. Educational programs for NPs have become more congruent as a result of the National Organization of Nurse Practitioner Faculties' (NONPF) *Advanced Nursing Curriculum Guidelines and Program Standards for Nurse Practitioner Education* (1995), the *Domains and Competencies of Nurse Practitioner Practice* (2002, 2006, 2011), the *Criteria for Evaluation of Nurse Practitioner Programs* (2008), and the *Nurse Practitioner Competencies in Specialty Areas* (2002). As more NPs entered master's programs, the indirect-role (e.g., consultation, education, research) content in NP programs increased. Currently, more than 90% of NPs are master's prepared, and virtually all NPs are educated in graduate-level programs (Berlin, Stennett, & Bednash, 2004). The concept of the NP tipped in the mid-1990s, to use Malcolm Gladwell's (2000) term, and is now mainstream within nursing education. Currently, 330 graduate programs in nursing offer NP programs, with a total of

706 tracks, and 60% of master's program graduates are enrolled in NP programs (Berlin et al., 2004).

Another factor to consider is the new master's entry option that is popular in nursing education today. The number of graduate nursing programs offering this option, which allows a person with a non-nursing degree to earn a master's in nursing as an NP or CNS in 2–3 years, increased threefold from 1990 to 2002 (AACN, 2003). This development is important because originally most advanced practice nurses had experience in nursing before entering the advanced roles.

Finally, the members of the AACN endorsed the *Position Statement on the Practice Doctorate in Nursing*, which recommended that educational preparation for advanced practice nursing be extended from master's degree preparation to the doctoral completion by 2015. Currently, there are 210 doctor of nursing practice (DNP) programs in the United States, with another 100 under development. This latest trend, which has the potential to revolutionize health care, is the topic of much debate among nursing leaders and members of other healthcare disciplines. Chapters 4, 5, and 6 discuss the role of the DNP in greater detail.

THEORETICAL ISSUES AND CHALLENGES

The latest shifts have been important factors in shaping the current nursing environment. The key issue is that there are now entry-level advanced practice nurses. However, our understanding of "advanced" has not moved with this paradigm shift. What has occurred is that many of the skills involved in advanced practice roles have moved into the mainstream. Most new nurses see these distinct skills as basic rather than being unique to advanced practice. For example, many baccalaureate nursing programs now integrate physical assessment, pathophysiology, pharmacology, and health promotion, similar to advanced practice program curricula. Currently, the CNS, the CRNA, and the CNM are still viewed within the advanced practice role in the United States. But in many countries, a clear precedent has been set for basic nurses to have the skills of the nurse–midwife.

Internationally, the advanced practice role is evolving in diverse ways depending on the historical, political, and social factors that have shaped the nursing role and educational programs in each country. The definition of advanced practice nursing being adopted by the International Council of Nurses (2002) is as follows:

> The Nurse Practitioner/Advanced Practice Nurse (NP/APN) is a registered nurse who has acquired the expert knowledge base, complex decision-making skills and clinical competencies for expanded practice, the characteristics of which are shaped by the context and/or country in which s/he is credentialed to practice. A Master's degree is recommended for entry level.

Many countries are beginning to develop advanced practice nursing programs. This role advancement is built on the strong role that nurses have in developing nations. The International Nurse Practitioner/Advanced Practice Nursing Network (INP/APNN), which is affiliated with the International Council for Nurses, has been instrumental in publishing definitions and scope and standards statements to guide nations in the development and expansion of advanced practice nursing. The challenge is to standardize practice definitions and educational standards while building and honoring the traditions of individual countries.

How do we, in 2011, reconceptualize the concept of advanced practice, given the current state of nursing education for APNs both in the United States and internationally? Is our old concept of advanced practice out of date? Can we reconceptualize what we consider to be the skills necessary for entry into nursing practice? If we have been operating with an outdated definition of advanced practice, what are the skills or competencies of advanced practice nurses that can be expected on entry into the profession? Does one need a specified number of years of experience before being called advanced, or are the skills that we once called advanced really mainstream or entry-level skills? If the latter is true, then we need to rethink the skills and competencies necessary for entry-level versus expert practice.

Grypdonck, Schuurmans, Gamel, and Goverde (2004) reconceptualize advanced practice nursing by making a distinction between nursing science and nursing practice. These authors point out that nursing science and nursing practice operate in different spheres and ways of thinking. For example, scientists base their decisions on the greatest possible degree of certainty, and clinicians deal with uncertainty every day. According to Grypdonck et al., expert advanced practice nurses effectively bridge that gap through their advanced education and practice experience. This is where the practice doctorate may really begin to fit into this complex continuum of advanced practice nurses.

In nursing, we have placed a great deal of weight on experience and position rather than on a specific level of knowledge. As we replace our current cadre of nurses with younger individuals, we would do best to see knowledge acquisition as forming a continuum, beginning with a set of basic practice skills and moving to expert practice that integrates scientific principles and research skills with ongoing teaching, mentoring, and expert consultation.

In the last 12 years, the cadre of generic master's programs or accelerated master's programs has grown threefold, and in many master's programs, these students account for the majority of graduates. We must welcome these relatively young nurses into the fold of advanced practice nurses rather than exclude them and continue to operate in old ways.

In our reconceptualization of advanced practice, we might consider some way to recognize advanced practice through internships or other mechanisms of recognition. We may want to reconsider career ladders or Benner's levels of novice to expert practice. An expert advanced practice nurse should effectively use and incorporate research-based practice with a goal toward engaging in independent or collaborative research. Requirements for advanced practice nurses to precept, teach, or mentor newer nurses could be part of the certification credential. High-level skills such as consultation or clinical teaching require a body of expert knowledge and mastery of the content and are clearly in the realm of expert advanced practice nursing. Certification itself could be reframed to recognize entry-level versus expert practices, as was its original intent.

As we progress in redefining advanced practice, new technologies and knowledge, such as genetics and informatics, will increasingly enhance the patient-centered approach. Clinicians now are guided by state-of-the-art knowledge, which can be at the clinician's fingertips at any moment in practice through technology. In this new paradigm, the needs and demands of knowledgeable patients as well as scientific evidence-based guidelines will guide practice.

CONCLUSION

The nursing profession is now in a period of change, a paradigm shift. Nursing educators and policy makers must recognize this shift in order to plan for the future. As in the past, societal healthcare needs will shape the future direction of advanced practice nursing, and it will be up to our profession to change to meet those needs (Thompson & Watson, 2003). Our profession's ability to manage change and to move to a new conceptualization of advanced practice nursing will determine our success or failure in meeting societal needs. It is time to revisit even basic documents, such as *The Essentials of Master's Education for Advanced Practice Nursing* (AACN, 2011) and *The Essentials of Baccalaureate Education for Professional Nursing Practice* (AACN, 2008), which set the baseline definition of levels of nursing education. Our challenge now is to redefine advanced and recognize what is truly basic to all nursing practice.

DISCUSSION QUESTIONS ———————

1. Using the definitions of advanced practice nursing, should nursing administration, education, and research be considered advanced practice nursing?

2. List the similarities and differences between each of the roles discussed in this chapter.

3. What is the policy in your state related to licensure, reimbursement, and MD supervision for advanced practice nursing?

4. How can we reconceptualize what we consider to be the skills and knowledge needed for entry into practice as compared to those needed for advanced practice?

REFERENCES ———————

American Association of Colleges of Nursing. (2003). Accelerated programs: The fast-track to careers in nursing. Retrieved September 19, 2007, from http://www.aacn.nche.edu/Publications/issues/Aug02.htm

American Association of Colleges of Nursing. (2004). Doctor of nursing practice. Retrieved August 14, 2011, from http://www.aacn.nche.edu/DNP/DNPPositionStatement.htm

American Association of Colleges of Nursing. (2008). *The essentials of baccalaureate education for professional nursing practice.* Washington, DC: Author.

American Association of Colleges of Nursing. (2011). *The essentials of master's education for advanced practice nursing.* Washington, DC: Author.

American Association of Nurse Anesthetists, Council on Accreditation of Nurse Anesthesia Programs. (2004). List of recognized educational programs by Council on Accreditation of Nurse Anesthesia Educational Programs. Retrieved September 19, 2007, from http://www.aana.com/WorkArea/linkit.aspx?LinkIdentifier=ID&ItemID=118

American College of Nurse Midwives, Division on Accreditation. (2004). Division of accreditation. Retrieved September 19, 2007, from http://www.midwife.org/about.cfm?id=54

American Heritage dictionary of the American language. (1980). Boston: Houghton-Mifflin.

American Nurses Association. (1995). *Nursing's social policy statement.* Washington, DC: Author.

Berlin, L., Stennett, J., & Bednash, G. (2004). *Enrollment and graduations baccalaureate and graduate programs in nursing.* Washington, DC: American Association of Colleges of Nursing.

Gladwell, M. (2000). *The tipping point: How little things make a big difference.* Boston, MA: Little Brown Co.

Grypdonck, M., Schuurmans, M., Gamel, C., & Goverde, K. (2004). *Uniting both worlds: Nursing science and advanced nursing practice.* Presented at the International Nurse Practitioner/Advanced Practice Nursing Network Conference, Groningen, The Netherlands.

Hamric, A., & Hanson, C. (2003). Educating advanced practice nurses for practice reality. *Journal of Professional Nursing, 19*(5), 262-268.

Hamric, A., Spross, J., & Hanson, C. (2005). *Advanced practice nursing: An integrative approach.* St. Louis, MO: Elsevier Saunders.

Heitkemper, M., & Bond, E. (2004). Clinical nurse specialists: State of the profession and challenges ahead. *Clinical Nurse Specialist, 18*(3), 135-140.

International Council of Nurses. (2002). Health policy/nurse practitioner/advanced practice: Definitions and characteristics of the role. Retrieved September 19, 2007, from http://www.aanp.org/INP%20APN%20network/practice%20issues/role%20definitions.asp

Lyons, B. (2004). The CNS regulatory quagmire: We need clarity about advanced nursing practice. *Clinical Nurse Specialist, 18*(1), 9-13.

National Association of Clinical Nurse Specialists. (2004). *Statement on clinical nurse specialist practice and education.* Harrisburg, PA: Author.

National Organization of Nurse Practitioner Faculties. (1995). *Advanced nursing practice curriculum guidelines and program standards for nurse practitioner education.* Washington, DC: Author.

National Organization of Nurse Practitioner Faculties. (2002). *Nurse practitioner competencies in specialty areas.* Washington, DC: Author.

National Organization of Nurse Practitioner Faculties. (2006). *Domains and competencies of nurse practitioner practice.* Washington, DC: Author.

National Organization of Nurse Practitioner Faculties. (2008). *Criteria for evaluation of nurse practitioner programs.* Washington, DC: Author.

Pearson, L. (2004). Sixteenth annual legislative update: How each state stands on legislative issues affecting advanced nursing practice. *The Nurse Practitioner, 29*(1), 26-51.

Pulcini, J., & Vampola, D. (2002). Tracking NP prescribing trends. *The Nurse Practitioner, 29,* 10.

Pulcini, J., Vampola, D., & Levine, J. (2005). NPACE nurse practitioner practice characteristics, salary, and benefits survey: 2003. *Clinical Excellence for Nurse Practitioners, 9*(1), 49–58.

Thompson, D., & Watson, R. (2003). Advanced practice nursing: What is it? *International Journal of Nursing Practice, 9,* 129–130.

Towers, J. (2004). Region one meeting of the American Academy of Nurse Practitioners, Portsmouth, NH, October 2004.

CHAPTER 3

The Evolution of Doctoral Education in Nursing

Michael Carter

CHAPTER OBJECTIVES

1. Discuss the history of doctoral education in general and nursing doctoral programs in particular.

2. Differentiate between the different titles and structures for doctoral degrees in nursing.

3. Discuss some of the controversies surrounding the pros and cons of doctoral degrees in nursing

4. List different approaches that will influence the future of nursing doctorates.

INTRODUCTION

One of the most important aspects of any profession is the appropriate educational preparation of the leaders of the discipline. Almost without exception, the professions require that their leaders must hold doctoral degrees. The broad purposes of doctoral educational programs are to provide preparation that leads to careers in government, business, and industry, as well as academia (CAGS, 1990). Doctoral programs have been in existence since the Middle Ages, but it was during the 20th century that the United States saw a dramatic proliferation of doctoral educational programs in almost every academic field. The model of education that was created in the United States was built on earlier models from European universities. However, doctoral programs in the United States took on their own unique characteristics.

Nursing doctoral programs began in the later part of the 20th century, after their development in most other fields.

Perhaps this delay was because of nursing's unique history among the professions. Nursing in the United States began outside the mainstream of higher education and was located almost exclusively in hospitals. These hospitals, and the later universities where nursing educational programs moved, were controlled by administrative structures that are best described as highly paternalistic. These paternalistic organizations, in juxtaposition with the fact that most nurses were and still are women, may have delayed the profession from adopting doctoral degrees as the required credential for professional leadership. The profession adopted the master's degree early as the appropriate degree for leaders, and this may have been a disservice to the profession. Currently, nursing is far from having a unified approach to doctoral education.

The purpose of this chapter is to briefly discuss the history of doctoral education in general and nursing doctoral programs in particular. Clearly, this discussion is not exhaustive but is intended to provide an introduction to understanding doctoral education. Other, better historical overviews are available on the general topic of doctoral degrees (Harris, Troutt, & Andrews, 1980). This chapter also includes discussion of some of the controversies that are swirling about how doctoral degrees in nursing should be titled and structured and concludes with some ideas that may portend the future of nursing doctorates.

A BRIEF HISTORY OF DOCTORAL EDUCATION

The academic degrees that we see today are an outgrowth of the trade guilds and teaching guilds that flourished in Europe during the Middle Ages (U.S. DHEW, 1971). These early programs were often a product of the educational institutions that were either controlled or heavily dominated by the Catholic Church. Higher education was designed for the elite and certainly not for the general masses. Given this early tie with the Church, we can understand that many of the symbols, traditions, and rituals of the modern university emerged from the Church's influence on these schools. The doctoral gowns and hoods worn at graduation can be traced back to the garb worn by the priests.

The English word *doctor* comes from the Latin word *doctus,* the past participle of *docere,* which means "to teach" (*Webster's New Collegiate Dictionary,* 1979). Italian schools awarded formal doctoral degrees by 1219. This was the only degree offered by the schools, because they were preparing teachers. French schools used a slightly different approach and chose the name *masters,* from the Latin word *magister,* for their college graduates. Graduates from these schools were awarded the respective title and were admitted to the guild of teachers (Martin, 1989). Obtaining a degree meant that the graduate was fully qualified to serve as a teacher and did not need additional evaluation to begin this profession.

In the United States, the early colleges were established to prepare clergy and for the most part were built on the English and German systems of higher education. Harvard College was founded in 1636, and from that time until the Civil War, a little more than 200 years later, the only degree that could be earned in the United States was the bachelor of arts. Alumni who paid fees were able to obtain the master's degree without further collegiate work. Scientists who wished to obtain additional education had to receive this training in Europe (U.S. DHEW, 1971).

Following the Civil War, American colleges began to change. Yale awarded the first PhDs in the United States in 1861 (Martin, 1989). For the first time, there was an emerging emphasis on graduate education and the underlying research that is a part of graduate education today. Many of the faculty had obtained their graduate degrees at German universities. The German graduate school model did not usually include required class attendance or examinations. Rather, students studied under the direction of a major professor, conducted an original piece of research, and were expected to successfully defend their work before the standing faculty of the university to be granted the degree. However, because graduate education was embedded in undergraduate colleges, graduate students in the United States were often required to earn grades and attend lectures.

In the latter half of the 1800s, several professional associations were formed to advance their respective professions. One of their early activities was to persuade state legislatures that the professional services offered by the various disciplines would be greatly improved by creating licensure or certification requirements. As a part of this effort, educational programs that led to the professional doctorate, including the doctor of medicine (MD) and the doctor of dental surgery (DDS) were developed. New medical schools began to offer limited instruction in allopathic or homeopathic medicine. Although offering a doctoral degree, most of these early schools were little more than diploma mills with few, if any, paid faculty, very limited instruction, and substantial reliance on clerkships with practicing physicians. By the late 1800s, there were many different types of professional schools, but there were no accreditation standards. Most had limited faculty and questionable curricula. Seldom were these programs more than a year in length, and admission depended more on the student's economic achievements than on the student's prior academic achievements (U.S. DHEW, 1971).

Efforts to standardize curricula began at the turn of the century and continued well into the 1900s. Calls went out to improve professional education as well as the quality of the PhD. By 1900, approximately 50 universities in the United States offered the PhD, but there was almost no quality control. At the best universities, the PhD was awarded after about 2 years of postbaccalaureate study. There were a number of calls to improve this situation. For example, Abraham Flexner (1930) argued that the American universities had become misguided by their focus on preparing PhD graduates for practice and not for pure learning. He contended that this had diminished the quality of the education. His work in graduate education came on the heels of his work on the reform of allopathic medical education. By 1935, a fairly standardized model for PhD education was in place, and the emergence of various accrediting bodies ensured that quality standards were met. Many PhD programs were closed or merged because their quality did not meet emerging national standards.

Following World War II, a clear link developed between building the knowledge base for a specialized field and the award of the PhD in that field. For the first time, the U.S. government allocated funds to the building of the research needed to create new knowledge. A large portion of this new money was directed toward science as a part of the country's national defense efforts (Berelson, 1960).

In the early 1950s, a new debate emerged over whether the PhD should be the degree for the professions or whether the professions should use a professional degree such as the doctor of education (EdD), the doctor of business administration (DBA), the doctor of public health (DPH), or the doctor of nursing science (DNSc). The professions believed that the PhD was the standard and was well understood and aspired toward that degree. Arts and sciences faculty believed that awarding a PhD with a specialty in the professions would diminish the degree. In general, the professions prevailed in this argument, and the PhD was selected as the appropriate degree. This degree did carry with it the concomitant requirement that the completion of a satisfactory piece of research was required for its award (Berelson, 1960).

Professions that wished to prepare their practitioners without this research requirement awarded a professional degree such as the doctor of osteopathy (DO), the doctor of medicine (MD), the doctor of dental surgery (DDS), the doctor of dental medicine (DMD), the doctor of pharmacy (PharmD), the doctor of veterinary medicine (DVM), the doctor of optometry (OD), the doctor of chiropractic medicine (DC), and the doctor of podiatric medicine (DPM). These professional programs were not considered graduate programs because few of them required an undergraduate degree for admission and most did not build on undergraduate learning in a specific discipline to prepare for the profession (CAGS, 1966).

DOCTORAL PROGRAMS IN AND FOR NURSING

Stevenson and Woods (1986) identified four phases in nursing doctoral programs. Doctoral programs in nursing can be thought of as having four generations. The first phase was between 1900 and 1940, in which the doctor of education (EdD) or another functional degree was available. The second phase was between 1940 and 1960, when the degree could be obtained in a basic or social science discipline with no nursing content. The third phase was between 1960 and 1970, when a basic or social science PhD was available with a minor in nursing. The fourth phase began around 1970 with the rapid proliferation of the DNSc and nursing PhD programs.

The first research-focused doctoral programs in the United States were in various areas of science and did not seek to recruit nurses specifically. Nurses, as well as any other student, could be considered for admission if they possessed the necessary prerequisites. The problem was that few nurses at the beginning of the 20th century held an undergraduate degree. Basic nursing education was hospital based and did not award degrees.

The first doctoral programs that specifically recruited nurses were at Columbia University and New York University. These began in the 1920s and 1930s in education departments and were tailored to prepare nursing faculty. The programs awarded the PhD or EdD, but offered little, if any, coursework in nursing.

In the 1940s and 1950s, baccalaureate programs in nursing were created at a number of universities. Along with this move came important questions about the qualifications of the faculty. Faculty qualifications were a minor issue when the program was located in a hospital, but most universities held rather strict standards for faculty. Few nurses held baccalaureate degrees, and even fewer held master's degrees. Almost none held doctoral degrees, and the doctoral degree was the standard for university faculty positions.

This change in locus of nursing education gave rise to often acrimonious discussions among faculty at several schools of nursing about the need for doctoral education. These discussions often raised the following questions: Should the program of study be focused on the discipline of nursing or a science-related discipline? Should the degree not be in education, since most of the graduates would be educators? Would the master's degree not be sufficient, particularly if the focus of the master's degree was clinical nursing? If the new doctoral programs were to focus on nursing, from where would the faculty be drawn, as the number of nurses with doctorates in nursing was not sufficient for one school faculty, let alone many schools?

Several schools did begin doctoral programs in nursing in the 1950s and 1960s. While the program at Teachers College continued in nursing education and nursing administration, the program at New York University reconfigured the curriculum to focus on nursing as the science of unitary humans (Rogers, 1966). Boston University designed the first program to deal with the clinical practice of nursing and created the doctor of nursing science degree, with the first graduate in 1963. The University of California at San Francisco and the Catholic University of America followed

Boston University's lead and established doctor of nursing science programs shortly thereafter. The University of Pittsburgh created a PhD in clinical nursing around this same time. The University of Alabama at Birmingham developed a doctor of science in nursing (DSN) shortly thereafter, and it was designed similarly to the DNSc (Kelly, 1978).

A serious problem remained, however, in that many of the key players concluded that nursing science was not of sufficient maturity to justify the PhD. Of course, no measure of scientific maturity was advocated. Perhaps this problem grew from the fact that most nurses with doctorates at this time had obtained their degrees in another discipline. Those disciplines had the appearance of maturity because they offered a doctorate. These nurses had not spent their doctoral study in nursing because such doctoral study was not widely available. Further, some of the writings of the period display a rather romantic and narrow view of what constituted science. Nursing research texts proposed that science was logical and orderly, when in practice this is seldom the case. Some called for nursing practice to be derived from science, and yet few scientists would argue that practice is derived from science (McManus, 1960).

Funds from the federal government helped a number of nurses to obtain doctoral degrees, which may have contributed to the continuing debate over whether the doctoral degree should be in nursing or a different field. In 1955, the United States Public Health Service started funding doctoral study through the federal Predoctoral Research Fellowship Program. Funds were awarded directly to the doctoral student, and several aspiring faculty members were able to fund their education through this mechanism. Between 1955 and 1970, 156 nurses were supported by Division of Nursing fellowships (Grace, 1978). Almost none of these were in nursing.

Beginning in 1959, the Division of Nursing also funded the Faculty Research Development Grants Program. The purpose of these grants was to increase the research capabilities of faculty in graduate nursing programs by providing seed money. Eighteen institutions qualified for these grants between 1959 and 1968. Of these 18 programs, only three offered doctoral programs in nursing during the grant-funding period (1 PhD, 1 EdD, and 1 DNSc) (Martin, 1989).

In another attempt to increase the number of nurses with doctoral degrees, the Division of Nursing began to fund the nurse scientist graduate training grants. The intent of this program was to build a cadre of nurses with doctoral degrees at universities and to increase the number of nursing doctoral programs. Funding was designed to assist nurses in obtaining doctoral degrees in fields that were viewed as related to nursing. These fields included such areas as sociology, psychology, anthropology, biology, and physiology, with the expectation that there would be coursework or a minor in nursing. Nine universities representing 34 different departments received these grants. Four of the nine universities had doctoral programs in nursing at the time, but these were not eligible for receipt of this funding (Martin, 1989).

Beginning in the early 1970s, several new doctoral programs in nursing emerged. These new programs were most often in the older, more established schools of nursing. Growth continued through the 1980s and 1990s, with several new programs opening each year. The pace of new program development was often faster than the available faculty would have predicted would be the case. In 1970, there were 20 programs, but by 2000 there were 78 (AACN, 2002). Most of the research being conducted in these schools was done by students. Funding for nursing research in these schools was rare. The most common degree offered was the PhD, but several schools offered the DNSc or the DSN. Doctoral education in nursing became widely available throughout the United States during this time.

New approaches to delivery of the curriculum became available as well. Some schools offered a summers option, in which courses were scheduled during the summer months when faculty in nursing schools who needed the doctoral degree could participate. Other schools offered weekend programs, and Web-based distance learning programs emerged as well. Interestingly, the rapid increase in the number of programs and the development of creative ways to deliver the curriculum did little to increase the number of graduates each year.

This rapid growth and creativity in curriculum delivery were partly responsible for the development of new standards for doctoral programs. The American Association of Colleges of Nursing created a set of quality indicators for research-focused doctoral programs in nursing (AACN, 1993). These indicators became the standard for evaluation of these programs.

The rapid proliferation of programs did not create a concomitant increase in the number of graduates. The new programs were small (averaging six graduates per year), and the length of time to obtain the degree continued to be long, primarily because of the number of part-time students. Even though the number of programs had increased from 20 to 78, there were only 200 more graduates in 1998 than in 1989, and most of that growth occurred prior to 1992 (AACN, 2003). Clearly, these research-focused doctoral programs could not be expected to meet the needs for nursing faculty because of the small numbers and the fact that all graduates did not assume faculty positions after graduation. Also, the median age of the graduates at completion of the doctorate was older than 45 years.

CLINICAL DOCTORAL PROGRAMS

In 1979, the Frances Payne Bolton School of Nursing at Case Western Reserve University began a new approach to doctoral education in nursing (Standing & Kramer, 2003). Originally conceived as a first professional degree, the doctor of nursing (ND) was open to college graduates and prepared them to be nurses at a level similar to other health professional doctoral programs, such as medicine, veterinary medicine, dentistry, optometry, and others. The creation of this clinical program at the very time that nursing was struggling with building the research enterprise and research-focused doctorates was not accepted with universal agreement. Of some concern was how this program would be different from the DNSc. Up to this time, there had been the assumption that the PhD was to focus on scholarly research and the DNSc was to be the practice-oriented, clinical degree. Yet, studies had shown that the DNSc could not be distinguished from the PhD on the basis of admission standards, curriculum, or dissertation topics (Flaherty, 1989). For the first time, nursing had a doctoral degree that was open to non-nurses and that prepared the beginning clinician at the doctoral level.

Additional clinical doctoral programs were developed at Rush University, the University of Colorado, and the University of South Carolina. Today, most of these programs provide multiple entry points reflective of the diverse nature of nursing practice. Each of these programs prepares the clinician at the doctoral level to exert leadership in evidence-based practice, health policy, and management or education. These new programs created quite a stir, and one that the profession has yet to resolve. In 1963, when the first DNSc was awarded, the profession had assumed that the first clinical doctorate had arrived. But close inspection of the program showed that the DNSc curriculum required mastery within a field of knowledge and demonstrated ability to perform scholarly research—the very characteristics of the PhD (Standing & Kramer, 2003). The ND, in contrast, focused exclusively on preparing a clinical leader, not a researcher.

The clinical doctoral programs to some extent reflected the tremendous changes that were taking place in the clinical practice of nursing. The early beginning of the nurse practitioner and clinical nurse specialist movements had taken place. New master's programs were opening each year, and the major thrust of these programs was on advanced nursing practice. State laws were changing, and advanced practice nurses were obtaining greatly expanded scopes of practice and prescriptive privileges. Most of these new master's programs were between 18 months and 2 years in length.

Concern among some faculty was building that the length and rigor of these master's programs needed to be improved and that the graduate should earn a doctorate. Yet, the doctorate needed to be focused in clinical practice. This position was consistent with the Council on Graduate Schools' position that "the professional doctor's degree should be the highest university award given in a particular field in recognition of completion of academic preparation for professional practice" (CAGS, 1966, p. 3). The schools that created the ND programs were noted for their outstanding clinical master's programs. This new degree could be viewed as a logical extension of their programs.

Nursing educators have not universally accepted the ND program. As Standing and Kramer (2003) point out, reviews of nursing doctoral graduates published in the literature almost always ignore the graduates of such programs even though nearly 700 nurses hold this degree. The basis for ignoring or discounting these programs is not clear. The need for the clinical doctorate is clearly documented, and the demand for the scarce slots in these programs is also clear.

Recently, the University of Kentucky began a new clinical doctoral program, the doctor of nursing practice (DNP). On close inspection, this program shares many of the same curricular components as the ND programs. An additional planning group has met for several years to build a consensus for the development of additional doctor of nursing practice programs at senior universities. However, the distinctions between the doctor of nursing practice and the doctor of nursing are far from clear.

FUTURE DOCTORAL EDUCATION

The future of research-based doctoral programs in nursing is not likely to be much different from the recent past. No mechanisms are in place to determine how many programs there should be or to enforce quality standards at these programs. The demand for nursing faculty in the future is acute, and this will likely drive the creation of many more programs. Nursing has not been susceptible to the requirement seen in other disciplines that the faculty should be engaged in funded research prior to offering a research degree. Most schools offering the nursing PhD cannot be considered research-intensive schools.

The decision of a school to offer the PhD versus the DNSc often has been primarily a political decision. The PhD is often governed by the rules of the graduate school in addition to the nursing school, and this may mean that approval would be more problematic. Some schools (such as the University of California at San Francisco, the University of Pennsylvania, and Indiana University) began their doctoral programs as DNSc programs and later converted them to the PhD. Only two schools have begun PhD programs and then added DNSc programs—the University of Tennessee Health Science Center and Johns Hopkins University. In general, faculty prefer the PhD; therefore, it will likely continue to be the preferred degree in the future.

However, the world of clinical doctorates is quite different. The other major health professions have offered the clinical doctor's degree for a number of years. For example, pharmacy is the most recent profession to mandate the doctorate as the single degree for its professional practice. Nursing, the largest health profession, continues to prepare its beginning practitioners at less than the baccalaureate level. Attempts to alter this situation, even in light of important evidence of the value of higher education, have failed. What is emerging, however, is a de facto second license for nursing, the advanced practice license. This new license may accelerate the development of the clinical doctorate.

Nursing chose the master's degree as the minimum preparation for advanced practice. The master's degree in the United States has always been an unusual degree—more than the baccalaureate but less than the doctorate, and usually discipline specific. This degree is uncommon in the major health professions, at least as a professional degree. This degree designation is used for the master of public health and the master of hospital administration, but the other health professions use a nondegree, postdoctoral training period to prepare their specialists. Reasons as to why nursing adopted the master's degree are somewhat obscure, but are likely related to political considerations. Nursing's history of hospital-based education rather than degree-based education meant that much of nursing was left out of the advances in higher education during the 20th century. While medicine, dentistry, and, to some extent, pharmacy were able to strengthen their educational programs within the university tradition, nursing was still knocking at the door. Few women were able to obtain a college education until well after World War II. The idea that nursing should have a clinical doctoral degree similar to the other health fields would not have entered the minds of most academics, and certainly not most nurses, until recently.

Today, however, we see advanced practice nurses in roles that were unthinkable just a few years ago. Independent nursing practices in institutions and communities are making substantial changes in the way health care is delivered. The kind of education that these clinicians will need for the future cannot be achieved in today's master's programs. The future advanced practice nurses will need a minimum of a clinical doctoral degree and most likely will require substantial postdoctoral training in narrow specialties.

Not every school that currently offers the master's degree will have the faculty, clinical material, or other requisite resources to offer the clinical doctoral program. These programs are faculty intensive, require interdisciplinary coursework with the other major health professions, and are costly to operate. Schools of nursing must have a substantial clinical practice operation to be able to mount such a program. These new programs will prepare highly competent clinicians for such roles as primary care provider for cross-site practice; midwifery practice that includes surgical abilities to perform cesarean sections; anesthesia providers to administer all forms of anesthesia, including intrathecal approaches; as well as national and international leaders in policy formulation, complex organizational administration, and master clinical teachers. These roles cannot be achieved by obtaining a research-focused doctoral degree, and certainly not by way of the master's degree.

CONCLUSION

Doctoral education in the United States underwent dramatic changes during the 20th century and will likely continue to evolve over the next century. Nurses were once educated outside the mainstream of higher education, but following World War II the locus of nursing education was moved to the university. This trend has brought with it the need for a faculty commensurate with that of the rest of the university. For the arts and sciences, that meant the PhD degree; for the professional schools, it has meant the clinical doctorate.

Nursing was a bit slow to embrace the idea that nursing faculty would need the research doctorate. But once the idea was adopted, many schools—some would argue too many schools—rapidly developed these programs. There is still a reluctance to move to the development of the clinical doctorate on a broad scale. The potential for this degree to alter the power and political relationships between nursing and other professions, however, is substantial.

The clinical doctorate can provide a skill and science base for the graduate that cannot be achieved in today's educational programs. This level of expertise will be critical as the nation focuses on improving patient care and the safety of the systems that deliver health care. Clearly, the clinical doctorate will bring with it a level of independent practice that cannot be achieved at less than the doctoral level. For the first time, nursing would have parity in educational preparation with other healthcare disciplines.

Nursing is the most comprehensive of all the health professions. Clinical practice demands of nursing clinicians an understanding of the human condition, the environments in which clients live, the systems of care delivery, and the political milieu of care. Preparation of clinical leaders fundamentally requires a doctoral degree. The time is now for the discipline to move to the clinical doctorate to complement the many substantial accomplishments that have taken place by the creation of the research-focused doctorates.

DISCUSSION QUESTIONS

1. Visit the website of the American Association of Colleges of Nursing and specialty organizations. Read the most recent update on the clinical doctorate. Visit the sites of several universities and compare and contrast the similarities and differences of doctoral programs throughout the United States.

2. What are the pros and cons of requiring doctoral education for advanced practice in nursing? Include personal, professional, healthcare, and societal perspectives.

REFERENCES

American Association of Colleges of Nursing (AACN). (1993). *AACN position statement: Indicators of quality in doctoral programs in nursing.* Washington, DC: Author.

American Association of Colleges of Nursing (AACN). (2002). Indicators of quality in research-focused doctoral programs in nursing. Retrieved September 19, 2007, from http://www.aacn.nche.edu/Publications/positions/qualityindicators.htm

American Association of Colleges of Nursing (AACN). (2003). Indicators of quality in research-focused doctoral programs in nursing. *Journal of Professional Nursing, 18*(5), 289–294.

Berelson, B. (1960). *Graduate education in the United States.* New York: McGraw-Hill.

Council of Graduate Schools (CGS) in the United States. (1966). *The doctor's degree in professional fields: A statement by the Association of Graduate Schools and the Council of Graduate Schools in the United States.* Washington, DC: Author.

Council of Graduate Schools (CGS) in the United States. (1990). *The doctor of philosophy degree: A policy statement.* Washington, DC: Author.

Flaherty, M. J. (1989). The doctor of nursing science degree: Evolutionary and societal perspectives. In S. E. Hart (Ed.), *Doctoral education in nursing: History, process, and outcome* (pp. 17–31). New York: National League for Nursing.

Flexner, A. (1930). *Universities: American, English, German.* New York: Oxford University Press.

Grace, H. (1978). The research doctorate in nursing. In *Proceedings of the 1978 Forum on Doctoral Education in Nursing* (pp. 40–59). Chicago: Rush University.

Harris, J., Troutt, W., & Andrews, G. (1980). *The American doctorate in the context of new patterns in higher education.* Washington, DC: Council on Post Secondary Accreditation.

Kelly, J. (1978). The professional doctorate in nursing from the viewpoint of nursing service. In *Proceedings of the 1978 Forum on Doctoral Education in Nursing* (pp. 10–39). Chicago: Rush University.

Martin, E. J. (1989). The doctor of philosophy degree: Evolutionary and societal perspectives. In S. E. Hart (Ed.), *Doctoral education in nursing: History, process and outcome* (pp. 1–16). New York: National League for Nursing.

McManus, L. (1960). Doctoral education in nursing: A nurse educator responds. *Nursing Outlook, 8,* 543–546.

Rogers, M. (1966). Doctoral education in nursing. *Nursing Forum, 5*(2), 75–82.

Standing, T. S., & Kramer, F. M. (2003). The ND: Preparing nurses for clinical and educational leadership. *Reflections on Nursing Leadership, 29*(4), 35–37, 44.

Stevenson, J. S., & Woods, N. F. (1986). Nursing science and contemporary science: Emerging paradigms. In G. E. Sorensen (Ed.), *Setting the agenda for the year 2000: Knowledge development in nursing* (pp. 6–20). Kansas City, MO: American Academy of Nursing.

U.S. Department of Health, Education, and Welfare (U.S. DHEW). (1971). *Future directions of doctoral education for nurses.* (U.S. DHEW Publication No. [NIH] 72–82). Bethesda, MD: Author.

Webster's New Collegiate Dictionary. (1979). Springfield, MA: Merriam-Webster.

CHAPTER 4

Overview of the Doctor of Nursing Practice Degree

Lisa Astalos Chism

CHAPTER OBJECTIVES

1. Discuss differences between the practice doctorates in nursing vs. the research doctorate.

2. Describe the evolution of the doctor of nursing practice curriculum and its potential impact on the future of nursing.

3. Identify different educational pathways to the doctor of nursing practice degree.

4. Analyze factors in our current healthcare delivery system that is driving the need for nurses prepared as expert clinicians.

"You cannot hope to build a better world without improving the individual. To that end each of us must work for his own improvement, and at the same time share a general responsibility for all humanity, our particular duty being to aid those to whom we think we can be most useful."

—*Marie Curie (1867–1934)*

What exactly is a Doctor of Nursing Practice (DNP) degree? As enrollment to this innovative practice doctorate program increases, this question is frequently posed by nurses, patients, and other healthcare professionals both in and out of the healthcare setting. Providing an explanation to this question requires not only defining the DNP degree but also reflecting on the rich history of doctoral education in nursing. Doctoral education in nursing is connected to our past and influences the directions we may take in the future (Carpenter & Hudacek, 1996). The development of the DNP degree is a tribute to where nursing has been and where we hope to be in the future of doctoral education in nursing.

Understanding what a DNP degree is requires developing an awareness of the rationale for a practice doctorate. This rationale illustrates the motivation behind the evolution of doctoral education in nursing and provides further explanation of this contemporary degree. The need for parity across the healthcare team, the Institute of Medicine's call for safer healthcare practices, and the need for increased preparation of advanced practice registered nurses to meet the changing demands of health care are all contributing antecedents of the development of the practice doctorate in nursing (American Association of Colleges of Nursing [AACN], 2006a; AACN, 2006b; Apold, 2008; Dracup, Cronenwett, Meleis, & Benner, 2005; Roberts & Glod, 2005). Becoming familiar with the motivating factors behind the DNP degree will add to the understanding of the development of this innovative degree.

This chapter provides a definition of the DNP degree as well as a discussion of the evolution of doctoral education in nursing. The rationale for a practice doctorate is also described. The recipe for the DNP degree, which includes the *Essentials of Doctoral Education for Advanced Nursing Practice* degree outlined by the American Association of Colleges of Nursing (AACN, 2006b) and the *Practice Doctorate Nurse Practitioner Entry-Level Competencies* outlined by

the National Organization of Nurse Practitioner Faculties (NONPF, 2006), is provided in this chapter as well. The pathway to the DNP degree is also discussed. Providing a discussion regarding these topics will equip one with the information necessary to become familiar with this innovative degree.

THE DOCTOR OF NURSING PRACTICE DEGREE DEFINED

The DNP degree has been adopted as the terminal practice degree in nursing (AACN, 2004; AACN, 2006b). The AACN (2004) position statement specifically defines the DNP degree as a "practice focused" doctorate degree with nursing practice defined as:

> any form of nursing intervention that influences health care outcomes for individuals or populations, including the direct care of individual patients, management of care for individuals and populations, administration of nursing and health care organizations, and the development and implementation of health policy. (p. 3)

Preparation at the practice doctorate level is considered to be the highest level of preparation for nursing practice, hence, the terminal degree for nursing practice (AACN, 2004).

The DNP degree curriculum is focused on, although not limited to, evidence-based practice, scholarship to advance the profession, organizational and systems leadership, information technology, healthcare policy and advocacy, interprofessional collaboration across disciplines of health care, and advanced nursing practice (AACN, 2006b). It is projected that by 2015, the DNP degree will be the terminal preparation for advanced practice nursing, and current master's degree options for advanced nursing practice will be replaced by the DNP degree (AACN, 2006a). A newly developed master's degree, the Clinical Nurse Leader (CNL) degree, will be offered for those who wish to provide healthcare services at the point of care to individuals and cohorts of clients within a healthcare unit or setting (AACN, 2007). This degree prepares the graduate as "a leader in the health care delivery system, not just in the acute care setting but in all settings in which health care is delivered" (AACN, 2007, p. 10). Details regarding the content of the DNP degree curriculum are provided later in this chapter.

THE RESEARCH-FOCUSED DOCTORATE AND THE PRACTICE-FOCUSED DOCTORATE DEFINED

The question, What is a Doctor of Nursing Practice degree? is often followed by the question, What is the difference between a Doctor of Philosophy (PhD) and a DNP degree? Nurses now have a choice between a practice-focused or research-focused doctorate as a terminal degree. Although the academic or research degree, once the only terminal preparation in nursing, has traditionally been the Doctor of Philosophy (PhD), the American Association of Colleges of Nursing has included the Doctor of Nursing Science (DNS, DNSc, DSN) as a research-focused degree as well (AACN, 2004). Further, the AACN Task Force on the Practice Doctorate in nursing has recommended that the practice doctorate be the DNP degree, which will replace the traditional Nursing Doctorate (ND) degree (AACN, 2006a). Currently, nursing doctorate programs are taking the necessary steps to adjust their programs to fit the curriculum criteria of DNP degree programs.

The practice- and research-focused doctorates in nursing share a common goal regarding a "scholarly approach to the discipline and a commitment to the advancement of the profession" (AACN, 2006b, p. 3). The differences in these programs include differences in preparation and expertise. The practice doctorate curriculum places more emphasis on practice and less on theory and research methodology (AACN, 2006b; AACN, 2004). The final scholarly project differs as well in that a dissertation required of a PhD degree should document development of new knowledge, and a final scholarly project required of a DNP degree should be grounded in clinical practice and demonstrate ways in which research has an impact on practice.

The focus of the DNP degree is expertise in clinical practice. Additional foci include the *Essentials of Doctoral Education for Advanced Nursing Practice* as outlined by the AACN (2006b), which includes leadership, health policy and advocacy, and information technology. The focus of a research degree is the generation of new knowledge for the discipline and expertise as a principal investigator. However, although the research degree prepares the expert researcher, it should be noted that frequently DNP research projects will also contribute to the discipline by generating new knowledge related to clinical practice as well as demonstrate the use of evidence-based practice.

Please refer to **Table 4-1** for AACN's comparison of DNP and PhD/DNS/DNSc programs.

THE EVOLUTION OF DOCTORAL EDUCATION IN NURSING

To appreciate the development of doctoral education in nursing, one must understand where nursing has been with regard to education at the doctoral level. Indeed, nursing has been unique in the approach to doctoral preparation since nurses began to earn doctoral degrees. Even today nurses are prepared at the doctoral level through varying degrees, which include Doctor of Education (EdD), Doctor of Philosophy (PhD), Doctor of Nursing Science (DNS), and more recently, the Doctor of Nursing Practice degree. Prior to the development of the DNP degree, the Nursing Doctorate was also offered as a choice for nursing doctoral education.

Examining the chronological development of doctoral education in nursing is somewhat complicated due to the fact that early doctorates were offered outside of nursing. These included the EdD degree and the PhD degree in basic science fields, such as anatomy and physiology (Carpenter & Hudacek, 1996; Marriner-Tomey,

TABLE 4-1	AACN Contrast Grid of the Key Differences Between DNP and PhD/DNS/DNSc Programs	
	DNP	PhD/DNS/DNSc
Program of study	*Objectives:* ■ Prepare nurse specialists at the highest level of advanced practice *Competencies:* ■ Based on *Essentials of Doctoral Education for Advanced Nursing Practice* (AACN, 2006b)	*Objectives:* ■ Prepare nurse researchers *Content:* ■ Based on *Indicators of Quality in Research-Focused Doctoral Programs in Nursing* (AACN, 2001)
Students	■ Commitment to a practice career ■ Oriented toward improving outcomes of care	■ Commitment to a research career ■ Oriented toward developing new knowledge
Program faculty	■ Practice doctorate and/or experience in area in which teaching ■ Leadership experience in area of specialty practice ■ High level of expertise in specialty practice congruent with focus of academic program	■ Research doctorate in nursing or related field ■ Leadership experience in area of sustained research funding ■ High level of expertise in research congruent with focus of academic program
Resources	■ Mentors and/or precepts in leadership positions across a variety of practice settings ■ Access to diverse practice settings with appropriate resources for areas of practice ■ Access to financial aid ■ Access to information and patient-care technology resources congruent with areas of study	■ Mentors/preceptor in research settings ■ Access to research settings with appropriate resources ■ Access to dissertation support dollars ■ Access to information and research technology resources congruent with program of research
Program assessment and evaluation	*Program outcome:* ■ Healthcare improvements contributions via practice, policy change, and practice scholarship ■ Oversight by the institution's authorized bodies (i.e., graduate school) and regional accreditors ■ Receives accreditation by specialized nursing accreditor ■ Graduates are eligible for national certification exam	*Program outcome:* ■ Contributes to healthcare improvements via the development of new knowledge and other scholarly projects that provide the foundation for the advancement of nursing science ■ Oversight by the institution's authorized bodies (i.e., graduate school) and regional accreditor

Source: Reprinted with permission from *AACN DNP Roadmap Task Force Report,* October 20, 2006.

1990). The first nursing-related doctoral program was originated in 1924 at Teachers College, Columbia University and was an EdD designed to prepare nurses to teach at the college level (Carpenter & Hudacek, 1996). Teachers College was unique in that its program was the first to combine both the "nursing and education needs of leaders in the profession" (Carpenter & Hudacek, 1996, p. 5). Doctor of Education (EdD) degrees continued well into the 1960s to be the mainstay of doctoral education for nursing (Marriner-Tomey, 1990).

The first PhD in nursing was offered in 1934 at New York University. Unfortunately, the next PhD in nursing was not offered until the 1950s at the University of Pittsburgh and focused on maternal and child nursing. Incidentally, this degree was the first to recognize the importance of clinical research for the development of the discipline of nursing (Carpenter & Hudacek, 1996). The PhD degrees earned elsewhere continued to be in nursing-related fields, such as psychology, sociology, and anthropology. This trend continued until actual nursing PhD degrees became more popular in the 1970s (Grace, 1978).

Grace (1978) summarized the progression of nursing education over time. During the time between 1924 and 1959, doctoral education in nursing focused on preparing nurses for "functional specialty" (p. 22). In other words, nurses were prepared to fulfill functional roles as teachers and administrators to lead the field of nursing toward advancement as a profession. The problem noted with these programs is that they lacked the substantive content necessary to develop nursing as a discipline, as well as a profession. The next shift in doctoral education attempted to fulfill this need and took place between 1960 and 1969. Within this time period, popularity increased for doctoral programs that were nursing related. This included doctorates (PhDs) that were related to disciplines such as sociology, psychology, and anthropology. Grace (1978) noted that the development of these types of programs provided

the basic science and research input necessary for the development of future nursing doctorate programs. Murphy (1981) concurred that this stage in the development of doctoral education in nursing led to pertinent questions for the discipline of nursing, such as: "(1) What is the essential nature of professional nursing? (2) What is the substantive knowledge base of professional nursing? (3) What kind of research is important for nursing as a knowledge discipline? As a field of practice? (4) How can the scientific base of nursing knowledge be identified and expanded?" (p. 646).

In response to these questions, nursing doctoral education again progressed in the 1970s to include doctorate degrees that are actually in nursing (Grace, 1978). This stage also supported the growth of nursing's substantive structure, hence, the growth of the discipline of nursing.

Now, this is where nursing's history of doctoral education becomes more complex. In 1960, the Doctor of Nursing Science (DNS) degree originated at Boston University and "focused on the development of nursing theory for a practice discipline" (Marriner-Tomey, 1990, p. 135), hence, the development of the first practice doctorate. The notion of a practice-focused doctorate in nursing is not new. Even as early as the 1970s, it was proposed that the research doctorate (PhD) should focus on preparing nurses to contribute to nursing science, and the practice (or professional) doctorate (DNS) should focus on expertise in clinical practice (Cleland, 1976). Newman (1975) also suggested a practice doctorate as the preparation of "professional practitioners" (p. 705) for entry into practice. Grace (1978) noted that it was not sufficient to have a core of nursing researchers building the knowledge base (discipline) without also giving attention to the clinical field. It was also suggested by Grace (1978) that nurses prepared through a practice doctorate be titled "social engineers" (p. 26). This seems appropriate given what expert clinicians in nursing are called upon to do.

Although the DNS degree was initially proposed as a practice or professional doctorate, over time the curriculum requirements have become very similar to those for a PhD degree (AACN, 2006a; Apold, 2008; Marriner-Tomey, 1990). Research requirements for this degree have eventually become indistinguishable from that of a PhD in nursing. Because of this, it is not surprising that the American Association of Colleges of Nursing has characterized all DNS degrees as research degrees (AACN, 2004).

With the DNS and PhD degrees so similar in content and focus, the challenge to develop a true practice doctorate remained. An attempt toward this was made in 1979 when the Nursing Doctorate (ND) originated at Case Western Reserve University, followed by the University of Colorado, Rush University, and South Carolina University. The first ND program was developed by Rozella M. Schlotfeldt, PhD, RN. The Nursing Doctorate was different in that the research component was not the general focus of the degree. This degree was designed to be a "pre-service nursing education which would orient nursing's approach to preparing professionals toward competent, independent, accountable nursing practice" (Carpenter & Hudacek, 1996, p. 42). This general theme for a practice doctorate remains consistent even today. Unfortunately, this program did not share the same popularity of DNS or PhD degrees in nursing, and it was less common to find a clinician with this preparation. Further, the curricula in these programs were varied and lacked a uniform approach toward a practice doctorate (Marion, et al., 2003).

In 2002, the AACN board of directors formed a task force to examine the current progress of practice doctorates in nursing. Their objective also included comparing proposed curriculum models and discussing recommendations for the future of a practice doctorate (AACN, 2004). To accomplish their mission, the AACN task force (2004) took part in the following activities:

- Reviewed the literature regarding practice doctorates in nursing and other disciplines.

- Established a collaborative relationship with the National Organization of Nurse Practitioner Faculties (NONPF).

- Interviewed key informants (deans, program directors, graduates, and current students) at the eight current or planned practice-focused doctoral programs in the United States.

- Held open discussions regarding issues surrounding practice-focused doctoral education at AACN's Doctoral Education Conference (January 2003 and February 2004).

- Participated in an open discussion with the NONPF along with representatives from key nursing organizations and schools of nursing that were offering or planning a practice doctorate.

- Invited an External Reaction Panel, which involved participation from 10 individuals from various disciplines outside of nursing. This panel responded to the draft of the *AACN Position Statement on the Practice Doctorate in Nursing*.

In 2004, the AACN published a *Position Statement on the Practice Doctorate in Nursing* and recommended that the Doctor of Nursing Practice degree would become the terminal degree for nursing practice by 2015. According to the NONPF, the purpose of the Doctor of Nursing Practice degree is to prepare nurses to meet the changing demands of health care today by becoming proficient at the following (Marion, et al., 2003):

- Evaluating evidence-based practices for care.
- Delivering care.
- Developing healthcare policy.
- Leading and managing clinical care and health systems.
- Developing interdisciplinary standards.
- Solving healthcare dilemmas.
- Reducing disparities in health care.

Not only is the development of the DNP degree a culmination of today's emerging healthcare demands, this degree also provides a choice for nurses who wish to focus their doctoral education on nursing practice.

Since its inception, the growth of this degree has been astonishing. The University of Kentucky's College of Nursing was the pioneer for this innovative degree and admitted the first DNP class in 2001. In spring of 2005, eight DNP programs were offered, with over 60 in development. By summer of 2005, 80 DNP programs were being considered. In the fall of 2005, 20 programs offered DNP degrees, and 140 programs were in development. Currently, approximately 130 DNP degree programs exist, and 100 are being considered (AACN, 2011a).

It should also be mentioned that in 1999, Columbia University's School of Nursing was formulating plans for a Doctor of Nursing Practice degree (DrNP) that would build on a model of "full-scope, cross-site primary care that Columbia had developed and evaluated over the past ten years" (Goldenberg, 2004, p. 25). This degree was spearheaded by Mary O. Mudinger, DrPH, RN, dean of Columbia University's School of Nursing. The curriculum of a DrNP program is clinically focused with advanced preparation designed to teach "cross-site, full-scope care with content in advanced differential diagnosis skills, advanced pathophysiology and microbiology, selected issues of compliance, management of health care delivery and reimbursement, advanced emergency triage and management, and professional role collaboration and referrals" (Goldenberg, 2004, p. 25). This expanded clinical component is what seems to differentiate a DrNP degree from a DNP degree. The first DrNP class graduated from Columbia University in 2003.

Since the development of the DrNP degree, the Commission on Collegiate Nursing Education (CCNE), the autonomous accrediting body of the American Association of Colleges of Nursing, has decided that only practice nursing doctorate degrees with the Doctor of Nursing Practice title will be eligible for CCNE accreditation (AACN, 2005). This decision was reached

unanimously by the CCNE Board of Directors on September 29, 2005 in an effort to develop a process for accrediting only clinically focused nursing doctorates (AACN, 2005). The CCNE's decision is consistent with accrediting organizations for other health professions and helps to ensure consistency with degree titling and criteria. Specific criteria for the DNP degree, including the AACN's *Essentials of Doctoral Education for Advanced Nursing Practice* (2006b) and the *Practice Doctorate Nurse Practitioner Entry-Level Competencies* (NONPF, 2006), are discussed later in this chapter.

WHY A PRACTICE DOCTORATE IN NURSING NOW?

It has already been mentioned that the notion of a practice doctorate is not new, so why the development of the DNP degree now? It has been noted that the development of the DNP is "more than a mere interruption but rather a response to the need within the healthcare system for expert clinical teachers and clinicians" (Marion, O'Sullivan, Crabtree, Price, & Fontana, 2005, p. 1). The needs of health care are also not new, yet the growth of this program has been escalating. The question is therefore posed, What are the drivers of this DNP degree, and why such urgency?

The Institute of Medicine's Report and Nursing's Response

In 2000, the Institute of Medicine (IOM) published a report titled *To Err Is Human*. This report summarized information regarding errors made in health care and offered recommendations to improve the overall quality of care. It was found that "preventable adverse events are a leading cause of death in the United States" (Kohn, Corrigan, & Donaldson, 2000, p. 26). Out of over 33.6 million admissions to U.S. hospitals in 1997, 44,000 to 98,000 people died as a result of medical-related errors (American Hospital Association, 1999). It was estimated that deaths in hospitals by preventable adverse events exceed the amount attributable to the eighth leading cause of death in America (Centers for Disease Control and Prevention, 1999b). These numbers also exceed the number of deaths attributable to motor vehicle accidents (43,458), breast cancer (42,297), or AIDS (16,516) (Centers for Disease Control and Prevention, 1999a). The total cost of health care is greatly affected by these errors as well, with estimated total national costs (lost income, lost household production, disability, healthcare costs) reported as being between $29 billion and $36 billion for adverse events and between $17 billion and $29 billion for preventable adverse events (Thomas, et al., 1999).

As a follow-up to the *To Err Is Human* report, in 2001 the IOM published *Crossing the Quality Chasm: A New Health System for the 21st Century*. In an effort to improve health care in the 21st century, the IOM proposed six specific aims for improvement. According to the IOM (2001), these six aims deem that health care should be:

1. Safe in avoiding injuries to patients from the care they receive.
2. Effective in providing services based on scientific knowledge to those who could benefit but refraining from providing services to those who may not benefit.
3. Patient centered in that provided care is respectful and responsive to individual patient preferences, needs, and values. Also, all patient values should guide all clinical decisions.
4. Timely in that wait time and sometimes harmful delays are reduced for those who give and receive care.
5. Efficient in that waste is avoided, particularly waste of equipment, supplies, ideas, and energy.
6. Equitable in that high-quality care is provided to all regardless of personal characteristics, such as gender, ethnicity, geographic location, and socioeconomic status.

The IOM (2001) emphasized that to achieve these aims, additional skills may be required of the healthcare team. This includes all individuals who care for patients. The new skills needed to improve health care and reduce errors are, ironically, many skills that nurses have long been known to exemplify. Some examples of these skills include using electronic communications, synthesizing evidence-based practice information, communicating with patients in an open manner to enable their decision making, understanding the course of illness that specifically relates to the patient's experience outside of the hospital, working collaboratively in teams, and understanding the link between health care and healthy populations (IOM, 2001). Developing expertise in these areas required curriculum changes in healthcare education as well as addressing how healthcare education is approached, organized, and funded (IOM, 2001).

In 2003, the Health Professions Education Committee responded to the IOM's *Crossing the Quality Chasm* report by publishing *Health Professions Education: A Bridge to Quality* (Greiner & Knebel, 2003). The committee recommended that "all health professionals should be educated to deliver patient-centered care as members of an interdisciplinary team, emphasizing evidence-based practice, quality improvement approaches, and informatics" (Greiner & Knebel, 2003, p. 45). To meet this goal, the committee proposed a set of competencies to be met by all healthcare clinicians, regardless of disciplines. These competencies include the following: provide patient-centered care, function in interdisciplinary teams, employ evidence-based practice, integrate quality improvement standards, and utilize various information systems (Greiner & Knebel, 2003).

As part of the continued effort to advance the education of healthcare professionals, the Robert Wood Johnson Foundation (RWJF) and the IOM specifically addressed advancing nursing education. In 2008, the RWJF and the IOM "launched a two-year initiative to respond to the need to access and transform the nursing profession" (IOM, 2010a, p. 1). The IOM appointed the Committee on the RWJF Initiative on the Future of Nursing. This committee published a report titled *The Future of Nursing: Focus on Education*.

Within this report, the IOM (2010a) concluded that "the ways in which nurses were educated during the 20th century are no longer adequate for dealing with the realities of healthcare in the 21st century" (p. 2). The IOM reiterated the need for the aforementioned competencies such as leadership, health policy, system improvement, research and evidence-based practice, and teamwork and collaboration. In response to the increasing demands of a complex healthcare environment, the IOM recommended higher levels of education for nurses as well as new ways to educate nurses to better meet the needs of this population.

The IOM (2010a) included recommendations within this report that specifically address the number of nurses with doctorate degrees. It was noted that, although 13% of nurses hold a graduate degree, less than 1% hold doctoral degrees (IOM, 2010a). The IOM (2010a) concluded that "nurses with doctorates are needed to teach future generations of nurses and to conduct research that becomes the basis for improvements in nursing science and practice" (p. 4). Therefore, Recommendation 5 states that "schools of nursing, with support from private and public funders, academic administrators and university trustees, and accreditation bodies, should double the number of nurses with a doctorate by 2020 to add to the cadre of nurse faculty and researchers, with attention to increasing diversity" (IOM, 2010b, p. 4).

The development of the DNP degree is one of the answers to the call proposed by both the IOM's Health Professions Education Committee and the IOM's and the RWJF's Initiative on the Future of Nursing Committee to redefine how healthcare professionals are educated. Nursing has always had a vested interest in improving quality of care and patient outcomes. Since Nightingale, "nursing education has been

directed toward the individualized, personalized care of the patient, not the disease" (Newman, 1975, p. 704). To further illustrate nursing's commitment to improve quality of care and patient outcomes, the competencies described by the Health Professions Education Committee are reflected in the AACN's *Essentials of Doctoral Education for Advanced Nursing Practice* and the NONPF's *Practice Doctorate Nurse Practitioner Entry-Level Competencies*. Preparing nurses at the practice doctorate level who are experts at using information technology, synthesizing and integrating evidence-based practices, and collaborating across healthcare disciplines will further enable nursing to meet the challenges of health care in the 21st century.

Additional Drivers for a Practice Doctorate in Nursing

In 2005, the National Academy of Sciences also recommended that nursing develop a nonresearch doctorate in a report entitled *Advancing the Nation's Health Needs: NIH Research Training Programs* (National Academy of Sciences, 2005). The rationale for this initiative included increasing the numbers of expert practitioners who can also fulfill clinical nursing faculty needs (AACN, 2011b). The report specifically states that "the need for doctorally prepared practitioners and clinical faculty would be met if nursing could develop a new non-research clinical doctorate, similar to the MD and PharmD in Medicine and Pharmacy, respectively" (National Academy of Sciences, 2005, p. 74). The initiatives of the National Academy of Sciences regarding doctoral education in nursing are reflected in the American Association of Colleges of Nursing's development of the DNP degree.

Additional rationale for a practice doctorate is reflected in nursing's educational history when the practice doctorate was first proposed. Newman (1975) noted that "nursing lacked the recognition for what it has to offer and authority for putting that knowledge into practice" (p. 704). Starck, Duffy, and Vogler (1993) stated that "for nursing to be accountable to the social mandate, the numbers as well as the type of doctorally prepared nurses need attention" (p. 214). The NONPF Practice Doctorate Task Force summarized the most frequently cited additional drivers for a practice doctorate in nursing (Marion, et al., 2005):

- Parity with other professionals who are prepared with a practice doctorate. Disciplines such as audiology, dentistry, medicine, pharmacy, psychology, and physical therapy require a practice doctorate for entry into practice.
- A need for longer programs that both reflect the credit hours invested in master's degrees as well as accommodate additional information needed to prepare nurses for the demands of health care. Most master's degrees require a similar number of credit hours for completion to the number required for that of practice doctoral degrees.
- Fulfill the current needs for nursing faculty shortages. The development of a practice doctorate will help meet the needs for clinical teaching in schools of nursing.
- The increasing complexity of healthcare systems requires additional information to be included in current graduate nursing programs. Rather than further burden the amount of information needed to prepare nurses at the graduate level for a master's degree, a practice doctorate allows for additional information to be provided as well as afford a practice doctorate to prepare nurses for the changing demands of society and health care.

WHAT IS A DNP DEGREE MADE OF? THE RECIPE FOR CURRICULUM STANDARDS

The standards of a DNP program have been formulated through a collaborative effort among various consensus-based standards. These standards reflect collaborative efforts

among the AACN as the *Essentials of Doctoral Education for Advanced Nursing Practice*, the NONPF as the *Practice Doctorate Nurse Practitioner Entry-Level Competencies*, and most recently, the National Association of Clinical Nurse Specialists (NACNS) as *Core Practice Doctorate Clinical Nurse Specialist (CNS) Competencies*. These organizations' strategies for setting the standards of a practice doctorate in nursing demonstrate interrelated criteria that are congruent with all rationales for a practice doctorate in nursing. It should be noted, however, that while maintaining these consensus-based standards, there may be some variability in content within DNP curricula.

The *Essentials of Doctoral Education for Advanced Nursing Practice*

In 2006, the AACN published the *Essentials of Doctoral Education for Advanced Nursing Practice*. These Essentials are the "foundational outcome competencies deemed essential for all graduates of a DNP program regardless of specialty or functional focus" (AACN, 2006b, p. 8). Nursing faculties have the freedom to creatively design course work to meet these Essentials, which are summarized as follows:

Essential I: Scientific Underpinnings for Practice

This Essential describes the scientific foundations of nursing practice, which are based on the natural and social sciences. These sciences may include human biology, physiology, and psychology. In addition, nursing science has provided nursing with a body of knowledge to contribute to the discipline of nursing. This body of knowledge or discipline is focused on the following (adapted from AACN, 2006b; Donaldson & Crowley, 1978; Fawcett, 2005; Gortner, 1980):

- The principles and laws that govern the life process, well-being, and optimal functioning of human beings, sick or well

- The patterning of human behavior in interaction with the environment in normal life events and critical life situations
- The processes by which positive changes in health status are affected
- The wholeness of health of human beings, recognizing that they are in continuous interaction with their environments

Nursing science has expanded the discipline of nursing and includes the development of middle-range nursing theories and concepts to guide practice. Understanding the practice of nursing includes developing an understanding of scientific underpinnings for practice (the science and discipline of nursing). Specifically, the DNP degree prepares the graduate to:

- Integrate nursing science with knowledge from the organizational, biophysical, psychological, and analytical sciences as well as ethics as the basis for the highest level of nursing practice.
- Develop and evaluate new practice approaches based on nursing theories and theories from other disciplines.
- Utilize science-based concepts and theories to determine the significance and nature of health and healthcare delivery phenomena, describe strategies used to enhance healthcare delivery, and evaluate outcomes

(Adapted from AACN, 2006b)

Essential II: Organizational and Systems Leadership for Quality Improvement and Systems Thinking

Preparation in organizational and systems leadership at every level is imperative for DNP graduates to have an impact on and improve healthcare delivery and patient care outcomes. DNP graduates are distinguished by their ability to focus on new healthcare delivery methods that are based on nursing science. Preparation in this area will provide DNP graduates with ex-pertise in "assessing organizations, identifying systems' issues, and facilitating organization-wide changes in practice delivery" (AACN, 2006b, p. 10). Specifically, the DNP graduate will be prepared to:

- Utilize scientific findings in nursing and other disciplines to develop and evaluate care delivery approaches that meet the current and future needs of patient populations.
- Guarantee accountability for the safety and quality of care for the patients they care for.
- Manage ethical dilemmas within patient care, healthcare organizations, and research, including developing and evaluating appropriate strategies.

(Adapted from AACN, 2006b)

Essential III: Clinical Scholarship and Analytical Methods for Evidence-Based Practice

DNP graduates are unique in that their contributions to nursing science involve the "translation of research into practice and the dissemination and integration of new knowledge" (AACN, 2006b, p. 11). Further, DNP graduates are in a distinctive position to merge nursing science, practice, human needs, and human caring. Specifically, the DNP graduate is expected to be an expert in the evaluation, integration, translation, and application of evidence-based practices. Additionally, DNP graduates are actively involved in nursing practice, which allows for practical, applicable research questions to arise from the practice environment. Working collaboratively with experts in research investigation, DNP graduates can also assist in the generation of new knowledge and affect evidence-based practice from the practice arena. To achieve these goals, the DNP program prepares the graduate to:

- Analytically and critically evaluate existing literature and other evidence to determine the best evidence for practice.

- Evaluate practice outcomes within populations in various arenas, such as healthcare organizations, communities, or practice settings.
- Design and evaluate methodologies that improve quality in an effort to promote "safe, effective, efficient, equitable, and patient-centered care" (AACN, 2006b, p. 12).
- Develop practice guidelines that are based on relevant, best-practice findings.
- Utilize informatics and research methodology to collect and analyze data, design databases, interpret findings to design evidence-based interventions, evaluate outcomes, and identify gaps within evidence-based practice, which will improve the practice environment.
- Work collaboratively with research specialists and act as a "practice consultant" (AACN, 2006b, p. 12).

(Adapted from AACN, 2006b)

Essential IV: Information Systems/ Technology and Patient Care Technology for the Improvement and Transformation of Health Care

DNP graduates are cutting edge in their ability to use information technology to improve patient care and outcomes. Knowledge regarding the designing and implementing of information systems to evaluate programs and outcomes of care is essential for preparation as a DNP graduate. Expertise is garnered in information technology, such as web-based communications, telemedicine, online documentation, and other unique healthcare delivery methods. DNP graduates must also develop expertise in utilizing information technologies to support practice leadership and clinical decision making. Specific to information systems, DNP graduates are prepared to:

- Evaluate and monitor outcomes of care and quality of care improvement by designing, selecting, using, and evaluating programs related to information technologies.
- Become proficient at the skills necessary to evaluate data extraction from practice information systems and databases.
- Attend to ethical and legal issues related to information technologies within the healthcare setting by providing leadership to evaluate and resolve these issues.
- Communicate and evaluate the accuracy, timeliness, and appropriateness of healthcare consumer information.

(Adapted from AACN, 2006b)

Essential V: Healthcare Policy for Advocacy in Health Care

Becoming involved in healthcare policy/ advocacy has the potential to affect the delivery of health care across all settings. Thus, knowledge and skills related to healthcare policy are central to nursing practice and therefore essential to the DNP graduate. Further, "health policy influences multiple care delivery issues, including health disparities, cultural sensitivity, ethics, the internalization of health care concerns, access to care, quality of care, health care financing, and issues of equity and social justice in the delivery of health care" (AACN, 2006b, p. 13). DNP graduates are uniquely positioned to be powerful advocates for healthcare policy through their practice experiences. These practice experiences provide rich influences for the development of policy. Nursing's interest in social justice and equality requires that DNP graduates become involved in and develop expertise in healthcare policy and advocacy.

Additionally, DNP graduates need to be prepared in leadership roles with regard to public policy. As leaders in the practice setting, DNP graduates frequently assimilate research, practice, and policy. Therefore, DNP preparation should include experience in recognizing the factors that influence the development of policy across various settings. The DNP graduate is prepared to:

- Decisively analyze health policies and proposals from the points of view of consumers, nurses, and other healthcare professionals.
- Provide leadership in the development and implementation of healthcare policy at the institutional, local, state, federal, and international levels.
- Actively participate on committees, boards, or task forces at the institutional, local, state, federal, and international levels.
- Participate in the education of other healthcare professionals, patients, or other stakeholders regarding healthcare policy issues.
- Act as an advocate for the nursing profession through activities related to healthcare policy.
- Influence healthcare financing, regulation, and delivery through the development of leadership in healthcare policy.
- Act as an advocate for ethical, equitable, and social justice policies across all healthcare settings.

(Adapted from AACN, 2006b)

Essential VI: Interprofessional Collaboration for Improving Patient and Population Health Outcomes

This Essential specifically relates to the IOM's mandate to provide safe, timely, equitable, effective, efficient, and patient-centered care. In a multitiered, complex healthcare environment, collaboration among all healthcare disciplines must exist to achieve the IOM's and nursing's goals. Nurses are experts at functioning as collaborators among multiple disciplines. Therefore, as nursing practice experts, DNP graduates must be prepared to facilitate collaboration and team building. This may include both participating in the work of the team and assuming leadership roles when necessary.

With regard to interprofessional collaboration, the DNP graduate must be prepared to:

- Participate in effective communication and collaboration throughout the development of "practice models, peer review, practice guidelines, health policy, standards of care, and/or other scholarly products" (AACN, 2006b, p. 15).
- Analyze complex practice or organizational issues through leadership of interprofessional teams.
- Act as a consultant to interprofessional teams to implement change in healthcare delivery systems.

(Adapted from AACN, 2006b)

Essential VII: Clinical Prevention and Population Health for Improving the Nation's Health

Clinical prevention is defined as health promotion and risk reduction/illness prevention for individuals and families, and population health is defined as including all community, environmental, cultural, and socioeconomic aspects of health (Allan, et al., 2004; AACN, 2006b). Nursing has foundations in health promotion and risk reduction and is therefore positioned to have an impact on the health status of people in multiple settings. The further preparation included in the DNP curriculum will prepare graduates to "analyze epidemiological, biostatistical, occupational, and environmental data in the development, implementation, and evaluation of clinical prevention and population health" (AACN, 2006b, p. 15). In other words, DNP graduates are in an ideal position to participate in health promotion and risk reduction activities from a nursing perspective with additional preparation in evaluating and interpreting data pertinent to improving the health status of individuals.

(Adapted from AACN, 2006b)

Essential VIII: Advanced Nursing Practice

Because one cannot become proficient in all areas of specialization, DNP degree programs "provide preparation within distinct specialties that require expertise, advanced knowledge, and mastery in one area of nursing practice" (AACN, 2006b, p. 16). This specialization is defined by a specialty practice area within the domain of nursing as well as a requisite of the DNP degree. Although the DNP graduate may function in a variety of roles, role preparation within the practice specialty, including legal and regulatory issues, is part of every DNP curriculum. With regard to advanced nursing practice, the DNP graduate is prepared to:

- Comprehensively assess health and illness parameters while incorporating diverse and culturally sensitive approaches.
- Implement and evaluate therapeutic interventions based on nursing and other sciences.
- Participate in therapeutic relationships with patients and other healthcare professionals to ensure optimal patient care and improve patient outcomes.
- Utilize advanced clinical decision-making skills and critical thinking, as well as deliver and evaluate evidence-based care to improve patient outcomes.
- Serve as a mentor to others in the nursing profession in an effort to maintain excellence in nursing practice.
- Participate in the education of patients, especially those in complex health situations.

(Adapted from AACN, 2006b)

A Note About Specialty-Focused Competencies According to the AACN

The purpose of specialty preparation within the DNP curricula is to prepare graduates to fulfill specific roles within health care. Specialty preparation, along with the DNP Essentials I–VIII, prepares DNP graduates for roles in two different domains. The first domain includes roles that involve specialization as advanced practice registered nurses who care for individuals (including, but not limited to: clinical nurse specialist, nurse practitioner, nurse anesthetist, nurse–midwife). The second domain includes roles that involve specialization in advanced practice at an organizational or systems level. Because of this variability, specialization content within DNP programs differs (AACN, 2006b).

The National Organization of Nurse Practitioner Faculties Practice Doctorate Nurse Practitioner Entry-Level Competencies

The NONPF has developed specific *Practice Doctorate Nurse Practitioner Entry-Level Competencies* for nurse practitioner/DNP graduates. These Competencies differ somewhat from the AACN's Essentials in that they are particular to nurse practitioner roles. However, these Competencies are also reflective of the AACN's Essentials. These Competencies are as follows:

I. Competency Area: Independent Practice
- Practices independently by assessing, diagnosing, treating, and managing undifferentiated patients.
- Assumes full accountability for actions as a licensed practitioner.

II. Competency Area: Scientific Foundation
- Critically analyzes data for practice by integrating knowledge from arts and sciences within the context of nursing's philosophical framework and scientific foundation.
- Translates research and data to anticipate, predict, and explain variations in practice.

III. Competency Area: Leadership
- Assumes increasingly complex leadership roles.

- Provides leadership to foster intercollaboration.
- Demonstrates a leadership style that uses critical and reflective thinking.

IV. Competency Area: Quality
- Uses best available evidence to enhance quality in clinical practice.
- Evaluates how organizational, structural, financial, marketing, and policy decisions affect cost, quality, and accessibility of health care.
- Demonstrates skills in peer review that promote a culture of excellence.

V. Competency Area: Practice Inquiry
- Applies clinical investigative skills for evaluation of health outcomes at the patient, family, population, clinical unit, systems, and/or community levels.
- Provides leadership in the translation of new knowledge into practice.
- Disseminates evidence from inquiry to diverse audiences using multiple methods.

VI. Competency Area: Technology and Information Literacy
- Demonstrates information literacy in complex decision making.
- Translates technical and scientific health information appropriate for user need.

VII. Competency Area: Policy
- Analyzes ethical, legal, and social factors in policy development.
- Influences health policy.
- Evaluates the impact of globalization on healthcare policy.

VIII. Competency Area: Health Delivery System
- Applies knowledge of organizational behavior and systems.
- Demonstrates skills in negotiating, consensus building, and partnering.

- Manages risks to individuals, families, populations, and healthcare systems.
- Facilitates development of culturally relevant healthcare systems.

IX. Competency Area: Ethics
- Applies ethically sound solutions to complex issues.[1]

Core Practice Doctorate Clinical Nurse Specialist (CNS) Competencies

In 2006, the National Association of Clinical Nurse Specialists (NACNS) consulted with various nursing organizations and nursing accrediting entities regarding the implications of the DNP degree for CNS practice and education (NACNS, 2009). A formal task force, including representatives from NACNS and 19 other nursing organizations, was charged with developing competencies for the CNS at the doctoral level (NACNS, 2009). Because traditional CNS education has included a master's degree, the *Core Practice Doctorate Clinical Nurse Specialist Competencies* should be used with the National CNS Competency Task Force Organizing Framework and Core Competencies (2008) and the AACN *Essentials of Doctoral Education for Advanced Nursing Practice* (2006) to inform educational programs and employer expectations" (NACNS, 2009, p. 10). The NACNS core competencies can be accessed at http://www.nacns .org/docs/CorePracticeDoctorate.pdf.

The foci of the *Core Practice Doctorate Clinical Nurse Specialist Competencies* are congruent with the AACN's *Essentials of Doctoral Education for Advanced Nursing Practice* and the NONPF's *Practice Doctorate Nurse Practitioner Entry-Level Competencies*. (See **Figure 4-1**.) Specifically, graduates of CNS-focused DNP programs

---

[1]Competencies provided courtesy of the National Organization of Nurse Practitioner Faculties (NONPF). Available at www.nonpf.org.

FIGURE 4-1	Relationship among the DNP Essentials, the NONPF Competencies, the NACNS Competencies, and the Core Competencies Needed for Healthcare Professionals per the Committee on Health Professions Education.

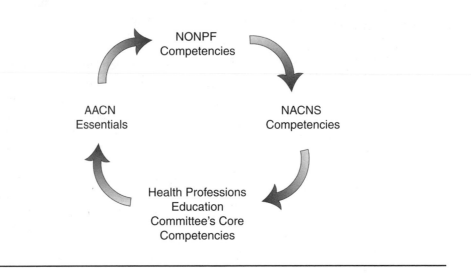

should be prepared beyond traditional CNS competencies to "strengthen the already significant contribution that CNSs make in ensuring quality patient outcomes through establishing a practice foundation based on advanced scientific, theoretical, ethical, and economic principles" (NACNS, 2009, p. 11). These competencies ensure that doctoral-prepared CNS graduates are prepared to:

- Generate and disseminate new knowledge

- Evaluate and translate evidence into practice

- Employ a broad range of theories from nursing and related disciplines

- Design and evaluate innovative strategies to improve quality of care and safety in all settings

- Improve systems of care

- Provide leadership that promotes interprofessional collaboration

- Influence and shape health policy

(Adapted from NACNS, 2009)

The Path to the DNP Degree: Follow the Academic Road

The path to the DNP degree is currently in transition. It should be mentioned that while the transition toward DNP preparation as entry into advanced nursing practice is taking place, current DNP programs are being offered as a post-master's degree. Many prospective students will have already fulfilled several of the criteria listed in the *Essentials of Doctoral Education for Advanced Nursing Practice* as well as the *Practice Doctorate Nurse Practitioner Entry-Level Competencies* in their master's degree curricula. Further, as mentioned earlier, the

| **FIGURE 4-2** | Pathways to the DNP degree. |

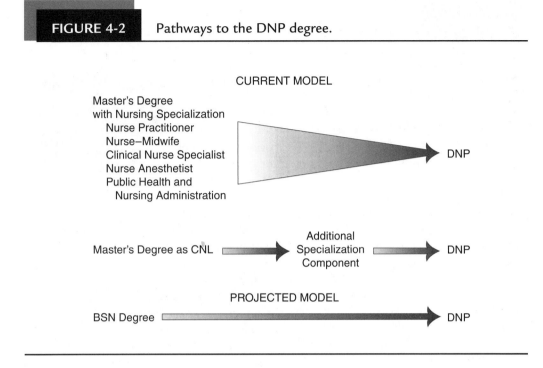

CURRENT MODEL

Master's Degree
with Nursing Specialization
   Nurse Practitioner
   Nurse–Midwife
   Clinical Nurse Specialist
   Nurse Anesthetist
   Public Health and
     Nursing Administration
→ DNP

Master's Degree as CNL → Additional Specialization Component → DNP

PROJECTED MODEL

BSN Degree → DNP

specialization content included in the DNP degree curriculum is currently being fulfilled within the master's degree curriculum. Therefore, each individual's path to the DNP degree may be unique. Prospective students' program content may be individualized to include the learning experiences necessary to incorporate the described requirements for the DNP degree. Please refer to **Figure 4-2** for an illustration of the pathways to the DNP degree.

ROLE TRANSITION INTRODUCED

As explained earlier in the chapter, the DNP is currently not a specialization degree but rather a practice doctorate for advanced nursing practice. This degree builds upon advanced nursing practice specialization and provides additional preparation in the formulation, interpretation, and utilization of evidence-based practices, health policy, information technology, and leadership. Although DNP graduates may function as evaluators and translators of research, health policy advocates, nursing leaders, educators or clinicians, it is entirely likely that these roles will be integrated as well. One DNP graduate may participate in research in addition to practicing as a nurse anesthetist. Another DNP graduate may be a nurse executive in addition to developing health policy. Nursing has always been a profession that involves juggling multiple roles (Dudley-Brown, 2006; Jennings & Rogers, 1988; Sperhac & Strodtbeck, 1997). Within these multiple roles, the fundamental goal of the DNP graduate remains the development of expertise in the delivery of high-quality, patient-centered care, which utilizes the necessary avenues to provide that care.

EXHIBIT 4-1 Interview with a DNP Co-Founder: Then and Now

Carolyn A. Williams, PhD, RN, FAAN, is Professor and Dean Emeritus of the University of Kentucky. She was president of the American Association of Colleges of Nursing from 2000 to 2002 and Scholar-in-Residence at the Institute of Medicine from 2007 to 2008.

Then . . . 2008

Dr. Williams, could you please describe your background and current position?

I began my nursing career as a public health nurse at a public health department in a rural area and practiced for 2 years before returning to graduate school. I then received my master's degree in public health nursing. This was a joint master's degree from both the School of Nursing and the School of Public Health from the University of North Carolina at Chapel Hill (UNC, CH). I then went on to earn a PhD in epidemiology from the School of Public Health at UNC, CH. This was met with some controversy in that I did not have a large amount of nursing experience before returning to graduate school. Interestingly, the School of Public Health was supportive of my doctoral studies whereas the School of Nursing seemed to think I needed more nursing experience. This is what I call a "pernicious pattern" in nursing education. I actually had to talk faculty (in nursing) into supporting me to earn a doctorate. However, faculty from other disciplines, e.g., medicine, psychology, and sociology in the School of Public Health, were very supportive. This is where nursing differs from medicine: We don't build in the experience into our educational programs.

Upon finishing my PhD in epidemiology, I took a faculty position at Emory University's School of Nursing. From there, I was asked to return to Chapel Hill to participate in the development and evaluation of a family nurse

practitioner program in the School of Nursing and to teach epidemiology in the School of Public Health. The program in the School of Nursing was one of the first 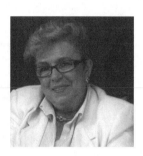 six federally funded family nurse practitioner programs in the country. I remained at Chapel Hill for 13 years before accepting an appointment as dean of the College of Nursing at the University of Kentucky. Last year I retired as dean after 22 years in that position and remained as a faculty member.

This year (2007 to 2008) I am a Scholar-in-Residence at the Institute of Medicine in Washington, DC. My role here includes development of a project, which happens to be interprofessional collaboration. This stems from the view that improvement in quality care depends on people working together in interprofessional teams. Interprofessional collaboration is happening around the margins of education for health care instead of in the mainstream, particularly core clinical components of undergraduate and graduate education for health care. It may be picked up in passing, but frequently it is not a formal part of the curriculum. Part of my project involves identifying the policy changes [that] are needed at the university level to integrate interprofessional collaboration as part [of] an integral component of education in the health professions. Interprofessional collaboration is a necessary part of practice and therefore needs to be integrated into the preparation of healthcare professionals. This leads me to an

| EXHIBIT 4-1 | Interview with a DNP Co-Founder: Then and Now *(continued)* |

issue I have always struggled with: Too few clinical faculty in nursing actually practice. This is a problem due to the fact that a practice culture is not as visible as I believe it needs to be in most schools of nursing. Some progress in having nursing faculty engaged in practice was achieved with the nurse practitioner movement that started in the 1970s, but it is still a struggle for nursing faculty to engage in practice as part of their faculty role in a manner similar to what happens in medical education. Some faculty attempt to practice on their own, not as a part of their faculty role, and usually faculty practice is not viewed as a priority in schools of nursing. I feel if we want nursing faculty to provide leadership in practice and develop leaders for practice, each school of nursing needs to have a core group of faculty who actually engage in practice as part of their faculty role.

Dr. Williams, could you please describe how your vision for a Doctor of Nursing Practice became a reality?
While on the faculty at the University of North Carolina at Chapel Hill and consulting with a number of individuals in practice settings, I developed some ideas of what nursing education to prepare nurse leaders needs to be. Initially, I viewed the degree as what public health nurses could earn to prepare them to face the challenges of public health nursing. I didn't feel that the master's degrees in nursing offered at that time (1970s through early 1980s) were sufficient for the kind of leadership roles nurses were moving into. I felt a true practice degree at the doctoral level was needed.

When I went to the University of Kentucky as the dean of nursing, I was charged with developing a PhD in nursing program. While at Chapel Hill I had been very involved in research

activity, doctoral education in epidemiology, and was active nationally in research development and advocacy in nursing as chair of the American Nurses Association's Commission on Nursing Research and as the president of the American Academy of Nursing. I proceeded to work with the faculty at the University of Kentucky, and we developed the PhD program in nursing. However, I was still interested in the concept of a practice doctorate and promoting stronger partnerships between nursing practice and nursing education.

As time went on it became clearer and clearer to me that to prepare nurses for leadership in practice, something more in tune with preparing nurses to utilize knowledge, not necessarily generate new knowledge, which was expected in PhD programs, was needed. Thus, I began to talk with and work with my faculty colleagues on the concept of a new practice degree for nurses to prepare for leadership in practice, not in education or research.

I saw practice as the focus with this degree, not research. Working with my University of Kentucky faculty colleagues, particularly Dr. Marcia K. Stanhope and Dr. Julie G. Sebastian, we developed the initial conceptualization of the degree. These foci included four themes that I feel should be central to a practice doctorate in nursing:

■ Leadership in practice, which included leadership at the point of care. This also includes leadership at the policy level to impact care.

■ A population approach and perspective. This involves a broader view of health care, which recognizes the importance of

(continues)

| EXHIBIT 4-1 | Interview with a DNP Co-Founder: Then and Now *(continued)* |

populations when planning and evaluating care processes.

- Integration of evidence-based practice to make informed decisions regarding care.
- The ability to understand change processes and institute positive changes in health care.

These four themes guided the development of the curriculum of the first DNP program at the University of Kentucky, which when we instituted it was the first in the United States. These themes also influenced and are incorporated in what became the AACN's Essentials of Doctoral Education in Advanced Nursing Practice.

To expand on the development of the DNP program at University of Kentucky, the following is the timeline:

1994–1998	Informal conversations among faculty, people in practice, and others regarding a practice doctorate in nursing.
1998	Professional Doctorate Task Force Committee formed.
May 1999	Approval of DNP program by total college faculty.
July 1999	Medical Center Academic Council approval.
January 2000	University of Kentucky Board of Trustees approved the program.
May 2000	Approval by the Kentucky Council of Postsecondary Education.
January 2001	The first national paper on the DNP degree at the AACN's National Doctoral Education Conference (Williams, Stanhope, & Sebastian, 2001).
Fall 2001	Students admitted to the first DNP program in the country.

In 1998, when the University of Kentucky's DNP task force was created, we decided we didn't want this degree to look like anything else currently in nursing education. We also decided on the name of this degree in this committee. We wanted the degree and the name to focus on nursing practice, and we did not want the degree to be limited to preparing for only one particular type of nursing practice. We decided on the Doctor of Nursing Practice because that describes what the degree is: a practice degree in nursing.

One of the most important things that happened during my presidency of the American Association of Colleges of Nursing was the appointment [of] a task force to look at the issue of a practice doctorate. The task force committee was carefully planned. I wanted to have a positive group of people as well as major stakeholders represented. These stakeholders were credible individuals who had an interest in the development of a practice doctorate. Members of the committee included representatives from Columbia University, the University of Kentucky, a representative from an ND program, as well as a representative from schools that did not have nursing doctoral programs. This committee was chaired by Dr. Elizabeth Lentz, who has written extensively on doctoral education in nursing. As this task force began sorting out the issues, it became the goal that by 2015, the DNP would become the terminal degree for specialization in nursing.

From this point, a group to develop both the essentials of doctoral education in nursing and a roadmap task force were formed. These committees worked together, and we presented together nationally in a series of regional forums. We invited others to engage in

EXHIBIT 4-1 Interview with a DNP Co-Founder: Then and Now *(continued)*

discourse regarding the essentials as well as ask questions about the DNP degree. As our presentations across the country came to a conclusion, we noticed an obvious transformation. The DNP degree was beginning to gain more acceptance. By the time we were done, the argument of whether to adopt a practice doctorate in nursing had given rise to how to put this degree in place.

Dr. Williams, are you surprised by the acceptance of the degree and speed with which programs are being developed?

Yes, I am surprised. I thought the DNP degree would be an important development for the field of nursing, and I thought some would adopt a practice doctorate. I certainly did not think things would move so fast. The idea of a DNP really struck a chord with many people.

Dr. Williams, do you think the history of doctoral education in nursing has influenced the development of a practice doctorate in nursing?

Well, we need to have scientists in our field. However, we also need to come to grips with the fact that we are a practice discipline. Over the years, since the late 1970s, many of the leading academic settings in nursing have become increasingly research intensive and [have] not spent as much effort on developing a complementary practice focus. I feel the development of a practice doctorate has more to do with our development as a discipline than the history of doctoral nursing education. Attraction and credibility from the university setting stem from involvement in research. Therefore, it becomes a struggle when handling this practice piece. If nursing wants acceptance as a discipline, we must have research. But we are a practice discipline, and all practice disciplines struggle to some extent in research-intensive university environments.

Dr. Williams, do you agree that nursing should have both a research- and a practice-focused doctorate?

Of course. The ratio between research-focused and practice-focused doctorates may be tipped toward the practice focused due to the practice focus of our discipline.

Dr. Williams, could you describe what you feel is the future of doctoral education in nursing?

Down the pike, some people may move into DNP programs and then discover they want to be researchers and end up also getting a PhD. This would be very healthy for our profession. Essentially, we have lost talented folks due to offering only a research-focused terminal degree. The DNP allows us to accommodate those folks who don't want a research-focused degree.

I also feel we need a more intensive clinical component integrated into the degree. This may be in the form of residency programs integrated within nursing degrees or as a post-doctorate option.

Dr. Williams, could you expand on the grandfathering of advanced practice registered nurses (APRN) who don't wish to pursue a DNP degree?

The DNP degree will not be required to practice anytime soon. It took a while to require a master's degree to practice as an APRN. There will be a similar transition regarding the DNP degree. If someone is certified and successful as an APRN without a DNP, they should continue to be successful.

Dr. Williams, do you believe the DNP will continue to flourish as a degree option for nursing? If so, what would your advice be regarding nurses earning a DNP degree?

Yes, I do. My advice regarding nurses earning a DNP degree is that it depends on their career

(continues)

EXHIBIT 4-1   Interview with a DNP Co-Founder: Then and Now *(continued)*

choice. Some have been looking for this option for a long time. This may be the right degree for some no matter where they are in practice.

Now . . . 2011

Dr. Williams, we discussed your nursing background and education last time we spoke. Could you please describe your current position and what types of projects you are currently involved in?

After leaving the deanship at the University of Kentucky I continued my role as a professor on the faculty. Throughout my time as dean of the college I always had a teaching assignment, although limited but usually one course a year. I now have a full-time teaching commitment and teach several courses in the DNP Program including one course that both DNP and PhD students take. In addition, I am working on a project to try to enhance the role of nursing faculty in clinical practice and decision-making roles in academic health science centers. This is the environment where many of our graduate students in nursing in North America are prepared, as well as a large proportion of our undergraduates. Yet, the way nursing education has been involved in clinical matters is very different from the role medicine plays. There are many reasons for this. I am evaluating this in an effort to understand and identify options for change.

Last time we talked, you were working at the Institute of Medicine on a special project regarding interprofessional collaboration. Did this project include any implications for DNP graduates?

While I was at the IOM I spent some time looking at interprofessional collaboration and how to enhance it. There is much written about preparing health professionals to value interprofessional collaboration and engage with other health professionals as they care for patients. However, innovative learning opportunities to expose students to interprofessional experiences represent a major challenge for educators in all of the health professions. Creating such experiences are particularly important for those preparing DNP students because of the role DNP graduates will play in working with and coordinating with other health professionals. But the educational model many DNP programs have developed involving distant learning strategies means that DNP faculty members have to be both highly committed to the importance of such learning experiences and extremely creative as they design them.

What is your impression of the progress of the DNP degree? How does the current progress of the DNP degree compare to your original vision of the DNP degree?

Our original vision at the University of Kentucky was that the DNP would be a doctoral degree for leadership in practice. The first program was set up as a post-master's offering. When AACN's Doctoral Task Force, that I appointed while I was AACN's President, proposed that preparation for specialization in nursing should be at the DNP level, I supported the proposal and worked to implement it as chair of the Roadmap Task Force and in other ways. I am still supportive of the concept.

I am surprised about how many programs have developed in a relatively short time. And, I admit to being somewhat concerned about what seems to be an effort in some programs to make the program as short as possible. Of course, we do not want to have unnecessarily long programs, but the DNP is a doctoral degree and there needs to be time for in-depth doctoral-level work. The challenge the discipline faces is to make sure that all DNP programs are high-quality doctoral programs. As more schools develop BSN to DNP programs,

| EXHIBIT 4-1 | Interview with a DNP Co-Founder: Then and Now *(continued)* |

this challenge will be felt to a greater extent. Faculty will be challenged to prepare, in a very limited time frame, beginning specialists in an area of practice who also possess the broader analytical skills necessary for leadership.

I am aware that there are those in nursing who argue we should retreat back to the master's in order to respond to human resources concerns. I do not agree. I believe the history of nursing is replete with examples of compromising the education of nurses to deal with human resources issues. I think the momentum of the DNP, a concept that has "clicked" with so many young nurses, is strong enough to overcoming the backtracking of some.

Why do you think the DNP degree continues to gain acceptance and momentum?

In my view the reason is that the DNP was conceived to prepare nurses to move with and lead the kind of system changes necessary in health care. The first DNP program at Kentucky had four key concepts which formed the foundation for the program: a population-system perspective, evidence-based decision making, leadership, and facilitating change. These concepts remain as important components of the DNP essentials and as curricular components in DNP programs. I believe that young nurses who want to make a difference in their career in nursing realize that they will need additional knowledge, skills, and approaches to be successful in the complex arena of health care and they see that the DNP program can help provide what is needed.

When we last spoke in 2008, you agreed that nursing needed both a research- and practice-focused doctorate. Do you still agree that a research- and practice-focused doctorate are beneficial to the profession?

Absolutely YES!!!! We are a practice discipline and we need some of those in practice to be prepared with a focus on practice at the doctoral level. Had we had a practice-focused second professional degree earlier in our history I believe our discipline would be in a very different place today. We have a lot of ground to make up when we consider that as a health professional group, professional nurses are the least educated of the health professionals and each year the majority of those who sit for the licensure examination are not prepared at the baccalaureate level. Yes, we desperately need as many nurses with a practice doctorate that we can produce in order to change the world of nursing practice.

Do you believe that a partnership is currently forming between PhD and DNP graduates?

I believe this is coming. I think it will be most evident in schools that offer both programs. I think it will become clear to thoughtful faculty in such schools that there are some commonalities to both programs and we will see some creative curricular plans that allow students in both programs to work together at various points in their programs of study. The faculty at the University of Iowa has developed an innovative curricular model that brings together both student groups for selected experiences and has excellent potential for facilitating collaboration. A key factor at Iowa is that the faculty who teach in both programs are modeling what collaboration looks like for the students of both programs. This is very innovative and very inspiring.

How would you recommend we continue to move forward with the AACN's recommended target date of the DNP for entry into practice by 2015?

My answer is very simple, KEEP PRESSING FORWARD, DON'T MISS A BEAT!

SUMMARY

- The DNP degree is defined as a practice-focused doctorate degree that prepares graduates as experts in nursing practice.

- Nursing practice is defined by the AACN as "any form of nursing intervention that influences health care outcomes for individuals or populations, including direct care of individual patients, administration of nursing and health care organizations, and the implementation of health policy" (AACN, 2004, p. 3).

- According to the AACN's (2004) position statement, the DNP degree is proposed to be the terminal degree for nursing practice by 2015.

- A nursing PhD degree is a research-focused degree, and the DNP degree is a practice-focused degree.

- The evolution of doctoral education in nursing illustrates where we have been in doctoral education and the direction nursing is taking in the development of doctoral education.

- The concept of a practice doctorate is not new. The idea began in the 1970s with the development of the DNS degree.

- The AACN now designates the DNS and PhD degrees as research-focused degrees, with the DNP/DrNP being the designated practice-focused degrees.

- In 2002, the AACN board of directors formed a task force to examine the current progress of proposed doctorates in nursing.

- In 2000, the Institute of Medicine published a report titled *To Err Is Human,* which summarized errors made in the healthcare system and proposed recommendations to improve the overall quality of care.

- In 2003, the Health Professions Education Committee published *Health Professions Education: A Bridge to Quality,* which outlined a specific set of competencies that should be met by all clinicians.

- In 2008, the IOM appointed the Committee on the RWJF Initiative on the Future of Nursing. This committee published a report in 2010 titled *The Future of Nursing: Focus on Education,* which concluded that the "the ways in which nurses were educated during the 20th century are no longer adequate for dealing with the realities of healthcare in the 21st century" (IOM, 2010, p. 2). This committee also recommended doubling the number of nurses with doctorates by the year 2020.

- In 2004, the AACN published a position statement regarding a practice doctorate in nursing and recommended that by 2015 all nurses pursuing advanced practice degrees will be prepared as DNP graduates.

- In 2005, the National Academy of Sciences also recommended that a nonresearch nursing doctorate be developed to meet nursing faculty needs.

- In 2006, the AACN described the *Essentials of Doctoral Education for Advanced Nursing Practice,* which represents the standards for DNP curricula.

- The NONPF outlined the *Practice Doctorate Nurse Practitioner Entry-Level Competencies* as standards for DNP curricula.

- In 2009, the NACNS developed *Core Practice Doctorate Clinical Nurse Specialist Competencies.*

- The DNP degree is currently a post-master's degree program while the transition to the doctoral preparation for advanced nursing practice is taking place.

- Graduate students may follow an individualized path to the DNP degree depending on their current master's degree preparation.

- DNP graduates may be involved in many different roles that may include, but are not limited to, evaluation and translation of research, leader, health policy advocate, educator, and clinician.

DISCUSSION QUESTIONS

1. How do you think nursing's history has contributed to the development of the DNP degree?

2. How do you think the IOM report *To Err Is Human*, along with the follow-up report *Crossing the Quality Chasm*, contributed to the development of the DNP degree?

3. Explain why you think the IOM and the RWJF concluded in their report *The Future of Nursing: Focus on Education* that nurses need improvement in their educational preparation.

4. Do you think a struggle still exists within nursing today regarding whether doctoral education should be research or practice focused?

5. Do you think nursing doctoral education should be research focused, practice focused, or both?

6. Do you think a DNP degree is the right degree for you?

REFERENCES

Allan, J., Barwick, T., Cashman, S., Cawley, J. F., Day, C., Douglass, C. W., et al. (2004). Clinical prevention and population health: Curriculum framework for health professions. *American Journal of Preventive Medicine, 27*(5), 471–476.

American Association of Colleges of Nursing (AACN). (2001). *Indicators of quality in research-focused doctoral programs in nursing.* Washington, DC: Author.

American Association of Colleges of Nursing (AACN). (2004). *AACN position statement on the practice doctorate in nursing.* Retrieved January 8, 2008, from http://www.aacn.nche.edu/DNP/pdf/DNP.pdf

American Association of Colleges of Nursing (AACN). (2005). *Commission on Collegiate Nursing Education moves to consider for accreditation only practice doctorates with the DNP degree title.* Retrieved from http://www.aacn.nche.edu/Media/NewsReleases/Archives/2005/CCNEDNP.htm

American Association of Colleges of Nursing (AACN). (2006a). *Doctor of nursing practice roadmap task force report.* Retrieved from http://www.aacn.nche.edu/dnp/roadmapreport.pdf

American Association of Colleges of Nursing (AACN). (2006b). *Essentials of doctoral education for advanced nursing practice.* Retrieved from http://www.aacn.nche.edu/publications/position/DNPEssentials.pdf

American Association of Colleges of Nursing (AACN). (2007). *AACN white paper on the education and role of the clinical nurse leader.* Retrieved from http://www.aacn.nche.edu/publications/white-papers/cnl

American Association of Colleges of Nursing (AACN). (2011a). *DNP program schools.* Retrieved from http://www.aacn.nche.edu/dnp/program-schools

American Association of Colleges of Nursing (AACN). (2011b). *Fact sheet: The doctor of nursing practice.* Retrieved from http://www.aacn.nche.edu/media-relations/fact-sheets/dnp

American Hospital Association. (1999). *Hospital statistics.* Chicago: Author.

Apold, S. (2008). The doctor of nursing practice: Looking back, moving forward. *Journal for Nurse Practitioners, 4*(2), 101–107.

Carpenter, R., & Hudacek, S. (1996). *On doctoral education in nursing: The voice of the student.* New York: National League for Nursing Press.

Centers for Disease Control and Prevention, National Center for Health Statistics. (1999a). Births and deaths: Preliminary data for 1998. *National Vital Statistics Reports, 47*(25), 1–45.

Centers for Disease Control and Prevention, National Center for Health Statistics. (1999b). Deaths: Final data for 1997. *National Vital Statistics Reports, 47*(19), 1–104.

Cleland, V. (1976). Developing a doctoral program. *Nursing Outlook, 24*(10), 631–635.

Donaldson, S., & Crowley, D. (1978). The discipline of nursing. *Nursing Outlook, 26*(2), 113–120.

Dracup, K., Cronenwett, L., Meleis, A., & Benner, P. (2005). Reflections on the doctorate of nursing practice. *Nursing Outlook, 53*(4), 177–182.

Dudley-Brown, S. (2006). Revisiting the blended role of the advanced practice nurse. *Gastroenterology Nursing, 29*(3), 249–250.

Fawcett, J. (2005). *Contemporary nursing knowledge: Analysis and evaluation of nursing models and theories* (2nd ed.). Philadelphia: F. A. Davis.

Goldenberg, G. (2004). The DrNP degree. *The Academic Nurse: The Journal of the Columbia University School of Nursing, 21*(1), 22–26.

Gortner, S. (1980). Nursing science in transition. *Nursing Research, 29*(3), 180–183.

Grace, H. (1978). The development of doctoral education in nursing: In historical perspective. *Journal of Nursing Education, 17*(4), 17–27.

Greiner, A. C., & Knebel, E. (Eds.). (2003). *Health professions education: A bridge to quality.* Washington, DC: National Academies Press.

Institute of Medicine (IOM). (2001). *Crossing the quality chasm: A new health system for the 21st century.* Washington, DC: National Academies Press.

Institute of Medicine. (2010a). *The future of nursing: Focus on education.* Retrieved from http://www.iom .edu/~/media/Files/Report%20Files/2010/The-Future-of-Nursing/Nursing%20Education%20 2010%20Brief.pdf

Institute of Medicine. (2010b). *The future of nursing: Leading change, advancing health.* Report recommendations. Retrieved from http://www.iom.edu /Reports/2010/The-Future-of-Nursing-Leading-Change-Advancing-Health.aspx

Jennings, B., & Rogers, S. (1988). Merging nursing research and practice: A case of multiple identities. *Journal of Advanced Nursing Research, 13*(6), 752–758.

Kohn, L. T., Corrigan, J. M., & Donaldson, M. S. (Eds). (2000). *To err is human: Building a safer health system.* Committee on Quality of Health Care in America, Institute of Medicine. Washington, DC: National Academies Press.

Marion, L., O'Sullivan, A., Crabtree, M. K., Price, M., & Fontana, S. (2005). Curriculum models for the practice doctorate in nursing. *Topics in Advanced Practice Nursing eJournal, 5*(1). Retrieved from http://www.medscape.com/viewarticle/500742 _print

Marion, L., Viens, D., O'Sullivan, A., Crabtree, M. K., Fontana, S., & Price, M. (2003). The practice doctorate in nursing: Future or fringe. *Topics in Advanced Practice Nursing eJournal, 3*(2). Retrieved from http://www.medscape.com/viewarticle/453247 _print

Marriner-Tomey, A. (1990). Historical development of doctoral programs from the middle ages to nursing education today. *Nursing and Health Care, 11*(3), 132–137.

Murphy, J. (1981). Doctoral education in, of, and for nursing: An historical analysis. *Nursing Outlook, 29*(11), 645–649.

National Academy of Sciences. (2005). *Advancing the nation's health needs: NIH Research Training Programs.* Washington, DC: National Academies Press. Retrieved from http://www.nap.edu/openbook .php?isbn=0309094275

National Association of Clinical Nurse Specialists (2009). *Core practice doctorate clinical nurse specialist competencies.* Retrieved from http://www.nacns.org /docs/CorePracticeDoctorate.pdf

National Organization of Nurse Practitioner Faculties (NONPF). (2006). *Practice doctorate nurse practitioner entry-level competencies.* Retrieved from http://www.nonpf.com/associations/10789/files /DNP%20NP%20competenciesApril2006.pdf

Newman, M. (1975). The professional doctorate in nursing: A position paper. *Nursing Outlook, 23*(11), 704–706.

Roberts, S., & Glod, C. (2005). The practice doctorate in nursing: Is it the answer? *The American Journal for Nurse Practitioners, 9*(11/12), 55–65.

Sperhac, A., & Strodtbeck, F. (1997). Advanced practice nursing: New opportunities for blended roles. *The American Journal of Maternal Child Nursing, 22*(6), 287–293.

Starck, P., Duffy, M., & Vogler, R. (1993). Developing a nursing doctorate for the 21st century. *Journal of Professional Nursing, 9*(4), 212–219.

Thomas, E., Studdert, D., Newhouse, J., Zbar, B., Howard, K., Williams, E., et al. (1999). Costs of medical injuries in Utah and Colorado. *Inquiry, 36*(3), 255–264.

Williams, C. A., Stanhope, M. K., & Sebastian, J. G. (2001). Clinical nursing leadership: One model of professional doctoral education in nursing. In *Envisioning Doctoral Education for the Future. Proceedings of the American Association of Colleges of Nursing's 2001 Doctoral Education Conference* (pp. 85–91). Washington, DC: AACN.

CHAPTER 5

Emerging Roles for the DNP: Nurse Educator, Nurse Administrator, Nursing Leaders, Nurse Entrepreneurs, and Community Health

Mary Zaccagnini

CHAPTER OBJECTIVES

1. Describe nursing leadership roles that are emerging from the doctor of nursing practice degree.

2. Explore the impact of the DNP on nursing education and healthcare outcomes.

3. Discuss the influence of the DNP on nursing administration and nurse executive roles.

4. Define the characteristics of a nurse entrepreneur.

5. Distinguish between public health and community health nursing and the role of the DNP as program developer and evaluator.

6. Analyze complementary healthcare modalities and discuss the role of the DNP as an integrative practitioner.

NURSE EDUCATOR: MICHELLE RILEY

Advances in the body of nursing knowledge promote educational development of professional nurses beyond entry-level practice to meet the increasing healthcare needs of society. Research to increase the body of nursing knowledge is important to improving the nation's health. There is also a significant need for advanced practice nurses (APNs) with clinical knowledge and skills to facilitate collaborative practice and leadership in the profession. Professional nurses require highly developed skill sets for continuous quality improvement in diverse systems and healthcare settings where APNs work (Heller, Oros, & Durney-Crowley, n.d.).

Nurses with a practice doctorate who have advanced their education in clinical practice and leadership can use specialized skills and clinical judgment to perform roles in complex healthcare systems (American Association of Colleges of Nursing [AACN], 2006). The doctor of nursing practice (DNP) degree is a doctoral degree that is different from a research doctorate, but no less important (Steefel, 2005, as cited in Stein, 2008). According to Stein (2008), the doctor of philosophy (PhD) focuses on theoretical developments leading to an advanced body of knowledge in nursing, whereas the DNP is more practice based. Furthermore, the PhD is the benchmark against which other forms of doctoral education are measured (Ellis, 2007).

According to the National League for Nursing (NLN), educator roles in nursing require preparation of leaders in higher education (NLN, 2007). Furthermore, "Educators who are not educated in pedagogy, evaluation, and educational theory will not be in a position to engage meaningfully in nursing education research or make evidence-based contributions to reform" (p. 2).

Strong proponents of the DNP understand the impact clinical expertise and education can have on client outcomes (AACN, 2008). Even though curricula may differ from state to state, educational programs that prepare doctoral-level clinicians offer courses in leadership and research translation (Fain, Asselin, & McCurry, 2008). In addition, doctorally prepared clinical experts can complete additional courses to acquire knowledge needed for academic positions (Long, 2006).

This section explores how DNP graduates, as expert clinicians, can use skills gained in their educational programs to perform effectively in the role of nurse educators in practice and academic settings. The section also explores the expanded role of the DNP nurse educator and suggests methods for seeking practice and leadership opportunities in a variety of settings.

DNP Nurse Educator Roles and Responsibilities

Practice Settings

Nurses with advanced education at the doctoral level can perform their roles at the bedside, at the table of college boards, or in community settings. In each of these scenarios and settings, a DNP graduate can perform the practice of nursing effectively. According to Riley, "The DNP will be the new standard for advancing practice nursing education" (2009, p. 12).

The clinical practice doctorate prepares nurses with advanced education to do research, apply new knowledge in practice, and educate nursing students (Stein, 2008). According to Ellis (2007), applying the knowledge nurses gain to clinical practice is at the heart of the clinical doctorate. This may explain why more clinicians are interested in pursuing this type of doctorate over the more traditional PhD.

Furthermore, graduates of DNP programs can seek leadership roles in settings that allow for enhancement, restructuring, and improvements in the quality of health services delivery (National Organization of Nurse Practitioner Faculties [NONPF], 2005). Clinically proficient, doctorally prepared nurses are needed as a result of increased demands for health professionals who are skilled in providing complex clinical care. Practice responsibilities in the clinical setting for DNPs may include overseeing medical centers, home care, and hospice services, as well as nursing education (Stein, 2008).

Academic Settings

Practice-focused doctorates allow practitioners to use clinical expertise at an advanced level in a variety of educational settings. Advanced practice nurses who are doctorally prepared and teach in baccalaureate and higher-degree programs can help to transform the education of nurses who will be practicing at the highest level of practice (Douglas, 2005). Developments in healthcare education and the demand for increasing the educational requirements in master's-level education have extended the credit requirements beyond conventional credits at the master's level, which has helped to increase interest in the practice doctorate (Douglas, 2005).

DNP graduates practicing in complex systems and organizational levels are called on to help define potential problems and to develop interventions to address these problems. Therefore, DNPs must be competent in identifying and developing interventions to facilitate healthcare delivery across multifaceted systems. DNP programs prepare expert clinicians who not only identify and implement systems changes, but also facilitate the expert clinical teaching needed for the communities and health systems they service: clients, students, families, communities, and expert colleagues (NONPF, 2005). Even though not all institutions offering the DNP are prepared to place faculty in tenure-track positions, students in bachelor, master, and doctoral programs will need access to faculty who are expert clinicians in various practice settings, which will increase the demand for DNP graduates (Yale Nursing, 2009). Furthermore, according to Loretta Ford, cofounder of the nurse practitioner role, since the DNP is the next appropriate step toward clinical excellence, it would seem that education

programs would have "expectations for translational research, clinical teaching and institutional leadership" from DNPs (Ford, 2009).

Nurses with practice doctorates will have a voice in research and have a bigger stage on which to show how they can positively affect client outcomes (Riley, 2009). DNPs in today's complex systems must maintain expert levels of clinical competence to make a positive impact on such systems. DNP-prepared individuals who participate in scholarship can reach beyond traditional definitions of teaching and research (Boyer, 1990, 1996). According to Boyer's concepts of scholarship, DNP-prepared faculty members can bring new perspectives to original research and can explore how research is applied to problems. Holland (2005) also speaks to the tradition of scholarship and balancing this with discovery, interpretation, and application by those with a practice doctorate.

More and more academic institutions are reviewing policies related to research scholarship and are trying to expand the definition of scholarship to support the work of faculty who bring practice-based experience to academia. In addition, educators are needed in nursing schools to teach students how to perform their roles as advanced practice nurses upon graduation by helping them to fill vacancies in educator and advocacy roles related to health, nursing policy, and client care outcomes within political and healthcare communities (Fain, Asselin, & McCurry, 2008).

Faculty members who have devoted their careers to research over practice cannot be expected to maintain the clinical competence needed to educate advanced practice students pursuing careers in clinical practice. Enrollment of students into PhD programs who want advanced clinical practice is controversial. Fitzpatrick (2003) postulates that "it is unethical to accept students into PhD programs that do not develop research careers" (p. 9). Since the introduction of the practice doctorate as a terminal degree allowing for permanent faculty roles in colleges and universities, students pursuing clinical practice or clinical teaching at the advanced level can now pursue careers in academia (Long, 2006).

Society will need educators with different doctorates to educate expert practitioners of the future. Given the complexity of health care, it is clear that master's-level education will no longer be sufficient to educate future nurses. The practice doctorate in nursing is evolving, and faculty members with doctoral preparation will need to move toward formal education beyond the master's level (Pennsylvania State Board of Nursing, 2005).

Nurses in clinical practice prepared at the doctoral level can also hold faculty appointments in academic settings, provide clinical oversight, and participate in teaching roles (AACN, 2005). With more and more DNP students graduating, the number of clinically prepared faculty holding a practice doctorate will continue to increase. The National Academy of Sciences supports the development of a "nonresearch" clinical doctorate to train advanced-level practitioners who will serve as clinical faculty (Long, 2006). More colleges and universities that offer the PhD are now offering the DNP as the terminal degree for clinical expertise. These clinical experts holding faculty roles can choose to take coursework to facilitate their transition to the academic educator role and add teaching skills to their clinical skill set (National League for Nursing, 2007).

Role Expansion Strategies for DNPs from a Nurse Educator Perspective

Nurses with practice doctorates have clinical, organizational, economic, and leadership skills to positively affect client outcomes at the systems level. These healthcare leaders can also use their considerable practice expertise to make management and policy decisions in health care while educating the interdisciplinary healthcare team on issues affecting the health of diverse client populations (Fain, Asselin, & McCurry, 2008).

Individuals who obtain the DNP degree will continue to seek faculty roles to educate future DNPs as more clinical doctorate programs for nurses are developed. It is estimated that approximately 60 schools with DNP programs are now admitting students to these programs, and more DNP programs are being developed (AACN, 2008).

It is important to remember that DNP curricula are not designed to prepare nurses to become educators necessarily, any more than PhD programs. However, in states such as Florida and Texas, graduates of doctoral programs who want to work in academia will be able to receive additional education to prepare and support their clinical expertise (Green, Starck, & Long, 2006).

For DNPs to continue to expand their roles in academia and contribute to the body of nursing knowledge, socializing them to their faculty roles through mentoring programs should be considered. Given the varied roles of faculty, supporting faculty members throughout their time in academia facilitates development of teaching research as well as service skills (National League for Nursing, 2007). The orientation and mentoring provided to DNP graduates who will work in academia are also essential to developing their ability to conduct research, apply empirical knowledge in practice, and educate future students (Stein, 2008).

The knowledge that DNP graduates gain in nursing programs will allow them to transition into practice and leadership roles with more confidence and skills to perform effectively in their new roles. As clinical leaders with nursing leadership, business, and healthcare management skills, these experts can use their knowledge of financial and business concepts to effect change on a global level.

Conclusions and Future Directions

Several demands in health care have provided momentum for the DNP degree. These demands include the changing complexity of our country's healthcare environments and improvements in the care of clients in clinical settings where advanced levels of practice expertise are needed at the bedside (Sperhac & Clinton, 2004; Williams, 2006). Parity with other healthcare professionals is another reason for the positive momentum behind the call for the DNP to be the highest degree for experts dedicated to the clinical role (Williams, 2006; Sperhac & Clinton, 2004).

Each nurse who completes the DNP degree can use that knowledge in a different way based on the individual's area of clinical expertise. Many will continue to fill faculty roles as more DNP programs are developed. Programs that offer practice doctorates will need DNP nurse educators in academic settings to educate students across all levels of nursing education to ensure that clinically competent faculty are educating students. Nurses who educate students and no longer practice in clinical care lose the connection to clinical care and tend to use more theoretical than clinical knowledge to educate students (Williams, 2006).

Improving communications channels in terms of how DNPs can help in practice and academic settings through mentoring relationships with experienced academic faculty will continue to be important to the transition of DNPs to academia (National League for Nursing, 2007). This key component of faculty transition is essential for faculty who are clinically competent and desire to have a career in academia because it affords the profession and society an opportunity to have clinical experts at clinical sites and in the classroom (Williams, 2006).

With the new emphasis on practice doctorates such as the DNP, nurse experts will continue to focus their work within areas of specialization that may not necessarily include the process of teaching. Some nurses with practice doctorates will be assuming needed roles in health care to meet various practice expectations, and others will remain in clinical work to facilitate healthcare policy changes (Riley, 2009). While working in various set-tings with other healthcare personnel with the title of "Doctor," DNPs will need to continue educating the public on the role and responsibilities related to their title (Green, Starck, & Long, 2006). Practice issues related to certification and reimbursement will continue to be a concern for some DNPs as the need for this level of clinical knowledge and expertise results in better client outcomes. It is essential that experts in clinical practice, academia, and research collaborate to facilitate changes in complex systems that lead to healthier outcomes for all of society.

NURSE ADMINISTRATOR/EXECUTIVE: DON R. HIRSCHMAN

Your goal is to become or be a better leader and administrator/executive. Which steps should you take to prepare yourself for the challenges and responsibilities of this role? This section posits the doctor of nursing practice, or DNP, as a major step toward your nursing leadership goal. Why go to the effort, expense, and commitment of earning a DNP? You have experience; the DNP is the education you need to help you reach your potential, become a better leader, and "Be all you can be," as the U.S. Army slogan says.

The University of California, San Francisco School of Nursing, defines nursing administration as "the specialty that integrates nursing science, business principles, organizational behavior, and resource management to prepare nurses to participate as full partners in managing and leading healthcare organizations." For our purposes, the term nurse administrator/executive will be used.

In the military, leaders are taught to balance the accomplishment of the mission with the welfare of the troops. The nurse administrator/executive must balance the welfare of patients and staff and the needs of the healthcare organization. Whatever the title, the nurse administrator/executive must not stray far from his or her role as patient advocate, because this is what distinguishes the role from the rest of the healthcare executive team—that is, the chief financial officer (CFO), chief executive officer (CEO), chief operating officer (COO), and the chief nursing officer (CNO). Of these important management team officers, only the nurse has ever had the primary role of patient advocate.

This section's goal is to answer some questions regarding the DNP. Is the DNP better prepared for the role of administrator/executive? If so, then in what ways? Several words are key to answering this question: leadership (University of Colorado, 2008; University of Tennessee, 2008; Wall, Novak, & Wilkerson, 2005), parity (i.e., similar to other professional doctorates) (Case Western Reserve University, 2008), commensurate, credibility, management, increased complexity (Fain, Asselin, & McCurry, 2008), and policy (Marion, Viens, O'Sullivan, Crabtree, Fontana, & Price, 2003).

Leadership

The DNP, as described by universities offering the degree, "educates students for leadership roles" (University of Tennessee, 2008). In addition to clinical and course work, the University of Tennessee requires a dissertation. Graduates of its rival, the University of Kentucky, "will be expert in designing, implementing, managing and evaluating health care delivery systems and will be prepared to lead at the highest clinical and executive ranks." DNP program graduates from the University of Colorado at Denver "will be prepared as leaders who will design models of health care delivery, evaluate clinical outcomes, identify and manage health care needs of populations, and use technology and information to transform health care systems" (University of Colorado, 2008). Case Western Reserve (2009) states, "Nurses with a DNP can move to the absolute pinnacle of their field: those with practice doctorates are the most highly educated and qualified practitioners in their profession. These advanced practice nurses apply their education and expertise in leadership roles on the front lines of nursing, in

clinical practice, teaching and research, and in health policy design and development."

Clearly, the stated intentions of DNP programs are to prepare nursing leaders. The programs cited are merely examples, because all programs cannot be mentioned in this text due to space limitations. As of December 2007, there were 45 programs offering the DNP, and at least 140 programs being considered (Partin, 2008).

The author's experience in the U.S. Army is relevant to this brief discussion of leadership. The Army defines leadership as "influencing, providing purpose, motivating and directing to accomplish the mission and improve an organization" (Department of the Army, 2004). The Army has been consistent in this definition since 1968 (Department of the Army, 1968). Although this section is specifically directed to nurse administrators/executives, the concept of leadership has many universal applications. The military has developed some great leaders. Nurse administrators/executives would be well advised to develop leadership skills by studying and learning from the captains of infantry as well as the captains of industry.

Parity

The *Merriam-Webster Online Dictionary* defines parity as "the quality or state of being equal or equivalent." Case Western Reserve University's Frances Payne Bolton School of Nursing (2009) describes its DNP program as "similar in concept [to] practice doctorates in other professions such as medicine (MD), law (JD) and dentistry (DDM)." Joyce Fitzpatrick of Case Western University further notes that the "practice doctorate allows both degree parity and additional strengthening of the educational program to assume full leadership roles in clinical practice, clinical teaching, and clinical action research" (Fitzpatrick, 2003). The entrance level of pharmacists is the PharmD. Psychologists earn a PhD. The professions of optometry, osteopathy, public health, physical therapy, audiology, chiropractic, and naturopathy all offer practice doctorates (Brown-Benedict, 2008), and the DNP offers parity with these professionals (Brown et al., 2006).

The Institute of Medicine (IOM) has suggested that all disciplines need to raise the bar in leadership training (IOM, 2003). The DNP degree is commensurate with more responsibility as a healthcare professional, and offers increased credibility to facilitate better management to meet the demands for delivery for modern health care and its increased complexity (Fain, 2008). The increased educational requirements of DNP-prepared nurses can improve the U.S. healthcare system.

Credibility and Personal Experience

Credibility is characterized by belief and trustworthiness. Knowledge, self-confidence, and reputation increase credibility. Does the DNP degree add to credibility? Jolley (2007) suggests the answer is yes. Clearly the title "Doctor" implies knowledge, academic achievement, scholarship, trust, and a list of other positives. The author's brother graduated from the University of Michigan Medical School in 1959. From then until 2002, whenever I heard "Dr. Hirschman," that always meant my brother. The first time I was introduced as "Dr. Hirschman" was as a speaker at the Ophthalmic Anesthesia Society. At that point the purpose of the sacrifice, expense, and efforts of the previous four years at Rush University became much clearer. A nursing doctorate paved the way for me to become part of a research team at Kansas University and the Department Veterans Affairs studying delayed cataract surgery and adverse effects on veterans. If funded, this study could reduce the time veterans wait to have sight-restoring cataract surgery through the Veterans Health Administration. The DNP will have opened the door to allow research to improve practice.

The percentages of DNP-prepared nurses are increasing, but this is still a very small group. DNPs, similar to those nurses who were motivated to earn master's degrees, are successful, productive nurses who have much to contribute. Nurses need to "be all we can be." Nurse want to be able to contribute at the highest levels of healthcare delivery. One of my fellow contributors is the administrator/president of Alterna-Care Home Health. No doubt there are many highly qualified, fine nurses working for this company, but the administrator/president is a DNP-prepared nurse.

The author's doctorate helped to secure an adjunct teaching appointment at Wichita State University. This enables teaching, motivating, and demonstration by example of what a doctor of nursing practice is and can do. My doctorate has not been to my financial advantage, earned me more vacation, gained me promotions, or had any other material benefit. Through doctoral studies I researched a question that had interested me for eight years. The question I studied was whether it was safe to continue anticoagulant therapy for cataract surgery patients. The common practice was to discontinue anticoagulants such as warfarin and aspirin for days or weeks before cataract surgery. This put patients at risk for developing the serious conditions the drugs were being used to prevent. Anecdotally, patients were reported to be experiencing embolisms, strokes, and other life-threatening conditions as a result of the withdrawal of anticoagulation therapy. There were no published data to confirm this, however. The study I led collected data from ophthalmic ambulatory surgery centers retrospectively. Without changing any medications pre- or postoperatively, we studied and compared the peri- and postoperative complications of patients on anticoagulation in more than 2,100 cases. There was no difference. We concluded that it was safe to continue anticoagulation therapy for cataract surgery patients (Hirschman & Morby, 2005).

To some, this is just another study. To some patients, however, it may mean the difference between continuing important medications or having them interrupted and putting them at unnecessary risk. The DNP you earn may touch lives, most of whom you will never know. The leadership you provide may touch many lives as well.

Management

A traditional master of science in nursing (MSN) may emphasize leadership and management. Advanced registered nurse practitioner programs also may or may not have a management track. Some DNP programs combine a healthcare leadership track using a combined faculty of nursing and business (Hardy, DeBasio, Warmbrodt, Gartland, Bassett, & Tansey, 2004).

The DNP manager can employ the techniques of the great management masters for better effectiveness. Some of the great names in management that DNP managers should study and emulate are W. Edwards Deming and Peter F. Drucker.

W. Edwards Deming, PhD, Yale University

Deming has written several books on management, productivity, and quality. One may ask how nursing relates to research on how post–World War II Japanese factories advanced from rubble to economic powerhouses so quickly. The answer is that the principles of building quality into the product at every stage rather than simply checking the end product can be adapted to healthcare delivery as well. Instead of inspecting a car as it rolls off the assembly line, Deming's method teaches quality to the designers and production workers and urges inspection during the process rather than simply at the end (Deming, 1986; Walton, 1986, 1991). In the realm of healthcare delivery, instead of relying on incident reports or chart reviews to discover problems, the DNP manager would develop a positive atmosphere of quality at every step of patient care.

Deming formulated 14 points for management, one of which is to "drive out fear" (Deming, 1986). All too often, incident reports are used punitively. Most nurses have been required to complete one after a real or perceived mistake. The DNP nurse administrator/executive would do well to drive out fear from his or her team and replace it with a "new philosophy" of leadership (Deming, 1986). DNP students should study Deming's management method. Do not limit your vision of leadership to only medical or nursing authors. Executive leadership by nurses must not be limited to the examples of nursing leadership.

Peter F. Drucker, Doctor of Law, University of Frankfurt

Peter Drucker has authored at least nine books on management and nine others on economics. His work is widely studied in graduate schools of business and management. Evidence of his timelessness is the fact that *The Practice of Management*, first published in 1954, is still in print. The DNP nurse administrator/executive has both the research and additional management training to face the increased expectations of staff and CEOs. The DNP administrator/executive is prepared to face the increased complexity of delivering modern health care.

Increased Complexity

Bob Dylan sang, "The times they are a-changin'." Nursing care is certainly becoming more complex (Draye, 2006). We have come a long way. The role of the nurse administrator/executive has come a long way as well. Nursing has come from the 1860s, when one sponge and one basin of water would be used to clean wounds on multiple patients, to the present use of disposables (Helmstadter, 2002). The nurse's role in leadership, management, and the boardroom has also evolved. The word "transformation" is often used to describe the changes (Draye, 2006). The DNP can help prepare nurses for the complex changes in clinical practice and leadership opportunities. Nurses could at one time aspire to be the "head nurse." Now complex healthcare delivery systems are led by doctorally prepared nurses. DNP nurses are trained to be community leaders and healthcare policy makers (Wall, Novak, & Wilkerson, 2005). Health policy administration is a very timely subject. Congress is continually debating health-care reform, and DNP nurses are well prepared to participate in that debate and form and implement policy (Acorn, Lamarche, & Edwards, 2009).

Experience dictates that doing well in a chosen field is one key to advancement to management. Salespersons are presumed to know how to train and motivate others to similar success. So, too, in nursing do exemplary nurses seek more knowledge and responsibility. A portion follow the clinical track, a portion the research track, and some gravitate to management and leadership. Master's-level nurses learn more to advance their clinical knowledge base and become nurse practitioners, clinical nurse specialists, certified registered nurse anesthetists, and certified nurse–midwives. Those nurses who choose the management track may earn a master of business administration, or MBA. The curriculum for the clinical master's degrees may not offer enough training for strategic planning. This nurse may not be ready for collaboration with the highest levels of corporate management (Marion et al., 2003). The DNP is uniquely prepared in strategic planning, organizational development, and systems.

Whatever path to graduate nursing education a nurse chooses, he or she is likely to study the concept of evidence-based practice.

Evidence-Based Practice

An important hallmark of doctoral programs is the focus on evidence-based practice. The term *evidence-based practice* (EBP) is now commonly used when discussing nursing practice. One very simple definition is that evidence-based practice examines all that we do to determine whether there is scientific evidence to support the practice. EBP means we do not do things just because we were taught to do so or because "we have always done it this way." It may well be that a common practice is a good one and should be continued, but not simply because

"that's the way we always do it." One practical example of EBP suggests a zero-based method, in which one starts with a blank policy and procedure manual and adds a procedure only after there is sound evidence to support it. Is this report, meeting, or process based on scientific evidence? Envision the savings of time, paper, and energy this would create. EBP must be the gold standard in every aspect of leadership, management, and administration.

Conclusions

The DNP prepares nurses for more responsibility in delivering health care. Having a doctoral preparation enhances the career path of nurses, whatever their specialty. The educational process is a component of this enhancement. The DNP-educated nurse will contribute to higher-quality health care with greater confidence gained from knowledge. The doctoral degree will help nurses gain parity when working with other doctorally prepared professionals as well as the leaders of healthcare organizations. It is reasonable to expect that CEOs, CFOs, and others who often are not doctorally prepared will give more credence to those who are. The DNP confers increased credibility. There will often be an assumption that the DNP-prepared individual is more knowledgeable and more credible than the individual with a master's degree.

The ideas and plans of DNP-prepared nurses are more likely to be tested than dismissed. The DNP program provides leadership training and the management emphasis track that will give the DNP enhanced skills. For those interested in management, executive leadership, patient care, and in making healthcare policy, the DNP is for you! As national government leaders continue to pursue healthcare reform, the DNP-prepared nurse will have strategic leverage to be at the table to determine and implement national healthcare policies. If in doubt about earning a DNP, remember and be guided by what may be the most appropriate and generally motivating ad slogan in current history: "Be all that you can be!"

NURSE ENTREPRENEUR: DEONNE J. BROWN BENEDICT

The nurse entrepreneur is at the forefront as a change leader. Innovative, creative, forward thinking, risk taking, visionary, strategic, emotionally intelligent, and persevering (Faugier, 2005; Kowal, 1988; Shirey, 2008; West, 2008) are all characteristics that have been ascribed to the nurse entrepreneur. "Entrepreneurship takes a lot of devotion and courage" (Grace Grymes Chapman, personal communication, July 10, 2009). "It requires compassion, passion for your specialty, and drive" to weather the unrelenting juggling act, frequent obstacles encountered, and multiple competencies required (Scharmaine Lawson-Baker, personal communication, July 21, 2009). "Entrepreneurs create something new, something different—they change values" (Drucker, 1985). What is less well known is that the ideal nurse entrepreneur also merges flexibility, patience, self-discipline, a customer service emphasis, and, in particular, planning and management expertise into his or her skill set (Castledine, 2006; Wilson, Averis, & Walsh, 2003). Strategic planning and process management tools are characteristics and competencies identified within the DNP.

Historically, nursing has often, but not always, been an employed occupation. The birth of nurse practitioners and advanced practice nursing in the 1960s set the stage for a new wave of innovative transformation in nursing, as nursing leaders such as Loretta Ford began to blaze new paths and take risks. Today, although exact figures on the numbers of nurse entrepreneurs are difficult to obtain, data from the U.S. Department of Health and Human Services (2004) indicate that 5.5% of RNs and 3% of nurse practitioners (NPs) are self-employed, a percentage that has been rising rapidly in recent years (Rollet & Lebo, 2007, 2008). Self-employed nurses report enhanced job satisfaction, especially in relation to empowerment for making a difference in the lives of the patients with whom they work (Wilson, Averis, & Walsh, 2003). Other benefits include autonomy, flexibility to work around personal and work schedules, control of quality improvements, improved patient satisfaction, and the ability to subspecialize (Caffrey, 2005; Elango, Hunter, & Winchell, 2007). Additionally, surveys of nurses have historically found that advanced practice nurses (APNs) who own their practice are more highly compensated than employed NPs (Rollet & Lebo, 2008).

At least as important as any one of the preceding factors is the reality that nurse entrepreneurs provide services not within the dominant medical model or under the oversight of other professionals, but in an interprofessional context within a distinctly nursing framework. Dr. Gregory Lind, owner of Lake Serene Clinic, an all–nurse practitioner practice in Washington State, says entrepreneurs recognize opportunity and apply their assets to a niche. When he started out as an NP in the late 1970s, local physicians transferred all of their nursing home patients to his practice. Through nursing interventions such as reducing overmedication and promoting safety and function, he was later rewarded with the responsibility of involvement in the development of a hospital birthing center. After obtaining his doctorate and briefly teaching at the university, he realized there was a need for an independent primary care open-access nurse practitioner practice. His walk-in clinic now employs seven nurse practitioners, with standard full time being three 11-hour days weekly alternating with four 11-hour days (personal communication, July 10, 2009).

Entrepreneurship provides the medium for an engaged and creative nursing populace without the subservience, sexism, inaccurate fettered public image, and other "cultural impediments" (Faugier, 2005, p. 50) that have historically tripped up nursing. Nurse entrepreneurship reminds the public that we are "far more than assistants to MDs," says Grace Grymes Chapman, owner of West Seattle Community Clinic (personal communication, July 10, 2009). Entrepreneurship provides the necessary conditions for "liberating" nurses to fulfill their professional promise (Howkins & Thornton, 2003, p. 219), while advancing technology and the growth of medical and nursing knowledge and in many ways continuing to aid the metamorphosis of nursing itself (Faugier, 2005). When Scharmaine Lawson-Baker, DNP and nurse practitioner, was asked why entrepreneurship is important for nursing, she responded, "Many patients are searching for affordable health care, and nurse entrepreneurs offer the holistic care, the quality care they need" (personal communication, July 21, 2009).

Although only recently identified as such through the use of the term *social entrepreneur* (Bishop, 2006), a contemporary term used to describe individuals who "bring about catalytic changes . . . in the perception of . . . social issues" (Waddock & Post, 1991), nursing history is replete with examples of entrepreneurship. Lillian Wald, together with Mary Brewster, founded the Henry Street Settlement. Lillian Wald coined the term "public health nursing," offering a new vision of a collaborative, problem-solving, community-based approach to social, economic, and mental health issues in addition to medical concerns (Abrams, 2008). Mary Breckenridge founded the Frontier Nursing Service, which introduced the first nurse–midwives to the United States, radically reducing pregnancy complications, maternal deaths, and stillborn rates in rural areas (Osborne & Dawley, 2005). Dorothea Dix became a champion for expanding appropriate, compassionate mental health care (Parry, 2006). In more recent times, there is Florence Wald, who changed the paradigm of care for the dying by introducing comprehensive hospice care services (Hoffmann, 2005), and others such as Loretta Ford, who founded the movement that became nurse practitioners (Houser & Player, 2004).

Nurse entrepreneurs pave new roads. They engage in novel healthcare delivery forms. Dr. Lawson-Baker pioneered comprehensive home visit services for elders, providing necessary health services in Louisiana after Hurricane Katrina when other healthcare providers left the state.

Nurse entrepreneurship changes public perceptions, as communities begin to better understand the capabilities of the profession. "NPs make decisions in concert with patients. As NPs become decision makers and not just decision-deliverers, clients see our worth and experience a different kind of care" (Gregory Lind, personal communication, July 22, 2009). Nurse entrepreneurs are found in legal consulting, care coordination services, camp nursing, continuing education provision, nursing staffing agencies, home care, stand-alone nurse anesthetist centers, adult day programs for elders, foot care services, energy work and complementary services, infection control, health writing, lactation consulting, medical coding, nursing informatics, nurse recruiting, occupational health, parish nursing, social programs for the uninsured, telehealth, telephone triage services, nursing marketing services, nursing research, wellness coaching, and vaccination services. They have private practices in psychiatric, family, and geriatric care, and subspecialty services as diverse as convenience care clinics, chronic disease home care, dermatologic services, integrative services, sexual assault services, palliative care, travel medicine, wound care, weight management, urgent care, urinary incontinence, and aesthetics (Bullock, 2009; Hardy, 2008; Kacel, 2008; Keyes, 2009; Marra, 2008; Moen, 2009; Pronsati, 2008; Rollet, 2008; Schiff, 2009; Smith, 2009; Veilleux, 2009).

Nurse entrepreneurship seems appropriately and inextricably linked to many of the DNP essentials (AACN, 2006). The second essential, organizational and systems leadership, identifies "practice management" (p. 10)—specifically, the need to balance productivity, quality of care, and budgetary issues. The development and evaluation of alternate delivery approaches and leading healthcare initiatives rings familiar to the ear of the entrepreneur. Dr. Lawson-Baker, owner of Advanced Clinical Consultants, a nurse practitioner house call service (personal interview, July 22, 2009), says the DNP promotes improved problem solving and education regarding the factors that promote successful change, but that additional content in business topics such as computer software, human resource management, billing, and accounting are needed because nurse entrepreneurs often still require seminars in these areas or experience learning through the school of hard knocks.

Clinical scholarship and evidence-based practice, the third essential, is also seen in the entrepreneur as she or he "designs and implements . . . [new] practice patterns and systems of care" (p. 12), using current research to improve healthcare outcomes for the population or populations she or he serves (AACN, 2006). Additionally, much entrepreneurship is being fueled by rapid gains in healthcare technologies (Essential IV) as entrepreneurs design or use existing technology to advance outcomes and assist consumers in understanding the vast amount of information available. At Charis Family Clinic, we use 100% electronic systems to coordinate care, bill claims, fax, strengthen patient education resources, and document visits, resulting in more space and time for the personalized human element of care.

Nurse entrepreneurs are advocates (Essential V) by nature. Often faced with barriers such as lack of reimbursement for nursing services and directly accountable to the clients they serve, they are often the nurses most involved in educating others about nursing and advocating for the advancement of the profession and the development of new policy. Dr. Lawson-Baker has been a regular visitor to lawmakers' offices in Washington, D.C., since 2006 to remove barriers to the care she and other NPs provide. The more entrepreneurs changing health care's landscape, the more nurses who will be calling for legislative change. Essential VI is often foundational for nurse entrepreneurs, as they lead interprofessional teams for the purpose of positive change and provide consultative services for individuals and other health entities

(AACN, 2006). "Nurse entrepreneurs need to understand hiring, firing, employee rights," and team concepts, says Dr. Lawson-Baker. Finally, the competency of advanced practice has laid the groundwork for much recent entrepreneurial activity.

Will the DNP facilitate nurse entrepreneurship? The answer is yes and no. "All professions have a practice base at the doctoral level. I applaud nursing for setting this standard instead of arguing for decades. . . . A recent presidential panel on health care lamented that medicine has abandoned primary care. [Fortunately,] there is no trouble finding nurses who want to become advanced practice nurses," said Dr. Gregory Lind. "I couldn't be more excited for the public, for nursing, or for countless advanced practice nurses to follow." The DNP places additional tools in the entrepreneurial toolbox. "[The DNP] helped me to practically apply evidence-based practice and to understand factors in addressing change," says Dr. Lawson-Baker. "The DNP will give more nurses the courage to follow their dream and go out on their own," says Grace Grymes Chapman. However, the DNP is a vital but insufficient condition for promoting nurse entrepreneurship. "It is the person with the degree, not the degree itself," that makes the entrepreneur, says Dr. Lind (personal communication, July 10, 2009).

As information technology continues to transform the delivery of care, clients continue to seek out customized wellness information and disease intervention, and organizations and skilled professionals continue to limit their long-term commitments to each other, opportunities for nursing entrepreneurship will grow and novel healthcare ventures will continue to flourish (Wilson, 1998). "Nursing must support entrepreneurship because medicine has abandoned setting up solo practices for the comfort of being employed . . . a true role reversal" (Gregory Lind, personal communication, June 12, 2009). The DNP will continue to provide the context for an adept nursing profession empowered to do what it was envisioned to do and what it does uniquely well—to radically alter and to deliver optimal health care.

Biosketches of Successful Nurse Entrepreneurs

Grace Grymes Chapman, MSN, FNP
West Seattle Community Clinic, PLLC

Grace Grymes Chapman, an advanced registered nurse practitioner, owns her own family practice clinic in West Seattle serving families of all ages, with a focus on women and adolescents. She has been an active presence on the boards of state and local nurse practitioner organizations. Chapman provides full-spectrum health care to people of all ages in West Seattle and surrounding communities. She provides health care to medically insured and the uninsured and is contracted with the Washington State Breast and Cervical Health Program, a state-funded program aimed at women without insurance between the ages of 40 and 65. Chapman is also contracted with the Vaccines for Children Program with the Public Health department, as well as the Washington State Take Charge Family Planning program.

Scharmaine Lawson-Baker, DNP, FNP-BC
Advanced Clinical Consultants, LLC, President/CEO

http://www.advancedclinicalconsultants.com, http://www.geriatricinitiatives.org

Scharmaine Lawson-Baker is the founder of Advanced Clinical Consultants. She is the family nurse practitioner for the only NP-owned house-call practice in New Orleans, Louisiana, established in 2004. House calls are made daily to elderly, disabled, and indigent patients who would otherwise not receive health care. In 2008, Lawson-Baker founded Geriatric Initiatives, a nonprofit organization formed to raise funds for medical supplies, diapers, pads, nutritional supplies, and other items not covered by Medicare or Medicaid. Lawson-Baker has been featured on CBS with Katie Couric, and in *Forbes*

magazine, *The Washington Post,* and countless other news sources. She is a frequent speaker on health disparities and elder care issues. Lawson-Baker has 19 years of experience as a registered nurse and nurse practitioner, providing care in almost every specialty from pediatrics to Level 1 trauma. She has also traveled on various mission trips, caring for the underserved in Puerto Rico and Dominican Republic. In 2007, she received the Housecall Clinician of the Year award from the American Academy of Home Care Physicians; she also received the 2008 NP Entrepreneur of the Year award from *Advance for Nurse Practitioners.*

Gregory A. Lind, PhD, ARNP
Lake Serene Clinic, Practice Owner

Gregory Lind is a nurse entrepreneur pioneer. He has graduate degrees from the University of Missouri in Columbia and the University of Kansas in Kansas City. In the 1970s, he worked with Missouri's School of Family and Community Medicine to start an NP role in a rural clinic. Lind later served for a short period of time as assistant director of a nurse practitioner program, but felt the pull toward reentering practice after Washington state changed its laws to allow independent NP practice with mandated insurance and prescriptive parity. In 1990, he founded Lake Serene Clinic, developing his vision of an all-NP urgent care practice that currently employs seven NPs. Lind developed the clinic to be open 9 a.m.–8 p.m. every day, and 11 a.m.–4 p.m. on holidays, allowing staff to work 3–11 shifts one week and 4–11 shifts the next week while also meeting a community need. His is still one of the oldest group FNP clinics owned and operated by an NP and has been featured in *Advance for Nurse Practitioners.*

PUBLIC AND COMMUNITY HEALTH PRACTITIONER: KATHLEEN SGRO

The doctor of nursing practice graduate specializing in public and community health nursing is able to take the advanced practice nursing role to a new level. Being able to identify systems problems in the delivery of health care and the promotion of wellness in our communities requires advanced training in evaluation of research, evidence-based nursing, and measurable outcomes. The DNP graduate possesses these skills and is able to apply them to these settings in many ways. Being able to measure responses to disasters, pandemic flu, treatment of chronic illnesses, women, infant, and children health programs, and so on will contribute to better care of populations, promotion of health, and prevention of illness.

Historical Development of Community and Public Health Nursing

> In essence, public health nursing requires specific educational preparation, and community health nursing denotes a setting for the practice of nursing.
> —*U.S. Department of Health and Human Services, 1985*

It is important for us to recognize the contribution of Lillian Wald to the profession of public health nursing. Wald was the originator of public health nursing and the founder of the Visiting Nurse Service in New York City. She focused her practice on caring for the poor on the Lower East Side. She established Henry House as a neighborhood program to provide care for those who were sick and at home. After the turn of the century, more than 90% of the sick stayed home. The poor had no money to pay physicians, and hospitals were reserved for extreme cases and generally did little good. Wald's influence on public health was felt worldwide through her visits to England, Germany, Italy, Mexico, and the Soviet Union (Falk, 2006). Modern public health nursing services emerged from the work of Lillian Wald.

Today public health nurses "provide population-focused care. Assessment, planning and evaluation occur at the population level. The nursing process is used in the planning and delivery of care to individuals, families, groups, populations, and communities" (ANA, 2007). The focus of the public health nurse is on promoting, restoring, and maintaining the health of the population or community, which is quite a different practice from what occurs in a facility or clinic. As our society has become more complex, so has public health nursing. Broad capabilities in systems thinking are foundational to the understanding of population health. The DNP graduate possesses the skills to identify these populations and incorporate evidence-based practice in addressing healthcare promotion and disease prevention for patient populations. In contrast, community health nursing is "the identification of needs, along with protection and improvement of collective health, within a geographically defined area" (Rector, 2010). The American Association of Colleges of Nursing supports the practice of doctoral education for public health and community nursing with Essential VII of doctoral education.

The DNP program prepares the graduate to:

1. Analyze epidemiological, biostatistical, environmental, and other appropriate scientific data related to individual, aggregate, and population health.

2. Synthesize concepts, including psychosocial dimensions and cultural diversity, related to clinical prevention and population health in developing, implementing, and evaluating interventions to address health promotion/disease prevention efforts, improve health status/access patterns, and/or address gaps in care of individuals, aggregates, or populations.

3. Evaluate care delivery models and/or strategies using concepts related to community, environmental and occupational health, and cultural and socioeconomic dimensions of health (AACN, 2006).

Measuring Progress in Population Health

Assessment of progress in population health is measured differently from that of an individual person's health. Progress is measured through collection and analysis of large data sets and the development of population wellness goals. This data collection and goal development is facilitated through the U.S. Department of Health and Human Services (DHHS). The current national goals are known as *Healthy People 2020*. An advisory committee developed these goals for the nation's health in an attempt to set national objectives and provide benchmarks against which progress can be measured toward the new goals (DHHS, 2008). It is thought that such objectives and benchmarks will focus actions toward the overall goal of improving the nation's health (see Figures 5-1 and 5-2).

Organizational Aspects of Public and Community Health

The Quad Council on Public Health Nursing Organizations is a group of member organizations that includes the Association of State and Territorial Directors of Nursing (ASTDN), the American Nurses Association (ANA) Council on Nursing Practice and Economics, the Association of Community Health Nursing Educators (ACHNE), and the Section of Public Health Nursing of the American Public Health Association (APHA). The purpose of the Quad Council is to provide a forum for developing ideas about issues. It also identifies public health nurse experts to advocate for public health nursing on national and other committees (ACHNE, n.d.). The DNP graduate has the skills and competencies to participate in the dialogue and present the perspective of public health nursing to legislators (AACN, 2006).

Community Health

The DNP graduate who practices in the community health role must integrate these initiatives into the planning and treatment of

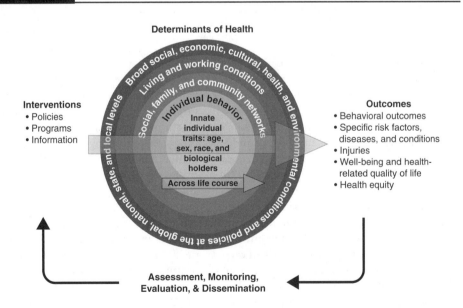

| FIGURE 5-1 | Action Model to Achieve *Healthy People 2020*'s Overarching Goals |

Source: U.S. Department of Health and Human Services, Secretary's Advisory Committee on Health Promotion and Disease Prevention Objectives for 2020. (2008). Phase I report: Recommendations for the framework and format of *Healthy People 2020* (p. 8). Retrieved from http://www.healthypeople.gov /hp2020/advisory/PhaseI/PhaseI.pdf.

FIGURE 5-2 *Healthy People 2020* Vision and Mission Statement

---

Vision

A society in which all people live long, healthy lives.

Mission

To improve health through strengthening policy and practice, Healthy People will:

- Identify nationwide health improvement priorities
- Increase public awareness and understanding of the determinants of health, disease, and disability and the opportunities for progress
- Provide measurable objectives and goals that can be used at the national, state, and local levels
- Engage multiple sectors to take actions that are driven by the best available evidence and knowledge
- Identify critical research and data collection needs

Source: Secretary's Advisory Committee on National Health Promotion and Disease Prevention Objectives for 2020. (2008). *Phase I report: Recommendations for the framework and format of Healthy People 2020*, p. 5. Retrieved from http://www.healthypeople.gov/HP2020/advisory/PhaseI/PhaseI.pdf.

---

patients within the community setting. There are many venues for community health nursing. Local county and city health departments, home health agencies, wellness programs, and government-sponsored community health programs are a few settings in which community and public health nurses focus on disease prevention and wellness promotion. The DNP's role in community health nursing is to maintain a knowledge base of the healthcare delivery system across the continuum of care and focus on evidence-based interventions when developing a comprehensive plan of care. The plan of care incorporates available community healthcare resources and established treatment guidelines in managing patients and clients. The DNP identifies illnesses that are being addressed through community health systems, develops interventions to improve the health of the patients and families

who are part of the community, and assists them in managing acute and chronic illnesses within the community setting. The community health nurse integrates outcomes and cost-control measures in the development and provision of nursing interventions. The DNP graduate in community health "has and continues to demonstrate great promise in reshaping nursing practice and health care management" (Cohen & Cesta, 2001). As more complex nursing interventions are provided to patients in settings outside the hospital, the need for doctorally prepared community health nurses will increase.

Another aspect of community nursing that the DNP graduate is well suited for is the development of disease management protocols that include the integration of technology in the delivery of community health services. Remote monitoring and electronic healthcare records are changing the delivery of healthcare services for the better. According to the AACN's Essentials of Doctoral Education, the DNP graduate has competencies in technology and information systems (AACN, 2006). The DNP's skills also promote the analysis of systems for cost-containment measures across the entire healthcare delivery system. Given the current financial climate, many local, state, and national legislatures are attempting to restructure the current system in the United States. The DNP is uniquely positioned to advocate for those who are unable to have a voice in the decision-making process. Vulnerable patient populations continue to need ongoing nursing care, and the DNP graduate has the skills to participate in policy formation to ensure that these patient populations have their needs addressed.

Community Healthcare Settings

County Health Departments

Disease prevention and control, emergency preparedness, maternal–child health, family health, clinic services, elder care, the homeless, and environmental health are all areas that government-operated health departments oversee. The DNP's expertise in identification of problems facing the community and development of evidence-based interventions contributes to continued preparedness in dealing with public health issues. County and city health departments vary in the number and types of services they offer. Some oversee the inspection and licensing of local restaurants. Many provide Medicare and Medicaid skilled home health services; women, infant, and children (WIC) programs; and wellness and prevention programs such as smoking cessation, disease management, and weight loss programs. The DNP graduate is well prepared to play a role as a member of the interdisciplinary team that plans and develops education programs that focus on disease prevention and health promotion.

The DNP graduate has a role in policy setting and in the tracking of illnesses in order to continue to improve the lives of these popula-tions. Identification of gaps in services to populations lies with the advanced practice nurse. Ongoing reevaluation of the effectiveness of these programs will lead to improved care, and the DNP must develop tracking and intervention criteria and outcome measures. The public health DNP uses evidence-based practice and research to develop needed programs for populations in the community. Since September 11, 2001, the focus on disaster preparedness has required the advanced practice nurse to develop strategic plans to deal with potential disasters such as bioterrorism and to work as a team member with other community resources in developing comprehensive response plans.

Pandemic Flu and Tuberculosis Prevention

Local county health departments are also the main distributors of flu vaccines and healthcare worker protective equipment during pandemic flu episodes. They usually provide tuberculosis testing for the public, and many provide annual flu vaccine clinics for the general public. Identification of public health concerns and potential infections requires the skills of the DNP. Development of action plans and coordination of dissemination of vaccines to communities requires advanced skills in developing strategic plans to have positive outcomes. Being able to measure these outcomes is also the role of the DNP in controlling the spread of disease, educating the community, and promoting health.

Disaster Preparedness

County and city health departments are a focal point in implementing community disaster responses. They work closely with area hospitals, the Red Cross, and law enforcement in providing services to the community during a disaster. The public health DNP's input is vital to the development of comprehensive disaster preparedness programs. Hurricane Katrina was a wake-up call to our country that more work on our national disaster preparedness is needed. Examining our past failures leads us toward improved systems for providing services to our communities during disasters. The DNP plays a significant role in development of policies and disaster preparedness plans, as well as educating the healthcare workforce on the proper response.

Clinics

County and city health departments provide for health clinics and dental clinics for the uninsured as well as immunization programs for school-aged children. The public health nurse who works at a county health department wears many hats. County and city health departments are funded through local taxes and grants. The DNP has a major role in program development, cost controls, and adherence to grant requirements and other funding sources. Identification of patient populations and needs is important for the advanced practice nurse to prepare grant applications that will have an impact on the prevention of illnesses. Advanced practice nurses in government-sponsored health programs must develop methodologies for measuring the success of many programs. Treatment programs must be evidence based, with measurable outcomes, to provide a continuing evaluation of the effectiveness of programs.

Home Healthcare Settings

Community nursing is provided through several venues. One of these venues is home health services. Home health agencies are licensed by state departments of public health. The licensing acts cover skilled intermittent and part-time services. Some states require a certificate of need (CON) before a license is issued. These states attempt to control costs and manage services through the licensing process. Many states are beginning to develop standards and licensing requirements for private-duty skilled and nonskilled hourly home services. The state of Illinois recently amended its home health licensing act to include these levels of home care services. This policy change was achieved through the work of community health nurses

and social workers in Illinois who requested oversight of the delivery of hourly home care to homebound patients in the state. Issues relating to unlicensed care were identified as a problem-prone area by community nurses. Through their efforts, the state now has oversight of the nursing care and home care services delivered to one of the most vulnerable patient populations, the homebound disabled and elderly. The advanced practice nurse can effect change through policy development and testifying before legislatures so as to meet the needs of the community.

Medicaid and Medicare Issues in Home Health Services

Skilled home health services are funded through the Medicare Part A benefit. Senior citizens aged 65 and older and disabled adults are covered under the Medicare home health benefit. When a patient is admitted to a home health agency, a plan of care is established by the community health nurse assigned to the patient and the patient's primary care physician. The community health nurse coordinates the care needed and develops a plan of care that may include other disciplines, such as therapy, social services, and home health aides for assistance with personal hygiene. Most home health agencies provide these services on an intermittent basis. Community health nurses and therapists make visits on a predetermined frequency. All services must be ordered by a medical doctor, doctor of osteopathy, or psychiatrist.

The DNP has a role as a program and treatment manager in a home health agency, as well as in identification of developing trends and gaps in services available to patient populations within the community. The advanced practice nurse is able to serve as a liaison to community healthcare nurses in directing disease management programs that will reduce hospitalization and emergency room usage for these patient populations. Evidence-based practice protocols need to be designed for home health nursing.

The DNP has the expertise to identify best practices that will lead to management of chronic illnesses that produces improved outcomes.

Disease Management and Evidence-Based Practice in Home Health

Development of disease management programs that are evidence based provides the DNP with a challenging role in the community setting. The Disease Management Association of America (DMAA) has established the following criteria for disease management programs:

- Population identification process
- Evidence-based practice guidelines
- Collaborative practice models to include physician support
- Patient self-management education
- Process outcomes measurement evaluation and management
- Routine reporting/feedback loop (DMAA, 2009)

Disease management programs are beginning to show evidence of improved quality of life for patients with chronic illnesses. Further research needs to be done in this area, and the DNP has the necessary tools to evaluate the effectiveness of disease management programs.

Home Hospice and Inpatient Services

Hospice services provided to terminally ill patients and their families focus on symptom management, pain control, medical equipment, and emotional and pastoral care services as well as bereavement follow-up for survivors. Hospice programs are home health based and are reimbursed under Medicare Part A. Coordinating care and managing patient symptoms must be designed to meet the individual needs of each patient. The advanced practice nurse specializing in hospice and palliative care collaborates with other healthcare providers in management of pain and symptoms related to the terminal illness.

Technology

Home healthcare agencies are incorporating technology into their practice. Electronic clinical records and telehealth vital sign monitoring devices are being used to provide accurate and immediate health status information to the community health nurse. Daily vital sign monitors transmit information such as pulse, weight, blood pressure, pulse oxygen levels, temperature, blood glucose readings, and prothrombin times to the agency so that community health nurses or therapists are able to intervene when a patient's condition fluctuates. The goal is to intervene early and prevent an emergency room visit or inpatient admission. DNPs collaborate with physicians and other healthcare professionals to develop standardized treatment protocols for chronic diseases. In the community health setting, DNPs also collaborate with other community resources and develop programs that incorporate technology to bridge the gap in information that is shared across the healthcare continuum.

Evidence-Based Practice and Community Health

It is the role of the community health nurse to provide evidence-based clinical treatments. Home health agencies are developing disease management programs in an attempt to prevent exacerbations of illnesses such as diabetes, congestive heart failure, and so forth, as well as implementing fall reduction programs. Outcome measurements provide nursing staff with measurable results to identify areas of success and areas needing improvement.

Case Study

In 2006, Alterna-Care Home Health Agency, located in Springfield, Illinois, completed a two-year project aimed at reducing emergency room visits and repeat hospitalizations among its diabetic and cardiac patient populations. Evidence-based treatments and a disease management model of care were implemented.

After the two-year project, repeat hospitalizations and emergency room visits were significantly reduced in these patients. Evidence-based practice that provides interventions to reduce acute care services will add cost savings to the Medicare program. Disease management using specialized nursing and collaboration with physician specialists are two components of the program that led to improved outcomes. This was a DNP project that showed successful results. The DNP must develop these types of programs that are replicable to other patient populations. The disease management model of care is easily replicable to other diagnoses, which is important for a DNP project (Sgro, 2007). The DNP identifies areas that need improvement or unmet needs of patient populations and develops a plan to improve the outcomes for this population. There is continued work to be done in the disease management arena.

Future and Proposed Legislation

In 2008 several states were chosen to pilot a pay-for-performance (P4P) reimbursement methodology for home health agencies. Value-based purchasing for services provided to Medicare beneficiaries will be the focus of P4P. The DNP must have the ability to track patient outcomes and efficacy of treatment to survive in the P4P environment. At this writing, the proposal is for home health agencies to receive a bonus if their outcome measures are in the top 10% of the national average and a penalty if their outcome measures are in the bottom 10%. This is an example of the type of outcomes-based payment strategies being proposed on a national level as a result of cost overruns and concerns about the sustainability of current Medicare and Medicaid benefits.

The need for long-term-care home- and community-based services is straining the Medicare system. By 2050, one in four Americans will be 65 years or older, making up 18.5% of the U.S. population by 2025 (U.S. Census Bureau, 1990). The DNP will need to focus on cost-effective and evidence-based interventions to meet the needs of the senior population in the community.

The Independence at Home Act (S.1131) was introduced on May 21, 2009. This bill would allow Medicare to authorize chronic care coordination programs for Medicare beneficiaries with multiple chronic conditions under the traditional fee-for-service program. The goal is to help patients to remain in their homes with additional support, at a lower cost than institutional care. The DNP graduate is well prepared to track legislation in order to prepare for the provision of nursing care to the large volume of aging baby boomers. "Research is needed to address and evaluate the effectiveness of our current public health system," and the DNP will play a major role in this research, American Academy of Home Care Physicians (AAHCP, 2009).

Wellness Programs in the Community

Insurance- and Employer-Sponsored Programs

Insurance payers are focusing on preventive care programs. For example, health insurance companies provide wellness programs to their beneficiaries. Employers are also developing these programs in an effort to decrease the cost of care for chronic illnesses such as diabetes, asthma, congestive heart failure, obesity, and smoking-related illnesses. Insurance companies use advanced practice nurses who provide phone teaching through case management to enrollees of the insurance program. The DNP is able to provide evidence-based preventive care programs while monitoring the cost effectiveness of interventions. Measuring the outcomes of a wellness program provides feedback to the organization on the benefits of preventive programs.

Government-Sponsored Community Health Programs

Specialized Services for Children

Each state receives federal money for home care services to support families who are caring for children with multiple handicaps. Many children who need complex nursing care are managed at home. Family members are taught to provide this type of care with support from community nursing services. These state grants use case managers to oversee and approve the care provided in the home. This vulnerable patient population needs ongoing evaluation by the advanced practice nurse to ensure the delivery of adequate community services in order for them to remain independent. Proper funding and policy making are the goals of the DNP in this setting.

Community Mental Health Services

Community-based case management systems for chronically mentally ill patients integrate the role of the case manager as a coordinator of community resources and as coordinator of care. Two models of community-based care to support the mentally ill have emerged. The assertive community treatment model and the intensive case management model both have a low patient-to-staff ratio, with services provided in the community rather than in mental health centers. The assertive community model uses a team approach with nurses and physicians sharing the caseload. The intensive case management model provides for a stronger relationship between the nurse and the patient (Cohen & Cesta, 2001). Further research is needed to measure the effectiveness of these programs.

Senior Community Care Programs

State-sponsored community care programs for senior citizens are similar to the services provided through the Department of Rehabilitative Services. The community care programs for seniors provide assistance with daily living. Clients must qualify financially to receive the services. A case coordination assessment is completed using a scoring system to determine the number of hours of assistance for which each applicant qualifies. The doctor of nursing practice must be aware of all the programs available in the community. The DNP needs to bring these services together to meet the needs of each individual.

Summary

The advanced practice nurse has numerous roles in public and community health nursing across the life span of individuals. Research into the efficacy of community programs is needed to provide the best evidence-based and cost-effective interventions. As the population ages, the provision of care in the home will become more common in an attempt to keep seniors in their own homes. Emerging technologies will provide much-needed improvements in communication and valuable outcome measurements. Implementing evidence-based care and using feedback and outcome measures to improve care provide direction for improvement of community-based healthcare services.

Healthcare issues such as pandemic flu outbreaks, natural disasters, and treatment of chronic illnesses require a global perspective. Nursing must be involved in policy making and the identification of trends and the needs of patient populations in the community. Advanced practice nurses are instrumental in developing programs, influencing policy, and providing research for evidence-based practice in community and public health nursing.

INTEGRATIVE PRACTITIONER: JOY ELWELL AND KATHRYN WAUD WHITE

Integrative health care is growing as a choice for Americans. According to the National Institutes of Health, in 2005 38% of American adults and 12% of children used alternative or complementary therapies of some type ("Americans Continue," 2009). Integrative health care is just that: the integration of the best concepts of traditional medicine with the best concepts of alternative therapies (Center for Spirituality and Healing, 2008). The skills gained in the DNP program will enhance the advanced nurse practitioner in integrative therapy. Essential III states that the DNP program prepares advanced practice nurses to "[c]ritically appraise existing literature and other evidence to implement the best evidence for practice" (AACN, 2006). Essential VI speaks to interprofessional collaboration, which is truly an essential for the practice of this specialty that reaches across so many different healthcare fields (AACN, 2006). Essential VII describes clinical prevention and population health, all facilitated through integrative health care (AACN, 2006). The DNP-prepared integrative health practitioner will have much to offer patients.

To address the DNP-prepared advanced practice nurse as an integrative practitioner, it is essential to explore integrative health as a specialty within health care. Integrative health, also known as holistic health, is described as "treating the whole person, helping the person to bring the mental, emotional, physical, social, and spiritual dimensions of his or her being into greater harmony, using the basic principles and elements of holistic healing and, as much as possible, placing reliance on treatment modalities that foster the self regenerative and self reparatory processes of natural healing" (Otto & Knight, 1979, p. 3). Nursing's approach to wellness from a holistic perspective makes nursing and integrative health perfect partners for the advanced practice nurse.

Nurses as Integrative Practitioners

Historically, Florence Nightingale may be considered one of the first professional integrative health practitioners in nursing. Nightingale "was a mystic, visionary, healer, reformer, environmentalist, feminist, practitioner, scientist, politician and global citizen" (Dossey, Selanders, Beck, & Attewell, 2005). She looked beyond the era's traditional medical and surgical treatment of disease and injury to include nutrition and sanitation, lighting, and activity. She addressed the mind, body, and spirit connection that would pave the way for modern professional integrative practitioners.

Since Nightingale's death in 1910, professional nursing has evolved in numerous ways, including the development of advanced practice nursing roles. Numerous nursing pioneers have explored integrative modalities to assist clients in achieving optimal levels of wellness, alleviating suffering, and facilitating healing. Founded in 1980, the American Holistic Nurses Association (AHNA) focuses on holistic nursing as "all nursing practice that has healing the whole person as its goal" (AHNA, 1998, cited in AHNA, n.d.).

New York University established the first holistic nurse practitioner program; other academic institutions have since followed suit. Within the United States, certain states (e.g., New York) identify holistic health as a specialty (New York State Office of the Professions, n.d.). There are also holistic clinical nurse specialists. The American Nurses Association now recognizes holistic nursing as a specialty, and certification can be obtained through the American Holistic Nurses' Certification Corporation (AHNCC). The American Holistic Nurses Organization (AHNO) has also articulated standards of practice, core values, a certification curriculum, and requirements for endorsement of holistic nursing programs. A current listing of nursing programs that are endorsed by the AHNCC can be found at http://ahncc.org/home/endorsedschools.html.

Nurses can pursue educational programs for integrative or holistic modalities at all levels of post-licensure preparation; generally, there is no prescribed level of degree preparation for an integrative practice. Certain roles within the realm of integrative practitioners, such as chiropractors, acupuncturists, and massage therapists, are licensed and do have educational requirements. Nurses who pursue these roles must fulfill those requirements in addition to any nursing curriculum.

That nurses practice integratively is not a novel concept. Major nursing theorists incorporate holism into their theories. Dr. Jean Watson's theory of human caring is one example. She identifies caring beliefs and behaviors that benefit not only the client but also the nurse.

Types of Integrative Healing Modalities

Integrative health care includes many healing modalities. There are five different approaches to care as organized by the National Center for Complementary and Alternative Medicine (NCCAM): whole medical systems, manipulative and body-based practices, mind–body medicine, biologically based practices, and energy medicine (NCCAM, 2007). The modalities described here are not intended to be an exhaustive list of every integrative healing modality known. Table 5-1 lists websites where further information can be found.

Whole Medical Systems

- Homeopathy: A medical discipline that facilitates healing through the administration of substances prescribed according to three principles: (1) like cures like, also known as the "law of similars"; (2) the more a remedy is diluted, the greater the potency; and (3) illness is specific to the individual. Homeopathy is based on the belief that symptoms are signs of the body's effort to get rid of disease; treatment is based on the whole person, rather than on the symptoms (NCCAM, 2009).

- Osteopathic medicine: A form of medicine focusing on the relationship between the structure of the body and its function, identifying that both structure and function are subject to a range of illnesses. In treating the client, osteopathic practitioners use various types of physical manipulation to stimulate the body's self-healing ability, as well as traditional allopathic medical modalities. Osteopathic physicians are licensed to diagnose, treat, and prescribe nationally.

Manipulative Modalities

- Acupressure: Pressure, by fingers and hands, over specific areas of the body, is used to alleviate pain and discomfort and to positively influence the function of internal organs and body systems. Various approaches are used to release tension and restore the natural flow of energy in the body.

- Acupuncture: Fine-gauged needles are inserted into specific points on the body to stimulate or disperse the flow of energy. This

---

TABLE 5-1   Websites for Further Information on Integrative Health

American Holistic Nurses' Certification Corporation

　http://www.ahncc.org

Center for Spirituality and Healing at the University of Minnesota

　http://www.csh.umn.edu

Life Science Foundation

　http://lifesciencefoundation.org

National Center for Complementary and Alternative Medicine (NCCAM)

　http://nccam.nih.gov/health/whatiscam

University of Michigan, Doctor of Nursing Practice Program

　http://www.nursing.umn.edu/dnp/ProspectiveStudent/Specialties/Integrative_Health_and_Healing/home.html

ancient Oriental technique is used to alleviate pain or increase immunity by balancing energy flow. Massage, herbal medicine, and nutritional counseling are often used in conjunction with acupuncture.

- Alexander technique: This technique, developed by the Australian actor Frederick Matthias Alexander, involves learning a series of lessons in rebalancing the body through awareness, movement, and touch. As the student explores new ways of reorganizing neuromuscular function, the body is reintroduced to healthy posture and direct, efficient movement (Trivieri & Anderson, 2002).

- AMMA therapy: AMMA therapy is a form of Oriental massage that focuses on the balance and movement of energy within the body.

- Applied kinesiology: Originated by chiropractic physician George Goodheart, Jr., in the 1960s, applied kinesiology incorporates the principles of a number of holistic therapies, "including chiropractic, osteopathic medicine and acupuncture, and involves manual manipulation of the spine, extremities, and cranial bones in performing its procedures" (Trivieri & Anderson, 2002, p. 71).

- Aromatherapy: Aromatherapy incorporates the use of essential oils extracted from plants and herbs to treat physical imbalances, as well as to achieve psychological and spiritual well-being. The oils are inhaled, applied externally, or ingested. According to Dr. Kurt Schnaubelt, "the chemical makeup of essential oils gives them a host of desirable pharmacological properties, ranging from antibacterial, antiviral, and antispasmodic, to uses as diuretics, vasodilators, and vasoconstrictors. Essential oils also act on the adrenals, ovaries, and thyroid, and can energize, pacify or detoxify, and facilitate the digestive process" (Trivieri & Anderson, 2002, p. 76).

- Breema bodywork: Breema bodywork incorporates simple, playful bodywork sequences along with stretch and movement exercises that help create greater flexibility, a relaxed body, a clear mind, and calm, supportive feelings. Developed by chiropractic physician Jon Schraiber, Breema bodywork is based on nine principles: body comfortable, no extra, firmness and gentleness, full participation, mutual support, no judgment, single moment/single activity, no hurry/no pause, and no force (Mann, 2009).

- Chiropractic medicine: This healthcare system emphasizes structural alignment of the spine. Adjustments involve the manipulation of the spine and joints to reestablish and maintain normal nervous system functioning. Some chiropractors employ additional therapies, such as massage, nutrition, and specialized kinesiology.

- Cranial osteopathy: Gentle and almost imperceptible manipulation of the skull is used to reestablish its natural configuration and movement. Such correction can have a positive influence on disorders manifested throughout the body.

- Craniosacral therapy: This therapy focuses on diagnosis and treatment of imbalances in the craniosacral system. Subtle adjustments are made to the system through light touch and gentle manipulations.

- Dance therapy: Dance therapy is a modality in which dance and music combine to allow the body, mind, soul, and spirit to be refreshed and uplifted and to experience the freedom that natural bodily movement allows.

- Feldenkrais method: The Feldenkrais method is a method of instruction, through movement and gentle manipulation, to enhance self-image and restore mobility. Students are taught to notice how they are using their bodies and how to improve their posture and move more freely.

- Jin shin jyutsu: This bodywork technique balances body energy as it travels along specific pathways. Specific combinations of healing points are held with the fingertips to restore balance and harmony.

- Lymphatic therapy: Lymphatic therapy is a vigorous form of massage that helps the body release toxins stored in the lymphatic system—excellent for the immune system and rebuilding the body.

- Massage: Massage involves the use of strokes and pressure on the body to dispel tension, increase circulation, and relieve muscular pain. Massage can provide comfort and increased body awareness and can facilitate the release of emotional as well as bodily tension.

- Movement therapy: This modality involves guided series of movements and body work to open energy pathways and facilitate healing.

- Neuromuscular therapy: Neuromuscular therapy is a massage therapy in which moderate pressure over muscles and nerves, as well as on trigger points, is used to decrease pain and tension.

- Physical therapy: Physical therapy includes the treatment of physical conditions of body malfunction, damage, or injury using procedures designed to reduce swelling, relieve pain, strengthen muscles, restore range of motion, and return functioning to the patient.

- Shiatsu: Shiatsu is an energy-based system of bodywork using a firm sequence of rhythmic pressure held on specific pressure points on the body, designed to awaken acupressure meridians.

- Trigger point therapy: This is a method of compression of sensitive points in the muscle tissue, along with massage and passive stretches, for the relief of pain and tension. Treatment decreases swelling and stiffness and increases range of motion. Exercises may be assigned.

Mind–Body Medicine

- Art therapy: Art therapy incorporates the use of basic art materials to discover how to restore, maintain, or improve physical and mental health. Through observation and analysis, the art therapist is able to formulate treatment plans specific to the individual.

- Color therapy: Color therapy involves the use of electronic instrumentation and color receptivity, according to the work of Jacob Lieberman (1993), to integrate the nervous system and body–mind. It increases well-being, and can be helpful for many acute and chronic ailments.

- Counseling/psychotherapy: This broad category includes therapies that treat individuals as a whole. Treatments and sessions are focused on integrated care on all levels, for individuals, families, or groups.

- Eye movement desensitization and reprocessing (EMDR): EMDR is an accelerated information-processing method using alternating stimuli—either eye movements or sounds—to desensitize and reprocess emotional wounds and install a healthier belief system. EMDR is effective with post-traumatic stress syndrome, childhood trauma, depression, addictions, compulsions, unhealthy patterns, and future-oriented solutions.

- Guided imagery: This holistic modality assists clients in connecting with their inner knowledge at the thinking, feeling, and sensing levels, thus promoting their innate healing abilities. Together, guide and client co-create an effective way to work with pain, symptom, grief, and stress management; conflict resolution; self-empowerment issues; and preparing for medical or surgical interventions.

- Hypnotherapy: A state of focused attention achieved through guided relaxation, hypnotherapy is used to access the unconscious mind. Hypnosis is used for memory recall, medical treatment, and skill enhancement or personal growth.

- Interactive imagery: Fostering active participation, disease prevention, and health promotion, interactive imagery returns the focus of wellness to the individual.

- Meditation: Meditation is a method of relaxing and quieting the mind to relieve muscle tension and facilitate inner peace. There are numerous forms of meditation, taught individually or in group settings, and it is thought that prayer for the self might have an effect similar to meditation. The nonsectarian form of prayer, which is akin to meditation and used for stress reduction, has long been recognized by clinicians to improve one's sense of well-being.

- Music therapy: This expressive art form is designed to help the individual move into harmony and balance. Through the use of music, individuals explore emotional, spiritual, and behavioral issues. Musical skill is not necessary, as the process, rather than technique, is emphasized.

- Neurolinguistic programming: This systematic approach seeks to change behavior by changing patterns of thinking. Its originators, Dilts, Grinder, and Bandler (1980), propose theoretical connections between neurological processes (neuro), language (linguistic), and behavioral patterns that have been learned through experience (programming) that can be organized to achieve specific goals in life.

- Stress management: Stress management includes any therapy or educational practice with the objective of decreasing stress and enhancing one's response to the elements of life that cannot be changed. This broad category may include bodywork, energy work, visualization, and counseling.

- Tai chi (chuan): This movement practice and Chinese martial art enhances coordination, balance and breathing, and promotes physical, emotional, and spiritual well-being. Tai chi is taught in classes or as private lessons, and requires home practice to be effective.

- Yoga therapy: The use of yoga postures, controlled breathing, relaxation, meditation, and nutrition facilitates the release of muscular and emotional tension, improves concentration, increases oxygen levels in the blood, and assists the body in healing itself.

Biologically Based Practices

- Biofeedback: this relaxation technique involves careful monitoring of vital functions (such as breathing, heart rate, and blood pressure) so as to improve health. By conscious thought, visualization, movement, or relaxation, one can learn which actions result in desirable changes in these vital functions. Biofeedback is used for medical problems related to stress and for management of many health problems, including pain syndrome, migraine, and irritable bowel syndrome.

- Herbal therapy: Herbs and their chemical properties are used to alleviate specific conditions or to support the function of various body systems. Herbal formulas have three basic functions: elimination and detoxification, health management and maintenance, and health building. The scope of herbal medicine is sometimes extended to include fungal and bee products, as well as minerals, shells, and certain animal parts (Acharya & Shrivastava, 2008).

- Hydrotherapy: Water, ice, steam, and hot and cold temperatures are used to relieve pain, fever, inflammation, and maintain and restore health. Treatments include full-body immersion, steam baths, saunas, and the application of hot or cold compresses or both.

- Nutritional counseling: Nutritional counseling is performed by a practitioner who uses diet and supplementation therapeutically as the primary or adjunctive treatment for illness, as well as for maintaining good health. Nutritionists employ a variety of approaches, including food combining, macrobiotics, and orthomolecular theory.

Energy Medicine

- Chi kung healing touch: An Eastern method of healing involving breath and gentle movements that follows the Chinese five-element theory and works with the meridian system.

- Energy work: A broad category of healing influencing the seven major energy centers (chakras) and the flow of energy around and through this field.

- Healing touch: A therapeutic approach in which touch is used to influence energy systems. Healing touch is employed to affect physical, emotional, mental, and spiritual health and healing.

- Magnetic therapy: A modality using magnets to generate controlled magnetic fields. Magnetic therapy is used to improve the functioning of bodily systems and facilitate healing.

- Reiki: Use of the hands and visualization by the Reiki practitioner to direct energy to affected areas of the client's body to facilitate healing and relaxation.

- Therapeutic touch: A technique for balancing energy flow in the body through human energy transfer.

The DNP as Integrative Practitioner: Unique Aspects of DNP Preparation

The question will be asked, What advantage is there to having DNP preparation for an advanced practice nurse specializing in integrative health? Any registered professional nurse who takes a course in holistic nursing at the post-RN level should be able to function competently and therapeutically as an integrative practitioner. What, then, does the DNP bring to integrative health? And what is the advantage to seeking DNP preparation for this role?

The AACN addresses the competencies of the doctorally prepared APN (AACN, 2006). The DNP, a practice-focused terminal degree, prepares the APN to serve as an expert in nursing practice. Compared with the PhD and DNS degrees, which are research-focused degrees, the DNP is unique in providing education in those components of advanced nursing practice essential to practice at the highest clinical level. The skills gained in the DNP course of study will not only prepare the nurse for clinical competence but also prepare him or her for establishing a successful practice or business.

As DNP programs proliferate in colleges and universities across the nation, and the world, certain states (e.g., Alabama and New York) are mandating that the curricula include a significant percentage of clinical content; indeed, some DNP programs (e.g., Columbia University, University of Wisconsin, University of Washington) include a clinical residency in the curriculum. Including clinical components in the DNP curriculum strengthens the DNP-prepared APN as a clinician. The University of Minnesota's Doctor of Nursing Practice Integrative Health and Healing area of concentration "prepares graduates with skills necessary for working with individuals, families, communities and health systems in developing holistic approaches to health promotion, disease prevention and chronic disease management, with a special emphasis on managing lifestyle changes and incorporating the use of complementary therapies" (University of Minnesota, n.d.). This program fully integrates the specialty courses relevant to integrative practice with those courses designed to meet the requirements of the AACN's Essentials competencies. These courses uniquely position the DNP graduate to succeed on many different fronts of integrative health.

DNP curricula are unique in other areas, in that they include coursework in the areas of business finance, health policy, human resource management, change, and leadership (Rush University, n.d.). The advanced practice nurse engaging in integrative health practice benefits from understanding past, current, and future trends in health policy. Healthcare legislation and regulation undergo frequent change, affecting the right to practice, scope of practice, definition of specialty, and related rights, privileges, and responsibilities. Legislation and regulation are influenced by many factors, including political, socioeconomic, and cultural. Advanced coursework in public policy provides the DNP with a firm foundation to clearly view the nuanced political landscape.

The number of APNs owning or directing solo practices remains small, due in part to the expensive and adventurous nature of being an entrepreneur. Because of the lack of research on APNs in private practice, it is not possible to quantify with any specificity the number of APNs who own their own businesses. However, one survey on nurse practitioners indicated that 3% are engaged in private practice (Rollet & Lebo, 2007). Given the nature and challenges of integrative health care (e.g., that health insurers do not consistently pay for holistic health services, that clients may be more inclined to pay for these services with disposable income, and that educated healthcare consumers are becoming increasingly interested in modalities that are more wellness oriented), it is reasonable to speculate that the numbers of APNs starting integrative health practices will increase. DNP programs provide the APN with education in health economics, financial management, budget creation and management, human resources, practice management, and business models.

In the case of the DNP as integrative or holistic practitioner, earning the DNP provides advantages in the areas of direct delivery of health care, practice development and management, and interpreting and synthesizing research. Although some will posit that enough is learned at the baccalaureate or master's levels, the competencies needed to provide health care to increasingly complex populations while managing a practice autonomously, using research for evidence-based care, and advocating for patient access to all relevant forms of interventions that promote wellness are all presented comprehensively in a DNP curriculum and provide the APN with the most optimal level of preparation for practice.

DISCUSSION QUESTIONS

1. After reflecting on all the possible roles of the doctor of nursing practice graduate can assume, where do you see your career in 5 years? In 10 years?

2. Select one of the *Healthy People 2020* healthcare goals and propose a community intervention program to meet a minimum of one of the objectives for that goal.

3. Give examples of barriers to and factors facilitating advanced practice nurses as entrepreneurs. How can the nurse entrepreneur influence healthcare outcomes?

4. Can an educator with a doctor of nursing practice degree influence curriculum development in nursing education? Give examples.

REFERENCES

Abrams, S. E. (2008). The best of public health nursing, circa 1941. *Public Health Nursing, 25*(3), 285–291.

Acharya, D., & Shrivastava, A. (2008). *Indigenous herbal medicines: Tribal formulations and traditional herbal practices.* Jaipur, India: Aavishkar Publishers.

Acorn, S., Lamarche, K., & Edwards, M. (2009). Practice doctorates in nursing: Developing nursing leaders. *Nursing Leadership, 22*(2), 85–91.

Alabama Commission on Higher Education, Division of Instruction, Planning, and Special Services. (2006). The doctor of nursing practice: A background paper for Alabama. Retrieved from http://www.ache.state.al.us/Reports/Nursing%20Study%2015%20June %202007%20Revision.pdf

American Academy of Home Care Physicians. (2009). The Independent at Home Act (S. 1131, H.R. 2560). Retrieved from www.aahcp.org/iahsummary.pdf

American Association of Colleges of Nursing. (2005). Frequently asked questions concerning the AACN position statement on the practice doctorate in nursing. Retrieved from http://www.aacn.nche.edu/DNP/AboutDNP.htm

American Association of Colleges of Nursing. (2006). The essentials of doctoral education for advanced nursing practice. Retrieved from http://www.aacn.nche.edu/DNP/pdf/Essentials.pdf

American Association of Colleges of Nursing. (2008). Doctor of nursing talking points. Retrieved from http://www.aacn.nche.edu/DNP/talkingpoints.htm

American Holistic Nurses Association. (n.d.). Who we are. Retrieved from http://www.ahna.org/Aboutus/tabid/1158/Default.aspx

American Nurses Association. (2007). *Public health nursing: Scope and standards of practice.* Silver Spring, MD: Author.

Americans continue to use complementary, alternative medicine. (2009, February 20). NIH Record, 61(4). Retrieved from http://nihrecord.od.nih.gov/newsletters/2009/02_20_2009/story8.htm

Association of Community Health Nursing Educators. (n.d.). The Quad Council of Public Health Nursing Organizations. Retrieved from http://www.achne.org/i4a/pages/index.cfm?pageid=3292

Bishop, M. (2006, February 25). The rise of the social entrepreneur. *The Economist, 76*(8466), 12.

Boyer, E. L. (1990). *Scholarship reconsidered: Priorities of the professoriate.* Princeton, NJ: Carnegie Foundation for the Advancement of Teaching.

Boyer, E. L. (1996). The scholarship of engagement. *Journal of Public Service and Outreach, 1*(1), 11-20.

Brown, M. A., Draye, M. A., Zimmer, P. A., Magyary, D., Woods, S. L., Whitney, J., et al. (2006). Developing a practice doctorate in nursing: University of Washington perspectives and experience. *Nursing Outlook, 54*(3), 130-138.

Brown-Benedict, D. (2008). The doctor of nursing practice degree: Lessons from the history of the professional doctorate in other health disciplines. *Journal of Nursing Education, 47*(10), 448-457.

Bullock, P. (2009). Practice snapshot: New genesis center. *Advance for Nurse Practitioners.* Retrieved from http://nurse-practitioners.advanceweb.com/Article/Practice-Snapshot-New-Genesis-Center.aspx

Caffrey, R. A. (2005). The rural community care gerontological nurse entrepreneur: Role development strategies. *Journal of Gerontological Nursing, 31,* 11-16.

Case Western Reserve University, Frances Payne Bolton School of Nursing. (2009). *Post-master's DNP* [Brochure]. Cleveland, OH: Author.

Castledine, G. (2006). The business habits of highly effective nurses. *British Journal of Nursing, 15*(20), 1143.

Center for Spirituality and Healing. (2008). About us. Retrieved from http://www.csh.umn.edu/about/home.html

Cohen, E., & Cesta, T. (2001). *Nursing case management* (3rd ed.). St. Louis, MO: Elsevier/Mosby.

Deming, W. (1986). *Out of the crisis.* Cambridge, MA: Massachusetts Institute of Technology, Center for Advanced Engineering Study.

Department of the Army. (1968). *FM 22-100.* Washington, DC: U.S. Government Printing Office.

Department of the Army. (2004). *The U.S. Army leadership field manual.* Washington, DC: U.S. Government Printing Office.

Dilts, R., Grinder, J., Delozier, J., & Bandler, R. (1980). *Neuro-linguistic programming. Volume I: The study of the structure of subjective experience.* Cupertino, CA: Meta Publications.

Disease Management Association of America. (2009). DMAA definition of disease management. Retrieved from http://www.dmaa.org/dm_definition.asp

Dossey, B. (1997). *Core curriculum for holistic nursing.* New York: Aspen.

Dossey, B., & Keegan, L. (2008). *Holistic nursing: A handbook for practice* (5th ed.). Sudbury, MA: Jones and Bartlett.

Dossey, B., Selanders, L., Beck, D. M., & Attewell, A. (2005). *Florence Nightingale today: Healing, leadership, global action.* Washington, DC: Nursesbooks.org.

Douglas, W. (2005). Nursing considers clinical practice doctorate degree. *Texas Nurse, 79*(8), 6-14.

Draye, M. A., Acker, M., Zimmer, P. A. (2006). The practice doctorate in nursing: Approaches to transform nurse practitioner education and practice. *Nursing Outlook, 54*(3), 123-129.

Drucker, P. (1954). *The practice of management.* New York: Harper & Row.

Drucker, P. F. (1985). *Innovation and entrepreneurship: Practice and principles.* New York: Harper & Row.

Elango, B., Hunter, G. L., & Winchell, M. (2007). Barriers to nurse entrepreneurship: A study of the process model of entrepreneurship. *Journal of the American Academy of Nurse Practitioners, 19,* 198-204.

Ellis, L. (2007). Academics' perceptions of the professional or clinical doctorate: Findings of a national survey. *Journal of Clinical Nursing, 16,* 2272-2279.

Fain, J. A., Asselin, M., & McCurry, M. (2008). The DNP. . . why now? *Nursing Management, 39*(7), 34-37.

Falk, G. (2006). Biography of Lillian Wald. Retrieved from http://jbuff.com/c042706.htm

Faugier, J. (2005). Developing a new generation of nurse entrepreneurs. *Nursing Standard, 19*(30), 49-53.

Fitzpatrick, J. J. (2003). The case for the clinical doctorate in nursing. *Reflections on Nursing Leadership, 29*(1), 8-9, 37.

Fitzpatrick, J., & Wallace, M. (2009). *The doctor of nursing practice and clinical nurse leader: Essentials of program development and implementation for clinical practice.* New York: Springer.

Ford, J. (2009). DNP coming into focus. *Advance for Nurse Practitioners*. Retrieved from http://nurse-practitioners.advanceweb.com/Editorial/Content/Editorial.aspx?CC=191346

Green, A., Starck, P., & Long, K. (2006). Doctorate of nursing practice (DNP): Talking points prepared for/responses to frequently asked questions. Texas DNP Roadmap Taskforce. Retrieved from http://tobgne.org/download/DNP_Texas_Talking_Points.pdf

Hardy, E. (2008). Practice snapshot: Holistic Family Healthcare. *Advance for Nurse Practitioners, 16*(6), 16.

Hardy, E., DeBasio, N., Warmbrodt, L., Gartland, M., Bassett, W., & Tansey, M. (2004). Collaborative graduate education: Executive nurse practice and health care leadership. *Nursing Leadership Forum, 8*(4), 123–127.

Heller, B. R., Oros, M. T., & Durney-Crowley, J. (n.d.). The future of nursing education: Ten trends to watch. Retrieved from http://www.nln.org/nln journal/infotrends.htm

Helmstadter, C. (2002). Early nursing reform in nineteenth-century London: A doctor-driven phenomenon. *Medical History, 46*(3), 325–350.

Hirschman, D., & Morby, L. (2006). A study of the safety of continued anticoagulation for cataract surgery patients. *Nursing Forum, 41*(1), 30–37.

Hoffmann, R. L. (2005). The evolution of hospice in America: Nursing's role in the movement. *Journal of Gerontological Nursing, 31*(7), 26–34, 53–54.

Holland, B. (2005). Community engagement and community-engaged scholarship: Clarifying our meanings when using these terms. Teleconference call to the Community-Engaged Scholarship for Health Collaborative.

Houser, B. P., & Player, K. N. (2004). Loretta Ford. In *Pivotal moments in nursing: Leaders who changed the path of a profession.* Indianapolis, IN: Sigma Theta Tau International.

Howkins, E., & Thornton, C. (2003). Liberating the talents: Whose talents, and for what purpose? *Journal of Nursing Management, 11*(4), 219.

Institute of Medicine. (2003). *Crossing the quality chasm: A new health system for the 21st century.* Washington, DC: National Academies Press.

Jolley, J. (2007). Choose your doctorate. *Clinical Nursing, 16*(2), 225–233.

Kacel, B. (2008). NP practice snapshot: New Image Body and Wellness Clinic. *Advance for Nurse Practitioners*. Retrieved from http://nurse-practitioners.advanceweb.com/Editorial/Content/Editorial.aspx?CC=115800

Keyes, L. (2009). Business opportunities for nurses. *Nurse Entrepreneur Network*. Retrieved from: http://www.nurse-entrepreneur-network.com/public/281.cfm?sd=49

Kowal, N. (1988). Specialty practice entrepreneur: The advanced practice nurse. *Nursing Economics, 16*(5), 277–278.

Lieberman, J. (1993). *Light: Medicine of the future—how we can use it to heal ourselves now.* Santa Fe, NM: Inner Traditions/Bear & Company.

Long, K. A. (2006). Background information: The DNP in Florida. Retrieved from http://www.flbog.org/documents_meetings/0043_0135_1157_16%20- %20Strat%20Plan%20Background%20Info—%20DNP%20bullet%20list-03-23-06.doc

Mann, J. D. (2009, January–February). Practicing presence through Breema. *Spirituality and Health,* 1–2.

Marion, L., Viens, D., O'Sullivan, A., Crabtree, K., Fontana, & Price, M. (2003). The practice doctorate in nursing: Future or fringe? *Topics in Advanced Practice Nursing eJournal, 3*(2).

Marra, J., Jr. (2008). NP practice snapshot: Urgent Care Center. *Advance for Nurse Practitioners*. Retrieved from http://nurse-practitioners.advanceweb.com/Editorial/Content/Editorial.aspx?CC=122664

Merriam-Webster Online Dictionary. (2009). Retrieved from http://www.merriam-webster.com

Miller, J. (2008). The doctor of nursing practice: Recognizing a need or graying the line between doctor and nurse? *Medscape Journal of Medicine, 10*(11), 253.

Moen, G. (2009). Practice snapshot: Eagan Child and Family Care. *Advance for Nurse Practitioners*. Retrieved from http://nurse-practitioners.advanceweb.com/Editorial/Content/Editorial.aspx?CC=194750

National Center for Complementary and Alternative Medicine. (2007). What is CAM? Retrieved from http://nccam.nih.gov/health/whatiscam/overview.htm

National Center for Complementary and Alternative Medicine. (2009). Homeopathy: An introduction. Retrieved from http://nccam.nih.gov/health/homeopathy

National League for Nursing. (2007). Reflection and dialogue: Doctor of nursing practice. Retrieved from http://www.nln.org/aboutnln/reflection_dialogue/refl_dial_1.htm

National Organization of Nurse Practitioner Faculties. (2005). The practice doctorate resource center: Recommendations. Retrieved from http://www

.nonpf.com/NONPF2005/PracticeDoctorate
ResourceCenter/PDrecommendations.htm

New York State Office of the Professions, State Education Department. (n.d.). License requirements for nurse practitioner. Retrieved from http://www.op.nysed.gov/np.htm

Osborne, K., & Dawley, K. (2005). Mary Breckenridge and the birth of the ACNM. *Journal of Midwifery and Women's Health, 50*(3), 257.

Otto, H. A., & Knight, J. W. (1979). *Dimensions in wholistic healing: New frontiers in the treatment of the whole person.* Chicago: Burnham.

Parry, M. S. (2006). Voices from the past: Dorothea Dix (1802–1887). *American Journal of Public Health, 96*(4), 622–624.

Partin, B. (2008). Update on the DNP degree. *Nurse Practice, 33*(3), 7.

Pennsylvania State Board of Nursing. (2005). Draft language for CRNP educational programs regulation. Regulations of the State Board of Nursing, 49 PA Code 21.1–21.607.

Pronsati, M. (2008). Some kinda miracle stuff. *Advance for Nurse Practitioners, 16*(12), 10.

Rector, C. (2010). The journey begins: Introduction to community health nursing. In J. Allender, C. Rector, & K. Warner (Eds.), *Community health nursing: Promoting and protecting the public's health* (7th ed., pp. 1–4). Philadelphia: Wolters Kluwer Health/Lippincott Williams & Wilkins.

Riley, E. (2009, March). New degree of doctor. *AZ Nurse Update.* Retrieved from http://view.digipage.net/?userpath=00000001/00005932/00037812/&page=12

Rollet, J. (2008). Restoring dignity through dryness. *Advance for Nurse Practitioners.* Retrieved from http://nurse-practitioners.advanceweb.com/Editorial/Content/Editorial.aspx?CC=190253

Rollet, J., & Lebo, S. (2007). 2007 salary survey results: A decade of growth. Results of the 2007 national salary and workplace survey of nurse practitioners. *Advance for Nurse Practitioners.* Retrieved from http://nurse-practitioners.advanceweb.com/Article/2007-Salary-Survey-Results-A-Decade-of-Growth-3.aspx

Rollet, J., & Lebo, S. (2008). A decade of growth: Salaries increase as profession matures. *Advance for Nurse Practitioners.* Retrieved from http://nurse-practitioners.advanceweb.com/Article/A-Decade-of-Growth.aspx

Rush University. (n.d.). Doctor of nursing practice degree program of study (beginning Winter 2009 for new matriculants). Retrieved from http://www.rushu.rush.edu/servlet/Satellite?MetaAttr Name=meta_university&ParentId=1221491470501&ParentType=RushUnivLevel3Page&c=content_block&cid=1211209856164&level1-p=3&level1-pp=1221491470093&level1-ppp=1221491470093&pagename=Rush%2Fcontent_block%2FContentBlockDetail

Schiff, L. (2009). Practice snapshot: Advanced Practice Solutions. *Advance for Nurse Practitioners.* Retrieved from http://nurse-practitioners.advanceweb.com/Editorial/Content/Editorial.aspx?CC=196584

Scott, E. S., & Craig, J. B. (2008). Analysis of ANA's draft scope and standards of practice for nurse administrators. *Journal of Nursing Administration, 38*(9), 361–365.

Sgro, K. (2007). Reducing acute care hospitalization and emergent care use through home health disease management: One agency's success story. *Home Healthcare Nurse, 25*(10), 622–627.

Shirey, M. R. (2008). Endurance and inspiration for the entrepreneur. *Clinical Nurse Specialist, 22*(1), 9–11.

Smith, E. (2009). NP practice snapshot: Senior Moment Consulting. *Advance for Nurse Practitioners.* Retrieved from http://nurse-practitioners.advanceweb.com/Editorial/Content/Editorial.aspx?CC=193894

Sperhac, A., & Clinton, P. (2004). Facts and fallacies: The practice doctorate. *Journal of Pediatric Health, 18*(6), 292–296.

Stanhope, M., & Lancaster, J. (2006). *Foundations of nursing in the community: Community-oriented practice* (2nd ed.). St. Louis, MO: Mosby.

Stein, J. V. (2008). Becoming a doctor of nursing practice: My story. *Nursing Forum, 43*(1), 38–42.

Trivieri, L., & Anderson, J. W. (2002). *Alternative medicine: The definitive guide.* Berkeley, CA: Celestial Arts.

University of California, San Francisco, School of Nursing. (2009). Leadership, nursing, and health systems (administration). Retrieved from http://nurseweb.ucsf.edu/www/spec-adm.htm

University of Colorado at Denver, Health Sciences Center. (2008). *School of Nursing* [Brochure].

University of Kentucky, School of Nursing. (2009). Post M.S.N.–doctor of nursing practice (D.N.P. degree). Retrieved from http://www.mc.uky.edu/Nursing/academic/dnp/default.html

University of Minnesota, Doctor of Nursing Practice Program. (n.d.). Integrative health and healing. Retrieved from http://www.nursing.unm.edu/DNP/ProspectiveStudent/Specialties/Integrative_Health_and_Healing/home.html

University of Tennessee. (2006). Doctor of nursing practice. Retrieved from http://www.utmem.edu/nursing/academic%20programs/DNP/index.php

U.S. Census Bureau. (1990). State population projections (based on 1990 Census released 1996). *U.S. Population Projections.* Retrieved from http://www.census.gov/population/www/projections/stproj1996.html

U.S. Department of Health and Human Services, Health Resources and Services Administration. (2004). The registered nurse population: Findings from the March 2004 national sample survey of registered nurses. Retrieved from ftp://ftp.hrsa.gov/bhpr/workforce/0306rnss.pdf

U.S. Department of Health and Human Services. (2008). Phase I report: Recommendations for the framework and format of *Healthy People 2020.* Retrieved from http://www.healthypeople.gov/hp2020/advisory/PhaseI/summary.htm

Veilleux, C. (2009). NP practice snapshot: Espanola Advanced Center for Healing. *Advance for Nurse Practitioners.* Retrieved from http://nurse-practitioners.advanceweb.com/Editorial/Content/Editorial.aspx?CC=19363

Waddock, S. A., & Post, J. E. (1991). Social entrepreneurs and catalytic change. *Public Administration Review, 51*(5), 393–401.

Wall, B. M., Novak, J. C., & Wilkerson, S. A. (2005). Doctor of nursing practice program development: Reengineering health care. *Journal of Nursing Education, 44*(9), 396–403.

Walton, M. (1986). *The Deming management method.* New York: Perigee.

Walton, M. (1991). *Deming management at work.* New York: Perigee.

West, W. D. (2008, March). Do you have to be a true entrepreneur to succeed? *Optometric Management.* Retrieved from http://www.optometric.com/article.aspx?article=101462

Williams, S. (2006, September 11). Game of strategy. Retrieved from http://news.nurse.com/apps/pbcs.dll/article?AID=2006609110343

Wilson, C. K. (1998). Mentoring the entrepreneur. *Nursing Administration Quarterly, 22*(2), 1–12.

Wilson, A., Averis, A., & Walsh, K. (2003). The influences on and experiences of becoming nurse entrepreneurs: A Delphi study. *International Journal of Nursing Practice, 9,* 236–245.

Yale Nursing. (2009). DNP: Doctor of nursing practice degree. Retrieved from http://nursing.yale.edu/Academics/DNP_FAQs.html

PART 2

Healthcare Delivery and Health Policy for Advanced Practice: Core Knowledge

For the advanced practice nurse, understanding the system in which one works is an essential foundation for successful practice. In acting simultaneously as an advocate for the consumer and as a provider and/or manager of care, nurses in advanced practice need basic knowledge of the following topics:

- The structure, operations, scope, and characteristics of the healthcare delivery system

- The means by which the healthcare delivery system is financed, including national healthcare expenditures and sources of payment

- The trends that will influence the future of the system

- Ways in which nurses can influence healthcare policy and, conversely, policy influences practice

The information provided in Part 2 can help the reader move beyond the perspective of the nursing profession to a broader understanding of the organization in which one works, relationships with other members of the multidisciplinary team, and the forces that affect current and future practices. The ultimate goal is to prepare the reader as an advanced practice nurse to provide high-quality, cost-effective care; to participate in the design and implementation of programs in a variety of systems; and to assume leadership roles.

In reviewing the information provided in this part, it is helpful to think of the issues as constituting a triad of cost, quality, and access. Any change to correct the issue in one component will have a significant and possibly negative effect on the other two. For instance, if the United States implemented policies and practices so that every citizen would be insured, costs would increase dramatically. This change could, in turn, have a negative effect on quality if this new policy were not funded correctly.

The chapters selected for Part 2 were selected from several books. Chapters 6, 7, and 8 are the first three chapters in *Delivering Health Care in America: A Systems Approach,* by Shi and Singh. These chapters provide a foundation for understanding the healthcare delivery system. In Chapter 6, Shi and Singh paint a realistic—albeit gloomy—portrait of a complex, massive healthcare "system" in the United States. Because of the diversity of stakeholders in the U.S. healthcare system, including multiple providers, multiple payers, and the government, they suggest revolutionary changes in health care will be difficult, if not impossible, to achieve in this country. In Chapter 7, the same authors discuss issues of beliefs, values, and health. Although much of the content is not new to nursing—whose theorists and writers have focused on health as a meta-paradigm for the profession for more than 60 years (see Part 4)—this chapter explores the concept of holistic health and values in depth from the perspective of policy and leadership. Chapter 8 goes back in time and discusses the historical developments that have shaped the U.S. healthcare delivery system. This knowledge provides the advanced practice nurse with an understanding of the current and future trends in health care and nursing.

Chapter 9, which was taken from the book *Health Care USA,* by Sultz and Young, was selected to provide greater depth of information about healthcare financing—in particular, data about the nation's healthcare expenditures and sources of payment. The data presented were reported by the Center for Medicaid and Medicare, which collects, analyzes, and disseminates this information annually. Besides the statistical data presented in multiple tables, summary information analyzes the current data and projections for the future. Additionally, the journal *Health Affairs* presents a summary of the data and analysis in the first quarter of each year. Both should be valuable resources for the present and future advanced practice nurse. In Chapter 10, Sullivan provides a practical foundational knowledge for managing financial resources, budgeting, and reducing healthcare expenditures.

Chapter 11 was selected to give an overview of the major concepts of the regulation of health professionals, with emphasis on the oversight of advanced practice nurses providing direct patient care. Understanding the process of licensure and credentialing and their effects on the practice of advanced practice nursing is fundamental to practicing as a competent practitioner. In this chapter, Loversidge reviews the historical roots of advanced practice nursing regulation at state and federal levels and provides the reader with the tools to navigate the regulatory process and become a confident spokesperson for issues critical to all advanced practice nurses.

In Chapter 12, Milstead provides a comprehensive definition of the various stages of healthcare policy formation and suggests roles that nursing should play in this arena. Readers are encouraged to gain an appreciation of how policy influences research, practice, and education. Emphasis on participating in professional nursing organizations provides a forum for building strong coalitions and gaining power in the political process.

CHAPTER 6

A Distinctive System of Healthcare Delivery

Leiyu Shi and Douglas A. Singh

CHAPTER OBJECTIVES

1. Understand the basic nature of the U.S. healthcare system.

2. Outline the four key functional components of a healthcare delivery system.

3. Discuss the primary characteristics of the U.S. healthcare system from a free market perspective.

4. Emphasize why it is important for healthcare managers to understand the intricacies of the healthcare delivery system.

5. Analyze healthcare systems in other countries.

6. Discuss the systems model as a framework for studying the health services system in the United States.

INTRODUCTION

The United States has a unique system of healthcare delivery that is unlike any other healthcare system in the world. Most developed countries have national health insurance programs run by the government and financed through general taxes. Almost all citizens in such countries are entitled to receive healthcare services, depending on the system's capacity to deliver needed services. Such is not yet the case in the United States, where not all Americans are automatically covered by health insurance.

The U.S. healthcare delivery system is really not a system in its true sense, even though it is called a system when reference is made to its various features, components, and services. Hence, it may be somewhat misleading to talk about the American healthcare delivery "system" because a true system does not exist (Wolinsky 1988). One main feature of the U.S. healthcare system is that it is fragmented because different people obtain health care through different means. The delivery system has continued to undergo periodic changes, mainly in response to concerns regarding cost, access, and quality.

Describing healthcare delivery in the United States can be a daunting task. To facilitate an understanding of the structural and conceptual basis for the delivery of health services, a systems framework is presented at the end of this chapter. Also, the mechanisms of health services delivery in the United States are collectively referred to as a system. The main objective of this chapter is to provide a broad understanding of how health care is delivered in the United States.

AN OVERVIEW OF THE SCOPE AND SIZE OF THE SYSTEM

Table 6-1 demonstrates the complexity of healthcare delivery in the United States. Many organizations and individuals are involved in health care, ranging from educational and research institutions, medical suppliers, insurers, payers, and claims processors to healthcare providers. Multitudes of providers are involved in the delivery of preventive, primary, subacute, acute, auxiliary, rehabilitative, and continuing care. An increasing number of managed care organizations (MCOs) and integrated networks now provide a continuum of care, covering many of the service components.

The U.S. healthcare delivery system is massive, with total employment in various health delivery settings exceeding 16 million people in 2009. This number included more than 822,000 professionally active doctors of medicine (MDs), 70,480 osteopathic physicians (DOs), and 2.5 million active nurses (U.S. Census Bureau 2011). The vast majority of healthcare and health services professionals (5.8 million) work in ambulatory health service settings, such as the offices of physicians, dentists, and other health practitioners, medical and diagnostic laboratories, and home healthcare service locations (U.S. Census Bureau 2011). A smaller number are employed by hospitals (4.7 million) and nursing and residential care facilities (3.1 million) (U.S. Census Bureau 2011). The vast array of healthcare institutions in the United States includes 5,815 hospitals, 15,730 nursing homes, and 13,513 substance abuse treatment facilities (U.S. Census Bureau 2011). In 2009, 1,131 federally qualified health center grantees, with 123,012 full-time employees, provided preventive and primary care services to approximately 18.8 million people living in medically underserved, rural and urban areas (HRSA 2011). Various types of healthcare professionals are trained in 159 medical and osteopathic schools, 61 dental schools, more than 100 schools of pharmacy, and more than 1,500 nursing programs located throughout the country (U.S. Bureau of Labor Statistics 2011). In 2008, there were 200.9 million Americans with private health insurance coverage, 43 million Medicare beneficiaries, and 42.6 million Medicaid recipients, but 46.3 million people (15.4%) remained without any health insurance (U.S. Census Bureau 2011). Multitudes of government agencies are involved with the financing of health care, medical and health services research, and regulatory oversight of the various aspects of the healthcare delivery system.

A BROAD DESCRIPTION OF THE SYSTEM

U.S. health care does not function as a rational and integrated network of components designed to work together coherently. To the contrary, it is a kaleidoscope of financing, insurance, delivery, and payment mechanisms that remain loosely coordinated. Each of these basic functional components—financing, insurance, delivery, and payment—represents an amalgam of public (government) and private sources. Thus, government-run programs

TABLE 6-1	The Complexity of Healthcare Delivery

Education/ Research	Suppliers	Insurers	Providers	Payers
Medical schools	Pharmaceutical companies	Managed care plans	*Preventive Care* Health departments	Blue Cross/ Blue Shield plans
Dental schools				
Nursing programs	Multipurpose suppliers	Blue Cross/ Blue Shield plans	*Primary Care* Physician offices	Commercial insurers
Physician assistant programs	Biotechnology companies	Commercial insurers	Community health centers	Employers
Nurse practitioner programs		Self-insured employers	Dentists	Third-party administrators
Physical therapy, occupational therapy, speech therapy programs		Medicare	Nonphysician providers	State agencies
		Medicaid	*Subacute Care* Subacute care facilities	
Research organizations		VA Tricare	Ambulatory surgery centers	
Private foundations			*Acute Care* Hospitals	
U.S. Public Health Service (AHRQ, ATSDR, CDC, FDA, HRSA, IHS, NIH, SAMHSA)			*Auxiliary Services* Pharmacists Diagnostic clinics X-ray units	
Professional associations			Suppliers of medical equipment	
Trade associations			*Rehabilitative Services* Home health agencies Rehabilitation centers Skilled nursing facilities	
			Continuing Care Nursing homes	
			End-of-Life Care Hospices	
			Integrated Managed care organizations Integrated networks	

finance and insure health care for select groups of people who meet each program's prescribed criteria for eligibility. To a lesser degree, government programs also deliver certain healthcare services directly to recipients, such as veterans, military personnel, and the uninsured, who may depend on city and county hospitals or limited services offered by public health clinics. However, the financing, insurance, payment, and delivery functions are largely in private hands.

The market-oriented economy in the United States attracts a variety of private entrepreneurs driven by the pursuit of profits obtained by carrying out the key functions of healthcare delivery. Employers purchase health insurance for their employees through private sources, and employees receive healthcare services delivered by the private sector. The government finances public insurance through Medicare, Medicaid, and the Children's Health Insurance Program (CHIP) for a significant portion of the very low-income, elderly, disabled, and pediatric populations. However, insurance arrangements for many publicly insured people are made through private entities, such as health maintenance organizations (HMOs), and healthcare services are rendered by private physicians and hospitals. The blend of public and private involvement in the delivery of health care has resulted in the following outcomes:

- A multiplicity of financial arrangements that enable individuals to pay for healthcare services
- Numerous insurance agencies or MCOs that employ varied mechanisms for insuring against risk
- Multiple payers that make their own determinations regarding how much to pay for each type of service
- A large array of settings where medical services are delivered
- Numerous consulting firms offering expertise in planning, cost containment, quality, and restructuring of resources

There is little standardization in a system that is functionally fragmented, and the various system components fit together only loosely. Such a system is not subject to overall planning, direction, and coordination from a central agency, such as the government. Duplication, overlap, inadequacy, inconsistency, and waste exist, leading to complexity and inefficiency, due to the missing dimension of system-wide planning, direction, and coordination. The system does not lend itself to standard budgetary methods of cost control. Each individual and corporate entity within a predominantly private entrepreneurial system seeks to manipulate financial incentives to its own advantage, without regard to its impact on the system as a whole. Hence, cost containment remains an elusive goal. In short, the U.S. healthcare delivery system is like a behemoth or an economic megalith that is almost impossible for any single entity to manage or control. The U.S. economy is the largest in the world, and, compared to other nations, consumption of healthcare services in the United States represents a greater proportion of the country's total economic output. Although the system can be credited for delivering some of the best clinical care in the world, it falls short of delivering equitable services to every American.

An acceptable healthcare delivery system should have two primary objectives:

1. It must enable all citizens to obtain healthcare services when needed,
2. The services must be cost-effective and meet certain established standards of quality.

On one hand, the U.S. healthcare delivery system falls short of both these ideals. On the other hand, certain features of U.S. health care are the envy of the world. The United States leads the world in the latest and the best in medical technology, training, and research. It offers some of the most sophisticated institutions, products, and processes of healthcare delivery. These achievements are indeed admirable, but much more remains unaccomplished.

BASIC COMPONENTS OF A HEALTH SERVICES DELIVERY SYSTEM

Figure 6-1 illustrates that a healthcare delivery system incorporates four functional components—financing, insurance, delivery, and payment—necessary for the delivery of health services. The four functional components make up the *quad-function model*. Healthcare delivery systems differ depending on the arrangement of these components. The four functions generally overlap, but the degree of overlap varies between a private and a government-run system and between a traditional health insurance and a

managed care-based system. In a government-run system, the functions are more closely integrated and may be indistinguishable. Managed care arrangements also integrate the four functions to varying degrees.

Financing

Financing is necessary to obtain health insurance or to pay for healthcare services. For most privately insured Americans, health insurance is employer based; that is, their employers finance health care as a fringe benefit. A dependent spouse or children may also be covered by

FIGURE 6-1   Basic Healthcare Delivery Functions

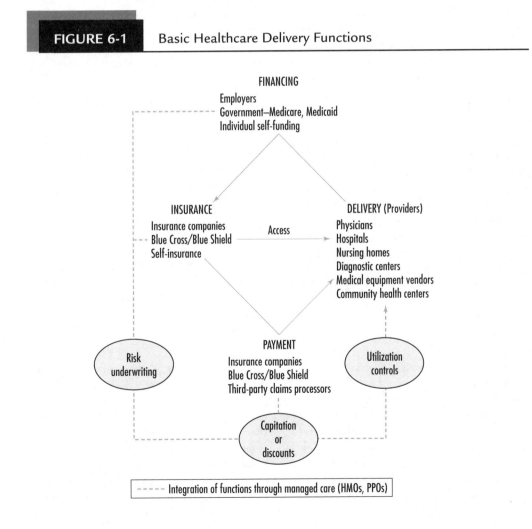

the working spouse's or working parent's employer. Most employers purchase health insurance for their employees through an MCO or an insurance company selected by the employer. Small employers may or may not be in a position to afford health insurance coverage for their employees.

Insurance

Insurance protects the insured against catastrophic risks when expensive healthcare services are needed. The insurance function also determines the package of health services the insured individual is entitled to receive. It specifies how and where healthcare services may be received. The MCO or insurance company also functions as a claims processor and manages the disbursement of funds to the healthcare providers.

Delivery

The term *delivery* refers to the provision of healthcare services by various providers. The term *provider* refers to any entity that delivers healthcare services and can either independently bill for those services or is tax supported. Common examples of providers include physicians, dentists, optometrists, and therapists in private practices, hospitals, and diagnostic and imaging clinics, and suppliers of medical equipment (e.g., wheelchairs, walkers, ostomy supplies, oxygen). With few exceptions, most providers render services to people who have health insurance.

Payment

The payment function deals with *reimbursement* to providers for services delivered. The insurer determines how much is paid for a certain service. Funds for actual disbursement come from the premiums paid to the MCO or insurance company. The patient is usually required, at the time of service, to pay a small out-of-pocket amount, such as $25 or $30, to see a physician. The remainder is covered by the MCO or insurance company. In government insurance plans, such as Medicare and Medicaid, tax revenues are used to pay providers.

UNINSURED AMERICANS

The United States has a significant number of *uninsured*—those persons without private or public health insurance coverage. A March 2009 report from Families USA found that 86.7 million Americans younger than the age of 65 (1 in every 3) were without health insurance for some period of time between 2008 and 2009 (Families USA 2009).

Given that the United States has an employer-based financing system, it is not difficult to see why the unemployed generally have no health insurance. However, even some employed individuals might not have health insurance coverage for two main reasons:

- In most states, employers are not mandated to offer health insurance to their employees; therefore, some employers, due to economic constraints, do not offer it. Some small businesses simply cannot get group insurance at affordable rates and, therefore, are not able to offer health insurance as a benefit to their employees.

- In many work settings, participation in health insurance programs is voluntary and does not require employees to join. Some employees choose not to sign up, mainly because they cannot afford the cost of health insurance premiums. Employers rarely pay 100% of the insurance premium; most require their employees to pay a portion of the cost, called *premium cost sharing*.

Employees who do not have health insurance offered by their employers or those who are self-employed have to obtain health insurance on their own. Individual rates are typically higher than group rates available to employers, and, in some instances, health insurance is unavailable when adverse health conditions are present.

In the United States, working people earning low wages are the most disenfranchised because most are not eligible for public benefits and cannot afford premium cost sharing. The U.S. government finances health benefits for certain special populations, including government employees, the elderly (people age 65 and older), people with disabilities, some people with very low incomes, and children from low-income families. The program for the elderly and certain disabled individuals is called *Medicare*. The program for the indigent, jointly administered by the federal government and state governments, is named *Medicaid*. The program for children from low-income families, another federal/state partnership, is called the Children's Health Insurance Program (CHIP). For such public programs, the government may function as both financier and insurer, or the insurance function may be carved out to an HMO. Private providers, with a few exceptions, render services to these special categories of people, and the government pays for the services, generally by establishing contractual arrangements with selected intermediaries for the actual disbursement of payments to the providers. Thus, even in government-financed programs, the four functions of financing, insurance, delivery, and payment can be quite distinct.

TRANSITION FROM TRADITIONAL INSURANCE TO MANAGED CARE

Under traditional insurance, the four basic health delivery functions have been fragmented; that is, the financiers, insurers, providers, and payers have often been different entities, with a few exceptions. During the 1990s, however, healthcare delivery in the United States underwent a fundamental change involving a tighter integration of the basic functions through managed care.

Previously, fragmentation of the functions meant a lack of control over utilization and payments. The quantity of health care consumed refers to *utilization* of health services. Traditionally, determination of the utilization of health services and the price charged for each service has been left up to the insured individuals and their physicians. Due to rising healthcare costs, however, current delivery mechanisms have instituted some controls over both utilization and price.

Managed care is a system of healthcare delivery that (1) seeks to achieve efficiencies by integrating the four functions of healthcare delivery discussed earlier, (2) employs mechanisms to control (manage) utilization of medical services, and (3) determines the price at which the services are purchased and, consequently, how much the providers get paid. The primary financier is still the employer or the government, as the case may be. Instead of purchasing health insurance through a traditional insurance company, the employer contracts with an MCO, such as an HMO or a preferred provider organization (PPO), to offer a selected health plan to its employees. In this case, the MCO functions like an insurance company and promises to provide healthcare services contracted under the health plan to the enrollees of the plan. The term *enrollee* (member) refers to the individual covered under the plan. The contractual arrangement between the MCO and the enrollee—including the collective array of covered health services that the enrollee is entitled to—is referred to as the *health plan* (or "plan," for short). The health plan uses selected providers from whom the enrollees can choose to receive services.

PRIMARY CHARACTERISTICS OF THE U.S. HEALTHCARE SYSTEM

In any country, certain external influences shape the basic character of the health services delivery system. These forces consist of the political climate of a nation; economic development; technological progress; social and cultural values; physical environment; population characteristics, such as demographic and health trends; and global influences (Figure 6-2). The combined interaction of these environmental forces influences the course of healthcare delivery.

FIGURE 6-2   External Forces Affecting Healthcare Delivery

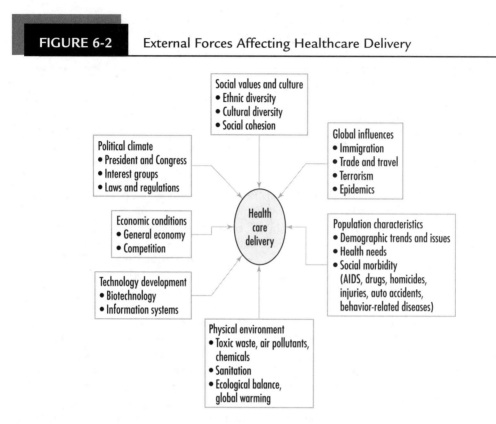

Ten basic characteristics differentiate the U.S. healthcare delivery system from that of other countries:

1. No central agency governs the system.
2. Access to healthcare services is selectively based on insurance coverage.
3. Health care is delivered under imperfect market conditions.
4. Third-party insurers act as intermediaries between the financing and delivery functions.
5. The existence of multiple payers makes the system cumbersome.
6. The balance of power among various players prevents any single entity from dominating the system.
7. Legal risks influence practice behavior of physicians.
8. Development of new technology creates an automatic demand for its use.
9. New service settings have evolved along a continuum.
10. Quality is no longer accepted as an unachievable goal in the delivery of health care.

No Central Agency

The U.S. healthcare system is not administratively controlled by a department or an agency of the government. Most other developed nations have national healthcare programs in which every citizen is entitled to receive a defined set of healthcare services. Availability of "free" services can break a system financially. To control costs, these systems use *global budgets* to determine total healthcare expenditures on a national scale and to allocate resources within budgetary limits. Availability of services, as well as payments to providers, is subject to such budgetary constraints. The government of these nations also controls the proliferation of healthcare services, especially costly medical technology. System-wide controls over the allocation of resources determine to what extent government-sponsored healthcare services are available to citizens. For instance, the availability of specialized services is restricted.

By contrast, the United States has mainly a private system of financing, as well as delivery. Private financing, predominantly through employers, accounts for approximately 54% of total healthcare expenditures; the government finances the remaining 46% (National Center for Health Statistics 2006). Private delivery of health care means that the majority of hospitals and physician clinics are private businesses, independent of the government. No central agency monitors total expenditures through global budgets or controls the availability and utilization of services. Nevertheless, the federal and state governments in the United States play an important role in healthcare delivery. They determine public-sector expenditures and reimbursement rates for services provided to Medicaid, CHIP, and Medicare beneficiaries. The government also formulates *standards of participation* through health policy and regulation, meaning providers must comply with the standards established by the government to be certified to provide services to Medicaid, CHIP, and Medicare beneficiaries. Certification standards are also regarded as minimum standards of quality in most sectors of the healthcare industry.

Partial Access

Access means the ability of an individual to obtain healthcare services when needed. In the United States, access is restricted to people who (1) have health insurance through their employers, (2) are covered under a government healthcare program, (3) can afford to buy insurance with their own private funds, or (4) are able to pay for services privately. Health insurance is the primary means for ensuring access.

Although the uninsured can access certain types of services, they often encounter barriers to obtaining needed health care. Federally supported community health centers, for example, provide physician services to anyone regardless of ability to pay. Such centers and other types of free clinics, however, are located only in certain geographic areas. Under U.S. law, hospital emergency departments are required to evaluate a patient's condition and render medically needed services for which the hospital does not receive any direct payments unless the patient is able to pay. Uninsured Americans, therefore, are able to obtain medical care for acute illness. On the hand, then, one can say that the United States does have a form of universal catastrophic health insurance even for the uninsured (Altman and Reinhardt 1996). On the other hand, the uninsured generally have to forego continual basic and routine care, commonly referred to as *primary care*.

Countries with national healthcare programs provide *universal coverage*; that is, health insurance is available to all citizens. However, access to services when needed may be restricted because no healthcare system has the capacity to deliver on demand every type of service the citizens may require. Hence, *universal access*—the ability of all citizens to obtain health care when needed—remains mostly a theoretical concept.

Experts generally believe that the inadequate access to basic and routine primary care services, particularly for the nation's vulnerable populations, is one of the main reasons why the United States, in spite of being the most economically advanced country, lags behind other developed nations in measures of population health, such as infant mortality and overall life expectancy. It remains to be seen whether the Patient Protection and Affordable Care Act of 2010 will be able to deliver on the promise of access to health care for all Americans by 2014.

Imperfect Market

In the United States, even though the delivery of services is largely in private hands, health care is only partially governed by free market forces. The delivery and consumption of health care in the United States does not quite pass the basic test of a *free market*, as subsequently described. Hence, the system is best described as a quasi-market or an imperfect market. Following are some key features characterizing free markets.

In a free market, multiple patients (buyers) and providers (sellers) act independently, and patients can choose to receive services from any provider. Providers do not collude to fix prices, nor are prices fixed by an external agency. Rather, prices are governed by the free and unencumbered interaction of the forces of supply and demand (Figure 6-3). *Demand*—that is, the quantity of health care purchased—in turn, is driven by the prices prevailing in the free market. Under free market conditions, the quantity demanded will increase as the price is lowered for a given product or service. Conversely, the quantity demanded will decrease as the price increases.

At casual observation, it may appear that multiple patients and providers do exist. Most

| **FIGURE 6-3** | Relationship Between Price, Supply, and Demand Under Free-Market Conditions |

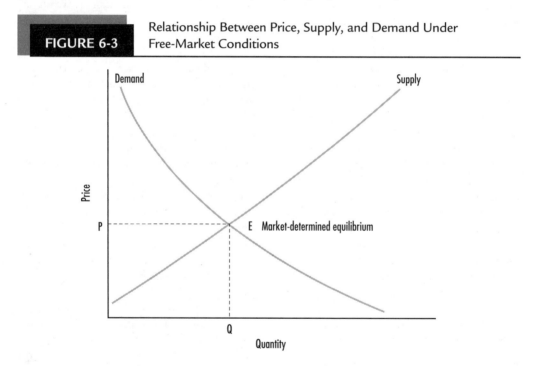

Under free market conditions, an inverse relationship exists between the quantity of medical services demanded and the price of medical services. That is, quantity demanded goes up when the prices go down, and vice versa. In contrast, there is a direct relationship between price and the quantity supplied by the providers of care. In other words, providers are willing to supply higher quantities at higher prices, and vice versa. In a free market, the quantity of medical care that patients are willing to purchase, the quantity of medical care that providers are willing to supply, and the price reach a state of equilibrium. This equilibrium is achieved without the interference of any nonmarket forces. It is important to keep in mind that these conditions exist only under free market conditions, which are not characteristic of the healthcare market.

patients, however, are now enrolled in either a private health plan or government-sponsored Medicare, Medicaid, or CHIP programs. These plans act as intermediaries for the patients, and the consolidation of patients into health plans has the effect of shifting the power from the patients to the administrators of the plans. The result is that the health plans, not the patients, are the real buyers in the healthcare services market. Private health plans, in many instances, offer their enrollees a limited choice of providers rather than an open choice.

Theoretically, prices are negotiated between the payers and providers. In practice, however, prices are determined by the payers, such as managed care, Medicare, and Medicaid. Because prices are set by agencies external to the market, they are not governed by the unencumbered forces of supply and demand.

For the healthcare market to be free, unrestrained competition must occur among providers based on price and quality. Generally speaking, free competition exists among healthcare providers in the United States. The consolidation of buying power in the hands of private health plans, however, has been forcing providers to form alliances and integrated delivery systems on the supply side. Integrated delivery systems are networks of health services organizations. In certain geographic sectors of the country, a single giant medical system has taken over as the sole provider of major healthcare services, thereby restricting competition. As the healthcare system continues to move in this direction, it appears that only in large metropolitan areas will there be more than one large integrated system competing to get the business of the health plans.

A free market requires that patients have information about the availability of various services. In reality, patients do not always have adequate information about services. Technology-driven medical care has become highly sophisticated. New diagnostic methods, intervention techniques, and drugs that are more effective fall in the domain of the professional physician. Also, medical interventions are commonly required in a state of urgency. Hence, patients have neither the skills nor the time and other resources to obtain necessary information when needed. Channeling all healthcare needs through a primary care provider is likely to reduce this information gap when the primary provider acts as a patient's advocate or agent. On the other hand, the Internet is becoming a prominent source of medical information. Pharmaceutical advertising is also having an impact on consumer expectations.

In a free market, patients have information on price and quality for each provider. The current system has other drawbacks that obstruct information-seeking efforts. Item-based pricing, instead of package pricing, is one such hurdle. Surgery is a good example to illustrate item-based pricing. Patients can generally obtain the fees the surgeon would charge for a particular operation. But the final bill, after the surgery has been performed, is likely to include charges for supplies, use of the hospital's facilities, and services performed by providers, such as anesthesiologists, nurse anesthetists, and pathologists. These providers, sometimes referred to as *phantom providers*, who function in an adjunct capacity, bill for their services separately. Item billing for such additional services, which sometimes cannot be anticipated, makes it extremely difficult to ascertain the total price before services have actually been received. Package pricing and capitated fees can help overcome these drawbacks, but they have made relatively little headway for pricing medical procedures. *Package pricing* refers to a bundled fee for a package of related services. In the surgery example, this would mean one all-inclusive price for the surgeon's fees, hospital facilities, supplies, diagnostics, pathology, anesthesia, and postsurgical follow-up. With *capitation*, all healthcare services are included under one set fee per covered individual.

In recent years, the quality of health care has received much emphasis. Performance ratings and report cards, however, furnish scant information on the quality of specific health-care providers.

In a free market, patients must directly bear the cost of services received. The purpose of insurance is to protect against the risk of unforeseen catastrophic events. Because the fundamental purpose of insurance is to meet major expenses when unlikely events occur, having insurance for basic and routine health care undermines the principle of insurance. When you buy home insurance to protect your property against the unlikely event of a fire, you do not anticipate the occurrence of a loss. The probability that you will suffer a loss by fire is very small. If a fire does occur and cause major damage, insurance will cover the loss, but the policy does not cover routine wear and tear on the house, such as chipped paint or a leaking faucet. Health insurance, however, generally covers basic and routine services that are predictable. Health insurance coverage for minor services, such as colds and coughs, earaches, and so forth, amounts to prepayment for such services. Health insurance has the effect of insulating patients from the full cost of health care. There is a *moral hazard* that, once enrollees have purchased health insurance, they will use healthcare services to a greater extent than if they were to bear the full cost of these services.

In a free market for health care, patients make decisions about the purchase of healthcare services. The main factors that limit patients' ability to make healthcare purchasing decisions have already been discussed. Even with the best intentions, the circumstances surrounding sickness and injury often prohibit comparative shopping based on price and quality. Further, such information is not easily available. At least two additional factors limit the ability of patients to make decisions.

First, decisions about the utilization of health care are often determined by need rather than by price-based demand. *Need* has been defined as the amount of medical care that medical experts believe a person should have to

remain or become healthy (Feldstein 1993). Need can also be based on self-evaluation of one's own health status.

Second, the delivery of health care can result in demand creation. This follows from self-assessed need, which, coupled with moral hazard, leads to greater utilization, creating an artificial demand because prices are not taken into consideration. Practitioners who have a financial interest in additional treatments also create artificial demand (Hemenway and Fallon 1985), commonly referred to as *provider-induced demand*, or supplier-induced demand. Functioning as patients' agents, physicians exert enormous influence on the demand for healthcare services (Altman and Wallack 1996). Research studies have pointed to physicians' behavior of creating demand to their own financial benefit (see, for instance, McGuire and Pauly 1991). Demand creation occurs when physicians prescribe medical care beyond what is clinically necessary. This can include practices such as making more frequent follow-up appointments than necessary, prescribing excessive medical tests, or performing unnecessary surgery (Santerre and Neun 1996).

Third-Party Insurers and Payers

Insurance often functions as the intermediary among those who finance, deliver, and receive health care. Delivery of health care is often viewed as a transaction between the patient and the provider, but insurance and payment functions introduce a *third party* into the transaction (Griffith 1995), the patient being the first party and the provider the second party. Apart from being the payer, the third-party insurer takes over most other administrative functions associated with the plan. The providers, as well as the enrollees, must comply with the policies set forth by the insurer in matters related to the delivery of health care and payment for services.

The intermediary role of insurance creates a wall of separation between the financing and delivery functions so that quality of care often remains a secondary concern. In normal economic markets, the consumer is armed with the power to influence demand based on the price and quality of goods and services. Another way to illustrate this concept is to say that, in a free market, consumers vote with their dollars for the best candidate among competing products, based on the price and quality of each product. The insurance intermediary does not have the incentive to be the patient's advocate on either price or quality. At best, employees can air their dissatisfactions with the plan to their employer, who has the power to discontinue the current plan and choose another company. In reality, however, employers may be reluctant to change plans if the current plan offers lower premiums compared to a new plan. National healthcare programs have even fewer incentives for promoting quality, although they can contain costs by artificially fixing prices.

Multiple Payers

A national healthcare system is sometimes referred to as a *single-payer system*, because there is one primary payer, the government. When delivering services, providers send the bill to an agency of the government, which subsequently sends payment to each provider.

By contrast, the United States has a multiplicity of health plans and insurance companies because each employer is free to determine the type of health plan it offers.

Each plan spells out the type of services the enrollee can receive. Some plans make an arbitrary determination of how much will be paid for a certain type of service. For Medicare and Medicaid recipients, the government has its own set of regulations and payment schedules.

Multiple payers often represent a billing and collection nightmare for the providers of services. Multiple payers make the system more cumbersome in several ways:

- It is extremely difficult for providers to keep tabs on the numerous health plans. For example, it is difficult to keep up with which services are covered under each plan and how much each plan will pay for those services.

- Providers must hire a battery of claims processors to bill for services and monitor receipt of payments. Billing practices are not always standardized, and each payer establishes its own format.

- Payments can be denied for not precisely following the requirements set by each payer.

- Denied claims necessitate rebilling.

- When only partial payment is received, some health plans may allow the provider to *balance bill* the patient for the amount the health plan did not pay. Other plans prohibit balance billing. Even when the balance billing option is available to the provider, it triggers a new cycle of billings and collection efforts.

- Providers must sometimes engage in lengthy collection efforts, including writing collection letters, turning delinquent accounts over to collection agencies, and finally writing off as bad debt amounts that cannot be collected.

- Government programs have complex regulations for determining whether payment is made for services actually delivered. Medicare, for example, requires that each provider maintain lengthy documentation on services provided. Medicaid is known for lengthy delays in paying providers.

It is generally believed that the United States spends far more on *administrative costs*—that is, the costs associated with billing, collections, bad debts, and maintaining medical records—than the national healthcare systems in other countries. However, estimates of cost differentials between the U.S. healthcare system and single-payer systems have been the subject of considerable controversy (Kahn et al. 2005).

Power Balancing

The U.S. health services system involves multiple players, not just multiple payers. The key players in the system have been physicians, administrators of health service institutions, insurance companies, large employers, and the government. Big business, labor, insurance companies, physicians, and hospitals make up the powerful and politically active special-interest groups represented before lawmakers by high-priced lobbyists. Each set of players has its own economic interests to protect. Physicians, for instance, want to maximize their incomes and have minimum interference with the way they practice medicine; institutional administrators seek to maximize reimbursement from private and public insurers. Insurance companies and MCOs are interested in maintaining their share of the healthcare insurance market; large employers want to minimize the costs they incur providing health insurance as a benefit to their employees. The government tries to maintain or enhance existing benefits for select population groups and simultaneously reduce the cost of providing these benefits.

The problem is that the self-interests of different players are often at odds. For example, providers seek to maximize government reimbursement for services delivered to Medicare, Medicaid, and CHIP beneficiaries, but the government wants to contain cost increases. Employers dislike rising health insurance premiums. Health plans, under pressure from the employers, may constrain fees for the providers, who resent any cuts in their incomes.

The fragmented self-interests of the various players produce countervailing forces within the system. One positive effect of these opposing forces is that they prevent any single entity from dominating the system. Conversely, each set of players has a large stake in health policy reforms. In an environment that is rife with motivations to protect conflicting self-interests, achieving comprehensive system-wide reforms has been next to impossible, and cost containment has remained a major challenge. Consequently, the approach to healthcare reform in the United States has been characterized as incremental or piece-meal, and the focus of reform initiatives has been confined to health insurance coverage and payment cuts to providers.

Legal Risks

The United States is a litigious society. Motivated by the prospects of enormous jury awards, Americans are quick to drag an alleged offender into a courtroom at the slightest perception of incurred harm. Private healthcare providers have become increasingly susceptible to litigation. By contrast, in national healthcare programs, governments are immune to lawsuits. Hence, in the United States, the risk of malpractice lawsuits is a real consideration in the practice of medicine. To protect themselves against the possibility of litigation, it is not uncommon for practitioners to engage in what is referred to as *defensive medicine* by prescribing additional diagnostic tests, scheduling return checkup visits, and maintaining copious documentation. Many of these additional efforts may be unnecessary; hence, they are costly and inefficient.

High Technology

The United States has been the hotbed of research and innovation in new medical technology. Growth in science and technology often creates demand for new services despite shrinking resources to finance sophisticated care. People generally equate high-tech care with high-quality care. They want "the latest and the best," especially when health insurance will pay for new treatments. Physicians and technicians want to try the latest gadgets. Hospitals compete on the basis of having the most modern equipment and facilities. Once capital investments are made, costs must be recouped through utilization. Legal risks for providers and health plans alike may also play a role in discouraging denial of new technology. Thus several factors promote the use of costly new technology once it is developed.

Continuum of Services

Medical care services are classified into three broad categories: curative (e.g., drugs, treatments, and surgeries), restorative (e.g., physical, occupational, and speech therapies), and preventive (e.g., prenatal care, mammograms, and immunizations). Healthcare service settings are no longer confined to the hospital and the physician's office, where many of the aforementioned services were once delivered. Several new settings, such as home health, subacute care units, and outpatient surgery centers, have emerged in response to the changing configuration of economic incentives. Table 6-2 depicts the continuum of healthcare services. The healthcare continuum in the United States remains lopsided, with a heavier emphasis on specialized services than on preventive services, primary care, and management of chronic conditions.

TABLE 6-2	The Continuum of Healthcare Services
Types of Health Services	**Delivery Settings**
Preventive care	Public health programs
	Community programs
	Personal lifestyles
	Primary care settings
Primary care	Physician's office or clinic
	Community health centers
	Self-care
	Alternative medicine
Specialized care	Specialist provider clinics
Chronic care	Primary care settings
	Specialist provider clinics
	Home health
	Long-term care facilities
	Self-care
	Alternative medicine
Long-term care	Long-term care facilities
	Home health
Subacute care	Special subacute units (hospitals, long-term care facilities)
	Home health
	Outpatient surgical centers
Acute care	Hospitals
Rehabilitative care	Rehabilitation departments (hospitals, long-term care facilities)
	Home health
	Outpatient rehabilitation centers

Quest for Quality

Even though the definition and measurement of quality in health care are not as clear cut as they are in other industries, the delivery sector of health care has come under increased pressure to develop quality standards and demonstrate compliance with those standards. There are higher expectations for improved health outcomes at the individual and broader community levels. The concept of continual quality improvement has also received much emphasis in managing healthcare institutions.

TRENDS AND DIRECTIONS

Since the 20th century, the U.S. healthcare delivery system has continued to undergo certain fundamental shifts in emphasis, summarized in Figure 6-4. Promotion of health at less cost has been the driving force behind these trends. An example of a shift in emphasis is the concept of health itself: The focus is changing from illness to wellness. Such a change requires new methods and settings for wellness promotion, although the treatment of illness continues to be the primary goal of the health services delivery system.

Significance for Healthcare Practitioners and Policymakers

An understanding of the healthcare delivery system is essential for managers and policymakers. In fact, an understanding of the intricacies within the health services system would be beneficial to all those who come in contact with the system. In their respective training programs, health professionals, such as physicians, nurses, technicians, therapists, dietitians, and pharmacists, as well as others, may understand their own individual roles but remain ignorant of the forces outside their profession that could significantly impact current and future practices. An understanding of the healthcare delivery system can attune health professionals to their relationship with the rest of the healthcare environment. It can help

them better understand changes and the potential impact of those changes on their own practice. Adaptation and relearning are strategies that can prepare health professionals to cope with an environment that will see ongoing change long into the future.

Policy decisions to address specific problems must also be made within the broader macro context because policies designed to bring about change in one healthcare sector can have wider repercussions, both desirable and undesirable, in other sectors of the system. Policy decisions and their implementation are often critical to the future direction of the healthcare delivery system. However, in a multifaceted system, future issues will be best addressed by a joint undertaking with a balanced representation of the key players in health services delivery: physicians, insurance companies, managed care organizations, employers, institutional representatives, and the government.

Significance for Healthcare Managers

An understanding of the healthcare system has specific implications for health services managers, who must understand the macro environment in which they make critical decisions in planning and strategic management, regardless of whether they manage a private institution or a public service agency. Such decisions and actions, eventually, affect the efficiency and quality of services delivered. The interactions among the system's key components and the implications of those interactions must be well understood because the operations of healthcare institutions are strongly influenced, either directly or indirectly, by the financing of health services, reimbursement rates, insurance mechanisms, delivery modes, new statutes and legal opinions, and government regulations.

The environment of healthcare delivery will continue to remain fluid and dynamic. The viability of delivery settings and, therefore, the success of healthcare managers often depend on how the managers react to the system dynamics. Timeliness of action is often a critical

| **FIGURE 6-4** | Trends and Directions in Healthcare Delivery |

◊ Illness ⟶ Wellness

◊ Acute care ⟶ Primary care

◊ Inpatient ⟶ Outpatient

◊ Individual health ⟶ Community well-being

◊ Fragmented care ⟶ Managed care

◊ Independent institutions ⟶ Integrated systems

◊ Service duplication ⟶ Continuum of services

factor that can make the difference between failure and success. Following are some more specific reasons why understanding the healthcare delivery system is indispensable for healthcare managers.

Positioning the Organization

Health services administrators need to understand their own organizational position within the macro environment of the system. Senior managers, such as chief executive officers, must constantly gauge the nature and impact of the fundamental shifts illustrated in Figure 6-4. Managers need to consider which changes in the current configuration of financing, insurance, payment, and delivery might affect their organization's long-term stability. Middle and first-line managers also need to understand their role in the current configuration, including how that role might change in the future. How should resources be realigned to effectively respond to those changes? For example, these managers need to evaluate whether certain functions in their departments will have to be eliminated, modified, or added. Will the changes involve further training? Which processes are likely to change and how? What do the managers need to do to maintain the integrity of their institution's mission, the good-

will of the patients they serve, and the quality of the services? Well-thought-out and appropriately planned change is likely to cause less turbulence for the providers, as well as the recipients of care.

Handling Threats and Opportunities

Changes in any of the functions of financing, insurance, payment, and delivery can present new threats or opportunities in the healthcare market. Healthcare managers are more effective if they proactively deal with any threats to their institution's profitability and viability. Managers need to find ways to transform certain threats into new opportunities.

Evaluating Implications

Managers are better able to evaluate the implications of health policy and new reform proposals when they understand the relevant issues and recognize how such issues link to the delivery of health services in the establishments they manage. With the expansion of health insurance coverage, more individuals will be brought into the healthcare system, creating further demand for health services. Planning and staffing for the right mix of healthcare workforce to meet this anticipated surge in demand is critical.

Planning

Senior managers are often responsible for strategic planning regarding which services should be added or discontinued, which resources should be committed to facility expansion, or what should be done with excess capacity. Any long-range planning must take into consideration the current makeup of health services delivery, the evolving trends, and the potential impact of these trends.

Capturing New Markets

Healthcare administrators are in a better position to capture new health services markets if they understand emerging trends in the financing, insurance, payment, and delivery functions. New opportunities must be explored before any newly evolving segments of the market get overcrowded. An understanding of the dynamics within the system is essential to forging new marketing strategies to stay ahead of the competition and often to finding a service niche.

Complying with Regulations

Delivery of healthcare services is heavily regulated. Healthcare managers must comply with government regulations, such as standards of participation in government programs, licensing rules, and security and privacy laws regarding patient information, and must operate within the constraints of reimbursement rates. The Medicare and Medicaid programs have periodically made drastic changes to their reimbursement methodologies that have triggered the need for operational changes in the way services are organized and delivered. Private agencies, such as The Joint Commission [formerly the Joint Commission on Accreditation of Healthcare Organizations (JCAHO)], also play an indirect regulatory role, mainly in the monitoring of quality of services. Healthcare managers have no choice except to play by the rules set by the various public and private agencies. Hence, it is paramount that healthcare managers acquaint themselves with the rules and regulations governing their areas of operation.

Following the Organizational Mission

Knowledge of the healthcare system and its development is essential for effective management of healthcare organizations. By keeping up-to-date on community needs, technological progress, consumer demand, and economic prospects, managers can be in a better position to fulfill their organizational missions to enhance access, improve service quality, and achieve efficiency in the delivery of services.

HEALTHCARE SYSTEMS OF OTHER COUNTRIES

Canada and most Western European countries have national healthcare programs that provide universal coverage. There are three basic models for structuring national healthcare systems:

1. In a system under *national health insurance* (NHI), such as in Canada, the government finances health care through general taxes, but the actual care is delivered by private providers. In the context of the quad-function model, NHI requires a tighter consolidation of the financing, insurance, and payment functions coordinated by the government. Delivery is characterized by detached private arrangements.

2. In a *national health system* (NHS), such as in Great Britain, in addition to financing a tax-supported NHI program, the government manages the infrastructure for the delivery of medical care. Under such a system, the government operates most of the medical institutions. Most healthcare providers, such as physicians, are either government employees or are tightly organized in a publicly managed infrastructure. In the context of the quad-function model, NHS requires a tighter consolidation of all four functions.

3. In a *socialized health insurance* (SHI) system, such as in Germany, government-mandated contributions by employers and employees

finance health care. Private providers deliver health care. Private not-for-profit insurance companies, called sickness funds, are responsible for collecting the contributions and paying physicians and hospitals (Santerre and Neun 1996). In a socialized health insurance system, insurance and payment functions are closely integrated, and the financing function is better coordinated with the insurance and payment functions than in the United States. Delivery is characterized by independent private arrangements. The government exercises overall control.

The terms "national healthcare program" and "national health insurance" are often used generically and interchangeably to refer to any type of government-supported universal health insurance program. Table 6-3 presents selected features of the national healthcare programs in Canada, Germany, and Great Britain compared to the United States. Following is a brief discussion of healthcare delivery in selected countries from various parts of the world, to illustrate the application of the three models discussed and to provide a sample of the variety of healthcare systems in the world.

Australia

In the past, Australia had switched from a universal national healthcare program to a privately financed system. Since 1984, it has returned to a national program—called Medicare—financed by income taxes and an income-based Medicare levy. The system is built on the philosophy of everyone contributing to the cost of health care according to his

TABLE 6-3	Healthcare Systems of Selected Industrialized Countries			
	United States	**Canada**	**Great Britain**	**Germany**
Type	Pluralistic	National health insurance	National health system	Socialized health insurance
Ownership	Private	Public/Private	Public	Private
Financing	Voluntary, multipayer system (premiums or general taxes)	Single payer (general taxes)	Single payer (general taxes)	Employer–employee (mandated payroll contributions and general taxes)
Reimbursement (hospital)	Varies (DRG, negotiated fee for service, per diem, capitation)	Global budgets	Global budgets	Per diem payments
Reimbursement (physicians)	RBRVS, fee for service	Negotiated fee for service	Salaries and capitation payments	Negotiated fee for service
Consumer copayment	Small to significant	Negligible	Negligible	Negligible

Note: RBRVS, resource-based relative value scale.

Source: Data from R.E. Santerre and S.P. Neun, *Health Economics: Theories, Insights, and Industry Studies*, p. 146, © 1996, Irwin.

or her capacity to pay. In addition to Medicare, approximately 43% of Australians carry private health insurance (Australian Government 2004) to cover gaps in public coverage, such as dental services and care received in private hospitals (Willcox 2001). Although private health insurance is voluntary, it is strongly encouraged by the Australian government through tax subsidies for purchasers and tax penalties for nonpurchasers (Healy 2002). Public hospital spending is funded by the government, but private hospitals offer better choices. Costs incurred by patients receiving private medical services, whether in or out of the hospital, are reimbursed in whole or in part by Medicare. Private patients are free to choose and/or change their doctors. The medical profession in Australia is composed mainly of private practitioners, who provide care predominantly on a fee-for-service basis (Hall 1999; Podger 1999).

Recent healthcare reform undertaken by the Australian government has focused mainly on creating a better primary care system with the aim of offsetting the growing prevalence of chronic diseases (Gregory 2010; National Health and Hospitals Reform Commission 2010). Efforts have been launched to improve access and quality. Another objective is to reform the public hospital system by increasing the number of beds and improving productivity.

As part of the reform efforts, information on safety and quality standards, as well as prices, will be accessible to the public and closely monitored to ensure transparency. The reform also created the Australian Commission on Safety and Quality in Health Care, the Independent Hospital Pricing Authority, and the National Performance Authority to help improve system performance. These three divisions have been established for continual improvement, well after the implementation of reform legislation, and to assist Australians in making more informed decisions about health services (Australian Government 2010).

Canada

Canada implemented its national health insurance system—referred to as Medicare—under the Medical Care Act of 1966. Currently, Medicare is composed of 13 provincial and territorial health insurance plans, sharing basic standards of coverage, as defined by the Canada Health Act (Health Canada 2006). The bulk of financing for Medicare comes from general provincial tax revenues; the federal government provides a fixed amount that is independent of actual expenditures. Taxes are used to pay for nearly 70% of total healthcare expenditures in Canada. The remaining 30%, which pays for supplementary services, such as drugs, dental care, and vision care, is financed privately (Canadian Institute for Health Information 2005). Many employers offer private insurance for supplemental coverage.

Provincial and territorial departments of health have the responsibility to administer medical insurance plans, determine reimbursement for providers, and deliver certain public health services. Provinces are required by law to provide reasonable access to all medically necessary services and to provide portability of benefits from province to province. Patients are free to select their providers (Akaho et al. 1998). Several provinces have established contracts with providers in the United States for certain specialized services. According to Canada's Fraser Institute, specialist physicians surveyed across 12 specialties and 10 Canadian provinces reported a total waiting time of 18.2 weeks between referral from a general practitioner and delivery of treatment in 2010, an increase from 16.1 weeks in 2009. Patients had to wait the longest to undergo orthopedic surgery (35.6 weeks) (Barua et al. 2010).

Nearly all the Canadian provinces (Ontario being one notable exception) have resorted to regionalization, by creating administrative districts within each province. The objective of regionalization is to decentralize authority and responsibility to more efficiently address local needs and to promote citizen participation in healthcare decision making (Church and Barker 1998). The majority of Canadian hospitals are operated as private nonprofit entities run by community boards of trustees, voluntary organizations, or municipalities, and most physicians are in private practice (Health Canada 2006). Most provinces use global budgets and allocate set reimbursement amounts for each hospital. Physicians are paid fee-for-service rates, negotiated between each provincial government and medical association (MacPhee 1996; Naylor 1999).

Over the years, federal financial support to the provinces has been drastically reduced. Under the increasing burden of higher costs, certain provinces, such as Alberta and Ontario, have started small-scale experimentation with privatization. However, in 2003, the Health Council of Canada, composed of representatives of federal, provincial, and territorial governments, as well as healthcare experts, was established to assess Canada's healthcare system performance and establish goals for improvement. The Council's 2003 First Ministers' Accord on Health Care Renewal created a 5-year, $16 billion Health Reform Fund targeted at improving primary health care, home care, and catastrophic drug coverage (Health Council of Canada 2005).

Although most Canadians are quite satisfied with their healthcare system, sustaining the current healthcare delivery and financing model remains a challenge. Spending on health care has increased from approximately 7% of program spending at the provincial level in the 1970s to almost 40% today. It is expected to surpass 50% in every province and territory within the next few years.

China

Since the economic reforms initiated in the late 1970s, health care in the People's Republic of China has undergone significant changes. In urban China, health insurance has evolved from a predominantly public insurance (either government or public enterprise) system to a multipayer system. Government employees are covered under government insurance as a part of their benefits. Employees for public enterprises are largely covered through public enterprise insurance, but the actual benefits and payments vary according to the financial well-being of the enterprises. Employees of foreign businesses or joint ventures are, for the most part, well insured through private insurance arrangements. Almost all of these plans contain costs through a variety of means, such as experience-based premiums, deductibles, co-payments, and health benefit dollars (i.e., pre-allocated benefit dollars for health care that can be converted into income if not fully used). The unemployed, self-employed, and employees working for small enterprises (public or private) are largely uninsured. They can purchase individual or family plans in the private market or pay for services out of pocket. In rural China, the New Cooperative Medical Scheme (NCMS) (discussed later) has become widespread, being supported by funds pooled from national and local government as well as from private citizens. Although the insurance coverage rate is high (reaching more than 90% of the Chinese population), the actual benefits available from China's healthcare system are still very limited.

Similar to the United States, China has been facing the growing problems of a large uninsured population and healthcare cost inflation. Although healthcare funding was increased by 87% in 2006 and 2007, the country has yet to reform its healthcare system into one that is efficient and effective. Employment-based insurance in China does not cover dependents, nor does it cover migrant workers, leading to high out-of-pocket cost sharing in total health spending. Rural areas in China are the most vulnerable because of a lack of true insurance plans and the accompanying comprehensive coverage. Healthcare cost inflation is also growing at a rate that is 7% faster than gross domestic product (GDP) growth of 16% per year (Yip and Hsia 2008).

Healthcare delivery has also undergone significant changes. The former three-tier referral system (primary, second, tertiary) has been largely abolished. Patients can now go to any hospital of their choice as long as they are insured or can pay out of pocket. As a result, large (tertiary) hospitals are typically overutilized, whereas smaller (primary and secondary) hospitals are underutilized. Use of large hospitals contributes to medical cost escalation and medical specialization.

Major changes in health insurance and delivery have made obtaining access to medical care more difficult for the poor, uninsured, and underinsured. As a result, wide and growing disparities in access, quality, and outcomes are becoming apparent between rural and urban areas, and between the rich and the poor. Since the severe acute respiratory syndrome (SARS) epidemic in 2003, the government created an electronic disease reporting system at the district level. In addition, each district in China now has a hospital dedicated to infectious disease. However, flaws still remain, particularly in monitoring infectious disease in the remote localities that constitute some districts (Blumenthal and Hsiao 2005).

To fix some of its problems, the Chinese government has pushed through health reform initiatives in five prominent areas: health insurance, pharmaceuticals, primary care, public health, and public/community hospitals. For example, it created the New Cooperative Medical Scheme to provide rural areas with a government-run voluntary insurance program. This program prevents individuals living in these areas from becoming impoverished due to illness or catastrophic health expenses (Yip and Hsia 2008). A similar program was established in urban areas in 2008, called the Urban Resident Basic Medical Insurance scheme. The scheme targets the uninsured children, elderly, and other nonworking urban residents and enrolls them into the program at the household level rather than at the individual level (Wagstaff et al. 2009).

To improve access to primary care, China has reestablished community health centers (CHCs) to provide preventive and primary care services to offset the expensive outpatient services at hospitals. The goal is to reduce hospital utilization in favor of CHCs that can provide prevention, home care, and rehabilitative services (Yip and Hsia 2008; Yip and Mahal 2008). The CHCs have not been very popular among the public because of their perceived lack of quality and reputation. It remains uncertain whether China will restore its previously integrated healthcare delivery system, aimed at achieving universal access, or continue its current course of medical specialization and privatization.

Germany

The German healthcare system is characterized by socialized health insurance (SHI) financed by pooling employer and employee premium contributions through payroll taxes. Nonprofit sickness funds manage the social insurance pool. About 88% of the population has been enrolled in a sickness fund; another 11% either have private health insurance or are government workers with special coverage provisions. Fewer than 0.2% of Germans are uninsured (Busse 2002). Sickness funds act as purchasing entities by negotiating contracts with hospitals. However, with an aging population, fewer people in the workforce, and stagnant wage growth during recessions, paying for the increasing cost of medical care has been challenging.

During the 1990s, Germany adopted legislation to promote competition among sickness funds (Brown and Amelung 1999). To further control costs, the system employs global budgets for the hospital sector and places annual limits on spending for physician services. Disease management programs have also been implemented to standardize care for ailments like diabetes, as well as fixed payments to hospitals that discourage overtreatment.

Great Britain

Great Britain follows the national health system (NHS) model. Coincidentally, the British health delivery system is also named NHS (National Health Service); it marked 60 years of existence in 2008. The NHS is founded on the principles of primary care and has strong focus on community health services. The system owns its hospitals and employs its hospital-based specialists and other staff on a salaried basis. The primary care physicians, referred to as general practitioners (GPs), are mostly private practitioners.

Delivery of primary care is through primary care trusts (PCTs) in England, local health groups in Wales, health boards in Scotland, and primary care partnerships in Northern Ireland. PCTs have geographically assigned responsibility for community health services, in which each person living in a given geographic area is assigned to a particular PCT. A typical PCT is responsible for approximately 50,000 to 250,000 patients (Dixon and Robinson 2002). PCTs function independently of the local health authorities and are governed by a consumer-dominated board. A fully developed PCT has its own budget allocations, used for both primary care and hospital-based services. In this respect, PCTs function like MCOs in the United States.

It is also of interest to note that 11.5% of the British population holds private healthcare insurance (Dixon and Robinson 2002), and approximately £2.2 billion is spent annually in the acute sector of private health care (Doyle and McNeilly 1999). Future "pro-market" reforms in the United Kingdom's National Health Service would likely shift decision making to general practitioners, let some hospitals become nonprofit entities, and give patients more control over their health care.

Israel

Until 1995, Israel had a system of universal coverage based on the German SHI model, financed through an employer tax and income-based contributions from individuals. When the National Health Insurance (NHI) Law went into effect in 1995, it made insurance coverage mandatory for all Israeli citizens. Adults are required to pay a health tax. General tax revenue supplements the health tax revenue, which the government distributes to the various health plans based on a capitation formula. Each year the government determines how much from the general tax revenue should be contributed toward the NHI. The employer tax for health care was abolished in 1997; as a result, the share of general tax revenue to finance health care rose from 26% in 1995 to 46% in 2000 (Rosen 2003).

Health plans (or sickness funds) offer a predefined basic package of healthcare services and are prohibited from discriminating against those who have preexisting medical conditions. The capitation formula has built-in incentives for the funds to accept a larger number of elderly and chronically ill members. Rather than relying on a single-payer system, the reform allowed the existence of multiple health plans (today there are four competing, nonprofit sickness funds) to foster competition among funds, under the assumption that competition would lead to better quality of care and an increased responsiveness to patient needs. The plans also sell private health insurance to supplement the basic package. The system is believed to provide a high standard of care (Rosen and Merkur 2009; Gross et al. 1998).

Unlike in Germany, approximately 85% of the general hospital beds in Israel are owned by the government and the General Sick Fund, the largest of the four sickness funds. Hospitals are reimbursed under the global budget model (Chinitz and Israeli 1997). There was a major effort, in the early 1990s, to shift hospitals from government ownership to independent, nonprofit trusts, but this endeavor failed because of opposition from labor unions. Despite this, government hospitals have been granted more autonomy in the intervening years (Rosen 2003).

Japan

Since 1961, Japan has been providing universal coverage to its citizens through two main health insurance schemes. The first one is an employer-based system, modeled after Germany's SHI program. The second is a national health insurance program. Generally, large employers (with more than 300 employees) have their own health programs. Nearly 2,000 private, nonprofit health insurance societies manage insurance for large firms. Smaller companies either band together to provide private health insurance or belong to a government-run plan. Day laborers, seamen, agricultural workers, the self-employed, and retirees are all covered under the national healthcare program. Individual employees pay roughly 8% of their salaries as premiums and receive coverage for about 90% of the cost of medical services, with some limitations. Dependents receive slightly less than 90% coverage. Employers and the national government subsidize the cost of private premiums. Coverage is comprehensive, including dental care and prescription drugs, and patients are free to select their providers (Akaho et al. 1998; Babazono et al. 1998). Providers are paid on a fee-for-service basis with little control over reimbursement (McClellan and Kessler 1999).

Several health policy issues have emerged in Japan in the past few years. First, since 2002, some business leaders and economists have urged the Japanese government to lift its ban on mixed public/private payments for medical services, arguing that private payments should be allowed for services not covered by medical insurance (i.e., services involving new technologies or drugs). The Japan Medical Association and Ministry of Health, Labor, and Welfare have argued against these recommendations, stating that such a policy would favor the wealthy, would create disparities in access to care, and could be a risk to patient safety. Although the ban on mixed payments has not been lifted, Prime Minister Koizumi expanded the existing "exceptional approvals system" for new medical technologies in 2004 to allow private payments for selected technologies not covered by medical insurance (Nomura and Nakayama 2005).

Another recent policy development in Japan is the hospitals' increased use of a new system of reimbursement for inpatient care services, called diagnosis–procedure combinations (DPCs). Using DPCs, hospitals receive daily fees for each condition and treatment, regardless of actual provision of tests and interventions, proportionate to patients' length of stay. It is theorized that the DPC system will incentivize hospitals to provide more-efficient, higher-quality care to patients (Nomura and Nakayama 2005).

Japan's economic stagnation in the last several years has led to an increased pressure to contain costs (Ikegami and Campbell 2004). In 2005, Japan implemented reform initiatives in long-term care (LTC) delivery to contain costs in a growing sector of health care with rapidly rising costs. The new policy required residents in LTC facilities to pay for room and board. It also established new preventive benefits for seniors with low needs, who are at risk of requiring care in the future. The preventive benefits were designed to maintain health and independence and to postpone the need for nursing home care. Charging nursing home residents a fee for room and board was a departure from past policies that promoted institutionalization (Tsutsui and Muramatsu 2007).

Singapore

Prior to 1984, Singapore had a British-style NHS program, in which medical services were provided mainly by the public sector and financed through general taxes. Since then, the nation has designed a system based on market competition and self-reliance. Singapore has achieved universal coverage through a policy that requires mandatory private contributions but little government financing. The program, known as Medisave, mandates every working person, including the self-employed, to deposit a portion of earnings into an individual Medisave account. Employers are required to match employee contributions. These savings can be withdrawn for only two reasons: (1) to pay for hospital services and some selected, expensive physician services or (2) to purchase a government-sponsored insurance plan, called Medishield, for catastrophic (expensive and major) illness. For basic and routine services, people are expected to pay out of pocket. Those who cannot afford to pay receive government assistance (Hsiao 1995). In 2002, the government introduced ElderShield, which defrays out-of-pocket medical expenses for the elderly and severely disabled requiring long-term care (Singapore Ministry of Health 2004). The fee-for-service system of payment is prevalent throughout Singapore (McClellan and Kessler 1999).

Developing Countries

Developing countries, although they contain 84% of the world's population, provide for only 11% of the world's health spending. At the same time, these countries account for 93% of the worldwide burden of disease. The six developing regions of the world are East Asia and the Pacific, Europe (mainly Eastern Europe) and Central Asia, Latin America and the Caribbean, the Middle East and North Africa, South Asia, and Sub-Saharan Africa. Of these areas, the latter two have the least resources and the greatest health burden. On a per capita basis, industrialized countries have six times as many hospital beds and three times as many physicians as developing countries. People with private financial means can find reasonably good health care in many parts of the developing world. The majority of the populations in these regions, however, have to depend on limited government services that are often of questionable quality, as evaluated by Western standards. As a general observation, government financing for health services increases in countries with higher per capita incomes (Schieber and Maeda 1999).

THE SYSTEMS FRAMEWORK

A *system* consists of a set of interrelated and interdependent, logically coordinated components designed to achieve common goals. Even though the various functional components of the health services delivery structure in the United States are, at best, only loosely coordinated, the main components can be identified using a systems model. The systems framework used here helps one understand that the structure of healthcare services in the United States is based on some foundations, provides a logical arrangement of the various components, and demonstrates a progression from inputs to outputs. The main elements of this arrangement are system inputs (resources), system structure, system processes, and system outputs (outcomes). In addition, system outlook (future directions) is a necessary feature of a dynamic system.

System Foundations

The current healthcare system is not an accident. Historical, cultural, social, and economic factors explain its current structure. These factors also affect forces that shape new trends and developments, as well as those that impede change.

System Resources

No mechanism for health services delivery can fulfill its primary objective without deploying the necessary human and nonhuman resources. Human resources consist of the various types and categories of workers directly engaged in the delivery of health services to patients. Such personnel—physicians, nurses, dentists, pharmacists, other doctoral trained professionals, and numerous categories of allied health professionals—usually have direct contact with patients. Numerous ancillary workers—billing and collection agents, marketing and public relations personnel, and building maintenance employees—often play important, but indirect, supportive roles in the delivery of health care. Healthcare managers are needed to manage various types of healthcare services.

Resources are closely intertwined with access to health care. For instance, in certain rural areas of the United States, access is restricted due to a shortage of health professionals within certain categories. Development and diffusion of technology also determine the caliber of health care to which people may have access. Financing for health insurance and reimbursement to providers affect access indirectly.

System Processes

System resources influence the development and change in the physical infrastructure—such as hospitals, clinics, and nursing homes—essential for the different processes of healthcare delivery. Most healthcare services are delivered in noninstitutional settings, mainly associated with processes referred to as *outpatient care*. Institutional health services provided in hospitals, nursing homes, and rehabilitation institutions, for example, are predominantly *inpatient services*. Managed care and integrated systems represent a fundamental change in the financing (including payment and insurance) and delivery of health care. Even though managed care represents an integration of the resource and process elements of the systems model, it may be discussed as a process for the sake of clarity and continuity. Special institutional and community-based settings have been developed for long-term care and mental health.

System Outcomes

System outcomes refer to the critical issues and concerns surrounding what the health services system has been able to accomplish, or not accomplish, in relation to its primary objective, to provide, to an entire nation, cost-effective health services that meet certain established standards of quality. The previous three elements of the systems model play a critical role in fulfilling this objective. Access, cost, and quality are the main outcome criteria to evaluate the success of a healthcare delivery system. Issues and concerns regarding these criteria trigger broad initiatives for reforming the system through health policy.

System Outlook

A dynamic healthcare system must be forward looking. In essence, it must project into the future the accomplishment of desired system outcomes in view of anticipated social, economic, political, technological, informational, and ecological forces of change.

CONCLUSION

The United States has a unique system of healthcare delivery. The basic features characterizing this system—or rather a patchwork of subsystems—include the absence of a central agency to govern the system; unequal access to healthcare services, mainly because of a lack of health insurance for all Americans; healthcare delivery under imperfect market conditions; the existence of multiple payers; third-party insurers functioning as intermediaries between the financing and delivery aspects of health care; a balancing of power among various players; legal risks influencing practice behavior; new and expensive medical technology; a continuum of service settings; and a focus on quality improvement.

No country in the world has a perfect system, and most nations with a national healthcare program also have a private sector that varies in size. Because of resource limitations, universal access remains a theoretical concept even in countries that offer universal health insurance coverage. The developing countries of the world also face serious challenges due to scarce resources and strong underlying needs for services.

Under free market conditions, an inverse relationship exists between the quantity of medical services demanded and the price of medical services. Conversely, there is a direct relationship between price and the quantity supplied by the providers of care. In a free market, the quantity of medical care that patients are willing to purchase, the quantity of medical care that providers are willing to supply, and the price reach a state of equilibrium. The equilibrium is achieved without interference of any nonmarket forces. These conditions exist only under free market conditions, which are not characteristic of the healthcare market.

Healthcare administrators must understand how the healthcare delivery system works and evolves. Such an understanding improves awareness of the position their organization occupies within the macro environment of the system. This awareness also facilitates strategic planning and compliance with health regulations, enabling them to deal proactively with both opportunities and threats, and enabling them to effectively manage healthcare organizations. The systems framework provides an organized approach to an understanding of the various components of the U.S. healthcare delivery system.

DISCUSSION QUESTIONS

1. Why does cost containment remain an elusive goal in U.S. health services delivery?

2. What are the two main objectives of a healthcare delivery system?

3. Name the four basic functional components of the U.S. healthcare delivery system. What role does each play in the delivery of health care?

4. What is the primary reason for employers to purchase insurance plans to provide health benefits to their employees?

5. Why is it that, despite public and private health insurance programs, some U.S. citizens are without healthcare coverage?

6. What is managed care?

7. Why is the U.S. healthcare market referred to as "imperfect"?

8. Discuss the intermediary role of insurance in the delivery of health care.

9. Who are the major players in the U.S. health services system? What are the positive and negative effects of the often-conflicting self-interests of these players?

10. What main roles does the government play in the U.S. health services system?

11. Why is it important for healthcare managers and policymakers to understand the intricacies of the healthcare delivery system?

12. What kind of a cooperative approach do the authors recommend for charting the future course of the healthcare delivery system?

13. What is the difference between national health insurance (NHI) and a national health system (NHS)?

14. What is socialized health insurance (SHI)?

REFERENCES

Akaho, E., et al. 1998. A proposed optimal health care system based on a comparative study conducted between Canada and Japan. *Canadian Journal of Public Health* 89, no. 5: 301–307.

Altman, S.H., and U.E. Reinhardt. 1996. Introduction: Where does health care reform go from here? An uncharted odyssey. In: *Strategic choices for a changing health care system.* S.H. Altman and U.E. Reinhardt, eds. Chicago: Health Administration Press. p. xxi–xxxii.

Altman, S.H., and S.S. Wallack. 1996. Health care spending: Can the United States control it? In: *Strategic choices for a changing health care system.* S.H. Altman and U.E. Reinhardt, eds. Chicago: Health Administration Press. p. 1–32.

Australian Government, Department of Health and Ageing. May 2004. *Australia: Selected health care delivery and financing statistics.* Available at: http://www.health.gov/au. Accessed December 15, 2010.

Australian Government, Department of Health and Ageing. 2010. *A national health and hospitals network for Australia's future: Delivering the reforms.* Commonwealth of Australia.

Babazono, A., et al. 1998. The effect of a redistribution system for health care for the elderly on the financial performance of health insurance societies in Japan. *International Journal of Technology Assessment in Health* Care 14, no. 3: 458–466.

Barua, B., et al. 2010. *Waiting your turn: Wait times for health care in Canada 2010 report.* Vancouver, Canada: The Fraser Institute.

Blue Cross Blue Shield Association. 2007. Available at: http://www.bcbs.com/coverage/find/plan. Accessed December 15, 2010.

Blumenthal, D., and W. Hsiao. 2005. Privatization and its discontents: The evolving Chinese health care system. *New England Journal of Medicine* 353, no. 11: 1165–1170.

Brown, L.D., and V.E. Amelung. 1999. "Manacled competition": Market reforms in German health care. *Health Affairs* 18, no. 3: 76–91.

Busse, R. 2002. Germany. In: *Health care systems in eight countries: Trends and challenges*. A. Dixon and E. Mossialos, eds. London: The European Observatory on Health Care Systems, London School of Economics & Political Science. p. 47–60.

Canadian Institute for Health Information. 2005. *National health expenditure trends, 1975–2005*. Ottawa, ON: The Institute. p. iii, 7.

Chinitz, D., and A. Israeli. 1997. Health reform and rationing in Israel. *Health Affairs* 16, no. 5: 205–210.

Church, J., and P. Barker. 1998. Regionalization of health services in Canada: A critical perspective. *International Journal of Health Services* 28, no. 3: 467–486.

Dixon, A., and R. Robinson. 2002. The United Kingdom. In: *Health care systems in eight countries: Trends and challenges*. A. Dixon and E. Mossialos, eds. London: The European Observatory on Health Care Systems, London School of Economics & Political Science. p. 103–114.

Doyle, Y.G., and R.H. McNeilly. 1999. The diffusion of new medical technologies in the private sector of the U.K. health care system. *International Journal of Technology Assessment in Health Care* 15, no. 4: 619–628.

Families USA. 2009. *Americans at risk*. Available at: http://www.familiesusa.org/resources /publications /reports/americans-at-risk-findings.html. Accessed January 2011.

Feldstein, P.J. 1993. *Health care economics*. 4th ed. New York: Delmar Publishing.

Gregory, G. 2010. A brief history of "health reform" in Australia, 2007-2009. *Australian Journal of Rural Health* 18: 49–55.

Griffith, J.R. 1995. *The well-managed health care organization*. Ann Arbor, MI: AUPHA Press/Health Administration Press.

Gross, R., et al. 1998. Evaluating the Israeli health care reform: Strategy, challenges, and lessons. *Health Policy* 45: 99–117.

Hall, J. 1999. Incremental change in the Australian health care system. *Health Affairs* 18, no. 3: 95–110.

Health Canada. 2006. Available at: http://www.hc-sc .gc.ca/hcs-sss/medi-assur/index_e.htmlwhich. Accessed September 2006.

Health Council of Canada. 2005. *Annual report 2005*. Available at: http://www.healthcouncilcanada.ca /en/index.php?option=com_content&task=view &id=51&Itemid=50. Accessed September 2006.

Health Resources and Services Administration (HRSA) 2011. *Health center snapshot 2009*. Available at: http://www.hrsa.gov/data-statistics/health-center-data/index.html. Accessed January 2011.

Healy, J. 2002. Australia. In: *Health care systems in eight countries: Trends and challenges*. A. Dixon and E. Mossialos, eds. London: The European Observatory on Health Care Systems, London School of Economics & Political Science. p. 3–16.

Hemenway, D., and D. Fallon. 1985. Testing for physician-induced demand with hypothetical cases. *Medical Care* 23, no. 4: 344–349.

Hsiao, W.C. 1995. Medical savings accounts: Lessons from Singapore. *Health Affairs* 14, no. 2: 260–266.

Ikegami, N., and J.C. Campbell. 2004. Japan's health care system: Containing costs and attempting reform. *Health Affair* 23: 26–36.

Kahn, J.G., et al. 2005. The cost of health insurance administration in California: Estimates for insurers, physicians, and hospitals. *Health Affairs* 24, no. 6: 1629–1639.

MacPhee, S. 1996. Reform the watchword as OECD countries struggle to contain health care costs. *Canadian Medical Association Journal* 154, no. 5: 699–701.

McClellan, M., and D. Kessler. 1999. A global analysis of technological change in health care: The case of heart attacks. *Health Affairs* 18, no. 3: 250–257.

McGuire, T.G., and M.V. Pauly. 1991. Physician response to fee changes with multiple payers. *Journal of Health Economics* 10, no. 4: 385–410.

National Association of Community Health Centers (NACHC). 2006. *A sketch of community health centers: Chart book, 2006*. Washington, DC: NACHC.

National Center for Health Statistics. 2006. *Health, United States, 2006: With chartbook on trends in the health of Americans*. Hyattsville, MD: Department of Health and Human Services.

National Health and Hospitals Reform Commission. 2010. *A Healthier Future for All Australians: Final Report June 2009*. Commonwealth of Australia. http://www.yourhealth.gov.au/internet/your health/publishing.nsf/Content/nhhrc-report-toc. Accessed April 22, 2011.

Naylor, C.D. 1999. Health care in Canada: Incrementalism under fiscal duress. *Health Affairs* 18, no. 3: 9–26.

Nomura, H., and T. Nakayama. 2005. The Japanese healthcare system. *BMJ* 331: 648–649.

Podger, A. 1999. Reforming the Australian health care system: A government perspective. *Health Affairs* 18, no. 3: 111–113.

Rosen, B. 2003. Israel: Health system review. In: *Health care systems in transition*. S. Tomson and E. Mossialos, eds. Copenhagen: European Observatory on Health Care Systems.

Rosen, B., and S. Merkur. 2009. Israel: Health system review. *Health Systems in Transition* 11: 1–226.

Santerre, R.E., and S.P. Neun. 1996. *Health economics: Theories, insights, and industry studies*. Chicago: Irwin.

Schieber, G., and A. Maeda. 1999. Health care financing and delivery in developing countries. *Health Affairs* 18, no. 3: 193–205.

Singapore Ministry of Health. 2004. *Medisave, Medishield and other subsidy schemes: Overview*. Available at: www.moh.gov.sg/corp/financing/overview.do. Accessed September 2006.

Tsutsui, T., and N. Muramatsu. 2007. Japan's universal long-term care system reform of 2005: Containing costs and realizing a vision. *Journal of the American Geriatrics Society* 55: 1458–1463.

U.S. Bureau of Labor Statistics. 2011. *Occupational outlook handbook, 2010–2011*. Available at: http://www.bls.gov/oco/home.htm. Accessed January 2011.

U.S. Census Bureau. 2011. The 2011 Statistical Abstract. Available at: http://www.census.gov/compendia/statab/cats/health_nutrition/health_care_resources.html. Accessed January 2011.

Wagstaff, A., et al. 2009. China's health system and its reform: A review of recent studies. *Health Economics* 18: S7–S23.

Willcox, S. 2001. Promoting private health insurance in Australia. *Health Affairs* 20, no. 3: 152–161.

Wolinsky, F.D. 1988. *The sociology of health: Principles, practitioners, and issues*. 2nd ed. Belmont, CA: Wadsworth Publishing Company.

Yip, W., and W.C. Hsia. 2008. The Chinese health system at a crossroads. *Health Affairs* 27: 460–468.

Yip, W., and A. Mahal. 2008. The health care systems of China and India: Performance and future challenges. *Health Affairs* 27: 921–932.

CHAPTER 7

Beliefs, Values, and Health

Leiyu Shi and Douglas A. Singh

CHAPTER OBJECTIVES

1. Understand the concepts of health and disease.

2. Examine the determinants of health.

3. Explore the American beliefs and values related to the delivery of health care.

4. Appreciate the implications of the meaning of health, its determinants, and beliefs and values for medical care delivery.

5. Develop a position on the equitable distribution of healthcare services.

6. Explore the efforts undertaken to integrate individual and community health.

7. Understand the basic measures of health status and health services utilization.

INTRODUCTION

From an economic perspective, curative medicine appears to produce decreasing returns in health improvement while increasing healthcare expenditures (Saward and Sorensen 1980). There has also been a growing recognition of the benefits to society from the promotion of health and prevention of disease, disability, and premature death. However, progress in this direction has been slow because of the prevailing social values and beliefs that still focus on curing diseases rather than promoting health. The common definitions of health, as well as measures for evaluating health status, reflect similar inclinations. This chapter proposes a holistic approach to health, although such an ideal would be quite difficult to fully achieve. For example, it is not easy for a system to enact a change in personal lifestyles and behaviors among the population. Regardless, the healthcare delivery system must allocate resources and take other measures to bring about a change in course. The 10-year *Healthy People* initiatives, undertaken by the U.S. Department of Health and Human Services (DHHS) since 1980, illustrate steps taken in this direction, even though these initiatives have been typically strong in rhetoric but weak in actionable strategies or the necessary funding.

Beliefs and values ingrained in the American culture have been influential in laying the foundations of a system that has remained predominantly private, as opposed to a tax-financed national healthcare program. Social norms also help explain how American society views illness and the expectations it has of those who are sick.

This chapter further explores the issue of equity in the distribution of health services, using the contrasting theories of market justice and social justice. The conflict between the principles of market and social justice is reflected throughout U.S. healthcare delivery. For the most part, strong market justice values prevail, although some components of healthcare delivery in the United States reflect social justice values. This chapter concludes with an overview of measures commonly used to understand the health status of a population.

SIGNIFICANCE FOR MANAGERS AND POLICYMAKERS

Materials covered in this chapter have several implications for health services managers and policymakers:

1. The health status of a population has tremendous bearing on the utilization of health services, assuming the services are readily available. Planning of health services must be governed by demographic and health trends and initiatives toward reducing disease and disability.

2. The basic meaning of health, determinants of health, and health risk appraisal should be used to design appropriate educational, preventive, and therapeutic initiatives.

3. There is a growing emphasis on evaluating the effectiveness of healthcare organizations based on the contributions they make to community and population health. The concepts discussed in this chapter can guide administrators in implementing programs of most value to their communities.

4. The exercise of justice and equity in making health care available to all Americans remains a lingering concern. This monumental problem requires a joint undertaking from providers, administrators, policymakers, and other key stakeholders.

5. Quantified measures of health status and utilization can be used by managers and policymakers to evaluate the adequacy and effectiveness of existing programs, plan new strategies, measure progress, and discontinue ineffective services.

BASIC CONCEPTS OF HEALTH AND HEALTH CARE

In the United States, the concepts of health and health care have largely been governed by the medical model, more specifically referred to as the biomedical model. The *medical model* defines health as the absence of illness or disease. This definition implies that optimal health exists when a person is free of symptoms and does not require medical treatment. However, it is not a definition of health in the true sense, but rather a definition of what ill health is not (Wolinsky 1988). This prevailing view of health emphasizes clinical diagnoses and medical interventions to treat disease or symptoms of disease, while prevention of disease and health promotion are relegated to a secondary status. Therefore, when the term "healthcare delivery" is used, in reality it refers to medical care delivery.

Medical sociologists have gone a step further in defining health as the state of optimal capacity of an individual to perform his or her expected social roles and tasks, such as work, school, and doing household chores (Parsons 1972). A person who is unable (as opposed to unwilling) to perform his or her social roles in society is considered sick. However, this concept also tends to view health negatively, because many people continue to engage in their social obligations despite suffering from pain, cough, colds, and other types of temporary disabilities, including mental distress. In other words, a person's engagement in social roles does not necessarily signify that the individual is in optimal health.

An emphasis on both physical and mental dimensions of health is found in the definition of health proposed by the Society for Academic Emergency Medicine, according to which health is "a state of physical and mental well-being that facilitates the achievement of individual and societal goals" (Ethics Committee, Society for Academic Emergency Medicine 1992). This view of health recognizes the importance of achieving harmony between the physiological and emotional dimensions.

The World Health Organization's (WHO) definition of health is most often cited as the ideal for healthcare delivery systems. WHO defines health as "a state of complete physical, mental and social wellbeing and not merely the absence of disease or infirmity" (WHO 1948). Since it includes the physical, mental, and social dimensions, WHO's model can be referred to as the biopsychosocial model of health. WHO's definition specifically identifies social well-being as a third dimension of health. In doing so, it emphasizes the importance of positive social relationships. Having a social support network is positively associated with life stresses, self-esteem, and social relations. The social aspects of health also extend beyond the individual level to include responsibility for the health of entire communities and populations. WHO's definition recognizes that optimal health is more than a mere absence of disease or infirmity.

WHO has also defined a healthcare system as all the activities whose primary purpose is to promote, restore, or maintain health (McKee 2001). As this chapter points out, health care should include much more than medical care. Thus, *health care* can be defined as a variety of services believed to improve a person's health and well-being.

In recent years, there has been a growing interest in *holistic health*, which emphasizes the well-being of every aspect of what makes a person whole and complete. Thus, *holistic medicine* seeks to treat the individual as a whole person (Ward 1995). For example, diagnosis and treatment should take into account the mental, emotional, spiritual, nutritional, environmental, and other factors surrounding the origin of disease (Cohen 2003).

Holistic health incorporates the spiritual dimension as a fourth element—in addition to the physical, mental, and social aspects—as necessary for optimal health (Figure 7-1). A growing volume of medical literature points to the healing effects of a person's religion and spirituality on morbidity and mortality (Levin 1994). Numerous studies have identified an inverse association between religious involvement and all-cause mortality (McCullough et al. 2000). Religious and spiritual beliefs and practices have shown a positive impact on a person's physical, mental, and social well-being. These

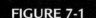

FIGURE 7-1   The Four Dimensions of Holistic Health

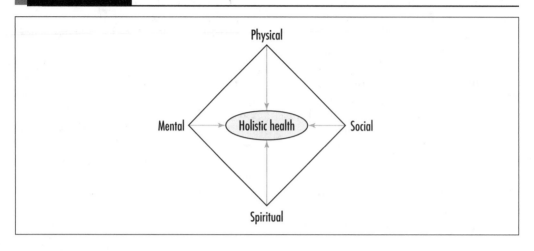

beliefs and practices may affect the incidences, experiences, and outcomes of several common medical problems (Maugans 1996). For instance, people with high levels of general religious involvement are likely to suffer less from depressive symptoms and disorders (McCullough and Larson 1999). Spiritual well-being has also been recognized as an important internal resource for helping people cope with illness. For instance, a study conducted at the University of Michigan found that 93% of the women undergoing cancer treatment indicated that their religious lives helped them sustain their hope (Roberts et al. 1997). Studies have found that a large percentage of patients want their physicians to consider their spiritual needs, and almost half have expressed a desire for the physicians to pray with them if they could (see Post et al. 2000). However, many physicians feel that spiritual matters fall outside their expertise or that they would be intruding into patients' private lives. Also, ethical issues and religious coercion are valid concerns, and referral to a chaplain or pastoral leader is often a more appropriate alternative (Post et al. 2000).

The spiritual dimension is frequently tied to one's religious beliefs, values, morals, and practices. Broadly, it is described as meaning, purpose, and fulfillment in life; hope and will to live; faith; and a person's relationship with God (Marwick 1995; Ross 1995; Swanson 1995). A clinically tested scale to measure spiritual well-being included categories such as belief in a power greater than oneself, purpose in life, faith, trust in providence, prayer, meditation, group worship, ability to forgive, and gratitude for life (Hatch et al. 1998).

Some of the nation's leading medical schools now offer courses that explore spiritual issues in health care, as well as ways to address such issues in patient care delivery (American Physical Therapy Association 1997). Spiritual assessment instruments have been developed to assist physicians and other clinicians in spiritual history taking (Maugans 1996; Puchalski and Romer 2000). The Committee on Religion and Psychiatry of the American Psychological Association has issued a position statement to emphasize the importance of maintaining respect for a patient's religious/spiritual beliefs. For the first time, "religious or spiritual problem" has been included as a diagnostic category in DSM-IV.[1] The holistic approach to health also alludes to the need for incorporating alternative therapies into the predominant medical model.

Tamm (1993) observes that different groups in society—including physicians, nurses, and patients—look at health and disease from partly different vantage points, those that are holistic and those that emphasize illness and disease. Such tensions can have significant implications for the delivery of health services, especially in a pluralistic society such as the United States. Although the medical model plays a key role in the delivery of health care, integration of the concepts of holistic health can optimize well-being and promote early recovery from sickness.

Quality of Life

The term *quality of life* is used in a denotative sense to capture the essence of overall satisfaction with life during and following a person's encounter with the healthcare delivery system. Thus the term is employed in two ways.

First, it is an indicator of how satisfied a person is with the experiences while receiving health care. Specific life domains, such as comfort factors, respect, privacy, security, degree of independence, decision-making autonomy, and attention to personal preferences are significant to most people. These factors are now regarded as rights that patients can demand during any type of healthcare encounter.

Second, quality of life can refer to a person's overall satisfaction with life and with self-perceptions of health, particularly after some medical intervention. The implication is that desirable processes during medical treatment and successful outcomes would, subsequently, have a positive effect on an individual's ability to function, carry out social roles and obligations, and have a sense of fulfillment and self-worth.

Risk Factors and Disease

The occurrence of disease involves more than just a single factor. For example, the mere presence of the tubercle bacillus does not mean the infected person will develop tuberculosis. Other factors, such as poverty, overcrowding, and malnutrition, may be essential for development of the disease (Friedman 1980). Hence, tracing *risk factors*—attributes that increase the likelihood of developing a particular disease or negative health condition in the future—requires a broad approach.

One useful explanation of disease occurrence (for communicable diseases, in particular) is provided by the tripartite model, sometimes referred to as the Epidemiology[2] Triangle (Figure 7-2). Of the three entities in this model, the *host* is the organism—generally, a human—that becomes sick. Factors associated with the host include genetic makeup, level of immunity, fitness, and personal habits and behaviors. However, for the host to become sick, an *agent* must be present, although presence of an agent does not ensure that disease will occur. In the previous example, tubercle bacillus is the agent for tuberculosis. Other examples are chemical agents, radiation, tobacco smoke, dietary indiscretions, and nutritional deficiencies. The third entity, *environment*, is external to the host and includes the physical, social, cultural, and economic aspects of the environment. Examples include sanitation, air pollution, cultural beliefs, social equity, social norms, and economic status. The environmental factors play a moderating role that can either enhance or reduce susceptibility to disease. Because the three entities often interact to produce disease, disease

---

[1] *Diagnostic and Statistical Manual of Mental Disorders* is the most widely recognized system of classifying mental disorders.

[2] Epidemiology is the study of the nature, cause, control, and determinants of the frequency and distribution of disease, disability, and death in human populations (Timmreck 1994, 2).

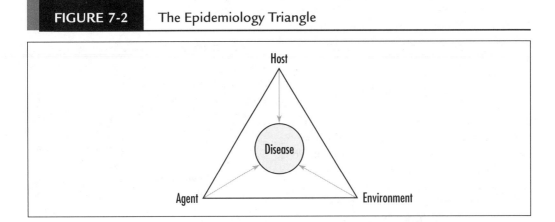

FIGURE 7-2 The Epidemiology Triangle

prevention efforts should focus on a broad approach to mitigate or eliminate risk factors associated with all three entities.

Behavioral Risk Factors

Certain individual behaviors and personal lifestyle choices represent important risk factors for illness and disease. For example, smoking has been identified as the leading cause of preventable disease and death in the United States, because it significantly increases the risk of heart disease, stroke, lung cancer, and chronic lung disease (DHHS 2004). Substance abuse, inadequate physical exercise, a high-fat diet, irresponsible use of motor vehicles, and unsafe sex are additional examples of behavioral risk factors. (Table 7-1 presents the percentage of the U.S. population with selected behavioral risks.)

Acute, Subacute, and Chronic Conditions

Disease can be classified as acute, subacute, or chronic. An *acute condition* is relatively severe, episodic (of short duration), and often treatable and subject to recovery. Treatments are generally provided in a hospital. Examples of acute conditions are a sudden interruption of kidney function or a myocardial infarction (heart at-

tack). A *subacute condition* is a less severe phase of an acute illness. It can be a postacute condition, requiring treatment after discharge from a hospital. Examples include ventilator and head trauma care.

A *chronic condition* is one that persists over time, is not severe, but is generally irreversible. A chronic condition may be kept under control through appropriate medical treatment, but if left untreated, the condition may lead to severe and life-threatening health problems. Examples of chronic conditions are hypertension, asthma, arthritis, heart disease, and diabetes. Contributors to chronic disease include ethnic, cultural, and behavioral factors and the social and physical environment, discussed later in this chapter.

In the United States, chronic diseases have become the leading cause of death and disability. According to the Centers for Disease Control and Prevention (CDC), almost 50% of Americans have at least one chronic illness, and 7 out of every 10 deaths are attributable to chronic disease (CDC 2010a). Among both the younger and older age groups (ages 18 and older), hypertension is ranked the most common chronic condition, followed by cholesterol disorders. Among children up to age 17, respiratory diseases and asthma are the most

TABLE 7-1	Percentage of U.S. Population with Behavioral Risks		
Behavioral Risk	**Percentage of Population**	**Year**	
Alcohol (12 years and older)	51.1	2007	
Marijuana (12 years and older)	5.8	2007	
Cocaine use (12th graders)	1.9	2008	
Cocaine use (10th graders)	1.2	2008	
Cocaine use (8th graders)	0.8	2008	
Cigarette smoking (18 years and older)	19.7	2007	
Hypertension (20 years and older)	31.3	2003–2006	
Overweight (20–74 years)	66.9	2003–2006	
Serum cholesterol (20 years and older)	15.6	2005–2006	

Note: Data are based on household interviews of a sample of the civilian noninstitutionalized population 12 years of age and older in the coterminous United States.

Source: Data from National Center for Health Statistics. *Health, United States, 2009.* Hyattsville, MD: Department of Health and Human Services, 2010, pp. 276, 281, 283, 292, 293, 301.

common chronic conditions (Agency for Healthcare Research and Quality 2006). The incidence of childhood chronic diseases has almost quadrupled over the past four decades, mostly due to a threefold increase in childhood obesity (PFCD 2009).

It is estimated that 75% of total health expenditures in the United States are attributable to the treatment of chronic conditions (PFCD 2009). In 2007, total healthcare costs associated with the treatment of chronic diseases were approximately $1.7 trillion. In addition, health disparities continue to be a serious threat to the health and well-being of some population groups. For example, African American, Hispanic, American Indian, and Alaskan Native adults are twice as likely as white adults to have diabetes (CDC 2010a).

There are three main reasons behind the rise of chronic conditions in the U.S. population:

1. New diagnostic methods, medical procedures, and pharmaceuticals have significantly improved the treatment of acute illnesses, survival rates, and longevity, but these achievements have come at the consequence of a larger number of people living with chronic conditions. The prevalence of chronic disease is expected to continue to rise with an aging population and longer life expectancy.

2. Screening and diagnosis have expanded in scope, frequency, and accuracy (Robert Wood Johnson Foundation 2010).

3. Lifestyle choices, such as high-salt and high-fat diets and sedentary lifestyles, are risk factors that contribute to the development of chronic conditions. To address these issues, the DHHS launched a comprehensive initiative with the aid of $650 million allocated under the American Recovery and Reinvestment Act of 2009. The goal of this initiative—Communities Putting Prevention to Work—is to "reduce risk factors, prevent/delay chronic disease, promote wellness in children and adults, and provide positive, sustainable health change in communities" (DHHS 2010a).

HEALTH PROMOTION AND DISEASE PREVENTION

A program of health promotion and disease prevention is built on three main principles:

1. An understanding of risk factors associated with host, agent, and/or environment. Risk factors and their health consequences are evaluated through a process called *health risk appraisal*. Only when the risk factors and their health consequences are known can interventions be developed to help individuals adopt healthier lifestyles.

2. Interventions for counteracting the key risk factors include two main approaches: (a) behavior modification geared toward the goal of adopting healthier lifestyles and (b) therapeutic interventions. Both are discussed later in this section.

3. Adequate public health and social services, as discussed later in this chapter, include all health-related services designed to minimize risk factors and their negative effects so as to prevent disease, control disease outbreaks, and contain the spread of infectious agents. The goal of public health is to maximize the health of a population.

Various avenues can be used for motivating individuals to alter behaviors that may contribute to disease, disability, or death. Behavior can be modified through educational programs and incentives directed at specific high-risk populations. In the case of cigarette smoking, for example, health promotion aims at building people's knowledge, attitudes, and skills to avoid or quit smoking. It also involves reducing advertisements and other environmental enticements that promote nicotine addiction. Financial incentives, such as a higher cigarette tax, are used to discourage purchase of cigarettes.

Therapeutic interventions fall into three areas of preventive effort: primary prevention, secondary prevention, and tertiary prevention. *Primary prevention* refers to activities undertaken to reduce the probability that a disease will develop in the future (Kane 1988). Its objective is to restrain the development of a disease or negative health condition before it occurs. Therapeutic interventions would include community health efforts to assist patients in smoking cessation and exercise programs to prevent conditions such as lung cancer and heart disease. Teen driver education can prevent disability and death from auto accidents. Safety training and practices can reduce serious workplace injuries. Prenatal care is known to lower infant mortality rates. Immunization has had a greater impact on prevention against childhood diseases and mortality reduction than any other public health intervention besides clean water (Plotkin and Plotkin 1999). Hand washing, refrigeration of foods, garbage collection, sewage treatment, and protection of the water supply are also examples of primary prevention (Timmreck 1994). There have been numerous incidents where emphasis on food safety and proper cooking could have prevented outbreaks of potentially deadly episodes, such as those caused by *E. coli*.

Secondary prevention refers to early detection and treatment of disease. Health screenings and periodic health examinations are just two examples. The main objective of secondary prevention is to block the progression of a disease or an injury from developing into an impairment or disability (Timmreck 1994). Screening tests, such as hypertension screening, Pap smears, and mammograms, have been instrumental in prescribing early treatment.

Tertiary prevention refers to interventions that could prevent complications from chronic conditions and prevent further illness, injury, or disability. For example, regular turning of bed-bound patients prevents pressure sores; rehabilitation therapies can prevent permanent disability; and infection control practices in hospitals and nursing homes are designed to prevent *iatrogenic illnesses*, that is, illnesses or injuries caused by the process of health care.

As shown in Table 7-2, prevention, early detection, and treatment efforts helped reduce

TABLE 7-2	Annual Percent Decline in U.S. Cancer Mortality, 1991–2007		
Type of Cancer	1991–1995	1994–2003	1998–2007
All cancers	3.0	1.1	1.4
Breast cancer	6.3	2.5	2.2
Cervical cancer	9.7	3.6	2.6
Ovarian cancer	4.8	0.5	0.8
Prostate cancer	6.3	3.5	3.1

Source: Data from National Center for Health Statistics of the Centers for Disease Control and Prevention, National Cancer Institute, *SEER Cancer Statistics Review, 1975–2007.*

cancer mortality quite significantly between 1991 and 2007. This decrease was the first sustained decline since record keeping was instituted in the 1930s. The decline in breast cancer has been credited to early detection and treatment advances. The drop in cervical cancer has been attributed to the widespread use of Pap screening. Later data, however, show that the declines in cancer death rates are moderating, most likely due to other factors, such as aging.

Promotion of Developmental Health

Development refers to growth in skill and capacity to function normally (Hancock and Mandle 1994). Early childhood development influences a person's health in later years. The foundations laid in the early years often determine the individual's future adjustments to life (Berger 1988) and shape individual behaviors. Children who fail to acquire certain skills in childhood often have real difficulties as adults (Wynder and Orlandi 1984). The importance of early childhood development has important implications for health services delivery in two main areas:

■ Expectant mothers need adequate prenatal care. The health promotion needs of the expectant mother and the fetus are so closely intertwined that the two must be considered one unit (Hancock and Mandle 1994).

■ Adequate child care is needed, especially during the first few years of growth. Immunization, nutrition, family and social interaction, and health care are key developmental elements until a child reaches adulthood. Preventable developmental disabilities impose an undue burden on the healthcare delivery system.

Public Health

Public health remains poorly understood by its prime beneficiaries, the public. For some people, the notion of public health evokes images of a massive social enterprise or welfare system. To others, the term means healthcare services for everyone. Still another image of public health is that of a body of knowledge and techniques that can be applied to health-related problems (Turnock 1997). However, none of these ideas adequately reflects what public health is.

The Institute of Medicine (IOM) proposed that the mission of public health is to fulfill "society's interest in assuring conditions in which people can be healthy" (IOM 1988). *Public health* deals with broad societal concerns about ensuring conditions that promote optimal health for the society as a whole. It involves the application of scientific knowledge to counteract disease outbreaks and protect the general population.

Three main distinctions can be seen between the practices of medicine and public health:

1. Medicine focuses on the individual patient—diagnosing symptoms, treating and preventing disease, relieving pain and suffering, and maintaining or restoring normal function. Public health, conversely, focuses on populations (Lasker 1997).

2. The emphases in modern medicine are on the biological causes of disease and developing treatments and therapies. Public health focuses on identifying the environmental, social, and behavioral risk factors that cause disease and on developing and implementing population-wide interventions to minimize those risk factors (Peters et al. 2001).

3. Medicine focuses on the treatment of disease and recovery of health, whereas public health deals with various efforts to prevent disease and promote health.

To promote and protect society's interest in health and well-being, public health activities can range from providing education on nutrition to passing laws that enhance automobile safety. For example, public health includes dissemination to the public and to health professionals of timely and appropriate information about important health issues, particularly when communicable diseases pose potential threats to large segments of a population.

Compared to the delivery of medical services, public health involves a broader range of professionals. The medical sector encompasses physicians, nurses, dentists, therapists, social workers, psychologists, nutritionists, health educators, pharmacists, laboratory technicians, health services administrators, and so forth. In addition to these professionals, public health involves professionals such as sanitarians, epidemiologists, statisticians, industrial hygienists, environmental health specialists, food and drug inspectors, toxicologists, and economists (Lasker 1997).

Health Protection and Environmental Health

Health protection is one of the main public health functions. In the 1850s, John Snow successfully traced the risk of cholera outbreaks in London to the Broad Street water pump (Rosen 1993). Since then, *environmental health* has specifically dealt with preventing the spread of disease through water, air, and food (Schneider 2000). Environmental health science, along with other public health measures, was instrumental in reducing the risk of infectious diseases during the 1900s. For example, in 1900, pneumonia, tuberculosis, and diarrhea, along with enteritis, were the top three killers in the United States (CDC 1999); that is no longer the case today (see Table 7-3). With the rapid industrialization during the 20th century, environmental health faced new challenges, due to serious health hazards from chemicals, industrial waste, infectious waste, radiation, asbestos, and other toxic substances.

Health Protection During Global Pandemics

In 2003, to prevent the introduction, transmission, and spread of severe acute respiratory syndrome (SARS)—a contagious disease that is accompanied by fever and symptoms of pneumonia or other respiratory illness—the White House designated SARS as a communicable disease for the apprehension, detention, or conditional release of individuals with the disease.

The global threat of avian influenza also solicited a public health and government response. The CDC launched a website dedicated to educating the public about avian influenza, how it is spread, and past and current outbreaks. The website contains specific information for health professionals, travelers, the poultry industry, state departments of health, and people with possible exposures to avian influenza (CDC 2007).

TABLE 7-3	Leading Causes of Death, 2006	
Cause of Death	Deaths	Percentage
All causes	2,426,264	100.0
Diseases of the heart	631,636	26.0
Malignant neoplasms	559,888	23.1
Cerebrovascular diseases	137,119	5.7
Chronic lower respiratory diseases	124,583	5.1
Unintentional injuries	121,599	5.0
Diabetes mellitus	72,449	3.0
Alzheimer's disease	56,326	2.3
Influenza and pneumonia	72,432	3.0
Nephritis, nephrotic syndrome, and nephrosis	45,344	1.9
Septicemia	34,234	1.4

Source: Data from National Center for Health Statistics. *Health, United States, 2009.* Hyattsville, MD: Department of Health and Human Services, 2010, p. 198.

After a novel H1N1 influenza virus emerged from Mexico in early April 2009, the first H1N1 influenza patient in the United States was confirmed by CDC on April 15, 2009 (DHHS 2009). Although U.S. health officials anticipated and prepared for an influenza pandemic, the H1N1 virus had strained the response capabilities of the public health system. The virus affected every U.S. state, and Americans were left unprotected in the outbreak, due to unavailability of antiviral medications. On April 26, 2009, DHHS declared a nationwide Public Health Emergency (PHE), which enabled the Food and Drug Administration (FDA) to issue Emergency Use Authorizations (EUAs) for certain antiviral medications, such as Tamiflu, Relenza, and Peramivir IV, in vitro diagnostic devices, and respiratory protection products (DHHS 2009). As of July 24, 2009, CDC had reported 43,771 confirmed and probable cases, with 5,011 hospitalizations and 302 deaths (DHHS 2009).

Bioterrorism and Disaster Preparedness

Since the horrific events of what is now commonly referred to as 9/11 (September 11, 2001), America has opened a new chapter in health protection. As the nation was still recovering from the shock of the attacks on New York's World Trade Center, attempts to disseminate anthrax through the U.S. Postal Service were discovered. In June 2002, former President George W. Bush signed into law the Public Health Security and Bioterrorism Response Act of 2002.

The term *bioterrorism* encompasses the use of chemical, biological, and nuclear agents to cause harm to relatively large civilian populations. Dealing with such a threat requires large-scale preparations, which include appropriate tools and training for workers in medical care, public health, emergency care, and civil defense agencies at the federal, state, and local levels. It requires national initiatives to develop countermeasures, such as new vaccines, a robust public health infrastructure, and coordination among numerous agencies. It requires an infrastructure to handle large numbers of casualties and isolation facilities for contagious patients. Hospitals, public health agencies, and civil defense must be linked together through information systems. Containment of infectious agents, such as smallpox, would require quick detection, treatment, isolation, and organized efforts to protect the unaffected population. Rapid cleanup, evacuation of the affected population, and transfer of victims to medical care facilities require detailed plans and logistics.

The Homeland Security Act of 2002, signed into law in November 2002 during the George W. Bush administration, created the Department of Homeland Security (DHS) and called for a major restructuring of the nation's resources with the primary mission of helping prevent, protect against, and respond to any acts of terrorism in the United States. It also provided better tools to contain attacks on the food and water supplies; protect the nation's vital infrastructures, such as nuclear facilities; and track biological materials anywhere in the United States.

Over the past several years, the United States has witnessed unprecedented efforts to prepare for and respond to natural and human-made disasters. Following the creation of DHS in 2002 and the establishment of the National Incident Management System (NIMS) and the National Response Framework (NRF) in 2008, the nation confronted major natural disasters, such as hurricanes Katrina, Rita, and Wilma in 2005. In December 2006, President Bush signed into law the Pandemic and All-Hazards Preparedness Act (PAHPA), which sought "to improve the nation's public health and medical preparedness and response capabilities for emergencies, whether deliberate, accidental, or natural" (DHHS 2010b). The Act authorized a new Assistant Secretary for Preparedness and Response (ASPR) within DHHS and called for the establishment of a quadrennial National Health Security Strategy (NHSS), with specific planning provisions that included National Preparedness Goal implementation and the Strategic National Stockpile (SNS).

In 2007, in response to a call from Homeland Security Presidential Directive 21 to enhance the nation's ability to detect and respond to health-related threats, CDC and DHHS developed the National Biosurveillance Strategy for Human Health. Six priority areas were established: electronic health information exchange, electronic laboratory information exchange, unstructured data, integrated biosurveillance information, global disease detection and collaboration, and biosurveillance workforce. A progress report shows that most states and localities have strong biological laboratory capabilities and capacities, with nearly 90% of laboratories in the Laboratory Response Network reachable around the clock (CDC 2010b).

Notable progress has also been made in the detection of hazardous substances. The Hazardous Substances Emergency Event Surveillance system (HSEES), which was established in 1998 to reduce injury and death among first responders, employees, and the general public, tracked 8,150 hazardous substance incidents, 2,290 injuries, and 67 fatalities sustained from hazardous substance incidents. In addition, 606 incidents led to the evacuation of 48,464 people in 14 states in 2008 (CDC 2010b).

DETERMINANTS OF HEALTH

Health determinants are major factors that, over time, affect the health and well-being of individuals. Individual health eventually determines, at an aggregate level, the health of communities and even larger populations. An understanding of health determinants is necessary for any positive interventions necessary to improve health and longevity at both the individual and population levels.

Blum's Model of Health Determinants

In 1974, Blum (1981) proposed an "Environment of Health" model, later called the "Force Field and Well-Being Paradigms of Health" (Figure 7-3). Blum proposed four major inputs that contributed to health and well-being. These main influences (called "force fields") are environment, lifestyle, heredity, and medical care, all of which must be considered simultaneously when addressing the health status of an individual or a population. In other words, there is no single pathway to better health, because health determinants interact in complex ways. Consequently, improvement in health requires a multipronged approach.

The four wedges in Figure 7-3 represent the four major force fields. The size of each wedge signifies its relative importance. Thus the most important force field, according to this model, is environment, followed by lifestyles and heredity. Medical care has the least impact on health and well-being.

Environment

Environmental factors encompass the physical, socioeconomic, sociopolitical, and sociocul-

tural dimensions. Among physical environmental factors are air pollution, food and water contaminants, radiation, toxic chemicals, wastes, disease vectors, safety hazards, and habitat alterations.

The relationship of socioeconomic status (SES) to health and well-being may be explained by the general likelihood that people who have better education will also have higher incomes. They tend to live in better homes and locations where they are less exposed to environmental risks. They have better access to health care and are more likely to avoid risky behaviors, such as smoking and drug abuse. The greater the economic gap between the rich and the poor in a given geographic area, the worse the health status of the population in that area is likely to be. It has been suggested that wide income gaps produce less social cohesion, greater psychosocial stress, and, consequently, poorer health (Wilkinson 1997). For example, social cohesion—

| FIGURE 7-3 | The Force Field and Well-Being Paradigms of Health |

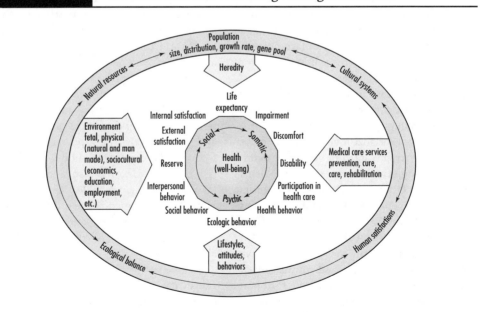

Source: Reprinted with permission from H.L. Blum, *Planning for Health,* © 1981, Human Sciences Press.

characterized by a hospitable social environment in which people trust one another and participate in communal activities—is linked to lower overall mortality and better self-rated health (Kawachi et al. 1997, 1999). Researchers have postulated that a political and policy context that creates income inequality is a precursor to health inequalities (Dye 1991). However, even countries with national health insurance programs, such as Britain, Australia, Denmark, and Sweden, experience persistent and widening disparities in health according to socioeconomic status (Pincus et al. 1998). The joint relationship of income inequality and availability of primary care has also been found to be significantly associated with individuals' self-rated health status (Shi et al. 2002).

The relationship between education and health status has been well established. Less-educated Americans die younger, compared to their better-educated counterparts. Unemployment may affect social health because of reduced social functioning; mental health because of increased levels of stress; and physical health due to various stress-related illnesses. Pincus and colleagues (1998) proposed that poor health in sociologically disadvantaged populations results more from unfavorable social conditions and ineffective self-management than from limitations in access to medical care.

The environment can also have a significant influence on developmental health. It has been shown, for example, that children who are isolated and do not socialize much with their peers tend to be overrepresented in groups of delinquents and adults with mental health problems (Wynder and Orlandi 1984). Research points out that the experiences that children have and the way adults interact with them in early years have a major impact on children's mental and emotional development. Neuroscientists have found that good nurturing and stimulation in the first 3 years of life—a prime time for brain development—activate neural pathways in the brain that might otherwise atrophy and may even permanently increase the number of brain cells. Hence, the importance of quality of child care provided in the first 3 years of life is monumental (Shellenbarger 1997).

Lifestyle

Lifestyle, or behavioral risk factors, were previously discussed. This section provides some illustrations of how lifestyle factors are related to health. Studies have shown that diet and foods, for example, play a major role in most of the significant health problems of today. Heart disease, diabetes, stroke, and cancer are but some of the diseases with direct links to dietary choices. Throughout the world, incidence and mortality rates for many forms of cancer are rising, yet research has clearly indicated that a significant portion of cancer is preventable. The role of diet and nutrition in cancer prevention has been one of the most exciting and promising research areas over the past few years. Researchers estimate that 40% to 60% of all cancers, and as many as 35% of cancer deaths, are linked to diet (American Institute for Cancer Research 1996). Current research also shows that a diet rich in fruits, vegetables, and low-fat dairy foods, and with reduced saturated and total fat, can substantially lower blood pressure (see, for example, the DASH Eating Plan recommended by DHHS; available at http://www.nhlbi.nih.gov/health /public/heart/hbp/dash /new_dash.pdf as of April 2011). Thus a nutritional approach can be effective in both preventing and treating hypertension and other diseases. The role of exercise and physical activity as a potentially useful, effective, and acceptable method for reducing the risk of colon cancer is also significant (Macfarlane and Lowenfels 1994). Research findings have also confirmed the association between recreational and/or occupational physical activity and a reduced risk of colon cancer (White et al. 1996).

Heredity

Genetic factors predispose individuals to certain diseases. For example, cancer occurs when the body's healthy genes lose their ability to suppress malignant growth or when other genetic processes stop working properly, although this does not mean that cancer is entirely a disease of the genes (Davis and Webster 2002).

A person can do little about the genetic makeup he or she has inherited. However, lifestyles and behaviors that a person may currently engage in can have significant influences on future progeny. Advances in gene therapy hold the promise of treating a variety of inherited or acquired diseases.

Medical Care

Even though the other three factors are more important in the determination of health, well-being, and susceptibility to premature death, medical care is, nevertheless, a key determinant of health. Both individual and population health are closely related to having access to adequate preventive and curative healthcare services. Despite the fact that medical care, compared to the other three factors, has the least impact on health and well-being, Americans' attitudes toward health improvement focus on more medical research, development of new medical technology, and spending more on high-tech medical care. Yet, significant declines in mortality rates were achieved well before the modernization of Western medicine and the escalation in medical care expenditures.

The availability of primary care may be one alternative pathway through which income inequality influences population-level health outcomes. Shi and colleagues (1999, 2001) examined the joint relationships among income inequality, availability of primary care, and certain health indicators. The results suggest that access to primary care physicians, in addition to income inequality, significantly correlates with reduced mortality, increased life expectancy, and improved birth outcome. In the United States, individuals living in states with a higher primary care physician-to-population ratio are more likely to report good health than those living in states with a lower ratio (Shi et al. 2002).

Contemporary Models of Health Determinants

Although Blum's model lays the foundation for understanding the determinants of health and wellness, more recent models have built upon this foundation. For example, the model proposed by Dahlgren and Whitehead (2006) states that age, sex, and genetic makeup are fixed factors, but other factors in the surrounding layers can be modified to positively influence population health. Individual lifestyle factors have the potential to promote or damage health, and social interactions can sustain people's health; but living and working conditions; food supplies; access to essential goods and services; and the overall economic, cultural, and environmental conditions have wider influences on individual and population health.

Ansari and colleagues (2003) proposed a public health model of the social determinants of health in which the determinants are categorized into four major groups: social determinants, healthcare system attributes, disease inducing behaviors, and health outcomes (Ansari et al. 2003).

The WHO Commission on Social Determinants of Health (WHOCSDH, 2007) concluded that "the social conditions in which people are born, live, and work are the single most important determinant of one's health status." The WHO model provides a conceptual framework for understanding the socioeconomic and political contexts; structural determinants; intermediary determinants (including material circumstances, social-environmental circumstances, behavioral and biological factors, social cohesion, and the healthcare system); and the impact on health equity and well-being measured as health outcomes.

In the United States, government agencies, such as CDC and DHHS, have recognized the need to address health inequities. CDC's National Center for HIV/AIDS, Viral Hepatitis, STD, and TB Prevention adopted the WHO framework on social determinants of health to use as a guide for its activities (see Figure 7-4). The Patient Protection and Affordable Care Act of 2010 and *Healthy People 2020* also focus on health determinants that may create new opportunities to apply a comprehensive approach to address health disparities.

Overarching Factors and Implications for Healthcare Delivery

The force fields illustrated in Blum's model (Figure 7-3) are affected by broad national and international factors, such as a nation's population characteristics, natural resources, ecological balance, human satisfactions, and cultural systems. Among these factors, the type of healthcare delivery system can also be included. In the United States, the preponderance of healthcare expenditures is devoted to the treatment of medical conditions rather than to the prevention and control of factors that produce those medical conditions in the first place. This misdirection can be traced to the conflicts that often result from the beliefs and values ingrained in the American culture.

CULTURAL BELIEFS AND VALUES

A value system orients the members of a society toward defining what is desirable for that society. It has been observed that even a society as complex and highly differentiated as in the United States can be said to have a relatively well-integrated system of institutionalized common values at the societal level (Parsons 1972). Although such a view may still prevail, American society now has several different subcultures that have grown in size due to a steady influx of immigrants from different parts of the world.

The current system of health services delivery traces its roots to the traditional beliefs and values espoused by the American people. The value and belief system governs the training and general orientation of healthcare providers, types of health delivery settings, financing and allocation of resources, and access to health care. Also, beliefs and values have historically led Americans to oppose any major reforms of the healthcare system. Healthcare systems in other countries also reflect deeply rooted beliefs and values. For example, Canadians prefer

FIGURE 7-4   WHO Commission on Social Determinants of Health's Conceptual Framework

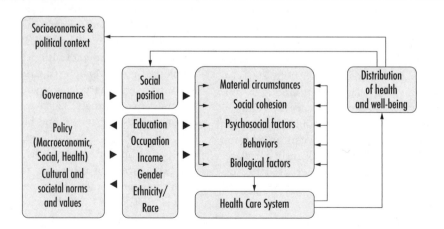

Source: Centers for Disease Control and Prevention. 2010a. *Establishing a Holistic Framework to Reduce Inequities in HIV, Viral Hepatitis, STDs, and Tuberculosis in the United States.*

increased spending on health and social programs to receiving a tax cut from the government. Conversely, Americans are skeptical of any heavy-handed government involvement in the healthcare system.

Some of the main beliefs and values predominant in the American culture are outlined as follows:

1. A strong belief in the advancement of science and the application of scientific methods to medicine were instrumental in creating the medical model that primarily governs healthcare delivery in the United States. In turn, the medical model has fueled the tremendous growth in medical science and technological innovation. As a result, the United States has been leading the world in medical breakthroughs. These developments have had numerous implications for health services delivery:

   a. They increase the demand for the latest treatments and raise patients' expectations for finding cures.

   b. Medical professionals have been preoccupied, almost exclusively, with clinical interventions, whereas the holistic aspects of health and use of alternative therapies have been deemphasized.

   c. Healthcare professionals have been trained to focus on physical symptoms rather than the underlying causes of disease.

   d. Few attempts have been made to integrate diagnosis and treatment with health education and disease prevention.

   e. The concern with diseases has funneled most research efforts away from the pursuit of health and toward the development of sophisticated medical technology. Commitment of resources to the preservation and enhancement of health and well-being has lagged far behind.

   f. Medical specialists, using the latest technology, are held in higher esteem and earn higher incomes than general practitioners and health educators.

   g. The desirability of healthcare delivery institutions, such as hospitals, is often evaluated based on their acquisition of advanced technology.

   h. Whereas biomedicine has taken central stage, diagnosis and treatment of mental health have been relegated to a lesser status.

   i. The biomedical model has isolated the social and spiritual elements of health.

2. America has been a champion of capitalism. Due to a strong belief in capitalism, health care has largely been viewed as an economic good (or service), not as a public resource.

3. A culture of capitalism promotes entrepreneurial spirit and self-determination. Hence, individual capabilities to obtain health services have largely determined the production and consumption of health care—which services will be produced, where and in what quantity, and who will have access to those services. Some key implications are as follows:

   a. Financing of health care largely through private health insurance has made access to health care a social privilege.

   b. A clear distinction exists between the types of services for poor and affluent communities and between those in rural and urban locations.

   c. The culture of individualism emphasizes individual health rather than population health. Medical practice, therefore, has been directed at keeping the individual healthy rather than keeping the entire community healthy.

4. A concern for the most underprivileged classes in society—the poor, the elderly, the disabled, and children—led to the creation of the public programs Medicare, Medicaid, and CHIP.

5. Principles of free enterprise and a general distrust of big government have kept the delivery of health care largely in private hands. Hence, a separation also exists between public health functions and the private practice of medicine.

EQUITABLE DISTRIBUTION OF HEALTH CARE

Scarcity of economic resources is a central economic concept. From this perspective, health care can be viewed as an economic good. Two fundamental questions arise with regard to how scarce healthcare resources ought to be used:

1. How much health care should be produced?
2. How should health care be distributed?

The first question concerns the appropriate combination in which health services ought to be produced in relation to all other goods and services in the overall economy. If more health care is produced, a society may have to do less with some other goods, such as food, clothing, and transportation. The second question affects individuals at a more personal level. It deals with who can receive which type of medical service, and how access to services will be restricted.

The production, distribution, and subsequent consumption of health care must be perceived as equitable. No society has found a perfectly equitable method to distribute limited economic resources. In fact, any method of resource distribution leaves some inequalities. Societies, therefore, try to allocate resources according to some guiding principles acceptable to each society. Such principles are ingrained in a society's value and belief system. It is recognized that not everyone can receive everything medical science has to offer. The fundamental question that deals with distributive justice or equity is who should receive the medical goods and services that society produces (Santerre and Neun 1996). By extension, this basic question about equity includes not only who should receive medical care, but also which type of services and in what quantity.

A just and fair allocation of health care poses conceptual and practical difficulties; hence, a theory of justice needs to resolve the problem of healthcare allocation (Jonsen 1986). The principle of justice derives from ethical theories, especially those advanced by John Rawls, who defined justice as fairness (Darr 1991). Even though various ethical principles can be used to guide decisions pertaining to just and fair allocation of health care in individual circumstances, the broad concern about equitable access to health services is addressed by the theories referred to as market justice and social justice. These two contrasting theories govern the production and distribution of healthcare services.

Market Justice

The principle of *market justice* ascribes the fair distribution of health care to the market forces in a free economy. Medical care and its benefits are distributed based on people's willingness and ability to pay (Santerre and Neun 1996). In other words, people are entitled to purchase a share of the available goods and services that they value. They are to purchase these valued goods and services by means of wealth acquired through their own legitimate efforts. This is how most goods and services are distributed in a free market. The free market implies that giving people something they have not earned would be morally and economically wrong.

Chapter 6 discussed several characteristics that describe a free market. Those market characteristics are a precondition to the distribution of healthcare services according to market justice principles. It should be added that health care in the United States is not delivered in a free market; rather, it is delivered in a quasi-market (see Chapter 6). Hence, market justice principles are only partially applicable to the U.S. healthcare delivery system. Distribution of health care according to market justice is based on the following key assumptions:

- Health care is like any other economic good or service, the distribution and consumption of which are determined by free market forces of supply and demand.
- Individuals are responsible for their own achievements. From the rewards of their achievements, people are free to obtain various economic goods and services, including

health care. When individuals pursue their own best interests, the interests of society as a whole are best served (Ferguson and Maurice 1970).

- People make rational choices in their decisions to purchase healthcare products and services. People demand health care because it can rectify a health problem and restore health, can reduce pain and discomfort and make people feel better, and can reduce anxiety about their health and well-being. Therefore, people are willing to purchase healthcare services. Grossman (1972) proposed that health is also an investment commodity; that is, people consider the purchase of health services as an investment. For example, the investment has a monetary payoff when it reduces the number of sick days, making extra time available for productive activities, such as earning a living. Alternatively, it can have a utility payoff—a payoff in terms of satisfaction—when it makes life more enjoyable and fulfilling.

- People, in consultation with their physicians, know what is best for them. This assumption implies that people place a certain degree of trust in their physicians and that the physician–patient relationship is ongoing.

- The marketplace works best with minimum interference from the government. In other words, the market, rather than the government, can allocate healthcare resources in the most efficient and equitable manner.

The classical ethical theory known as *deontology* may be applied to market justice. Deontology asserts that it is an individual's duty (from the Greek word "deon") to do what is right. The results are not important. Deontology emphasizes individual responsibilities, as in a physician–patient relationship. A physician is duty bound to do whatever is necessary to restore a patient's health. The patient is responsible for compensating the physician for his or her services. The destitute and poor may be served by charity, but deontology largely tends

to ignore the importance of societal good. It does not address what responsibilities people have toward the society.

Market justice may also be associated with the libertarian view that equity is achieved when resources are distributed according to merits. That is, health care should be distributed according to minimum standards and financed according to willingness to pay. According to this view, equality in health status need not be a central priority (Starfield 1998).

Under market justice, the production of health care is determined by how much the consumers are willing and able to purchase at the prevailing market prices. It follows that, in a free market system, individuals without sufficient income face a financial barrier to obtaining health care (Santerre and Neun 1996). Thus prices and ability to pay ration the quantity and type of healthcare services people consume. The uninsured and those who lack sufficient income to pay privately face barriers to obtaining health care. Such limitations to obtaining health care are referred to as "rationing by ability to pay" (Feldstein 1994), *demand-side rationing*, or price rationing.

The key characteristics and their implications under the system of market justice are summarized in Table 7-4. Market justice emphasizes individual, rather than collective, responsibility for health. It proposes private, rather than government, solutions to social problems of health.

Social Justice

The idea of social justice is at odds with the principles of capitalism and market justice. The term "social justice" was invented in the 19th century by the critics of capitalism to describe the "good society" (Kristol 1978). According to the principle of *social justice*, the equitable distribution of health care is a societal responsibility, which is best achieved by letting a central agency, generally the government, take over the production and distribution of health care. Social justice regards health care as a social

TABLE 7-4	Comparison of Market Justice and Social Justice

Market Justice	Social Justice
Characteristics	
Views health care as an economic good	Views health care as a social resource
Assumes free market conditions for health services delivery	Requires active government involvement in health services delivery
Assumes that markets are more efficient in allocating health resources equitably	Assumes that the government is more efficient in allocating health resources equitably
Production and distribution of health care determined by market-based demand	Medical resource allocation determined by central planning
Medical care distribution based on people's ability to pay	Ability to pay is inconsequential for receiving medical care
Access to medical care viewed as an economic reward of personal effort and achievement	Equal access to medical services viewed as a basic right
Implications	
Individual responsibility for health	Collective responsibility for health
Benefits based on individual purchasing power	Everyone is entitled to a basic package of benefits
Limited obligation to the collective good	Strong obligation to the collective good
Emphasis on individual well-being	Community well-being supersedes that of the individual
Private solutions to social problems	Public solutions to social problems
Rationing based on ability to pay	

good—as opposed to an economic good—that should be collectively financed and available to all citizens regardless of the individual recipient's ability to pay for that care. Canadians and Europeans, for example, long ago reached a broad social consensus that health care is a social good (Reinhardt 1994). Public health also has a social justice orientation (Turnock 1997). Under the social justice system, inability to obtain medical services because of a lack of financial resources is considered inequitable. A just distribution of health care must be based on

need, not simply on one's ability to purchase in the marketplace

DISCUSSION QUESTIONS

1. Discuss the differences between health, illness, and disease. How are these concepts related to the role of the advanced nurse practitioner in the delivery of health care?

2. What is the role of the advanced practice nurse in health promotion and disease prevention? Discuss how the advanced practice nurse's responsibilities differ for each of the roles.

3. Health promotion and disease prevention may require both behavioral modification and therapeutic intervention. Discuss the role of the advanced practice nurse in both approaches to care.

4. What are the main objectives of public health related to the role of the advanced practice nurse?

5. The Blum model points to four key determinants of health. Discuss their implications for healthcare delivery.

6. Discuss the main cultural beliefs and values in U.S. society that have influenced healthcare delivery, including how they have shaped the healthcare delivery system.

7. Briefly describe the concepts of market justice and social justice. In what way do these two principles complement each other, and in what way are they in conflict in the U.S. system of healthcare delivery?

8. To what extent do you think the objectives set forth in *Healthy People* initiatives can achieve the vision of an integrated approach to healthcare delivery in the United States? What is the role of the advanced nurse practitioner in advancing these initiatives?

REFERENCES

Agency for Healthcare Research and Quality. 2006. The Medical Expenditure Panel Survey. Available at: http://www.ahrq.gov/. Accessed December 2008.

American Institute for Cancer Research. 1996. *Food, nutrition and the prevention of cancer: A global perspective*. Washington, DC. Available at: http://www.aicr.org/site/PageServer. Accessed December 2000.

American Physical Therapy Association. 1997. Religion called valuable health tool. *PT Bulletin*, 10 October, p. 7.

Ansari, Z. et al. 2003. A public health model of the social determinants of health. *Sozial und Präventivmedizin/Social and Preventive Medicine* 48, no. 4: 242–251.

Berger, K.S. 1988. *The developing person through the lifespan*. 2nd ed. New York: Worth Publishers.

Blum, H.L. 1981. *Planning for health*. 2nd ed. New York: Human Sciences Press.

Breslow, L. 1972. A quantitative approach to the World Health Organization definition of health: Physical, mental and social well-being. *International Journal of Epidemiology* 1, no. 4: 347–355.

Centers for Disease Control and Prevention (CDC). 1999. *Morbidity and mortality weekly report* 48, no. 29.

Centers for Disease Control and Prevention (CDC). 2007. Avian influenza (bird flu). Available at: http://www.cdc.gov/flu/avian/. Accessed January 2007.

Centers for Disease Control and Prevention (CDC). 2010a. Establishing a holistic framework to reduce inequities in HIV, Viral Hepatitis, STDs, and Tuberculosis in the United States. Available at: www.cdc.gov/socialdeterminants. Accessed November 2010.

Centers for Disease Control and Prevention (CDC). 2010b. Office of Public Health Preparedness and Response. Public health preparedness: Strengthening the Nation's emergency response state by state. Available at: http://www.bt.cdc.gov/publications/2010phprep. Accessed November 2010.

Cohen, M.H. 2003. *Future medicine*. Ann Arbor: University of Michigan Press.

Dahlgren, G., and M. Whitehead. 2006. European strategies for tackling social inequities in health: Concepts and principles for tackling social inequities in health: Levelling up (part 2). Denmark: World Health Organization: Studies on Social and Economic Determinants of Population Health no. 3. Available at: http://www.euro.who.int/__data/assets/pdf_file/0018/103824/E89384.pdf. Accessed December 2010.

Darr, K. 1991. *Ethics in health services management*. Baltimore, MD: Health Professions Press.

Davis, D.L., and P.S. Webster. 2002. The social context of science: Cancer and the Environment. *The Annals of the American Academy of Political and Social Science* 584, November 13–34.

de Leeuw, E. 1989. Concepts in health promotion: The notion of relativism. *Social Science and Medicine* 29, no. 11: 1281–1288.

Department of Health and Human Services (DHHS). 1998. *Healthy People 2010 objectives: Draft for public comment*. Washington, DC: US Government Printing Office.

Department of Health and Human Services (DHHS). 2004. *The Health consequences of smoking:*

A report of the Surgeon General. Available at: http ://www.surgeongeneral.gov/library/smoking consequences/. Accessed December 2010.

Department of Health and Human Services (DHHS). 2009. *Testimony on 2009-H1N1* influenza: *HHS* preparedness and response *efforts.* Available at: http://www.hhs.gov/asl/testify/2009/07/t200907 29b.html. Accessed November 2010.

Department of Health and Human Services (DHHS). 2010a. *Summary of the prevention and wellness initiative.* Available at: http://www.hhs.gov/recovery /programs/cdc/chronicdisease.html. Accessed November 2010.

Department of Health and Human Services (DHHS). 2010b. *Office of the Assistant Secretary for Preparedness and Response. 2010. Pandemic and All Hazards Preparedness Act.* Available at: http://www .phe.gov/Preparedness/legal/pahpa/Pages/default .aspx. Accessed November 2010.

Department of Health and Human Services (DHHS). 2010c. Healthy People 2020. Available at: http ://healthypeople.gov/2020. Accessed December 2010.

Dever, G.E. 1984. *Epidemiology in health service management.* Gaithersburg, MD: Aspen Publishers, Inc.

Dye, T.R. 1991. *Politics in states and communities.* 7th ed. Englewood Cliffs, NJ: Prentice-Hall.

Ethics Committee, Society for Academic Emergency Medicine. 1992. An ethical foundation for health care: An emergency medicine perspective. *Annals of Emergency Medicine* 21, no. 11: 1381–1387.

Feldstein, P.J. 1994. *Health policy issues: An economic perspective on health reform.* Ann Arbor, MI: AUPHA/ HAP.

Ferguson, C.E., and S.C. Maurice. 1970. *Economic analysis.* Homewood, IL: Richard D. Irwin.

Friedman, G.D. 1980. *Primer of epidemiology.* New York: McGraw-Hill.

Grossman, M. 1972. On the concept of health capital and the demand for health. *Journal of Political Economy* 80, no. 2: 223–255.

Hancock, L.A., and C.L. Mandle. 1994. Overview of growth and development framework. In: *Health promotion through the lifespan.* C.L. Edelman and C.L. Mandle, eds. St. Louis, MO: Mosby–Year Book.

Hatch, R.L. et al. 1998. The spiritual involvement and beliefs scale: Development and testing of a new instrument. *Journal of Family Practice* 46: 476–486.

Henry, R.C. 1993. Community partnership model for health professions education. *Journal of the American Podiatric Medical Association* 83, no. 6: 328–331.

Holahan, J. 2011. The 2007-09 recession and health insurance coverage. *Health Affairs* 30, no. 1:145–152.

Ibrahim, M.A. 1985. *Epidemiology and health policy.* Gaithersburg, MD: Aspen Publishers, Inc.

Institute of Medicine, National Academy of Sciences (IOM). 1988. *The future of public health.* Washington, DC: National Academy Press.

Jonsen, A.R. 1986. Bentham in a box: Technology assessment and health care allocation. *Law, Medicine, and Health Care* 14, no. 3–4: 172–174.

Kaiser Family Foundation. 2010. *Summary of New Health Reform Law.* Available at: http://www.kff .org/healthreform/upload/8061.pdf. Accessed November 2010.

Kane, R.L. 1988. Empiric approaches to prevention in the elderly: Are we promoting too much? In: *Health promotion and disease prevention in the elderly.* R. Chernoff and D.A. Lipschitz, eds. New York: Raven Press. pp. 127–141.

Katz, S., and C.A. Akpom. 1979. A measure of primary sociobiological functions. In: *Sociomedical health indicators.* J. Elinson and A.E. Siegman, eds. Farmingdale, NY: Baywood Publishing Co. pp. 127–141.

Kawachi, I. et al. 1997. Social capital, income inequality, and mortality. *American Journal of Public Health* 87: 1491–1498.

Kawachi, I. et al. 1999. Social capital and self-rated health: A contextual analysis. *American Journal of Public Health* 89: 1187–1193.

Kristol, I. 1978. A capitalist conception of justice. In: *Ethics, free enterprise, and public policy: Original essays on moral issues in business.* R.T. De George and J.A. Pichler, eds. New York: Oxford University Press. pp. 57–69.

Lasker, R.D. 1997. *Medicine and public health: The power of collaboration.* New York: The New York Academy of Medicine.

Levin, J.S. 1994. Religion and health: Is there an association, is it valid, and is it causal? *Social Science and Medicine* 38, no. 11: 1475–1482.

Long, M.J. 1994. *The medical care system: A conceptual model.* Ann Arbor, MI: Health Administration Press.

Macfarlane, G.J., and A.B. Lowenfels. 1994. Physical activity and colon cancer. *European Journal of Cancer Prevention* 3, no. 5: 393–398.

Marwick, C. 1995. Should physicians prescribe prayer for health? Spiritual aspects of well-being considered. *Journal of the American Medical Association* 273, no. 20: 1561–1562.

Maugans, T.A. 1996. The SPIRITual history. *Archives of Family Medicine* 5, no. 1:11–16.

McCullough, M.E., and D.B. Larson. 1999. Religion and depression: A review of the literature. *Twin Research 2*: 126–136.

McCullough, M.E. et al. 2000. Religious involvement and mortality: A meta-analytic review. *Health Psychology* 19, no. 3: 211–222.

McKee, M. 2001. Measuring the efficiency of health systems. *British Medical Journal* 323, no. 7308: 295–296.

Ostir, G.V. et al. 1999. Disability in older adults 1: Prevalence, causes, and consequences. *Behavioral Medicine* 24, no. 4: 147–156.

Parsons, T. 1972. Definitions of health and illness in the light of American values and social structure. In: *Patients, physicians and illness: A sourcebook in behavioral science and health*. 2nd ed. E.G. Jaco, ed. New York: Free Press.

Partnership to Fight Chronic Disease (PFCD). 2009. *Almanac of Chronic Disease.*

Pasley, B.H. et al. 1995. Excess acute care bed capacity and its causes: The experience of New York State. *Health Services Research* 30, no. 1: 115–131.

Peters, K.E. et al. 2001. *Cooperative actions for health programs: Lessons learned in medicine and public health collaboration*. Chicago: American Medical Association. Available at: http://fightchronicdisease.ward health.com/resources/almanac-chronic-disease-0. Accessed April 25, 2011.

Pincus, T. et al. 1998. Social conditions and self-management are more powerful determinants of health than access to care. *Annals of Internal Medicine* 129, no. 5: 406–411.

Plotkin, S.L., and S.A. Plotkin. 1999. A short history of vaccination. In: *Vaccines*, 3rd ed. S.A. Plotkin and W.A. Orenstein, eds. Philadelphia, PA: W.B. Saunders.

Post, S.G. et al. 2000. Physicians and patient spirituality: Professional boundaries, competency, and ethics. *Annals of Internal Medicine* 132, no. 7: 578–583.

Puchalski, C., and A.L. Romer. 2000. Taking a spiritual history allows clinicians to understand patients more fully. *Journal of Palliative Medicine* 3, no. 1: 129–137.

Reinhardt, U.E. 1994. Providing access to health care and controlling costs: The universal dilemma. In: *The nation's health*, 4th ed. P.R. Lee and C.L. Estes, eds. Boston: Jones & Bartlett Publishers. pp. 263–278.

Robert Wood Johnson Foundation. 2010. *Chronic care: Making the case for ongoing care*. Available at: http://www.rwjf.org/pr/product.jsp?id=50968. Accessed April 25, 2011.

Roberts, J.A. et al. 1997. Factors influencing the views of patients with gynecologic cancer about end-of-life decisions. *American Journal of Obstetrics and Gynecology* 176: 166–172.

Rosen, G. 1993. *A history of public health*. Baltimore, MD: Johns Hopkins University Press.

Ross, L. 1995. The spiritual dimension: Its importance to patients' health, well-being and quality of life and its implications for nursing practice. *International Journal of Nursing Studies* 32, no. 5: 457–468.

Santerre, R.E., and S.P. Neun. 1996. *Health economics: Theories, insights, and industry studies*. Chicago: Irwin.

Saward, E., and A. Sorensen. 1980. The current emphasis on preventive medicine. In: *Issues in health services*. S.J. Williams, ed. New York: John Wiley & Sons. pp. 17–29.

Schneider, M.J. 2000. *Introduction to public health*. Gaithersburg, MD: Aspen Publishers, Inc.

Shellenbarger, S. 1997. Good, early care has a huge impact on kids, studies say. *The Wall Street Journal*, 9 April, B1.

Shi, L., and B. Starfield. 2001. Primary care physician supply, income inequality, and racial mortality in US metropolitan areas. *American Journal of Public Health* 91, no. 8: 1246–1250.

Shi, L. et al. 1999. Income inequality, primary care, and health indicators. *Journal of Family Practice* 48, no. 4: 275–284.

Shi, L. et al. 2002. Primary care, self-rated health, and reduction in social disparities in health. *Health Services Research* 37, no. 3: 529–550.

Shortell, S.M. et al. 1995. Reinventing the American hospital. *The Milbank Quarterly* 73, no. 2:131–160.

Smith, B.C. 1979. *Community health: An epidemiological approach*. New York: Macmillan Publishing Co. pp. 197–213.

Starfield, B. 1998. *Primary care and health services*. Oxford: Oxford University Press.

Swanson, C.S. 1995. A spirit-focused conceptual model of nursing for the advanced practice nurse. *Issues in Comprehensive Pediatric Nursing* 18, no. 4: 267–275.

Tamm, M.E. 1993. Models of health and disease. *British Journal of Medical Psychology* 66, no. 3: 213–228.

Timmreck, T.C. 1994. *An introduction to epidemiology*. Boston: Jones & Bartlett Publishers.

Turnock, B.J. 1997. *Public health: What it is and how it works*. Gaithersburg, MD: Aspen Publishers, Inc.

Vella-Brodrick, D.A., and F.C. Allen. 1995. Development and psychometric validation of the mental, physical, and spiritual well-being scale. *Psychological Reports* 77, no. 2: 659–674.

Ward, B. 1995. Holistic medicine. *Australian Family Physician* 24, no. 5: 761–762, 765.

White, E. et al. 1996. Physical activity in relation to colon cancer in middle-aged men and women. *American Journal of Epidemiology* 144, no. 1: 42–50.

Wilkinson, R.G. 1997. Comment: Income, inequality, and social cohesion. *American Journal of Public Health* 87: 1504–1506.

Wolinsky, F. 1988. *The sociology of health: Principles, practitioners, and issues.* 2nd ed. Belmont, CA: Wadsworth Publishing.

WHO Commission on Social Determinants of Health. 2007. V. CSDH framework for Action. In: *A Conceptual Framework for Action on the Social Determinants of Health.* Geneva, Switzerland: World Health Organization, 15–49, 71–75. Available at: http://www.who.int/social_determinants/resource /csdh_framework_action_05_07.pdf. Accessed November 4, 2009.

World Health Organization (WHO). 1948. *Preamble to the constitution.* Geneva, Switzerland: Author.

Wynder, E.L., and M.A. Orlandi. 1984. *The American Health Foundation guide to lifespan health: A family program for physical and emotional well-being.* New York: Dodd, Mead & Company.

CHAPTER 8

The Evolution of Health Services in the United States

Leiyu Shi and Douglas A. Singh

CHAPTER OBJECTIVES

1. Discover historical developments that have shaped the nature of the U.S. healthcare delivery system.

2. Evaluate why the system has been resistant to national health insurance reforms.

3. Explore developments associated with the corporatization of health care.

4. Speculate on whether the era of socialized medicine has dawned in the United States.

INTRODUCTION

The healthcare delivery system of the United States evolved quite differently from the systems in Europe. American values and the social, political, and economic antecedents on which the U.S. system is based have led to the formation of a unique system of healthcare delivery. This chapter discusses how these forces have been instrumental in shaping the current structure of medical services and how they are likely to shape its future. The evolutionary changes discussed here illustrate the American beliefs and values in action, within the context of broad social, political, and economic changes. Because social, political, and economic contexts are not static, their shifting influences lend a certain dynamism to the healthcare delivery system. Conversely, beliefs and values remain relatively stable over time. Consequently, in the American healthcare delivery experience, initiatives toward a national healthcare program have failed to make significant inroads. However, social, political, and economic forces have led to certain compromises, as seen in the creation of Medicare, Medicaid, and other public programs to extend health insurance to certain defined groups of people.

Could major social or economic shifts eventually usher in a national healthcare system? It is anyone's guess. Given the right set of conditions, a national healthcare system could become a reality in the United States, as recently seen with the passage of the Patient Protection and Affordable Care Act (ACA) of 2010, which promises to reduce the number of uninsured by 32 million (Henry J. Kaiser Family Foundation 2011). Cultural beliefs and values are strong forces against attempts to initiate fundamental changes in the financing and delivery of health care. Therefore, enactment of major health system reforms requires consensus among Americans on basic values and ethics (Kardos and Allen 1993). Ironically, American beliefs and values were not allowed a chance to play out in the political maneuvering that led to the passage of the ACA of 2010.

The growth of medical science and technology has also played a key role in shaping the U.S. healthcare delivery system. Stevens (1971) points out that the technological revolution has been primarily responsible for bringing medicine into the public domain. Advancement of technology has influenced other factors as well, such as medical education, growth of institutions, and urban development. Hence, American medicine did not emerge as a professional entity until the beginning of the 20th century, with the progress in biomedical science. Since then, the U.S. healthcare delivery system has been a growth enterprise. Debates over issues such as methods of financing health care, quality improvement, and the appropriate role of government have also been rooted in the presumed importance of gaining access to ever-rising levels of scientific medicine (Somers and Somers 1977).

This chapter traces the evolution of healthcare delivery through three major historical phases, each demarcating a major change in the structure of the delivery system. The first phase is the preindustrial era from the middle of the 18th century to the latter part of the 19th century. The second phase is the postindustrial era beginning in the late 19th century. The third, most recent and current phase, is marked by the growth of managed care, organizational integration, the information revolution, and globalization, called the corporate era.

The practice of medicine is central to the delivery of health care; therefore, a major portion of this chapter is devoted to tracing the transformations in medical practice from a weak and insecure trade to an independent, highly respected, and lucrative profession. Delivery of medical services through managed care and the corporatization of physician practices, however, have made a significant impact on practice styles and have compromised the autonomy that physicians have historically enjoyed. The medical profession has also consolidated into larger organizational units, away from the solo practice of medicine that had once prevailed.

MEDICAL SERVICES IN PREINDUSTRIAL AMERICA

From Colonial times to the beginning of the 20th century, American medicine lagged behind the advances in medical science, experimental research, and medical education that were taking place in Britain, France, and Germany. While London, Paris, and Berlin were flourishing as major research centers, Americans had a tendency to neglect research in basic sciences and to place more emphasis on applied science (Shryock 1966). In addition, American attitudes toward medical treatment placed strong emphasis on natural history and conservative common sense (Stevens 1971). Consequently, the practice of medicine in the United States had a strong domestic, rather than professional, character. Medical services, when deemed appropriate by the consumer, were purchased out of one's private funds, because there was no health insurance. The healthcare market was characterized by competition among providers, and the consumer decided who the provider would be. Thus the consumer was sovereign in the healthcare market and health care was delivered under free market conditions.

Five main factors explain why the medical profession remained largely an insignificant trade in preindustrial America:

1. Medical practice was in disarray.
2. Medical procedures were primitive.
3. An institutional core was missing.
4. Demand was unstable.
5. Medical education was substandard.

Medical Practice in Disarray

The early practice of medicine could be regarded more as a trade than as a profession. It did not require the rigorous course of study, clinical practice, residency training, board exams, or licensing, without which it is impossible to practice today. At the close of the Civil War (1861–1865), "anyone who had the inclination to set himself up as a physician could do so, the exigencies of the market alone determining who would prove successful in the field and who would not" (Hamowy 1979). The clergy, for example, often combined medical services and religious duties. The generally well-educated clergyman or government official was more learned in medicine than physicians were at the time (Shryock 1966). Tradesmen, such as tailors, barbers, commodity merchants, and those engaged in numerous other trades, also practiced the healing arts by selling herbal prescriptions, nostrums, elixirs, and cathartics. Midwives, homeopaths, and naturalists could also practice medicine without restriction. The red-and-white striped poles (symbolizing blood and bandages) seen outside barbershops are reminders that barbers

also functioned as surgeons at one time, using the same blade to cut hair, shave beards, and bleed the sick.

This era of medical pluralism has been referred to as a "war zone" by Kaptchuk and Eisenberg (2001) because it was marked by bitter antagonism among the various practicing sects. Later, in 1847, the American Medical Association (AMA) was founded with the main purpose of erecting a barrier between orthodox practitioners and the "irregulars" (Rothstein 1972).

In the absence of minimum standards of medical training, entry into private practice was relatively easy for both trained and untrained practitioners, creating intense competition. Medicine as a profession was weak and unorganized. Hence, physicians did not enjoy the prestige, influence, and incomes that they later earned. Many physicians found it necessary to engage in a second occupation because income from medical practice alone was inadequate to support a family. It is estimated that most physicians' incomes in the mid-19th century placed them at the lower end of the middle class (Starr 1982). In 1830, there were approximately 6,800 physicians serving primarily the upper classes (Gabe et al. 1994). It was not until 1870 that medical education was reformed and licensing laws were passed in the United States.

Primitive Medical Procedures

Up until the mid-1800s, medical care was based more on primitive medical traditions than science. In the absence of diagnostic tools, a theory of "intake and outgo" served as an explanation for all diseases (Rosenberg 1979). It was believed that diseases needed to be expelled from the body. Hence, bleeding, use of emetics (to induce vomiting) and diuretics (to increase urination), and purging with enemas and purgatives (to clean the bowels) were popular forms of clinical therapy.

When George Washington became ill with an inflamed throat in 1799, he, too, was bled by physicians. One of the attending physicians argued, unsuccessfully, in favor of making an incision to open the trachea, which today would be considered a more enlightened procedure. The bleeding most likely weakened Washington's resistance, and historians have debated whether it played a role in his death (Clark 1998).

Surgeries were limited because anesthesia had not yet been developed and antiseptic techniques were not known. Stethoscopes and X-rays had not been discovered, clinical thermometers were not in use, and microscopes were not available for medical diagnosis. Physicians relied mainly on their five senses and experience to diagnose and treat medical problems. Hence, in most cases, physicians did not possess any technical expertise greater than that of the mothers and grandparents at home or experienced neighbors in the community.

Missing Institutional Core

In the United States, no widespread development of hospitals occurred before the 1880s. A few isolated hospitals were either built or developed in rented private houses in large cities, such as Philadelphia, New York, Boston, Cincinnati, New Orleans, and St. Louis. By contrast, general hospital expansion began much before the 1800s in France and Britain (Stevens 1971). In Europe, medical professionals were closely associated with hospitals. New advances in medical science were being pioneered, which European hospitals readily adopted. The medical profession came to be supremely regarded because of its close association with an establishment that was scientifically advanced. In contrast, American hospitals played only a small part in medical practice because most hospitals served a social welfare function by taking care of the poor, those without families, or those who were away from home on travel.

The Almshouse and the Pesthouse

In the United States, the *almshouse* was the precursor of hospitals, but it was not a hospital in the true sense. Almshouses, also called poorhouses because they served primarily the poor, existed in almost all cities of moderate size and were run by the local governments. These institutions served, primarily, general welfare functions by providing food and shelter to the destitute. Therefore, the main function of the almshouse was custodial. Caring for the sick was incidental because some of the residents would inevitably become ill and would be cared for in an adjoining infirmary. Almshouses were unspecialized institutions that admitted poor and needy persons of all kinds: the elderly, the orphaned, the insane, the ill, and the disabled. Hence, the early hospital-type institutions emerged mainly to take care of indigent people whose families could not care for them.

Another type of institution, the *pesthouse*, was operated by local governments to quarantine people who had contracted a contagious disease, such as cholera, smallpox, typhoid, or yellow fever. Located primarily in seaports, the primary function of a pesthouse was to isolate people with contagious diseases so disease would not spread among the inhabitants of a city. These institutions were the predecessors of contagious disease and tuberculosis hospitals.

The Dispensary

Dispensaries were established to provide free care to those who could not afford to pay. Urban workers and their families often depended on such charity (Rosen 1983). Dispensaries operated independently of hospitals; hence, medical practice in the United States was not legitimized because it lacked organizational affiliation.

Starting with Philadelphia in 1786, dispensaries gradually spread to other cities. They were private institutions, financed by bequests and voluntary subscriptions. Their main function was to provide basic medical care and to dispense drugs to ambulatory patients (Raffel 1980). Generally, young physicians and medical students desiring clinical experience staffed these dispensaries, as well as hospital wards, on a part-time basis for little or no income (Martensen 1996), which served a dual purpose. It provided needed services to the poor and enabled both physicians and medical students to gain experience diagnosing and treating a variety of cases. Later, as the practice of specialized medicine, as well as teaching and research, was transferred to hospital settings, many dispensaries were gradually absorbed into hospitals as outpatient departments. Indeed, outpatient or ambulatory care departments became an important locale for specialty consultation services within large hospitals (Raffel 1980).

The Mental Asylum

Mental health care was seen, primarily, as the responsibility of state and local governments. At this time, little was known about what caused mental illness or how to treat it. Although almshouses were used to accommodate some mental health patients, asylums were built by states for patients with untreatable, chronic mental illness. The first such asylum was built around 1770 in Williamsburg, Virginia. When the Pennsylvania Hospital opened in Philadelphia in 1752, its basement was used as a mental asylum. Attendants in these asylums employed physical and psychological techniques in an effort to return patients to some level of rational thinking. Techniques such as bleeding, forced vomiting, and hot and ice-cold baths were also used.

Between 1894 and World War I, the State Care Acts were passed, centralizing financial responsibility for mentally ill patients in every state government. Local governments took advantage of this opportunity to send all those with a mental illness, including dependent, older citizens, to the state asylums. The quality of care in public asylums deteriorated rapidly, as overcrowding and underfunding ran rampant (U.S. Surgeon General 1999).

The Dreaded Hospital

Not until the 1850s were hospitals similar to those in Europe developed in the United States. These early hospitals had deplorable conditions due to a lack of resources. Poor sanitation and inadequate ventilation were hallmarks of these hospitals. Unhygienic practices prevailed because nurses were unskilled and untrained. These early hospitals had an undesirable image of being houses of death. The mortality rate among hospital patients, both in Europe and America, stood around 74% in the 1870s (Falk 1999). People went into hospitals because of dire consequences, not by personal choice. It is not hard to imagine why members of the middle and upper classes, in particular, shunned such establishments.

Unstable Demand

Professional services suffered from low demand in the mainly rural, preindustrial society, and much of the medical care was provided by people who were not physicians. The most competent physicians were located in more populated communities (Bordley and Harvey 1976). In the small communities of rural America, a spirit of strong self-reliance prevailed. Families and communities were accustomed to treating the sick, often using folk remedies passed from one generation to the next. It was also common to consult books and published pamphlets on home remedies (Rosen 1983).

The market for physicians' services was also limited by economic conditions. Many families could not afford to pay for medical services. Two factors contributed to the high cost associated with obtaining professional medical care:

- The indirect costs of transportation and the "opportunity cost" of travel (i.e., forgone value of time that could have been used for something more productive) could easily outweigh the direct costs of physicians' fees.
- The costs of travel often doubled because two people, the physician and an emissary, had to make the trip back and forth. For a farmer, a trip of 10 miles into town could mean an entire day's work lost.

Physicians passed much of their day traveling along backcountry roads. Farmers had to cover travel costs and the opportunity cost of time spent traveling. Mileage charges amounted to four or five times the basic fee for a visit if a physician had to travel 5 to 10 miles. Hence, most families obtained only occasional intervention from physicians, generally for nonroutine and severe conditions (Starr 1982).

Personal health services had to be purchased without the help of government or private insurance. Private practice and *fee for service*—the practice of billing separately for each individual type of service performed—was firmly embedded in American medical care. Similar to physicians, dentists were private entrepreneurs who made their living by private fee-for-service dental practice, but their services were not in great demand because there was little public concern about dental health (Anderson 1990).

Substandard Medical Education

From about 1800 to 1850, medical training was largely received through individual apprenticeship with a practicing physician, referred to as a preceptor, rather than through university education. Many of the preceptors were themselves poorly trained, especially in basic medical sciences (Rothstein 1972). By 1800, only four small medical schools were operating in the United States: College of Philadelphia (which was established in 1756 and later became the University of Pennsylvania), King's College (which was established in 1768 and later became Columbia University), Harvard University (opened in 1783), and Dartmouth College (started in 1797).

American physicians later initiated the establishment of medical schools in large numbers. This was partly to enhance professional status and prestige and partly to enhance income. Medical schools were inexpensive to operate and often quite profitable. All that was required was a faculty of four or more physicians, a classroom, a back room to conduct dissections, and legal authority to confer degrees. Operating expenses were met totally out of student fees that were paid directly to the physicians (Rothstein 1972). Physicians would affiliate with a local col-

lege for the conferral of degrees and use of classroom facilities. Large numbers of men entered medical practice as education in medicine became readily available and unrestricted entry into the profession was still possible (Hamowy 1979). Gradually, as physicians from medical schools began to outnumber those from the apprenticeship system, the doctor of medicine (MD) degree became the standard of competence. The number of medical schools tripled between 1800 and 1820 and tripled again between 1820 and 1850, numbering 42 in 1850 (Rothstein 1972). Academic preparation gradually replaced apprenticeship training.

At this point, medical education in the United States was seriously deficient in science-based training, unlike European medical schools. Medical schools in the United States did not have laboratories, and clinical observation and practice were not part of the curriculum. In contrast, European medical schools, particularly those in Germany, were emphasizing laboratory-based medical research. At the University of Berlin, for example, professors were expected to conduct research as well as teach, and were paid by the state. In American medical schools, students were taught by local practitioners, who were ill equipped in education and training. Unlike Europe, where medical education was financed and regulated by the government, proprietary medical schools in the United States set their own standards (Numbers and Warner 1985). A year of medical school in the United States, generally, lasted only 4 months and only 2 years of study were required for graduation. In addition, American medical students customarily repeated the same courses they had taken during their first year again during their second year (Numbers and Warner 1985; Rosner 2001). The physicians' desire to keep their schools profitable also contributed to low standards and a lack of rigor. It was feared that higher standards in medical education would drive enrollments down, which could lead the schools into bankruptcy (Starr 1982).

MEDICAL SERVICES IN POSTINDUSTRIAL AMERICA

In the postindustrial period, American physicians, unlike other physicians in the world, were highly successful in retaining private practice of medicine and resisting national health care. Physicians also became an organized medical profession and delivered scientifically and technically advanced services to insured patients. Notably, much of this transformation occurred in the aftermath of the Civil War. Social and scientific changes in the period following the war were accompanied by a transition from a rural, agricultural economy to a system of industrial capitalism. Mass production techniques used in the war were applied to peacetime industries. Railroads linked the east and west coasts, and small towns became cities (Stevens 1971).

The American system for delivering health care took its current shape during this period. Private practice of medicine became firmly entrenched as physicians grew into a cohesive profession and gained power and prestige. The well-defined role of employers in providing workers' compensation for work-related injuries and illnesses, together with other economic considerations, was instrumental in the growth of private health insurance. Rising costs of health care, however, prompted Congress to create the publicly financed programs, such as Medicare and Medicaid, for the most vulnerable members of the population. Cost considerations also motivated the formation of prototypes for modern managed care organizations (MCOs).

Growth of Professional Sovereignty

The 1920s may well mark the consolidation of physicians' professional power. During and after World War I, physicians' incomes grew sharply, and their prominence as a profession finally emerged. This prestige and power, however, did not materialize overnight. Through the years, several factors interacted in the gradual transformation of medicine from a weak, insecure, and isolated trade into a profession of power and authority. Seven key factors contributed to this transformation:

1. Urbanization
2. Science and technology
3. Institutionalization
4. Dependency
5. Cohesiveness and organization
6. Licensing
7. Educational reform

Urbanization

Urbanization created increased reliance on the specialized skills of paid professionals. First, it distanced people from their families and neighborhoods where family-based care was traditionally given. Women began working outside the home and could no longer care for sick members of the family. Second, physicians became less expensive to consult as telephones, automobiles, and paved roads reduced the opportunity cost of time and travel and medical care became more affordable. Urban development attracted more and more Americans to the growing towns and cities. In 1840, only 11% of the U.S. population lived in urban areas; by 1900, the proportion of the U.S. population living in urban areas grew to 40% (Stevens 1971). The trend away from home visits to office practice also began to develop around this time (Rosen 1983). Physicians moved to cities and towns in large numbers to be closer to their growing markets. Better geographic proximity of patients enabled physicians to see more patients in a given amount of time. Whereas physicians in 1850 only saw an average of 5 to 7 patients a day, by the early 1940s, the average patient load of general practitioners had risen to 18 to 22 patients a day (Starr 1982).

Science and Technology

Exhibit 8-1 summarizes some of the groundbreaking scientific discoveries in medicine. Advances in bacteriology, antiseptic surgery, anesthesia, immunology, and diagnostic techniques,

| EXHIBIT 8-1 | Groundbreaking Medical Discoveries |

- The discovery of anesthesia was instrumental in advancing the practice of surgery. Nitrous oxide (laughing gas) was first employed as an anesthetic around 1846 for tooth extraction by Horace Wells, a dentist. Ether anesthesia for surgery was first successfully used in 1846 at the Massachusetts General Hospital. Before anesthesia was discovered, strong doses of alcohol were used to dull the sensations. A surgeon who could do procedures, such as limb amputations, in the shortest length of time was held in high regard.

- Around 1847, Ignaz Semmelweis, a Hungarian physician practicing in a hospital in Vienna, implemented the policy of hand washing. Thus an aseptic technique was born. Semmelweis was concerned about the high death rate from puerperal fever among women after childbirth. Even though the germ theory of disease was unknown at this time, Semmelweis surmised that there might be a connection between puerperal fever and the common practice by medical students of not washing their hands before delivering babies and right after doing dissections. Semmelweis's hunch was right.

- Louis Pasteur is generally credited with pioneering the germ theory of disease and microbiology around 1860. Pasteur demonstrated sterilization techniques, such as boiling to kill microorganisms and withholding exposure to air to prevent contamination.

- Joseph Lister is often referred to as the father of antiseptic surgery. Around 1865, Lister used carbolic acid to wash wounds, and popularized the chemical inhibition of infection (antisepsis) during surgery.

- Advances in diagnostics and imaging can be traced to the discovery of X-rays in 1895 by Wilhelm Roentgen, a German professor of physics. Radiology became the first machine-based medical specialty. Some of the first training schools in X-ray therapy and radiography in the United States attracted photographers and electricians to become doctors in roentgenology (from the inventor's name).

- Alexander Fleming discovered the antibacterial properties of penicillin in 1929.

along with an expanding repertoire of new drugs, gave medicine an aura of legitimacy and complexity, and the therapeutic effectiveness of scientific medicine became widely recognized.

When advanced technical knowledge becomes essential to practice a profession and the benefits of professional services are widely recognized, a greater acceptance and a legitimate need for the services of that profession are simultaneously created. *Cultural authority* refers to the general acceptance of and reliance on the judgment of the members of a profession (Starr 1982) because of their superior knowledge and expertise. Cultural authority legitimizes a profession in the eyes of common people. Advances in medical science and technology bestowed this legitimacy on the medical profession because medical practice could no longer remain within the domain of lay competence.

Scientific and technological change also required improved therapeutic competence of physicians in the diagnosis and treatment of disease. Developing these skills was no longer possible without specialized training. Science-based medicine created an increased demand for advanced services that were no longer available through family and neighbors.

Physicians' cultural authority was further bolstered when medical decisions became necessary in various aspects of healthcare delivery. For example, physicians decide whether a person should be admitted to a hospital or nursing home and for how long, whether surgical or nonsurgical treatments should be used, and which medications should be prescribed. Physicians' decisions have a profound impact on other providers and nonproviders alike. The judgment and opinions of physicians even affect aspects of a person's life outside the delivery of health care. For example, physicians often evaluate the fitness of persons for jobs during pre-employment physicals many employers demand. Physicians assess the disability of the ill and the injured in workers' compensation cases. Granting of medical leave for sickness and release back to work require authorizations from physicians. Payment of medical claims requires physicians' evaluations. Other healthcare professionals, such as nurses, therapists, and dietitians, are expected to follow physicians' orders for treatment. Thus, during disease and disability, and sometimes even in good health, people's lives have become increasingly governed by decisions made by physicians.

Institutionalization

The evolution of medical technology and the professionalization of medical and nursing staff enabled advanced treatments that necessitated the pooling of resources in a common arena of care (Burns 2004). Rapid urbanization was another factor that necessitated the institutionalization of medical care. As had already occurred in Europe, in the United States, hospitals became the core around which the delivery of medical services was organized. Thus development of hospitals as the center for the practice of scientific medicine and the professionalization of medical practice became closely intertwined.

Indeed, physicians and hospitals developed a symbiotic relationship.

For economic reasons, as hospitals expanded, their survival became increasingly dependent on physicians to keep the beds filled because the physicians decided where to hospitalize their patients. Therefore, hospitals had to make every effort to keep the physicians satisfied, which enhanced physicians' professional dominance, even though they were not employees of the hospitals. This gave physicians enormous influence over hospital policy. Also, for the first time, hospitals began conforming to both physician practice patterns and public expectations about medicine as a modern scientific enterprise. The expansion of surgery, in particular, had profound implications for hospitals, physicians, and the public. As hospitals added specialized facilities and staff, their regular use became indispensable to physicians and surgeons, who earlier had been able to manage their practices with little reference to hospitals (Martensen 1996). Affiliation with establishments symbolizing the scientific cutting edge of medicine lent power and prestige to the medical profession.

Hospitals in the United States did not expand and become more directly related to medical care until the late 1890s. However, as late as the 1930s, hospitals incurred frequent deaths due to infections that could not be prevented or cured. Nevertheless, hospital use was on the rise due to the great influx of immigrants into large American cities (Falk 1999). From only a few score in 1875, the number of general hospitals in the United States expanded to 4,000 by 1900 (Anderson 1990) and to 5,000 by 1913 (Wright 1997).

Dependency

Patients depend on the medical profession's judgment and assistance. First, dependency is created because society expects a sick person to seek medical help and try to get well. The patient is then expected to comply with medical instructions. Second, dependency is created by the profession's cultural authority because its medical judgments must be relied on to (1) legitimize a person's sickness; (2) exempt the individual from social role obligations, such as work or school; and (3) provide competent medical care so the person can get well and resume his or her social role obligations. Third, in conjunction with the physician's cultural authority, the need for hospital services for critical illness and surgery creates dependency when patients are transferred from their homes to a hospital or surgery center.

Once physicians' cultural authority became legitimized, the sphere of their influence expanded into nearly all aspects of healthcare delivery. For example, laws were passed that prohibited individuals from obtaining certain classes of drugs without a physician's prescription. Health insurance paid for treatments only when they were rendered or prescribed by physicians. Thus beneficiaries of health insurance became dependent on physicians to obtain covered services. More recent, the referral role (gatekeeping) of primary care physicians in managed care plans has increased patients' dependency on primary care physicians for referral to specialized services.

Cohesiveness and Organization

Toward the end of the 1800s, social and economic changes brought about greater cohesiveness among medical professionals. With the growth of hospitals and specialization, physicians needed support from one another for patient referrals and for access to facilities to admit their patients. Standardization of education also advanced a common core of knowledge among physicians. They no longer remained members of isolated and competing medical sects. Greater cohesiveness, in turn, advanced their professional authority (Starr 1982).

For a long time, physicians' ability to remain free of control from hospitals and insurance companies remained a prominent feature of American medicine. Hospitals and insurance companies could have hired physicians on salary to provide medical services, but individual physicians who took up practice in a corporate setting were castigated by the medical profession and pressured to abandon such practices. In some states, courts ruled that corporations could not employ licensed physicians without engaging in the unlicensed practice of medicine, a legal doctrine that became known as the "corporate practice doctrine" (Farmer and Douglas 2001). Independence from corporate control enhanced private entrepreneurship and put American physicians in an enviable strategic position in relation to hospitals and insurance companies. Later, a formally organized medical profession was in a much better position to resist control from outside entities.

The AMA was formed in 1847, but it had little strength during its first half-century of existence. Its membership was small, with no permanent organization and scant resources. The AMA did not attain real strength until it was organized into county and state medical societies and until state societies were incorporated, delegating greater control at the local level. As part of the organizational reform, the AMA also began, in 1904, to concentrate attention on medical education (Bordley and Harvey 1976). Since then, it has been the chief proponent for the practitioners of conventional medicine in the United States. Although the AMA often stressed the importance of raising the quality of care for patients and protecting the uninformed consumer from "quacks" and "charlatans," its principal goal—like that of other professional associations—was to advance the professionalization, prestige, and financial well-being of its members. The AMA vigorously pursued its objectives by promoting the establishment of state medical licensing laws and the legal requirement that, to be licensed to practice, a physician must be a graduate of an AMA-approved medical school. The concerted activities of physicians through the AMA are collectively referred to as *organized medicine*, to distinguish them from the uncoordinated actions of individual physicians competing in the marketplace (Goodman and Musgrave 1992).

Licensing

Under the Medical Practice Acts established in the 1870s, medical licensure in the United States became a function of the states (Stevens 1971). By 1896, 26 states had enacted medical licensure laws (Anderson 1990). Licensing of physicians and upgrading of medical school standards developed hand in hand. At first, licensing required only a medical school diploma. Later, candidates could be rejected if the school they had attended was judged inadequate. Finally, all candidates were required to present an acceptable diploma and pass an independent state examination (Starr 1982).

Through both licensure and upgrading of medical school standards, physicians obtained a clear monopoly on the practice of medicine (Anderson 1990). The early licensing laws served to protect physicians from the competitive pressures posed by potential new entrants into the medical profession. Physicians led the campaign to restrict the practice of medicine. As biomedicine gained political and economic ground, the biomedical community expelled providers such as homeopaths, naturopaths, and chiropractors from medical societies; prohibited professional association with them; and encouraged prosecution of such providers for unlicensed medical practice (Rothstein 1972). In 1888, in a landmark Supreme Court decision, *Dent v. West Virginia*, Justice Stephen J. Field wrote that no one had the right to practice "without having the necessary qualifications of learning and skill" (Haber 1974). In the late 1880s and 1890s, many states revised laws to require all candidates for licensure, including those holding medical degrees, to pass an examination (Kaufman 1980).

Educational Reform

Advanced medical training was made necessary by scientific progress. Reform of medical education started around 1870, with the affiliation of medical schools with universities. In 1871,

Harvard Medical School, under the leadership of a new university president, Charles Eliot, completely revolutionized the system of medical education. The academic year was extended from 4 to 9 months, and the length of medical education was increased from 2 to 3 years. Following the European model, laboratory instruction and clinical subjects, such as chemistry, physiology, anatomy, and pathology, were added to the curriculum.

Johns Hopkins University took the lead in further reforming medical education when it opened its medical school in 1893, under the leadership of William H. Welch, who trained in Germany. Medical education, for the first time, became a graduate training course, requiring a college degree, not a high school diploma, as an entrance requirement. Johns Hopkins had well-equipped laboratories, a full-time faculty for the basic science courses, and its own teaching hospital (Rothstein 1972). Standards at Johns Hopkins became the model of medical education in other leading institutions around the country. The raising of standards made it difficult for proprietary schools to survive, and, in time, proprietary schools were closed.

The Association of American Medical Colleges (AAMC) was founded in 1876 by 22 medical schools (Coggeshall 1965). Later, the AAMC set minimum standards for medical education, including a 4-year curriculum, but it was unable to enforce its recommendations. In 1904, the AMA created the Council on Medical Education, which inspected the existing medical schools and found that less than half provided acceptable levels of training. The AMA did not publish its findings but obtained the help of the Carnegie Foundation for the Advancement of Teaching to provide a rating of medical schools (Goodman and Musgrave 1992). The Foundation appointed Abraham Flexner to investigate medical schools located in both the United States and Canada. The Flexner Report, published in 1910, had a profound effect on medical education reform. The report was widely accepted by both the profession and the public. Schools that did not meet the proposed standards were forced to close. State laws were established, requiring graduation from a medical school accredited by the AMA as the basis for a license to practice medicine (Haglund and Dowling 1993).

Once advanced graduate education became an integral part of medical training, it further legitimized the profession's authority and galvanized its sovereignty. Stevens (1971) noted that American medicine moved toward professional maturity between 1890 and 1914, mainly as a direct result of educational reform.

Specialization in Medicine

Specialization has been a key hallmark of American medicine. Consider that, in 1931, 17% of all physicians in the United States were specialists, whereas today, the ratio of specialists to generalists is approximately 58 to 42 (Bureau of Labor Statistics 2011), and many generalists also have a subspecialty focus. The growth of allied healthcare professionals has also diversified, both in medical specialization—such as laboratory and radiological technologists, nurse anesthetists, and physical therapists—and in new or expanded specialist fields—such as occupational therapists, psychologists, dietitians, and medical social workers (Stevens 1971).

Lack of a rational coordination of medical care in the United States has been one consequence of the preoccupation with specialization. The characteristics of the medical profession in various countries often shape and define the key attributes of their healthcare delivery systems. The role of the primary care physician (PCP), the relationship between generalists and specialists, the ratio of practicing generalists to specialists, the structure and nature of medical staff appointments in hospitals, and the approach to group practice of medicine have all been molded by the evolving structure and ethos of the medical profession. In Britain, for example, the medical profession has divided itself into general practitioners (GPs) practicing

in the community and consultants holding specialist positions in hospitals. This kind of stratification did not develop in American medicine. PCPs in America were not assigned the role that GPs had in Britain, where patients could consult a specialist only by referral from a GP. Unlike Britain, where GPs hold a key intermediary position in relation to the rest of the healthcare delivery system, the United States has lacked such a gatekeeping role. Only since the early 1990s, under health maintenance organizations (HMOs), has the *gatekeeping* model requiring initial contact with a generalist and the generalist's referral to a specialist gained prominence. The distinctive shaping of medical practice in the United States explains why the structure of medicine did not develop around a nucleus of primary care.

From the Asylum to Community Mental Health

At the turn of the 20th century, the scientific study and treatment of mental illnesses, called neuropathology, had just begun. Later, in 1946, federal funding was made available under the National Mental Health Act for psychiatric education and research. This Act led to the creation, in 1949, of the National Institute of Mental Health (NIMH). Early treatment of mental disorders was championed, and the concept of community mental health was born. By this time, new drugs for treating psychosis and depression had become available. Reformers of the mental health system argued that long-term institutional care had been neglectful, ineffective, and even harmful (U.S. Surgeon General 1999). Passage of the Community Mental Health Centers Act of 1963 lent support to the joint policies of "community care" and "deinstitutionalization." From 1970 to 2000, state-run psychiatric hospital beds dropped from 207 to 21 beds per 100,000 persons (Manderscheid et al. 2004). The deinstitutionalization movement further intensified after the 1999 U.S. Supreme Court decision in *Olmstead v. L.C.,* which directed

U.S. states to provide community-based services to people with mental illness.

The Development of Public Health

Historically, public health practices in the United States have concentrated on sanitary regulation, the study of epidemics, and vital statistics. The growth of urban centers for the purpose of commerce and industry, unsanitary living conditions in densely populated areas, inadequate methods of sewage and garbage disposal, limited access to clean water, and long work hours in unsafe and exploitative industries led to periodic epidemics of cholera, smallpox, typhoid, tuberculosis, yellow fever, and other diseases. Such outbreaks led to arduous efforts to protect the public interest. For example, in 1793, the national capital had to be moved out of Philadelphia due to a devastating outbreak of yellow fever. This epidemic prompted the city to develop its first board of health that same year. In 1850, Lemuel Shattuck outlined the blueprint for the development of a public health system in Massachusetts. Shattuck also called for the establishment of state and local health departments. A threatening outbreak of cholera in 1873 mobilized the New York City Health Department to alleviate the worst sanitary conditions within the city. Previously, cholera epidemics in 1832 and 1848–1849 had swept through American cities and towns within a few weeks, killing thousands (Duffy 1971).

Until about 1900, infectious diseases posed the greatest health threat to society. The development of public health played a major role in curtailing the spread of infection among populations. Simultaneously, widespread public health measures and better medical care reduced mortality and increased life expectancy.

By 1900, most states had health departments that were responsible for a variety of public health efforts, such as sanitary inspections, communicable disease control, operation of state laboratories, vital statistics, health educa-

tion, and regulation of food and water (Turnock 1997; Williams 1995). Public health functions were later extended to fill gaps in the medical care system. Such functions, however, were limited mainly to child immunizations, care of mothers and infants, health screening in public schools, and family planning. Federal grants were also made available to state and local governments for programs in substance abuse, mental health, and community prevention services (Turnock 1997).

Public health has remained separate from the private practice of medicine because of the skepticism of private physicians that the government could take control of the private practice of medicine. Physicians realized that the boards of health could be used to control the supply of physicians and to regulate the practice of medicine (Rothstein 1972). Fear of government intervention, loss of autonomy, and erosion of personal incomes created a wall of separation between public health and private medical practice. Under this dichotomous relationship, medicine has concentrated on the physical health of the individual, whereas public health has focused on the health of whole populations and communities. The extent of collaboration between the two has been largely confined to the requirement by public health departments that private practitioners report cases of contagious diseases, such as sexually transmitted diseases, human immunodeficiency virus (HIV) infection, and acquired immune deficiency syndrome (AIDS), and any outbreaks of cases such as West Nile virus and other types of infections.

Health Services for Veterans

Shortly after World War I, the government started to provide hospital services to veterans with service-related disabilities and for nonservice-related disabilities if the veteran declared an inability to pay for private care. At first, the federal government contracted for services with voluntary hospitals, but, over time, the

Department of Veterans Affairs (formerly called Veterans Administration) built its own hospitals, outpatient clinics, and nursing homes.

Birth of Workers' Compensation

The first broad-coverage health insurance in the United States emerged in the form of workers' compensation programs initiated in 1914 (Whitted 1993). Workers' compensation was originally concerned with cash payments to workers for wages lost due to job-related injuries and disease. Compensation for medical expenses and death benefits to the survivors were added later. Between 1910 and 1915, workers' compensation laws made rapid progress in the United States (Stevens 1971). Looking at the trend, some reformers believed that, since Americans had been persuaded to adopt compulsory insurance against industrial accidents, they could also be persuaded to adopt compulsory insurance against sickness. Workers' compensation served as a trial balloon for the idea of government-sponsored, universal health insurance in the United States. However, the growth of private health insurance, along with other key factors discussed later, has prevented any proposals for a national healthcare program from taking hold.

Rise of Private Health Insurance

Private health insurance was commonly referred to as *voluntary health insurance*, in contrast to proposals for a government-sponsored compulsory health insurance system. The initial role of private health insurance was income protection during sickness and temporary disability. Some private insurance coverage limited to bodily injuries had also been available since approximately 1850. By 1900, health insurance policies had become available, but their primary purpose was to protect against loss of income during sickness (Whitted 1993). Later, coverage was added for surgical fees, but emphasis remained on replacing lost income due to sickness or injury. Thus the coverage was, in reality,

disability insurance rather than health insurance (Mayer and Mayer 1984).

As detailed in subsequent sections, technological, social, and economic factors created a general need for health insurance. However, certain economic conditions that prompted private initiatives, self-interests of a well-organized medical profession, and the momentum of a successful health insurance enterprise, gave private health insurance a firm footing in the United States. Coverage for hospital and physician services began separately and was later combined under the auspices of Blue Cross and Blue Shield. Later, economic conditions during the World War II period laid the foundations for health insurance to become an employment-based benefit.

Technological, Social, and Economic Factors

The health insurance movement of the early 20th century was the product of three converging developments: the technological, the social, and the economic. From a technological perspective, medicine offered new and better treatments. Because of its well-established healing values, medical care had become individually and socially desirable, which created a growing demand for medical services. From an economic perspective, people could predict neither their future needs for medical care nor the costs, both of which had been gradually increasing. In short, scientific and technological advances made health care more desirable but less affordable. These developments pointed to the need for some kind of insurance that could spread the financial risks over a large number of people.

Early Blanket Insurance Policies

In 1911, insurance companies began to offer blanket policies for large industrial populations, usually covering life insurance, accidents and sickness, and nursing services. A few industrial and railroad companies set up their own medical plans, covering specified medical benefits, as did several unions and fraternal orders; however, the total amount of voluntary health insurance was minute (Stevens 1971). Between 1916 and 1918, 16 state legislatures, including New York and California, attempted to enact legislation compelling employers to provide health insurance, but these efforts were unsuccessful (Davis 1996).

Economic Necessity and the Baylor Plan

The Great Depression, which started at the end of 1929, forced hospitals to turn from philanthropic donations to patient fees for support. Patients now faced not only loss of income from illness but also increased debt from medical care costs when they became sick. People needed protection from the economic consequences of sickness and hospitalization. Hospitals also needed protection from economic instability (Mayer and Mayer 1984). During the Depression, occupancy rates in hospitals fell, income from endowments and contributions dropped sharply, and the charity load almost quadrupled (Richardson 1945).

In 1929, the blueprint for modern health insurance was established when J. F. Kimball began a hospital insurance plan for public school teachers at the Baylor University Hospital in Dallas, Texas. Kimball was able to enroll more than 1,200 teachers, who paid 50 cents per month for a maximum of 21 days of hospital care. Within a few years, it became the model for Blue Cross plans around the country (Raffel 1980). At first, other independent hospitals copied Baylor and started offering single-hospital plans. It was not long before communitywide plans, offered jointly by more than one hospital, became more popular because they provided consumers a choice of hospitals. The hospitals agreed to provide services in exchange for a fixed monthly payment by the plans. Hence, in essence, these were prepaid plans for hospital services. A *prepaid plan* is a contractual arrangement under which a provider must provide all needed services to a group of members (or enrollees) in exchange for a fixed monthly fee paid in advance.

Successful Private Enterprise: The Blue Cross Plans

A hospital plan in Minnesota was the first to use the name Blue Cross in 1933 (Davis 1996). The American Hospital Association (AHA) lent support to the hospital plans and became the coordinating agency to unite these plans into the Blue Cross network (Koch 1993; Raffel 1980). The Blue Cross plans were nonprofit—that is, they had no shareholders who would receive profit distributions—and covered only hospital charges, so as not to infringe on the domain of private physicians (Starr 1982).

Later, control of the plans was transferred to a completely independent body, the Blue Cross Commission, which later became the Blue Cross Association (Raffel 1980). In 1946, Blue Cross plans in 43 states served 20 million members. Between 1940 and 1950 alone, the proportion of the population covered by hospital insurance increased from 9% to 57% (Anderson 1990).

Self-Interests of Physicians: The Birth of Blue Shield

Voluntary health insurance had received the AMA's endorsement, but the AMA had also made it clear that private health insurance plans should include only hospital care. It is, therefore, not surprising that the first Blue Shield plan designed to pay for physicians' bills was started by the California Medical Association, which established the California Physicians Service in 1939 (Raffel 1980). By endorsing hospital insurance and by actively developing medical service plans, the medical profession committed itself to private health insurance as the means to spread the financial risk of sickness and to ensure that its own interests would not be threatened.

From the medical profession's point of view, voluntary health insurance, in conjunction with private fee-for-service practice by physicians, was regarded as a desirable feature of the evolving health system (Stevens 1971). Throughout the Blue Shield movement, physicians dominated the boards of directors not only because they underwrote the plans but also because the plans were, in a very real sense, their response to the challenge of national health insurance. In addition, the plans met the AMA's stipulation of keeping medical matters in the hands of physicians (Raffel and Raffel 1994).

Combined Hospital and Physician Coverage

Even though Blue Cross and Blue Shield developed independently and were financially and organizationally distinct, they often worked together to provide hospital and physician coverage (Law 1974). In 1974, the New York Superintendent of Insurance approved a merger of the Blue Cross and Blue Shield plans of Greater New York (Somers and Somers 1977). Since then, similar mergers have occurred in most states, and in nearly every state Blue Cross and Blue Shield plans are joint corporations or have close working relationships (Davis 1996).

The for-profit insurance companies were initially skeptical of the Blue Cross plans and adopted a wait-and-see attitude. Their apprehension was justified because no actuarial information was available to predict losses. But within a few years, lured by the success of the Blue Cross plans, commercial insurance companies also started offering health insurance.

Employment-Based Health Insurance

Three main factors explain how health insurance in the United States became employment based:

■ To control high inflation in the economy during the World War II period, Congress imposed wage freezes. In response, many employers started offering health insurance to their workers in lieu of wage increases.

■ In 1948, the Supreme Court ruled that employee benefits, including health insurance, were a legitimate part of the union-management bargaining process. Health insurance then became a permanent part of employee benefits in the postwar era (Health Insurance Association of America 1991).

■ According to a 1954 revision to the Internal Revenue Code, employer contributions for the purchase of employee health insurance became exempt from taxable income for the employee. In other words, employees could get noncash income without having to pay taxes on this income.

Employment-based health insurance expanded rapidly. The economy was strong during the postwar years of the 1950s, and employers started offering more extensive benefits. This led to the birth of "major medical" expense coverage to protect against prolonged or catastrophic illness or injury (Mayer and Mayer 1984). Thus private health insurance became the primary vehicle for the delivery of healthcare services in the United States.

Failure of National Healthcare Initiatives: A Historical Overview

Starting with Germany in 1883, compulsory sickness insurance had spread throughout Europe by 1912. Health insurance in European countries was viewed as a natural outgrowth of insurance against industrial accidents. Hence, it was considered logical that Americans would also be willing to espouse a national healthcare program to protect themselves from the high cost of sickness and accidents occurring outside employment.

The American Association of Labor Legislation (AALL) was founded in 1906. Although the AALL took no official position on labor unions, its membership did include prominent labor leaders (Starr 1982). Its relatively small membership, however, was mainly academic, including some leading economists and social scientists, whose all-important agenda was to bring about social reform through government action. The AALL was primarily responsible for leading the successful drive for workers' compensation. It then spearheaded the drive for a government-sponsored health insurance system for the general population (Anderson 1990) and supported the Progressive movement headed by former President Theodore Roosevelt, who was again running for the presidency in 1912 on a platform of social reform. Roosevelt, who might have been a national political sponsor for compulsory health insurance, was defeated by Woodrow Wilson, but the Progressive movement for national health insurance did not die.

The AALL continued its efforts toward a model for national health insurance by appealing to both social and economic concerns. The reformers argued that national health insurance would relieve poverty because sickness usually brought wage loss and high medical costs to individual families. Reformers also argued that national health insurance would contribute to economic efficiency by reducing illness, lengthening life, and diminishing the causes of industrial discontent (Starr 1982). Leadership of the AMA, at the time, showed outward support for a national plan, and the AALL and the AMA formed a united front to secure legislation. A standard health insurance bill was introduced in 15 states in 1917 (Stevens 1971).

As long as compulsory health insurance was only under study and discussion, potential opponents paid no heed to it; once bills were introduced into state legislatures, however, opponents expressed vehement disapproval. Eventually, support for the AMA's social change proved only superficial.

Historically, repeated attempts to pass national health insurance legislation in the United States have failed for several reasons, which can be classified under four broad categories: political inexpediency, institutional dissimilarities, ideological differences, and tax aversion.

Political Inexpediency

Before embarking on their national health programs, countries in Western Europe, notably Germany and England, were experiencing labor unrest that threatened political stability. Social insurance was seen as a means to obtain workers' loyalty and ward off political instability. Political conditions in the United States were quite different. There was no threat to political stability. Unlike the governments in countries in Europe, the American government was highly decentralized and engaged in little direct regulation of the economy or social welfare. Although Congress had set up a system of compulsory hospital insurance for merchant seamen as far back as 1798, it was an exceptional measure.* Matters related to health and welfare were typically left to state and local governments, and as a general rule, these levels of government left as much as possible to private and voluntary action.

The entry of America into World War I in 1917 provided a final political blow to the health insurance movement as anti-German feelings were aroused. The U.S. government denounced German social insurance, and opponents of health insurance called it a Prussian menace, inconsistent with American values (Starr 1982).

After attempts to pass compulsory health insurance laws failed at the state levels in California and New York, by 1920, the AALL itself lost interest in an obviously lost cause. Also in 1920, the AMA's House of Delegates approved a resolution condemning compulsory health insurance that would be regulated by the government (Numbers 1985). This AMA resolution opposing

---

*Important seaports, such as Boston, were often confronted with many sick and injured seamen, who were away from their homes and families. Congress enacted a law requiring that 20 cents per month be withheld from the wages of each seaman on American ships to support merchant marine hospitals (Raffel and Raffel 1994).

national health insurance solidified the profession against government interference with the practice of medicine.

Institutional Dissimilarities

The preexisting institutions in Europe and America were dissimilar. Germany and England had mutual benefit funds to provide sickness benefits. These benefits reflected an awareness of the value of insuring against the cost of sickness among a sector of the working population. Voluntary sickness funds were less developed in the United States than in Europe, reflecting less interest in health insurance and less familiarity with it. More important, American hospitals were mainly private, whereas in Europe they were largely government operated (Starr 1982).

Dominance of private institutions of healthcare delivery is not consistent with national financing and payment mechanisms. For instance, compulsory health insurance proposals of the AALL were regarded by individual members of the medical profession as a threat to their private practice because such proposals would shift the primary source of income of medical professionals from individual patients to the government (Anderson 1990). Any efforts that would potentially erode the fee-for-service payment system and let private practice of medicine be controlled by a powerful third party—particularly the government—were opposed.

Other institutional forces were also opposed to government-sponsored universal coverage. The insurance industry feared losing the income it derived from disability insurance, some insurance against medical services, and funeral benefits* (Anderson 1990). The pharmaceutical industry feared the government as a monopoly buyer, and retail pharmacists feared that hospitals would establish their own pharmacies

under a government-run national healthcare program (Anderson 1990). Employers also saw the proposals as contrary to their interests. Spokespersons for American business rejected the argument that national health insurance would add to productivity and efficiency. It may seem ironic, but the labor unions—the American Federation of Labor in particular—denounced compulsory health insurance at the time. Union leaders were afraid they would transfer over to the government their own legitimate role of providing social benefits, thereby weakening the unions' influence in the workplace. Organized labor was the largest and most powerful interest group at that time, and its lack of support is considered instrumental in the defeat of national health insurance (Anderson 1990).

Ideological Differences

The American value system is based largely on the principles of market justice (as discussed in Chapter 7). Individualism and self-determination, distrust of government, and reliance on the private sector to address social concerns are typical American ideologies that have stood as a bulwark against anything perceived as an onslaught on individual liberties. The cultural and ideological values represent the sentiments of the American middle class, whose support is necessary for any broad-based reform. Without such support, a national healthcare program was unable to withstand the attacks of its well-organized opponents (Anderson 1990). Conversely, during times of national distress, such as the Great Depression, pure necessity may have legitimized the advancement of social programs, such as the New Deal programs of the Franklin Roosevelt era (for example, Social Security legislation providing old-age pensions and unemployment compensation).

In the early 1940s, during Roosevelt's presidency, several bills on national health insurance were introduced in Congress, but all the proposed bills died. Perhaps the most notable bill was the Wagner-Murray-Dingell bill, drafted in

---

*Patients admitted to a hospital were required to pay a burial deposit so the hospital would not have to incur a burial expense if they died (Raffel and Raffel 1994). Therefore, many people bought funeral policies from insurance companies.

1943 and named after the bill's congressional sponsors. However, this time, World War II diverted the nation's attention to other issues, and without the president's active support the bill died quietly (Numbers 1985).

In 1946, Harry Truman became the first president to make an appeal for a national healthcare program (Anderson 1990). Unlike the Progressives, who had proposed a plan for the working class, Truman proposed a single health insurance plan that would include all classes of society. At the president's behest, the Wagner-Murray-Dingell bill was redrafted and reintroduced. The AMA was vehement in opposing the plan. Other healthcare interest groups, such as the AHA, also opposed it. By this time, private health insurance had expanded. Initial public reaction to the Wagner-Murray-Dingell bill was positive; however, when a government-controlled medical plan was compared to private insurance, polls showed that only 12% of the public favored extending Social Security to include health insurance (Numbers 1985).

During this era of the Cold War,* any attempts to introduce national health insurance were met with the stigmatizing label of *socialized medicine*, a label that has since become synonymous with any large-scale government-sponsored expansion of health insurance or intrusion in the private practice of medicine. The Republicans took control of Congress in 1946, and any interest in enacting national health insurance was put to rest. However, to the surprise of many, Truman was reelected in 1948, promising national health insurance if the Democrats would be returned to power (Starr 1982). Fearing the inevitable, the AMA levied a $25 fee on each of its members toward a war chest of $3.5 million (Anderson 1990). It hired the public relations firm of Whitaker and Baxter and spent $1.5 million, in 1949 alone, to launch one of the most expensive lobbying efforts in American history. The campaign directly linked national health insurance with Communism until the idea of socialized medicine was firmly implanted in the public's minds. Republicans proposed a few compromises in which neither the Democrats nor the AMA was interested. By 1952, the election of a Republican president, Dwight Eisenhower, effectively ended any further debate over national health insurance. Failure of government-sponsored universal healthcare coverage is often presented as a classic case of the tremendous influence of interest groups in American politics, especially in major health policy outcomes.

Tax Aversion

An aversion to increased taxes to pay for social programs is another reason why many middle-class Americans, who are typically already insured, have opposed national initiatives to expand health insurance coverage. According to polls, Americans have been found to support the idea that the government ought to help people who are in financial need to pay for their medical care. However, most Americans have not favored an increase in their own taxes to pay for such care. This is perhaps why health reform failed in 1993.

While seeking the presidency in 1992, Governor Bill Clinton made health system reform a major campaign issue. Not since Harry Truman's initiatives in the 1940s had such a bold attempt been made by a presidential candidate. As long as the electorate had remained reasonably satisfied with health care—with the exception of uninsured Americans, who have not been politically strong—elected officials had feared the political clout of big interest groups and had refrained from raising tough reform issues. In the Pennsylvania U.S. Senate election in November 1991, however, the victory of Democrat Harris Wofford over Republican Richard Thornburgh sent a clear signal that the time for a national healthcare program might be ripe. Wofford's call for national health insurance was widely supported by middle-class Pennsylvanians.

---

*Rivalry and hostility after World War II between the United States and the then Soviet Union.

Election results in other states were not quite as decisive on the health reform issue, but various public polls seemed to confirm that, after the economy (the United States was in a brief recession at the time), health care was the second most pressing concern on the minds of the American people. One national survey, conducted by Louis Harris and Associates, reported some disturbing findings about healthcare delivery. Substantial numbers of insured and relatively affluent people said they had not received the services they needed. The poll also suggested that the public was looking to the federal government, not the states or private sector, to contain rising healthcare costs (Smith et al. 1992). In other opinion polls, Americans expressed concerns that they might not be adequately insured in the future (Skocpol 1995). Against this backdrop, both Bill Clinton and the running incumbent, President George H. W. Bush, advanced healthcare reform proposals.

After taking office, President Clinton made health system reform one of his top priorities. Policy experts and public opinion leaders have since debated over what went wrong. Some of the fundamental causes for the failure of the Clinton plan were no doubt historical in nature, as discussed previously in this chapter. One seasoned political observer, James J. Mongan, however, remarked that reform debates in Congress have never been about the expansion of healthcare services but rather have been about the financing of the proposed services:

> Thus, the most important cause of health care reform's demise was that avoiding tax increases and their thinly veiled cousin, employer mandates, took priority over expanding coverage. . . . There undoubtedly would have been pitched legislative battles over other issues—how to pay doctors and hospitals, the role of health insurers, the structure of (regional health) alliances—but these debates never happened in detail. The first and only battle . . . was how to pay for reform. . . . What explains this unwillingness to pay for expanded coverage, on the part of citizens and government alike? Any answer must take into

account the economic, social, and political context of the past two decades. . . . The social context is that people tend to take for granted the progress achieved through social insurance programs such as Medicare and Social Security, and they perceive little progress or achievement from welfare expenditures targeted on low-income people. Politically, politicians from the courthouse to the White House have played to an anti-tax sentiment and have convinced Americans and American businesses that they are staggering under an oppressive burden of taxation that saps most productive effort. Although there is little evidence from other countries to support this belief, it is widely held. This climate fosters a self-centeredness—a focus more on the individual's needs than on the community's needs. Some liberals might use a harsher, more grating word—selfishness—to describe this state of mind. But many conservatives would use the phrase *rugged individualism* to describe the same phenomenon. . . . Somewhere in here is where health reform died. . . . Until we as a nation make the right diagnosis and begin an honest dialogue about our national values, about the balance between self-interest and community interests, we will not see our nation join almost all others in guaranteeing health coverage to all of its citizens. (Mongan 1995, 99–101)

When American polls indicated that a fundamental reform was needed, the people did not have in mind more government regulation or any significant redistribution of income through increased taxes. Most important, they did not wish to have a negative effect on their own access to care or the quality of care they were receiving (Altman and Reinhardt 1996).

Creation of Medicaid and Medicare

Before 1965, private health insurance was the only widely available source of payment for health care, and it was available primarily to middle-class working people and their families. The elderly, the unemployed, and the poor had to rely on their own resources, on limited public programs, or on charity from hospitals and individual physicians. Often, when charity care was provided, private payers were charged more to make up the difference, a practice referred to as *cost shifting* or *cross-subsidization*. In 1965, Congress passed the amendments to the Social Security Act and created the Medicare and Medicaid programs. Thus, for the first time in U.S. history, the government assumed direct responsibility to pay for some of the health care on behalf of two vulnerable population groups—the elderly and the poor (Potter and Longest 1994).

Through the debates over how to protect the public from rising costs of health care and the opposition to national health insurance, one thing had become clear: Government intervention was not desired insofar as it pertained to how most Americans received health care, with one exception. Less opposition would be encountered if reform initiatives were proposed for the underprivileged classes. In principle, the poor were considered a special class who could be served through a government-sponsored program. The elderly—those 65 years of age and older—were another group who started to receive increased attention in the 1950s. On their own, most of the poor and the elderly could not afford the increasing costs of health care. Also, because the health status of these population groups was significantly worse than that of the general population, they required a higher level of healthcare services. The elderly, in particular, had higher incidence and prevalence of disease compared to younger groups. It was also estimated that less than half of the elderly population was covered by private health insurance. By this time, the growing elderly middle class was also becoming a politically active force.

Government assistance for the poor and the elderly was sought once it became clear that the market alone would not ensure access for these vulnerable population groups. A bill introduced in Congress by Aime Forand, in 1957, provided momentum for including necessary hospital and nursing home care as an extension of Social Security benefits (Stevens 1971). The AMA,

however, undertook a massive campaign to portray a government insurance plan as a threat to the physician–patient relationship. The bill was stalled, but public hearings around the country, which were packed by the elderly, produced an intense grassroots support to push the issue onto the national agenda (Starr 1982).

A compromise reform bill, the Medical Assistance Act (Public Law 86–778), also known as the Kerr-Mills Act, went into effect in 1960. Under the Act, federal grants were given to the states to extend health services provided by the state welfare programs to those low-income elderly who previously did not qualify (Anderson 1990). Because the program was based on a *means test* that confined eligibility to people below a predetermined income level, it was opposed by liberal congressional representatives as a source of humiliation to the elderly (Starr 1982). Within 3 years, the program was declared ineffective because many states did not even implement it (Stevens 1971). In 1964, health insurance for the aged and the poor became top priorities of President Lyndon Johnson's Great Society programs.

During the debate over Medicare, the AMA developed its own "Eldercare" proposal, which called for a federal–state program to subsidize private insurance policies for hospital and physician services. Representative John W. Byrnes introduced yet another proposal, dubbed "Bettercare." It proposed a federal program based on partial premium contributions by the elderly, with the remainder subsidized by the government. Other proposals included tax credits and tax deductions for health insurance premiums.

In the end, a three-layered program emerged. The first two layers constituted Part A and Part B of *Medicare*, or *Title XVIII* of the Social Security Amendment of 1965 to provide publicly financed health insurance to the elderly. Based on Forand's initial bill, the administration's proposal to finance hospital insurance providing hospital care and partial nursing home coverage for the elderly through Social Security became *Part A* of Medicare. The Byrnes proposal to cover physicians' bills through government-subsidized insurance became *Part B* of Medicare. An extension of the Kerr-Mills program of federal matching funds to the states, based on each state's financial needs, became *Medicaid*, or *Title XIX* of the Social Security Amendment of 1965. The Medicaid program was for the indigent, based on means tests established by each state, but it was expanded to include all age groups, not just the poor elderly (Stevens 1971).

Although adopted together, Medicare and Medicaid reflected sharply different traditions. Medicare was upheld by broad grassroots support and, being attached to Social Security, had no class distinction. Medicaid, however, was burdened by the stigma of public welfare. Medicare had uniform national standards for eligibility and benefits; Medicaid varied from state to state in terms of eligibility and benefits. Medicare allowed physicians to *balance bill*—that is, charge the patient the amount above the program's set fees and recoup the difference. Medicaid prohibited balance billing and, consequently, had limited participation from physicians (Starr 1982). Medicaid, in essence, has created a two-tier system of medical care delivery because some physicians refuse to accept Medicaid patients due to the low fees set by the government.

Not long after Medicare and Medicaid were in operation, national spending for health services began to rise, as did public outlays of funds in relation to private spending for health services (Anderson 1990). For example, national health expenditures (NHE), which had increased by 50% from 1955 to 1960, and again from 1960 to 1965, jumped by 78% from 1965 to 1970, and by 71% from 1970 to 1975. Similarly, public expenditures for health care, which were stable at 25% of NHE for 1955, 1960, and 1965, increased to 36.5% of NHE in 1970, and to 42.1% of NHE in 1975 (based on data from Bureau of the Census 1976).

Regulatory Role of Public Health Agencies

With the expansion of publicly financed Medicare and Medicaid programs, the regulatory powers of government have increasingly encroached upon the private sector. This is because the government provides financing for the two programs, but services are delivered by the private sector. After the federal government developed the standards for participation in the Medicare program, states developed regulations in conjunction with the Medicaid program. The regulations often overlapped, and the federal government delegated authority to the states to carry out the monitoring of regulatory compliance. As a result, the regulatory powers assigned to state public health agencies increased dramatically. Thus most institutions of healthcare delivery are subject to annual scrutiny by public health agencies under the authority delegated to them by the federal and state governments.

Prototypes of Managed Care

Even though the early practice of medicine in the United States was mainly characterized by private solo practice, three subsequent developments in medical care delivery are noteworthy: contract practice, group practice, and prepaid group practice. All three required some sort of organizational integration, which was a departure from solo practice. These innovative arrangements can also be regarded as early precursors of managed care and integrated organizations.

Contract Practice

In 1882, Northern Pacific Railroad Beneficial Association was one of the first employers to provide medical care expense coverage (Davis 1996). Between 1850 and 1900, other railroad, mining, and lumber enterprises developed extensive employee medical programs. Such companies conducted operations in isolated areas where physicians were unavailable.

Inducements, such as a guaranteed salary, were commonly offered to attract physicians. Another common arrangement was to contract with independent physicians and hospitals at a flat fee per worker per month, referred to as *capitation*. The AMA recognized the necessity of contract practice in remote areas, but elsewhere contract practice was regarded as a form of exploitation because it was assumed that physicians would bid against one another and drive down the price. Offering services at reduced rates was regarded by the AMA as an unethical invasion of private practice. When group health insurance became common in the 1940s through collective bargaining, the medical profession was freed from the threat of direct control by large corporations. Health insurance also enabled workers to go to physicians and hospitals of their choice (Starr 1982).

Corporate practice of medicine—that is, provision of medical care by for-profit corporations—was generally prohibited by law. It was labeled as commercialism in medicine. In 1917, however, Oregon passed the Hospital Association Act, which permitted for-profit corporations to provide medical services. Whereas health insurance companies, functioning as insurers and payers, acted as intermediaries between patients and physicians, the hospital associations in Oregon contracted directly with physicians and exercised some control over them. Utilization was managed by requiring second opinions for major surgery and by reviewing length of hospital stays. The corporations also restricted medical fees, refusing to pay prices deemed excessive. In short, they acted as a countervailing power in the medical market to limit physicians' professional autonomy. Even though physicians resented controls, they continued to do business with the hospital associations due to guaranteed payments (Starr 1982).

Early contract practice arrangements and the Oregon hospital associations can be viewed as prototypes of managed care. Since the 1980s and 1990s, MCOs have successfully replaced the traditional fee-for-service payment arrangements by capitation and discounted fees. Mechanisms to control excessive utilization are another key feature of managed care.

Group Practice

Group medicine represented another form of corporate organization for medical care. Group practice changed the relationship among physicians by bringing them together with business managers and technical assistants in a more elaborate division of labor (Starr 1982). The Mayo Clinic, started in Rochester, Minnesota, in 1887, is regarded as a prototype of the consolidation of specialists into group practice.

The concept of a multispecialty group presented a threat to the continuation of general practice. It also presented competition to specialists who remained in solo practice. Hence, the development of group practice met with widespread professional resistance (Stevens 1971). Although specialist group practice did not become a movement, sharing of expenses and incomes, along with other economic advantages, has caused group practices to continue to grow.

Prepaid Group Plans

In time, the efficiencies of group practice led to the formation of prepaid group plans, in which an enrolled population received comprehensive services for a capitated fee. The HIP Health Plan of New York, started in 1947, stands as one of the most successful programs, providing comprehensive medical services through organized medical groups of family physicians and specialists (Raffel 1980). Similarly, Kaiser-Permanente, started in 1942, has grown on the West Coast. Other examples are the Group Health Cooperative of Puget Sound in Seattle, operating since 1947, which is a consumer-owned cooperative prepaid group practice (Williams 1993), and the Labor Health Institute in St. Louis, started in 1945, which is a union-sponsored group practice scheme (Stevens 1971).

The idea of prepaid group practice had limitations. It required the sponsorship of large organizations. HIP, for example, was created by New York's Mayor Fiorello La Guardia for city employees. Industrialist Henry Kaiser initially set up his prepaid plan to provide comprehensive healthcare services to his own employees, but the health plan was later extended to other employers.

In 1971, President Richard Nixon singled out prepaid group practice organizations as the model for a rational reorganization in the delivery of health services. They became the prototype of HMOs (Somers and Somers 1977). During the Nixon administration, the use of HMOs in the private sector was encouraged by federal legislation, the Health Maintenance Organization Act (HMO Act) of 1973. The HMO Act required employers to offer an HMO alternative to conventional health insurance (Goodman and Musgrave 1992). MCOs still attempt to combine the efficiencies of contract and group arrangements with the objective of delivering comprehensive healthcare services at predetermined costs.

MEDICAL CARE IN THE CORPORATE ERA

The latter part of the 20th century and start of the 21st century have been marked by the growth and consolidation of large business corporations and tremendous advances in global communications, transportation, and trade. These developments are starting to change the way health care is delivered in the United States and, indeed, around the world. The rise of multinational corporations, the information revolution, and globalization have been interdependent phenomena. The World Trade Organization's General Agreement on Trade in Services (GATS), which came into effect in 1995, aims to gradually remove all barriers to international trade in services. In healthcare services, GATS may regulate health insurance, hospital services, telemedicine, and acquisition of medical treatment abroad. GATS negotiations, however, have met with controversy, as various countries fear that it may shape their domestic healthcare systems (Belsky et al. 2004), although most analysts predict that GATS is likely to produce future market liberalization (Mutchnick et al. 2005).

Corporatization of Healthcare Delivery

Corporatization refers to the ways in which healthcare delivery in the United States has become the domain of large organizations. These corporations may operate either on a for-profit or nonprofit basis, yet they are driven, for the most part, by the common goal of maximizing their revenues. At least one benefit of this corporatization has been the ability of these organizations to deliver sophisticated modern health care in comfortable and pleasant surroundings. Nevertheless, one main expectation—that of delivering the same quality of health care at lesser cost—remains largely unrealized.

On the supply side, until the mid-1980s, physicians and hospitals clearly dominated the medical marketplace. Since then, managed care has emerged as a dominant force by becoming the primary vehicle for insuring and delivering health care to the majority of Americans. The rise of managed care consolidated immense purchasing power on the demand side. To counteract this imbalance, providers began to consolidate, and larger, integrated healthcare organizations began forming. A second, influential factor behind healthcare integration was reimbursement cuts for inpatient acute care hospital services in the mid-1980s. To make up for lost revenues in the inpatient sector, hospitals developed various types of outpatient services, such as primary care, outpatient surgery, and home health care, and expanded into other differentiated healthcare services, such as long-term care and specialized rehabilitation. Together, managed care and integrated delivery organizations have, in reality, corporatized the delivery of health care in the United States.

In a healthcare landscape that has been increasingly dominated by corporations, individual physicians have struggled to preserve their autonomy. As a matter of survival, many physicians consolidated into large clinics, formed strategic partnerships with hospitals, or started their own specialty hospitals. A growing number of physicians have become employees of large medical corporations. Proliferation of these new models of healthcare delivery has made it increasingly difficult for states to maintain outright bans on the employment of physicians (Farmer and Douglas 2001).

Both managed care and corporate delivery of medicine have made the healthcare system extremely complex from the consumer's standpoint. Managed care was supposed to be a market-based reform, but it has stripped the primary consumer—the patient—of practically all marketplace power. Dominance by any entity, whether organized medicine or integrated health organizations, subverts the sovereignty of the healthcare consumer. In this so-called market-driven integration, the consumer continues to wonder, "Where's the market?"

Information Revolution

The delivery of health care is being transformed in unprecedented and irreversible ways by telecommunication. The use of telemedicine and telehealth is on the rise. These technologies integrate telecommunication systems into the practice of protecting and promoting health, which may or may not incorporate actual physician–patient interactions.

Telemedicine dates back to the 1920s, when shore-based medical specialists were radio-linked to address medical emergencies at sea (Winters 1921). Telemedicine came to the forefront in the 1990s, with the technological advances in the distant transmission of image data and the recognition that there was inequitable access to medical care in rural America. Federal dollars were poured into rural telemedicine projects.

Telehealth consultations can occur in real time. Videoconferencing is now replacing telephone consultation as the preferred vehicle for behavioral telehealth or telepsychiatry. *E-health* has also become an unstoppable force that is driven by consumer demand for healthcare information and services offered over the Internet by professionals and nonprofessionals alike (Maheu et al. 2001). The Internet has created a new revolution that is increasingly characterized by patient empowerment. Access to expert information is no longer strictly confined to the physician's domain, which in some ways has led to a dilution of the dependent role of the patient.

Globalization

Globalization refers to various forms of cross-border economic activities. It is driven by global exchange of information, production of goods and services more economically in developing countries, and increased interdependence of mature and emerging world economies. It confers many advantages but also has its downsides.

From the standpoint of cross-border trade in health services, Mutchnick and colleagues (2005) identified four different modes of economic interrelationships:

1. Use of advanced telecommunication infrastructures in telemedicine transfers information cross-border for instant answers and services. For example, teleradiology (the electronic transmission of radiological images over a distance) now enables physicians in the United States to transmit radiological images to Australia, where they are interpreted and reported back the next day (McDonnell 2006). Innovative telemedicine consulting services in pathology and radiology are being delivered to other parts of the world by cutting-edge U.S. medical institutions, such as Johns Hopkins.

2. Consumers travel abroad to receive medical care. Specialty hospitals, such as the Apollo chain in India and Bumrungrad International

Hospital in Thailand, offer state-of-the-art medical facilities to foreigners at a fraction of the cost for the same procedures done in the United States or Europe. Physicians and hospitals outside the United States have clear competitive advantages: reasonable malpractice costs, minimum regulation, and lower costs of labor. As a result of these efficiencies, Indian specialty hospitals can do quality liver transplants for one-tenth of the cost in U.S. hospitals (Mutchnick et al. 2005). Some health insurance companies have also started to explore cheaper options for their covered members to receive certain costly services overseas. Conversely, dignitaries and other wealthy foreigners come to multispecialty centers in the United States, such as the Mayo Clinic, to receive highly specialized services.

3. Foreign direct investment in health services enterprises benefits foreign citizens. For example, Chindex International, a U.S. corporation, provides medical equipment, supplies, and clinical care in China. Chindex opened the Beijing United Family Hospital and Clinics in 1997 (Mutchnick et al. 2005).

4. Health professionals move to other countries that present high demand for their services and better economic opportunities than their native countries. For example, nurses from other countries are moving to the United States to relieve the existing personnel shortage. Migration of physicians from developing countries helps alleviate at least some of the shortage in underserved locations in the developed world.

To the preceding list, we can add two more factors:

1. Corporations based in the United States have increasingly expanded their operations overseas. As a result, an increasing number of Americans are now working overseas as expatriates. Health insurance companies based in the United States are, in turn, having to develop benefit plans for these expatriates. According to a survey of 87 insurance companies, health care is also becoming one of the most sought-after employee benefits worldwide, even in countries that have national health insurance programs. Also, the cost of medical care overseas is rising at a faster rate than the rate of inflation in the general economy (Cavanaugh 2008). Hence, the cost-effective delivery of health care is becoming a major challenge worldwide.

2. Medical care delivery by U.S. providers is in demand overseas. American providers, such as Johns Hopkins, Cleveland Clinic, Mayo Clinic, Duke University, and several others, are now delivering medical services in various developing countries.

Globalization has also produced some negative effects. The developing world pays a price when emigration leaves these countries with shortages of trained professionals. The burden of disease in these countries is often greater than it is in the developed world, and emigration only exacerbates the inability of these countries to provide adequate health care to their own populations (Norcini and Mazmanian 2005). Tobacco use is on the decline in many developed countries, yet economic development in emerging markets provides new targets for multinational tobacco companies. In addition, as developing countries become more prosperous, they acquire Western tastes and lifestyles. In some instances, negative health consequences follow. For example, increased use of motorized vehicles results in a lack of physical exercise, which, along with changes in diet, greatly increases the prevalence of chronic diseases, such as heart disease and diabetes, in the developing world. Conversely, better information about health promotion and disease prevention, as well as access to gyms and swimming pools, in developing countries is making a positive impact on the health and well-being of their middle-class citizens.

Globalization has also posed some new threats. For instance, the threat of infectious diseases has increased, as diseases appearing in one country can spread rapidly to other countries. HIV/AIDS, hepatitis B, and hepatitis C infections have spread worldwide. New viral infections, such as avian flu and SARS, have at times threatened to create worldwide pandemics.

Has the Era of Socialized Medicine Arrived?

Perhaps it has arrived, but only time can tell. Despite the obstacles to national health insurance, on March 21, 2010, the House Democrats in Congress successfully passed, by a 219 to 212 vote, the Patient Protection and Affordable Care Act, which was signed into law 2 days later by President Barack Obama. Not a single Republican voted in favor of the legislation.

Among his many campaign promises to bring change to America, Obama had included the goal of drastically reducing the number of Americans who had no health insurance coverage. Details of any "plan" to accomplish this goal, however, were left unstated. President Obama was sworn into office in January 2009. His inauguration marked the first time a Democratic president also had Democrat majority in both houses of Congress since 1993, the year in which President Clinton had proposed a massive overhaul of the U.S. healthcare system. Unlike with the defeat of Clinton's reform proposals, which were criticized by some congressional leaders in his own party, Obama was able to maneuver the passage of his healthcare agenda by uniting his party behind a common cause. Support for the bill required backroom deals with waffling members of the Democratic party and with interest groups representing the hospital and pharmaceutical industries. Surprisingly, the AMA sheepishly pledged its support for the legislation, which was a complete reversal of its historical stance toward national health insurance. According to one commentator, the AMA has tried to protect itself. The AMA is no longer the powerful organization it once was; it now represents only 17% of the physicians in the United States. It is plausible that the AMA has tried to protect its monopoly over the medical coding system that healthcare providers must use to get paid, which generates an annual income of more than $70 million for the organization (Scherz 2010). The American public was also kept in the dark about the details buried in the 2,700-page document that represented the final legislation.

Over half of the states and some private parties filed lawsuits challenging the constitutionality of the new law. In December 2010, a federal judge in Virginia ruled that at least certain provisions of the law were unconstitutional because they force individuals to purchase health insurance. In January 2011, a federal judge in Florida ruled in a lawsuit, joined by 26 states, that the entire law was unconstitutional. Many legal scholars think the matter will be finally settled by the U.S. Supreme Court.

Polls showed that nearly two-thirds of Americans opposed the legislation as too ambitious and too costly (Page 2010). A more current Gallup poll showed that 46% of Americans were in favor of repealing the law; 40% opposed repealing it (Jones 2011).

In the 2010 midterm elections, Republicans gained control of the U.S. House of Representatives, whereas the Democrats held their majority in the Senate. The balance of power shifted. The Republicans, taking advantage of their majority in the House, voted to repeal the healthcare law, but the Senate rejected this measure by a vote of 51 to 47 in favor of not repealing the law. Miller (2010) describes the stalemate in health reform as a "ceasefire in a political hundred years' war." The cease-fire may not last for too long.

CONCLUSION

Figure 8-1 provides a snapshot of the historical developments in U.S. healthcare delivery. The evolution of healthcare services has been

FIGURE 8-1 — Evolution of the U.S. Healthcare Delivery System

Development of Science and Technology

Mid-18th to Late 19th Century	Late 19th to Late 20th Century	Late 20th to 21st Century
Open entry into medical practice	Scientific basis of medicine	*Corporatization*
Intense competition	Urbanization	Managed care
Weak and unorganized profession	Emergence of the modern hospital	Healthcare integration
Apprenticeship training	Emergence of organized medicine	Diluted physician autonomy
Undeveloped hospitals	Emergence of scientific medical training	Complexity for the patient
Private payment for services	Licensing	*Information revolution*
Low demand for services	Development of public health	Telemedicine
Private medical schools providing only general education	Specialization in medicine	E-health
	Emergence of workers' compensation	Patient empowerment
	Emergence of private insurance	*Globalization*
	Failure of national health insurance	Global telemedicine
	Medicaid and Medicare	Medical travel
	Prototypes of managed care	Foreign investment in health care
		Migration of professionals
		Exportation of lifestyles
		Challenge of new diseases
		Bioterrorism
Consumer sovereignty	**Professional dominance**	**Corporate dominance**

Beliefs and values/Social, economic, and political constraints

strongly influenced by the advancement of scientific research and technological development. Early scientific discoveries were pioneered in Europe, but they were not readily adopted in the United States.

Therefore, medicine had a largely domestic, rather than professional, character in preindustrial America. The absence of standards of practice and licensing requirements allowed the trained and untrained alike to deliver medical care. Hospitals were more akin to places of refuge than centers of medical practice. The demand for professional services was relatively low because services had to be purchased privately, without the help of government or health insurance.

Medical education was seriously deficient in providing technical training based on scientific knowledge. The medical profession faced intense competition; it was weak, unorganized, and insecure.

Scientific and technological advances led to the development of sophisticated institutions, where better-trained physicians could practice medicine. The transformation of America from a mainly rural, sparsely populated country to one with growing centers of urban population created increased reliance on the specialized skills that only trained professionals could offer. Simultaneously, medical professionals banded together into a politically strong organization, the AMA. The AMA succeeded in controlling the practice of medicine, mainly through its influence on medical education, licensing of physicians, and political lobbying.

In Europe, national health insurance has been an outgrowth of generous social programs. In the United States, by contrast, the predominance of private institutions, ideologies founded on the principles of market justice, and an aversion to tax increases have been instrumental in maintaining a health care delivery system that is mainly privately financed and operated. The AMA and other interest groups have also wielded enormous influence in opposing efforts to initiate comprehensive reforms based on national health insurance. Access to health services in the United States is achieved, primarily, through private health insurance; however, two major social programs, Medicaid and Medicare, were expediently enacted to provide affordable health services to vulnerable populations.

The corporate era in health care dawned in the latter part of the 20th century. The rise of multinational corporations, the information revolution, and globalization have marked this current era. Managed care represents corporatization of healthcare delivery on the demand side. On the supply side, providers have been integrated into various types of consolidated arrangements. The information revolution is characterized by the growth of telemedicine and e-health. Globalization has made the mature and the emerging world economies more interdependent, which has both advantages and disadvantages.

In 2010, thanks to control of Congress and the presidency by the Democratic party, a sweeping healthcare reform legislation was passed in the United States. However, amid legal challenges, loss of control of the House of Representatives by the Democratic Party, and public opposition, the fate of this new law remains uncertain.

DISCUSSION QUESTIONS

1. Why did the professionalization of medicine start later in the United States than in some Western European nations?

2. Why did medicine have a domestic, rather than professional, character in the preindustrial era? How did urbanization change that?

3. Which factors explain why the demand for the services of a professional physician was inadequate in the preindustrial era? How did scientific medicine and technology change that?

4. How did the emergence of general hospitals strengthen the professional sovereignty of physicians?

5. Discuss the relationship of dependency within the context of the medical profession's cultural and legitimized authority. What role did medical education reform play in galvanizing professional authority?

6. How did the organized medical profession manage to remain free of control by business firms, insurance companies, and hospitals until the latter part of the 20th century?

7. In general, discuss how technological, social, and economic factors created the need for health insurance.

8. Which conditions during the World War II period lent support to private health insurance in the United States?

9. Discuss, with particular reference to the roles of (a) organized medicine, (b) the middle class, and (c) American beliefs and values, why reform efforts to bring in national health insurance have historically been unsuccessful in the United States.

10. Which particular factors that earlier may have been somewhat weak in bringing about national health insurance later led to the development of Medicare and Medicaid?

11. On what basis were the elderly and the poor regarded as vulnerable groups for whom special government-sponsored programs needed to be created?

12. Discuss the government's role in the delivery and financing of health care, with specific reference to the dichotomy between public health and private medicine.

13. Explain how contract practice and prepaid group practice were the prototypes of today's managed care plans.

14. Discuss the main ways in which current delivery of health care has become corporatized.

15. How has the information revolution affected the practice of medicine?

16. In the context of globalization in health services, what main economic activities are discussed in this chapter?

REFERENCES

Altman, S.H., and U.E. Reinhardt, eds. 1996. *Strategic choices for a changing health care system.* Chicago: Health Administration Press.

Anderson, O.W. 1990. *Health services as a growth enterprise in the United States since 1875.* Ann Arbor, MI: Health Administration Press.

Belsky, L. et al. 2004. The general agreement on trade in services: Implications for health policymakers. *Health Affairs* 23, no. 3: 137–145.

Bordley, J., and A.M. Harvey. 1976. *Two centuries of American medicine 1776–1976.* Philadelphia, PA: W.B. Saunders Company.

Bureau of the Census. 1976. *Statistical abstract of the United States, 1976.* Washington, DC: U.S. Department of Commerce.

Bureau of Labor Statistics. 2011. *Occupational outlook handbook, 2010-11.* Available at: http://www.bls.gov/oco/home.htm. Accessed January 2011.

Burns, J. 2004. Are nonprofit hospitals really charitable? Taking the question to the state and local level. *Journal of Corporate Law* 29, no. 3: 665–683.

Cavanaugh, B.B. 2008. Building the worldwide health network. *Best's Review* 108, no. 12: 32–37.

Clark, C. 1998. A bloody evolution: Human error in medicine is as old as the practice itself. *The Washington Post,* 20 October, Z10.

Coggeshall, L.T. 1965. *Planning for medical progress through education.* Evanston, IL: Association of American Medical Colleges.

Davis, P. 1996. The fate of Blue Shield and the new blues. *South Dakota Journal of Medicine* 49, no. 9: 323–330.

Duffy, J. 1971. Social impact of disease in the late 19th century. *Bulletin of the New York Academy of Medicine* 47: 797–811.

Falk, G. 1999. *Hippocrates assailed: The American health delivery system.* Lanham, MD: University Press of America, Inc.

Farmer, G.O., and J.H. Douglas. 2001. Physician "unionization": A primer and prescription. *Florida Bar Journal* 75, no. 7: 37–42.

Gabe, J. et al. 1994. *Challenging medicine.* New York: Routledge.

Goodman, J.C., and G.L. Musgrave. 1992. *Patient power: Solving America's health care crisis.* Washington, DC: CATO Institute.

Haber, S. 1974. The professions and higher education in America: A historical view. In: *Higher education and labor markets.* M.S. Gordon, ed. New York: McGraw-Hill Book Co.

Haglund, C.L., and W.L. Dowling. 1993. The hospital. In: *Introduction to health services.* 4th ed. S.J. Williams and P.R. Torrens, eds. New York: Delmar Publishers. pp. 135–176.

Hamowy, R. 1979. The early development of medical licensing laws in the United States, 1875–1900. *Journal of Libertarian Studies* 3, no. 1: 73–119.

Health Insurance Association of America. 1991. *Source book of health insurance data.* Washington, DC: Health Insurance Association of America.

Henry J. Kaiser Family Foundation. 2011. *Summary of coverage provisions in the Patient Protection and Affordable Care Act.* Available at: http://kff.org/healthreform/upload/8023-R.pdf. Accessed April 2011.

Jones, J.M. 2011. In U.S., 46% favor, 40% oppose repealing healthcare law. Available at: http://www.gallup.com/poll/145496/Favor-Oppose-Repealing-Healthcare-Law.aspx. Accessed April 2011.

Kaptchuk, T.J., and D.M. Eisenberg. 2001. Varieties of healing 1: Medical pluralism in the United States. *Annals of Internal Medicine* 135, no. 3: 189–195.

Kardos, B.C., and A.T. Allen. 1993. Healthy neighbors: Exploring the health care systems of the United States and Canada. *Journal of Post Anesthesia Nursing* 8, no. 1: 48–51.

Kaufman, M. 1980. American medical education. In: *The education of American physicians: Historical essays.* R.L. Numbers, ed. Los Angeles: University of California Press.

Koch, A.L. 1993. Financing health services. In: *Introduction to health services.* 4th ed. S.J. Williams and P.R. Torrens, eds. New York: Delmar Publishers. pp. 299–331.

Law, S.A. 1974. *Blue Cross: What went wrong?* New Haven, CT: Yale University Press.

Maheu, M.M. et al. 2001. *E-health, telehealth, and telemedicine: A guide to start-up and success.* San Francisco: Jossey-Bass.

Manderscheid, R.W. et al. 2004. Highlights of organized mental health services in 2000 and major national and state trends. In: *Mental health, United States, 2002.* R.W. Manderscheid and M.J. Henderson, eds. Washington, DC: U.S. Government Printing Office.

Martensen, R.L. 1996. Hospital hotels and the care of the "worthy rich." *Journal of the American Medical Association* 275, no. 4: 325.

Mayer, T.R., and G.G. Mayer. 1984. *The health insurance alternative: A complete guide to health maintenance organizations.* New York: Putnam Publishing Group.

McDonnell, J. 2006. Is the medical world flattening? *Ophthalmology Times* 31, no. 19: 4.

Miller, T.P. 2010. Health reform: Only a cease-fire in a political hundred years' war. *Health Affairs* 29, no. 6: 1101–1105.

Mongan, J.J. 1995. Anatomy and physiology of health reform's failure. *Health Affairs* 14, no. 1: 99–101.

Mutchnick, I.S. et al. 2005. Trading health services across borders: GATS, markets, and caveats. *Health Affairs* – Web Exclusive 24, suppl. 1: W5-42–W5-51.

Norcini, J.J., and P.E. Mazmanian. 2005. Physician migration, education, and health care. *Journal of Continuing Education in the Health Professions* 25, no. 1: 4–7.

Numbers, R.L. 1985. The third party: Health insurance in America. In: *Sickness and health in America: Readings in the history of medicine and public health.* J.W. Leavitt and R.L. Numbers, eds. Madison, WI: The University of Wisconsin Press.

Numbers, R.L., and J.H. Warner. 1985. The maturation of American medical science. In: *Sickness and health in America: Readings in the history of medicine and public health.* J.W. Leavitt and R.L. Numbers, eds. Madison, WI: The University of Wisconsin Press.

Page, S. 2010. Health care law too costly, most say. *USA Today.* Available at: http://www.usatoday.com/news/washington/2010-03-29-health-poll_N.htm. Accessed January 2011.

Potter, M.A., and B.B. Longest. 1994. The divergence of federal and state policies on the charitable tax exemption of nonprofit hospitals. *Journal of Health Politics, Policy and Law* 19, no. 2: 393–419.

Raffel, M.W. 1980. *The U.S. health system: Origins and functions.* New York: John Wiley & Sons.

Raffel, M.W., and N.K. Raffel. 1994. *The U.S. health system: Origins and functions.* 4th ed. Albany, NY: Delmar Publishers.

Richardson, J.T. 1945. *The origin and development of group hospitalization in the United States, 1890–1940.* University of Missouri Studies XX, no. 3.

Rosen, G. 1983. *The structure of American medical practice 1875–1941.* Philadelphia, PA: University of Pennsylvania Press.

Rosenberg, C.E. 1979. The therapeutic revolution: Medicine, meaning, and social change in nineteenth-century America. In: *The therapeutic revolution.* M.J. Vogel, ed. Philadelphia, PA: The University of Pennsylvania Press.

Rosner, L. 2001. The Philadelphia medical marketplace. In: *Major problems in the history of American medicine and public health.* J.H. Warner and J.A. Tighe, eds. Boston: Houghton Mifflin Company.

Rothstein, W.G. 1972. *American physicians in the nineteenth century: From sect to science.* Baltimore, MD: Johns Hopkins University Press.

Scherz, H. 2010. Why the AMA wants to muzzle your doctor (*The Wall Street Journal*). Available at: http://online.wsj.com/article/SB10001424052748703961104575226323909364054.html. Accessed April 2011.

Shryock, R.H. 1966. *Medicine in America: Historical essays.* Baltimore, MD: The Johns Hopkins Press.

Skocpol, T. 1995. The rise and resounding demise of the Clinton plan. *Health Affairs* 14, no. 1: 66–85.

Smith, M.D. et al. 1992. Taking the public's pulse on health system reform. *Health Affairs* 11, no. 2: 125–133.

Somers, A.R., and H.M. Somers. 1977. *Health and health care: Policies in perspective.* Germantown, MD: Aspen Systems.

Starr, P. 1982. *The social transformation of American medicine.* Cambridge, MA: Basic Books.

Stevens, R. 1971. *American medicine and the public interest.* New Haven, CT: Yale University Press.

Turnock, B.J. 1997. *Public health: What it is and how it works.* Gaithersburg, MD: Aspen Publishers, Inc. pp. 3–38.

U.S. Surgeon General. 1999. *Mental health: A report of the Surgeon General. Overview of mental health services.* Available at: http://www.surgeongeneral.gov/library/mentalhealth/chapter2 /sec2.html. Accessed February 2011.

Whitted, G. 1993. Private health insurance and employee benefits. In: *Introduction to health services.* 4th ed. S.J. Williams and P.R. Torrens, eds. New York: Delmar Publishers. pp. 332–360.

Williams, S.J. 1993. Ambulatory health care services. In: *Introduction to health services.* 4th ed. S.J. Williams and P.R. Torrens, eds. New York: Delmar Publishers.

Williams, S.J. 1995. *Essentials of health services.* Albany, NY: Delmar Publishers. pp. 108–134.

Winters, S.R. 1921. Diagnosis by wireless. *Scientific American* 124: 465.

Wright, J.W. 1997. *The New York Times almanac.* New York: Penguin Putnam, Inc.

CHAPTER 9

Financing Health Care

Harry A. Sultz and Kristina M. Young

CHAPTER OBJECTIVES

1. Develop an understanding of how health care is financed.

2. Analyze national healthcare expenditures and sources of payment.

3. Discuss the historical development of the national healthcare reimbursement infrastructure.

4. Identify the major factors that impact healthcare costs and the significant trends in healthcare spending.

5. Discuss the role of government as a payer and provider of services and the associated cost.

INTRODUCTION

This chapter reviews the most currently available data on national healthcare expenditures and sources of payment and provides a historical overview of the developments that played major roles in creating the national healthcare financing infrastructure. Major factors that affect healthcare costs are identified and discussed. Significant trends in healthcare spending are reviewed, along with underlying reasons for evolving changes. The roles of the private sector and government as payers are presented with an overview of continuing efforts to link costs with quality.

Healthcare expenditures in the United States are financed through a combination of private and public sources. Most working Americans younger than the age of 65 have private health insurance coverage provided by their employers.[1] The primary sources of public funding are Medicare, covering healthcare services for most individuals older than 65 years of age and disabled individuals, and Medicaid, which supports services for the low-income population.[1]

Financing of the U.S. healthcare system continues to evolve owing to a variety of influences, including provider, employer, purchaser, consumer, and political factors. As pointedly reflected in the national healthcare reform debates, these influences produce major tensions about the role and responsibility of the government as payer, the financial responsibilities of employers as the primary purchasers of health insurance, consumers, the relationships of costs to quality, and the impact of payment systems on quality. Controlling the rising costs of health care and dealing with the estimated 47 million uninsured or underinsured Americans remain two of the most challenging issues.

HEALTHCARE EXPENDITURES IN PERSPECTIVE

National health expenditures and trends are reported annually by the National Center for Health Statistics of the Centers for Disease Control and Prevention, the Office of the Actuary, National Health Statistics Group, and the U.S. Department of Health and Human Services, Centers for Medicare & Medicaid Services. Expenditures are reported and tracked over time using a standard format that identifies both the private and public sources of funds and the objects of expense. Table 9-1 provides an example of one such report for 2008.[2]

National healthcare expenditures in 2008 totaled $2.33 trillion, 16.2% of the gross domestic product and $7,681 per person[3] (Figure 9-1). Expenditures for personal healthcare services currently represent 83.6%, or $1.95 billion of the national total.[2] The three top expenses for personal health care in overall national healthcare expenditures are hospital care at $718.4 billion, physician services at $496.2 billion, and prescription drugs at $234.1 billion[2] (Figure 9-2). Private health insurance is the primary source of payment for healthcare services, with an outlay of $783.2 billion. Medicare, with expenditures of $469.2 billion, is the next highest source, and Medicaid ranks as third highest at $344.3 billion.[2] Together, all public sources of funding represent 48% of total payments (Figure 9-3).

With the nation in an economic recession in 2008, growth in healthcare spending slowed to 4.4% over the prior year, the slowest rate of growth in the past 48 years.[3] Historically, the rate of growth in healthcare expenditures has been an overarching concern of both the private and government sectors as healthcare expenditure growth outstripped general inflation by significant margins.[4,5] And although insured Americans view the U.S. healthcare delivery system as superior to that of other developed nations, all of which have some form of universal health care, serious questions have loomed regarding the value returned for U.S. costs that are much higher, while the citizens of those other nations experience better health outcomes.[5] Despite the largest increase in its percentage of gross domestic product devoted to health care among 29 Organization for Economic Cooperation and Development (OECD) countries in the period 1970–2005, the United States had a lower life expectancy than predicted based on per capita income and was just as likely to rank in the bottom half as in the top half on a series of health status indicators.[5] According to these data published by the OECD, the United States spent more than double the median spending per person among OECD countries in 2005, and despite having the third highest level of public source spending for health care, public insurance covered only 26.5% of the U.S. population.[5] The United States also has lower healthcare utilization rates in terms of factors such as hospital days and physician visits per capita than most other OECD countries and a lower supply of expensive technology. Extensive comparative studies have concluded that the U.S. higher per capita income and much higher U.S. prices for

TABLE 9-1 National Health Expenditures, 2008, by Type of Expenditure and Source of Payment

Year and Type of Expenditure	Total	Private					Public		
		All Private Funds	Total	Consumer		Other	Total	Federal	State and Local
				Out-of-Pocket Payments	Private Health Insurance				
2008									
National Health Expenditures	2,338.7	1,232.0	1,060.9	277.8	783.2	171.1	1106.7	816.8	289.8
Health Services and Supplies	2181.3	1,138.1	1,060.9	277.8	783.2	77.2	1,043.1	774.0	269.1
Personal Health Care	1,952.3	1,044.5	969.0	277.8	691.2	75.5	907.8	718.0	189.8
Hospital Care	718.4	309.3	282.2	23.2	259.0	27.1	409.0	330.7	78.3
Professional Services	731.2	457.7	425.5	111.1	314.3	42.2	263.5	202.3	61.1
Physician and Clinical Services	496.2	323.9	291.9	50.1	241.8	31.9	172.3	144.6	27.7
Other Professional Services	65.7	43.3	39.8	16.4	23.4	3.5	22.4	17.9	4.5
Dental Services	101.2	93.9	93.8	44.8	49.2	0.1	7.3	4.5	2.8
Other Personal Health Care	68.1	6.6	—	—	—	6.6	61.5	35.3	26.2
Nursing Home and Home Health	203.1	65.8	59.8	43.5	16.1	6.2	137.3	101.9	35.4
Home Health Care	64.7	13.5	12.4	6.6	5.8	1.2	51.1	39.8	11.3
Nursing Home Care	138.4	52.3	47.2	38.9	10.3	5.1	86.2	62.1	24.1
Retail Outlet Sales of Medical Products	299.6	201.7	201.7	100.0	101.7	0.0	97.9	83.0	14.9
Prescription Drugs	234.1	147.0	147.0	48.5	98.5	0.0	87.0	72.5	14.5
Other Medical Products	65.5	54.6	54.6	51.4	3.2	0.0	10.9	10.5	0.4
Durable Medical Equipment	26.6	18.1	18.1	14.9	3.2	0.0	8.4	8.0	0.4
Other Non-Durable Medical Products	39.0	38.5	36.5	36.5	0.0	0.0	2.5	2.5	0.0
Government Administration and Net Cost of Private Health Care	159.6	93.6	92.0	—	92.0	1.7	65.9	45.5	20.4
Government Public Health Activities	69.4	—	—	—	—	—	69.4	10.5	59.0
Investment	157.5	93.9	—	—	—	93.9	63.6	43.0	20.6
Research	43.8	4.7	—	—	—	4.7	38.9	33.5	5.4
Structures and Equipment	113.9	89.2	—	—	—	89.2	24.7	9.5	15.2

Note: Research and development expenditures of drug companies and other manufacturers and providers of medical equipment and supplies are excluded from research expenditures. These research expenditures are implicitly included in the expenditures class in which the product falls, in that they are covered by the payment received for that product. Numbers may not add to totals because of rounding. The figure 0.0 denotes amounts less than $50 million. Dashes (—) indicate "not applicable."

Source: Centers for Medicare & Medicaid, Office of Actuary, National Health Statistics Group.

| FIGURE 9-1 | National Health Expenditures per Capita and Their Share of the Gross Domestic Product, 1960–2008 |

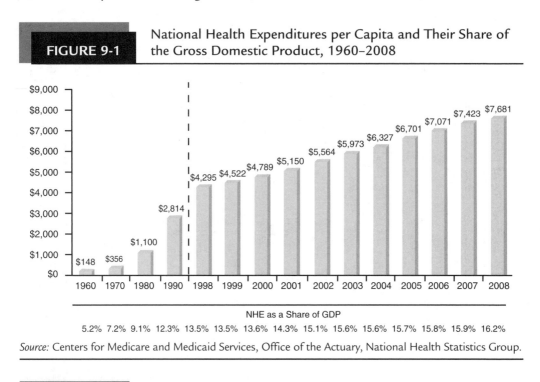

NHE as a Share of GDP

5.2% 7.2% 9.1% 12.3% 13.5% 13.5% 13.6% 14.3% 15.1% 15.6% 15.6% 15.7% 15.8% 15.9% 16.2%

Source: Centers for Medicare and Medicaid Services, Office of the Actuary, National Health Statistics Group.

| FIGURE 9-2 | The U.S. Healthcare Dollar, 2008: Where It Went |

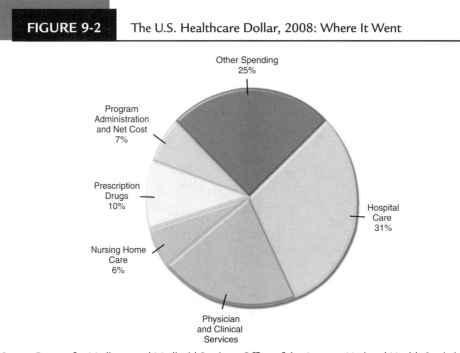

Source: Centers for Medicare and Medicaid Services, Office of the Actuary, National Health Statistics Group.

FIGURE 9-3	The U.S. Healthcare Dollar, 2008: Where It Came From

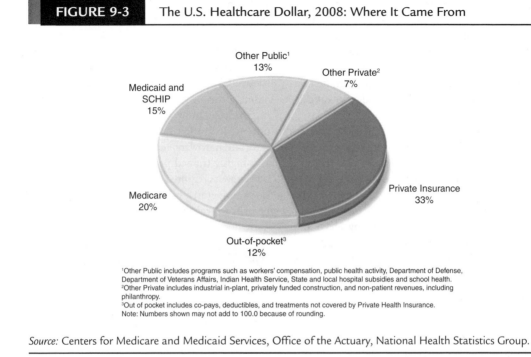

[1]Other Public includes programs such as workers' compensation, public health activity, Department of Defense, Department of Veterans Affairs, Indian Health Service, State and local hospital subsidies and school health.
[2]Other Private includes industrial in-plant, privately funded construction, and non-patient revenues, including philanthropy.
[3]Out of pocket includes co-pays, deductibles, and treatments not covered by Private Health Insurance.
Note: Numbers shown may not add to 100.0 because of rounding.

Source: Centers for Medicare and Medicaid Services, Office of the Actuary, National Health Statistics Group.

medical care account for much of the spending differences, not superior health care that yields better health outcomes.[6]

Studies indicate that 30% to 40% of U.S. health spending is "waste," in that it provides services of no discernible value and inefficiently produces valuable services; this is another important dimension of U.S. healthcare spending.[7] One of these studies was reported in a mid-2008 statement by Peter R. Orszag, Director of the Congressional Budget Office at the Health Reform Summit of the Committee on Finance of the U.S. Senate, "Opportunities to Increase Efficiency in Health Care."[8] In his statement Mr. Orszag noted that "future health care spending is the single most important factor determining the nation's long-term fiscal condition" and that changing physician practice norms through the use of evidence-based practices to decrease variability in costs and re-

vised economic incentives are needed to decrease waste.[8]

It is no surprise that a $2 trillion–plus enterprise invites fraud and abuse. The Federal Bureau of Investigation estimated that "fraudulent billings to public and private health care programs [were] 3–10% of total health spending, or $75–250 billion in fiscal year 2009."[9] There is a decade-long history of collaboration among the U.S. Department of Justice and the Office of the Inspector General of the Department of Health and Human Services to fight healthcare fraud, which has had impressive results including hundreds of convictions and exclusions of providers from federal healthcare programs.[9] However, complex, sophisticated criminal schemes involving providers, patients, drug dealers, and others continue to evolve.[9] Recognizing that fraud and abuse drain critical and substantial resources from the healthcare delivery system, in 2009 the U.S. Attorney General and Health and Human Services Secretary announced a multifaceted new approach to curbing fraud and abuse through creation of a Health Care Fraud Prevention and Enforcement Action Team that will use "cutting edge technology to identify and analyze suspected fraud and to build complex healthcare fraud cases quickly and efficiently."[9]

A well-rounded perspective on healthcare financing in the United States requires a grasp of much more than just the numbers. It requires an appreciation for the complexity of the human aspects of the multiple players in the healthcare delivery system, the financing system's historical roots, and the many social, political, and economic characteristics that now intertwine in an industry that encompasses one-sixth of the total U.S. economy.

DRIVERS OF HEALTHCARE EXPENDITURES

Major drivers of healthcare expenditures include advancing medical and diagnostic technology, growth in the population of older adults, emphasis on specialty medicine, the uninsured and underinsured, labor intensity, and reimbursement system incentives.

Beginning in the 1950s, healthcare technology expanded rapidly. Hospitals became high-technology centers, consuming increasing resources in care delivery and capital to expand capacity and add technology. In 1960 national hospital care expenditures totaled $9.2 billion; by 1970 they had increased threefold to $27.6 billion,[2] a growth rate vastly outstripping overall inflation and growth in the gross domestic product. The array of medical interventions and diagnostic modalities continued to increase exponentially in succeeding decades. Examples include the development and several refinements of angioplasty as a routine treatment for blocked coronary blood vessels, and diagnostic modalities such as computed tomography, magnetic resonance imaging, and positron emission

tomography, which are continuously upgraded and enhanced through new technology that is significantly expanding applications to an ever-wider variety of clinical situations.

Many other diagnostic, therapeutic, and surgical techniques require changes resulting from the availability of new equipment and computer-aided technologies. Such advances come at a high price.[10] Information technology and computer-aided innovations require expensive software and hardware, new patient care equipment, and highly trained personnel. The large capital investments required drive economic and professional imperatives for their use. Historically, the healthcare reimbursement system did not require documentation of the necessity for the use of technologic interventions or estimates of their benefit. The tendency to favor broad, rather than discretionary, use has grown with the number of interventions available.

The addition of new pharmacologic agents, increased access to drug coverage through Medicare and managed care, and "direct to consumer" marketing of prescription drugs via television, radio, and print media have combined to make the rise in prescription drug spending a focal point of national attention.[11] Recent data indicate that growth in prescription drug spending has slowed due to several factors, including the economic recession, few new product introductions, and safety concerns.[3] However, spending for prescription drugs remains among the top three expenses in total national healthcare expenditures.[2]

Growth in the number of older adults is another major factor in rising healthcare expenditures. Current estimates place the population 65 years of age and older at 37.9 million, 12.6% of the population, or about one of every eight Americans. The number of persons aged 65 years or older is expected to grow to 19.3% of the population by 2030, totaling 72.1 million.[12] The population 85 years of age and older is expected to grow from 5.5 million in 2007 to 6.6 million by 2020.[13]

Persons older than the age of 65 years are the major consumers of inpatient hospital care. These individuals account for more than one-third of all hospital stays and one-half of all days of care in hospitals.[14,15] In addition, the aging of the baby boomers (born between 1946 and 1964) is expected to have a profound effect on healthcare services consumption beginning with the second decade of the 21st century.[16]

Growth in specialized medicine occurred as medical science and technology advanced. Americans' preference for specialty care resulted in high utilization and rapidly rising costs. Unlike other developed nations, where physician specialists represent half or fewer of physicians in general practice, approximately 60% of practicing physicians in the United States are specialists.[17] Since the 1940s, when employers offset post–World War II wage controls with fully paid health insurance benefits, working Americans were insulated from healthcare costs. They grew to expect and demand what they perceived as the "best" care, placing a high value on the use of specialists and advanced technology, sometimes resulting in inappropriate use and expense. For most, the costs of treatment were irrelevant, and physicians' recommendations were uninhibited by economic considerations among their well-insured patients. Historically, U.S. health insurance models carried no prohibitions against patient self-referrals to specialty care. Patients freely referred themselves to specialists based on their own interpretations of symptoms. Initially, managed care plans placed strong restrictions on patient self-referrals to specialists. However, consumer backlash in subsequent years significantly loosened restrictions against such self-referrals.

Among all developed countries of the world, the United States has the highest proportion of its population without health insurance coverage. In 2009 the U.S. Bureau of the Census estimated that approximately 47 million Americans had no health insurance.[18] Lacking health insurance or having insufficient coverage carries major consequences by affecting the ability of individuals to receive timely preventive, acute, and chronic care. A lack of insurance coverage drives individuals to seek care in hospital emergency departments at costs higher than care provided at the physician's office or other ambulatory settings. Furthermore, uninsured or underinsured individuals tend to be low users of preventive services and are known to delay seeking care, even for acute conditions. These behaviors often result in increased illness severity and more complications, adding to diagnostic and treatment costs. Uninsured Americans are much more likely than insured individuals to enter care in the late stages of disease and require avoidable hospitalizations.[19] Providers absorb increased costs as free care. Insurers pass costs on to the insured in the form of higher premiums, and citizens pay higher taxes to support public hospitals or public insurance programs.[20]

Health care is a labor-intensive industry. It is one of the largest industries in the United States, employing approximately 14.3 million workers, many of whom represent some of the most highly educated, trained, and compensated individuals in the workforce.[21] The U.S. Department of Labor predicts that the healthcare industry will generate approximately 3.2 million new jobs by 2014.[21] Among the most important factors that continue to produce high employment demands are technologic advances and continued growth in the aging population with more intense and diverse healthcare needs.

Both private and government healthcare financing mechanisms are recognized as major contributors to rising costs. Until the widespread introduction of prospective payment and managed care in the 1980s, government and private third-party payers reimbursed largely on a piecework, fee-for-service, retrospective basis. This system created economic incentives favoring high utilization among both physicians and hospitals. In combination with other factors fueling increased consumption of healthcare resources, the economic incentives created by the healthcare financing system played major roles in the rapid rate of expenditure growth. Later sections of this chapter review the history of attempts to change the healthcare financing system, providing a foundation for managed care's emergence as the predominant form of healthcare financing in the United States.

EVOLUTION OF PRIVATE HEALTH INSURANCE

As early as the mid-1800s, a movement began to insure workers against lost wages resulting from work-related injuries. Later, insurance to cover lost wages resulting from catastrophic illness was added to accident policies. It was not until the 1930s that health insurance began paying part or all costs of medical treatment to providers. The basic concept of health insurance is antithetical to the central premise by which "insurance" was historically defined. Whereas insurance originally guarded against the low risk of rare occurrences such as premature death and accidents, the health insurance model that evolved provided coverage for predictable and discretionary uses of the healthcare system as well as unforeseen and unpredictable health events. With indemnity insurance (so called because it protected individuals from financial risk associated with the costs of care), the insurance company set allowable charges for services, and providers could bill the patient for any excess.[22] Indemnity coverage prevailed until the advent of managed care in the 1970s.

Development of Blue Cross and Blue Shield and Commercial Health Insurance

In 1930 a group of Baylor University teachers contracted with Baylor Hospital in Dallas, Texas, to provide coverage for hospital expenses.[23] This arrangement created a model for the development of what was to become Blue Cross, a private, not-for-profit insurance empire that grew over the succeeding four decades into the dominant form of health insurance in the United States. The Blue Shield plans providing physician payments began shortly after Blue Cross, and by the early 1940s numerous Blue Shield plans were operating across the country. In 1946 the American Medical Association (AMA) financed the Association Medical Care Plans, which later became the National Association of Blue Shield Plans.

These developments, through which health insurance was transformed from a mechanism to reimburse individuals for lost wages resulting from injury or illness to one that reimbursed providers for the costs of medical care, carried major implications. The basic concept of health insurance is antithetical to the central premise of insurance. Whereas insurance originally guarded against the low risk of a rare occurrence, such as premature death, and unpredictable events such as accidents, the new medical care insurance model provided coverage for predictable, routine uses of the healthcare system as well as unforeseen and unpredictable illnesses or injuries. Coverage for routine use of healthcare services added a new dimension to the concept of insurance.

The establishment and subsequent proliferation of the "Blues" signaled a new era in U.S. healthcare delivery and financing. They played a significant role in establishing hospitals as the centers of medical care proliferation and technology, and by reimbursing for expensive services they put hospital care easily within the reach of middle-class working Americans for the first time. The insulation from costs of care provided by the Blues had a major impact on utilization. By the late 1930s annual hospital admission rates for Blue Cross enrollees were 50% higher on average than for the nation as a whole.[24] In addition to contributing to increased utilization of hospital services by removing financial barriers, the Blue Cross movement had other lasting impacts on national policymaking. Rosemary Stevens noted, "In the United States, the brave new world of medicine was specialized, interventionist, mechanistic and expensive—at least as interpreted, through prepayment, for workers in major organizations" (p. 190).[24] By 1940 the Blue Cross movement represented a major financing alternative, countering forces that had long lobbied politically for a form of national health insurance, a concept opposed vehemently by private medicine. The plans also stimulated the American Hospital Association and local hospitals to consider providing similar forms of reimbursement for low-income populations, modeled after the Blue Cross benefits recognizing private, semiprivate, and ward care. This latter movement, which continued for the next 20 years, focused attention on government as a potential source of insurance that was designed for low-income populations, the unemployed, or sporadic seasonal workers modeled along Blue Cross lines.[24]

Uniform features of all Blue Cross plans included not-for-profit status, supervision by state insurance departments, direct payments through contract arrangements with providers, and the use of community rating, in which all individuals in a defined group pay single premiums without regard to age, gender, occupation, or health status. Community rating helped ensure nondiscrimination against groups with varying risk characteristics to provide coverage at reasonable rates for the community as a whole; however, as commercial insurers entered the healthcare insurance marketplace, using "experience rating," basing premiums on historically documented patterns of utilization, Blue Cross plans, to remain competitive, began offering a variety of benefit packages. Ultimately, the Blue Cross plans were compelled to switch to experience-rating schemes to avoid attracting a disproportionate share of high-risk individuals for whom commercial insurance was prohibitively expensive.[24] During a

period of insurance consolidations and mergers, beginning in the mid-1990s, Blue Cross plans in several states converted from not-for-profit to for-profit status. The effects of these conversions on costs of coverage and access to care remain under study.[25]

For-profit commercial health insurers entered the market in significant numbers in the decade after start-up of Blue Cross and Blue Shield. Unbounded by the requirement for community-rating by the not-for-profit Blues, they used experience-rating to charge higher premiums to less healthy individuals and successfully competed for the market of healthier individuals by offering lower premiums than the Blues. By the early 1950s commercial insurers had enrolled more subscribers than the Blues.[26]

Managed Care

By the 1960s rapidly increasing Medicare expenditures accompanied by quality concerns captured the attention of health and government policymakers and of industry as the major purchasers of healthcare benefits, and a proposal was designed by the Nixon administration and Congress that resulted in enactment of the Health Maintenance Organization (HMO) Act of 1973.[22] Although many employer groups had used principles of managed care for prior decades through contracts with healthcare providers to serve employees on a prepaid basis, provisions of the HMO Act opened participation to the employer-based market, allowing the rapid proliferation of managed care plans.[22]

The HMO Act of 1973 provided loans and grants for the planning, development, and implementation of combined insurance and healthcare delivery organizations and required that a comprehensive array of preventive and primary care services be included in the HMO arrangement.

The legislation also mandated that employers with 25 or more employees offer an HMO option if one was available in their area and required employers to contribute to employees' HMO premiums in an amount equal to what they contributed to indemnity plan premiums. Initially, this employer mandate helped stimulate the growth of HMO membership in regions where federally funded and qualified plans were first established.

As authorized by the 1973 legislation, HMOs were organizations that combined providers and insurers into one organizational entity. As originally established, members of HMOs usually were required to obtain all their medical care within the organization.

Initially, there were two major types of HMOs. The first was a staff model and was the type most commonly established from the initial HMO legislation. It employed groups of physicians to provide most healthcare services needed by the HMO's members. HMOs often provided some specialty services within the organization or contracted for services with community specialists. In the staff model the HMO also operated the facilities in which its physicians practiced, providing on-site ancillary support services, such as radiology, laboratory, and pharmacy services. The HMO usually purchased hospital care and other services for its members through fee-for-service or prepaid contracted arrangements. Staff model HMOs were referred to as "closed panel" because they employed the physicians who provided the majority of their members' care, and those physicians did not provide services outside the HMO membership. Similarly, community-based physicians could not participate in HMO member care without authorization by the HMO.

The second type of HMO stimulated by the 1973 legislation was the individual practice association (IPA). IPAs are physician organizations composed of community-based independent physicians in solo or group practices who provide services to HMO members. An IPA HMO, therefore, did not operate facilities in which members received care but rather provided its members services through private physician office practices. Like the staff model HMO, the IPA HMO purchased hospital care and specialty

services not available through IPA-participating physicians from other area providers on a prepaid or fee-for-service basis. Some IPA HMOs allowed physicians to have a nonexclusive relationship that permitted treatment of nonmembers as well as members; however, HMO relationships with an IPA also could be established on an exclusive basis. In this scenario an HMO took the initiative in recruiting and organizing community physicians into an IPA to serve its members. Because the HMO was the organizing force in such an arrangement, it was common for the HMO to require exclusivity by the IPA, limiting its services only to that HMO's membership.[27]

The staff model and IPA-type organizations illustrate two major types of HMOs, but each type spawned several hybrids. Other forms of managed care organizations (MCOs) emerged throughout the 1980s in response to national cost and quality concerns. Peter Kongstvedt identified three additional HMO models as the most common: group practice, network, and direct contract.[27] In a group practice model an HMO contracts with a multispecialty group practice to provide all the physician services required by HMO enrollees. The physicians remain independent—employed by their group rather than by the HMO. In the network model the HMO contracts with more than one group practice and maintains contracts with several physician groups representing both primary care and specialty practices. The direct contract model HMOs maintain contractual relationships with individual physicians, in contrast to the physician groups as in the IPA and network models. The direct contract approach gives the HMO the advantages of maintaining a higher level of control over fee arrangements by reducing physicians' negotiating power to an individual basis and avoiding the risk of lost services to its members by contractual termination of a large group of providers.

All forms of managed care entail interdependence between the provision of and payment for health care. Managed care is population, rather than individual, oriented. It is a system through which care-providing groups or networks take responsibility and share financial risk with an insurer for a specified population's medical care and health maintenance. The population basis enables the insurer to determine actuarially, projected use of services related to age, gender, and other factors. Service utilization estimates provide a basis for expected costs over a defined period. Estimates enable the insurer to establish premiums for benefit coverage.

By linking the insurance and delivery of services, managed care reverses the financial incentives of providers in the fee-for-service model. Fee-for-service is essentially a piecework, pay-as-you-go system in which the care provider is financially rewarded for high service utilization. Managed care uses the concept of prepayment, in which providers are paid a preset amount in advance for all services their insured population is projected to need in a given period. Capitation, a method that pays providers for services on a per-member-per-month basis, is a common form of prepayment. The provider receives payment whether or not services are used. If a physician exceeds the predetermined payment level, he or she may suffer a financial penalty. Similarly, if the physician uses fewer resources than predicted, he or she may retain the excess as profit.

Withholds are another form of payment device that seeks to provide financial incentives for efficient resource management. In the withhold scheme a percentage of the monthly capitated fee is withheld from payment to accommodate potential cost overruns for referrals or hospitalizations; all, part, or none of the withholds may be returned to the physician at the end of an annual period, depending on financial performance.[22] The key element of all physician prepayment arrangements is to encourage cost-conscious, efficient, and effective care.

Managed care plans also rely on transferring some measure of financial risk from the insurers to beneficiaries. Transfers of financial risk to beneficiaries most commonly take the form of copayments and deductibles. Copayments require that beneficiaries pay a set fee each time they receive a covered service, such as a copayment for each physician office visit. A deductible requires beneficiaries to meet a predetermined, out-of-pocket expenditure level before the MCO assumes payment responsibility for the balance of charges.

Today, managed care is synonymous with health insurance in the United States, and its principles have been adopted by the Medicare and Medicaid programs. Employers provide the primary source of health insurance, covering approximately 159 million Americans younger than age 65 years.[28] Sixty percent of employers offered health benefits in 2009, as did almost all firms with at least 50 employees.[28] Most employees in companies offering healthcare coverage subscribe to one or more managed care plans, with only 1% now enrolled in conventional plans.

As enrollment in managed care accelerated throughout the 1980s and 1990s, concerns emerged about MCO restrictions on consumer choice of providers and services. In response, MCOs spawned point-of-service plans that allow members to use providers outside the MCOs' approved provider networks. To exercise this choice, point-of-service members are charged copayments and deductibles higher than those charged for in-network services. In 2009 point-of-service plans represented 10% of covered employee enrollment.[28]

Another form of managed care arrangement, preferred provider organizations (PPOs), were formed by physicians and hospitals to serve the needs of private, third-party payers and self-insured firms. Through these arrangements PPOs guarantee a certain volume of business to hospitals and physicians in return for a negotiated discount in fees. PPOs offer attractive features to both physicians and hospitals. Physicians are not required to share in financial risk as a condition of participation, and PPOs reimburse physicians on a fee-for-service basis.

By providing predictable admission volume, PPOs help hospitals to shore up declining occupancy rates and attenuate the competition for admissions with other hospitals. To control costs, PPOs use negotiated discount fees, requirements that members receive care exclusively from contracted providers (or incur financial penalty), requirements for pre-authorization of hospital admission, and second opinions for major procedures. PPOs maintain systems of utilization review to control costs and advocate for more efficient service utilization by hospitals and physicians. Currently, PPOs are the most popular managed care plans, encompassing 60% of employer-covered workers.[28]

The organizational forms of managed care have continued evolving because of changing marketplace conditions, including purchaser preferences, beneficiary demands, and other factors. The emergence of PPOs as the most popular employee choice and the decline of staff model HMOs are notable trends. PPOs represented a means to involve payers and providers in negotiating fees and monitoring utilization while giving beneficiaries more choice. The decline of the staff model HMO resulted from many factors, including beneficiary demands for more choice among providers, large capital outlays associated with facility maintenance and expansion, and increased competition from IPA models. In 1988 staff models constituted about 42% of MCO membership. Currently, they represent less than 0.5% of managed care enrollment.[29]

Another trend has been MCOs' increased use of evidence-based clinical practice guidelines contained in programs of disease management for subscribers with potentially medically high-risk and high-cost conditions. The Disease Management Association of America describes disease management as a system of coordinated healthcare interventions and communications for populations in which patient self-care efforts are significant.[22] Candidates for these programs are identified from claims data and enrolled in services through which they are periodically contacted by professional staff of the insurer or a contracted disease management company to ensure compliance with physician orders and monitor their condition status between physician visits. The goal is to prevent complications, thereby controlling costs.[22] For very-high-risk conditions such as heart failure, disease management programs may equip subscribers with electronic devices connected to the Internet that allow real-time condition monitoring from the subscribers' homes.[22]

Because physicians are the predominant influence over the use of virtually all patient care resources, managed care emphasizes the primary physician's role as the "gatekeeper" who controls patient entry to all other levels of care. In response to patient demands for easier access to specialty services, some MCOs have relented on specialty referral requirements, but all continue to encourage avoidance of unnecessary use of high-cost services by appropriate and timely treatment at the primary level and, when indicated, participation in disease management programs.

Managed Care Backlash

In what is termed the managed care "backlash" that began in the late 1990s, organized medicine, other healthcare providers, and consumers railed against MCO policies on choice of providers, referrals, and other practices that were viewed as unduly restrictive.[22] A federal commission was established to review the need for guidelines in the managed care industry.[30] In 1998, President Bill Clinton imposed patient protection requirements on private insurance companies providing health coverage to federal workers.[31] Public dissatisfaction with constraints over the right to receive care deemed necessary and the freedom of physicians to refer patients to specialists received wide publicity. Public concerns driving sentiments toward more government regulation of the managed care industry included the belief that managed care was hurting the quality of patient care and that the managed care industry was not doing as good a job for patients as other sectors of the healthcare industry. Ultimately, the states took the lead in the patients' rights arena. Beginning in 1998, state legislatures have enacted more than 900 laws and regulations addressing both consumer and provider protections.[32]

In another response to the managed care backlash, increasing numbers of employers began allowing employees to make personal decisions about their coverage, dubbed consumer-driven health plans (CDHPs). The ultimate goals of the CDHP are to have employees take more responsibility for healthcare decisions and exercise more cost consciousness. The typical CDHP consists of either a health reimbursement arrangement or a health savings account (HSA).[33] Eligibility for an HSA requires the employee's enrollment in a high-deductible health insurance plan. Employers and employees may contribute to the HSA up to a qualified amount. CDHPs provide comparative information to employees in Web-based and traditional formats to increase knowledge about their healthcare choices and associated costs. In the HSA high deductible arrangement, the employee draws on the HSA to purchase care until the account is exhausted, when the policy's major medical provision activates. The second type of plan allows employees to design their own provider networks and benefits, based on anticipated needs and costs. The third uses Web-based information to enable employees to choose from established groupings of provider networks and benefits to "customize" coverage. In 2009, 8% of those persons obtaining health benefits from their employers participated in CDHPs.[28] Predictions vary widely regarding the future of such arrangements in the health insurance marketplace.

Trends in Managed Care Costs

Beginning in the 1980s, restrictions imposed on hospital and physician practices through prospective payment and restrictive fee schedules contributed to a decline in healthcare expenditure growth. Throughout the 1990s

market factors that enabled large health insurance purchasers to aggressively negotiate provider arrangements contributed to the impact of expenditure-cutting managed care initiatives.

The surge in managed care enrollment in the 1990s with decreases in premiums significantly contributed to a decline in the average annual growth of national healthcare expenditures[34]; however, after 4 years of decline health insurance premiums increased 8.2% in 1998, more than double the increase of the 3 previous years.[35] The insurance "underwriting cycle," in which insurers under-price during periods of market development and then increase premiums later to restore profitability, was noted as a major reason for increases.

Since 1999, average premiums for family coverage have increased 131% to a 2009 level of $13,375.[28] On average in 2009, covered workers contributed 17% of total premiums for single coverage and 27% for family coverage[28] (Figure 9-4). Higher premiums and requirements for larger employee contributions often cause workers to drop coverage. This effect increases in severity as the annual earnings of employees decrease, meaning that lower-wage workers who can least afford the risk of high healthcare costs are the most likely to become uninsured. Employers also seek to control costs through "benefit buy-downs." Methods include reducing the scope of benefits, increasing copayments and/or coinsurance, and increasing copayments for prescription drugs.[36] Some experts estimate that every 1% increase in premiums produces a net increase of 164,000 uninsured individuals.[37]

Since the mid-1990s, MCOs have undergone many changes. Company mergers and consolidations have been among the most prominent. A mere five publicly traded managed care companies now have enrollments totaling more than 103 million members,[38] representing 82% of all managed care subscribers.[39] Changes in managed care company operating policies have responded to provider and consumer demands reflected by state-enacted patient protection

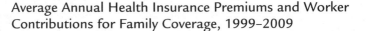

FIGURE 9-4   Average Annual Health Insurance Premiums and Worker Contributions for Family Coverage, 1999–2009

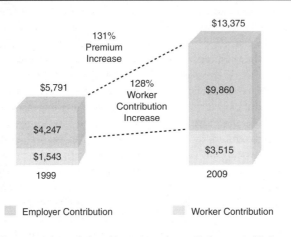

Note: The average worker contribution and the average employer contribution may not add to the average total premium due to rounding.

Source: Employer Health Benefits 2009 Annual Survey—Summary of Findings (#7937), The Henry J. Kaiser Family Foundation, September, 2009. This information was reprinted with permission from the Henry J. Kaiser Family Foundation. The Kaiser Family Foundation is a non-profit private operating foundation, based in Menlo Park, California, dedicated to producing and communicating the best possible analysis and information on health issues.

legislation, a loosening of early restrictions on patient provider choice and specialty referrals, and patient access to information about operating policies, especially regarding denials of payment.[22] A 5-year literature analysis of MCO performance indicates that MCOs overall did not accomplish their early promises to change clinical practice and improve quality while lowering costs. Findings suggest that a systematic revamping of information systems, coupled with appropriate incentives and revised clinical processes, will be required to produce the desired changes in cost and quality performance.[40]

MCOs and Quality

The most influential managed care quality assurance organization is the National Committee on Quality Assurance (NCQA). The NCQA formed in 1979 as two managed care trade organizations, the American Managed Care and Review Association and Group Health Association of America, merged under the title of the American Association of Health Plans. The title was later changed to the NCQA. In 1990, the NCQA became an independent, not-for-profit organization deriving its revenue primarily from fees for accreditation services.[41] The organization also publishes and markets a compendium of quality indicators on 250 health plans serving 50 million Americans.[42]

The NCQA evaluates participating organizations on a voluntary request basis. NCQA programs include accreditation for MCOs, PPOs, managed behavioral healthcare organizations, new health plans, and disease management programs. The NCQA also provides certification for organizations that verify provider credentials, physician organizations, utilization management organizations, and disease management organizations and programs. In addition, it provides physician recognition programs for performance excellence in several areas of condition management.[43] Accreditation of MCOs entails rigorous reviews of all aspects of the respective organizations, including online surveys and onsite reviews of key clinical and administrative processes. The review focuses on six major areas: management, physician credentials, member rights and responsibilities, preventive health services, utilization, and medical records. Beginning in 1999, the NCQA began including outcomes of care and measures of clinical processes in accreditation reviews, increasing the likelihood that accreditation status accurately reflects the quality of care delivered.[44]

In 1989 a partnership among the NCQA, health plans, and employers developed the Health Plan Employer Data and Information Set (HEDIS).[45] The HEDIS (now the Health Care Effectiveness Data and Information Set) provides a standardized method for MCOs to collect, calculate, and report information about their performance to allow employers, other purchasers, and consumers to compare different plans. It has evolved through several stages of development and continuously refines its measurements through a rigorous review and independent audits. The data set contains measures of MCO performance, divided among eight domains[46]:

1. Effectiveness of care
2. Access/availability of care
3. Satisfaction with the experience of care
4. Health plan stability
5. Use of services
6. Cost of care
7. Informed healthcare choices
8. Health plan descriptive information

The Centers for Medicare & Medicaid Services requires that all Medicare–managed care plans publicly report HEDIS data, and the NCQA requires all accredited plans to allow public reporting of their clinical quality data. A number of states also require plans providing Medicaid-managed care to report HEDIS data.[47]

The NCQA/HEDIS data provide an important avenue of accountability to the employer purchasers and consumers of health care and provide feedback to the providers that is critical in efforts to achieve improvement. The 2009 NCQA report "The State of Health Care Quality" noted an all-time high submission of audited HEDIS data representing 116 million Americans.[48] Benchmarked against the performance of the top 10% of all participating health plans, these data disclose quality disparities and gaps that inform purchasers, plan administrators, and policymakers. Comparisons allow the calculation of numbers of avoidable illnesses and deaths for several of the most common, costly, and life-threatening health conditions.[48]

MCOs also apply several internal techniques to manage quality, many of which directly or indirectly relate to physician performance. They focus attention on the quality of the institutional providers, especially on the hospitals with which they contract for services. Data systems that monitor claims information track the use of services to provide feedback to monitor resource use and quality. Through disease management programs, MCOs are attempting to control costs and improve care quality for individuals with chronic and costly conditions through methods such as the use of evidence-based clinical guidelines, patient self-management education, disease registries, risk stratification, proactive patient outreach, and performance feedback to providers. Programs may also use clinical specialists who provide monitoring and support to patients with disease management issues. Employer purchasers, several states, and the federal government are endorsing disease management programs for their employees and Medicaid and Medicare recipients.[49,50]

Self-Funded Insurance Programs

Since the late 1970s self-funding (full or partial) and self-insurance of employee health benefits have become increasingly common among large employers.[51] Through the self-funded mechanism, the employer (or other group, such as a union or trade association) collects premiums and pools these into a fund or account from which it pays claims against medical benefits instead of using a commercial carrier. Self-funded plans often use the services of an actuarial firm to set premium rates and a third-party administrator to administer benefits, pay claims, and collect data on utilization.[52] Many third-party administrators also provide case management services for potentially extraordinarily expensive cases to help coordinate care and control employer risk of catastrophic expenses.

Self-funded plans offer significant advantages to employers, such as avoiding additional administrative and other charges made by commercial carriers. By self-funding benefits, employers also can avoid premium taxes and accrue interest on the cash reserves held in the benefit account. A major stimulus to the development of self-insurance programs has been their exemption from the Employee Retirement and Income Security Act of 1974 (ERISA), which mandates minimum benefits under state law. This exemption allowed employers much greater flexibility in designing benefit packages and provided one mechanism to control benefit costs.

Major controversies continue to arise from the ERISA exemption of self-insured employer plans. One controversy is based in states' interpretation of their responsibilities for consumer protection through regulation of the types and scope of required coverage in employer-provided plans. ERISA has historically preempted such regulation. Another major area of dispute centers on the states' losses of premium revenue taxes as they struggle with growing financial burdens of uncompensated care and caring for uninsured populations. An additional area of controversy and legal actions surrounding ERISA is its prohibition against employees suing employer-provided health plans over matters involving coverage decisions. Under ERISA, organizations that administer employer-based health benefit plans maintain a degree of legal immunity from litigation and liability for withholding coverage or failing to provide necessary care. In 2004 the U.S. Supreme Court upheld an Appeals Court decision that beneficiaries of employment-related managed care plans cannot hold the plans accountable for damages when patients are injured as a result of coverage denial decisions.[53]

GOVERNMENT AS A SOURCE OF PAYMENT: A SYSTEM IN NAME ONLY

Federal and state government—and, to a lesser extent, local government—finance healthcare services as well. Federal funding originally focused on specific population groups, providing health care for those in government service, their dependents, and particular population groups, such as Native Americans. Today, a combination of public programs, chief among them the federal Medicare program and joint federal–state Medicaid program, constitutes almost half of total national care expenditures.[2]

Government payment for health services includes federal support of U.S. Public Health Service hospitals, the Indian Health Service, state and local inpatient psychiatric and other long-term care facilities, services of the Veterans Affairs hospitals and health services, services provided by the Department of Defense to military personnel and their dependents, workers' compensation, public health activities, and other government-sponsored service grants and initiatives.

In the absence of a comprehensive national health and social services policy, government's role in financing healthcare services can be described as a system only in the loosest interpretation of that term. It may be more accurate to describe government's various roles in healthcare financing as a mosaic of individual programs of reimbursement, direct payments to vendors, grants, matching funds, and subsidies.

As a source of healthcare service payments, the system of financing operates primarily in a vendor–purchaser relationship, with government contracting with healthcare services providers rather than providing services directly. A prime example is the Medicare program in which the federal government purchases hospital, home health, nursing home, physician, and other medical services under contract with suppliers. The Medicaid system operates similarly.

America's history of fierce resistance from the private sector—both organized medicine and, to an extent, the voluntary medicine and hospital systems—has prevented enactment of a comprehensive national healthcare system. Private sector lobby resistance can be traced from attempts in the early 20th century to provide some form of national health insurance through the current debates of the Obama administration and Congress.

Medicare and Medicaid, which account for the majority of U.S. public spending on health, are discussed next.

Medicare

Were it not for the successful opposition of the private sector led by the AMA, the Social Security Act of 1935, the most significant piece of social legislation ever enacted by the federal government, would have included a form of national health insurance. It was not to be for another 30 years, during which time many presidential and congressional acts for national health insurance had been proposed and defeated, that Congress enacted Medicare, "Health Insurance for the Aged," Title XVIII of the Social Security Act, in 1965. Medicare became only the second mandated health insurance program in the United States, after workers' compensation. When Medicare was enacted, approximately one-half of the elderly had any health insurance that usually covered only inpatient hospital costs, and much of healthcare spending was paid for out-of-pocket.[54] Today, the Medicare program covers 46 million Americans, including most 65 years of age and older, younger individuals who receive Social Security Disability Insurance benefits, and individuals with end-stage kidney disease and Lou Gehrig's disease following their eligibility for Social Security Disability Insurance. Projected 2010 expenditures total $504 billion, approximately 15% of the federal budget.[55]

The enactment of Medicare legislation was an historical benchmark, signaling government's entry into the personal healthcare financing arena. The Medicare program was established under the aegis of the Social Security Administration, and hospital payment was contracted to local intermediaries chosen by hospitals. More than 90% of hospitals chose their local Blue Cross association as the intermediary. In response to organized medicine's opposition to government certification, the Social Security Administration agreed to accreditation by the private Joint Commission on Accreditation of Hospitals as meeting the certification requirement for Medicare participation. Describing the enactment of Medicare as a "watershed," Rosemary Stevens wrote the following (pp. 281–282)[24]:

> Thus with the stroke of a pen, the elderly acquired hospital benefits, the hospitals acquired cost reimbursement for these benefits, the Blue Cross Association was precipitated into prominence as a major national organization (since the national contract was to be with the association, with subcontracting to local plans), and the Joint Commission was given formal government recognition.

The Medicare amendment stated that there should be "prohibition against any federal interference with the practice of medicine or the way medical services were provided" (pp. 286–287).[24] Ultimately, however, the government's acceptance of responsibility for payment for the care of older adults generated a flood of regulations to address cost and quality control of the services and products for which it was now a major payer.

As originally implemented, the Medicare program consisted of two parts, which differed in sources of funding and benefits. Part A provided benefits for hospital care, limited skilled nursing care, short-term home health care after hospitalization, and hospice care.[55] This portion of coverage was mandatory and was funded by Social Security payroll taxes.[54] Part B, supplementary medical insurance, was structured as a voluntary program covering physician services and services ordered by physicians, such as outpatient diagnostic tests, medical equipment and supplies, and home health services.[55] This portion was funded from benefi-

ciary premium payments, matched by general federal revenues.[54]

The Balanced Budget Act of 1997 added Part C, Medicare + Choice, allowing private health plans to administer Medicare contracts, with beneficiary enrollment on a voluntary basis. In 2003 the Medicare Prescription Drug, Improvement, and Modernization Act changed Part C to "Medicare Advantage," revising the administration of Medicare managed care programs to entice additional participation.[55] Since passage of the Medicare Prescription Drug, Improvement, and Modernization Act beneficiary enrollment in private health plans has increased substantially (Figure 9-5). Today, approximately 10 million beneficiaries participate in private health plans. The Medicare Prescription Drug, Improvement, and Modernization Act also added

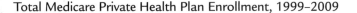

FIGURE 9-5   Total Medicare Private Health Plan Enrollment, 1999–2009

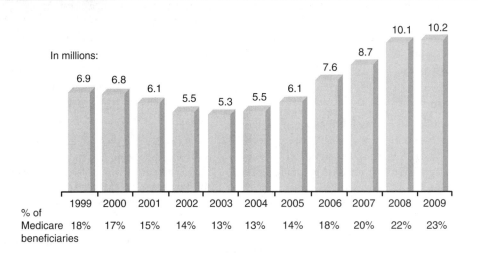

Note: Includes local HMOs, PSOs, PPOs, regional PPOs, PFFS plans, 1876 Cost Plans, Demonstrations, HCPP and PACE Plans.

Source: Medicare Advantage Fact Sheet (#2052-13), The Henry J. Kaiser Family Foundation, November, 2009. This information was reprinted with permission from the Henry J. Kaiser Family Foundation. The Kaiser Family Foundation is a non-profit private operating foundation, based in Menlo Park, California, dedicated to producing and communicating the best possible analysis and information on health issues.

a new Part D for prescription drug coverage to provide financial relief from these costs, particularly for low-income individuals.

From its inception, Medicare coverage was not fully comprehensive, and that remains true today. Beneficiaries are required to share costs through a system of deductibles and coinsurance, and there is no limit on out-of-pocket expenditures. For Part A, the deductible requires beneficiaries to reach a set amount in personal outlays for hospitalization each 12-month period, and coinsurance requires that patients cover 20% of hospitalization costs. The program also limits total compensated days of hospital care on a lifetime pool of days. For Part B coverage, monthly premiums are deducted from Social Security payments. These limitations gave rise to a variety of private supplemental, or "Medi-gap," policies, designed to assist with cost-sharing requirements and benefit gaps.[55] Also, the prescription drug benefit contains a gap in which beneficiaries are fully exposed to costs between designated levels of expenditures.[56]

Medicare Cost Containment and Quality Initiatives

Within a few years after implementation, Medicare spending was significantly exceeding projections. Although hospital costs for the growing older adult population increased more rapidly than expected, the rise over projected Medicare expenses could not be explained by that phenomenon. A 1976 study by the U.S. Human Resources Administration reviewed the first 10 years of Medicare hospital expenses and attributed less than 10% of increases to utilization by the older adult population. Almost one-fourth of the increase over projected hospital costs was attributed to general inflation and two-thirds to huge growth in hospital payroll and nonpayroll expenses, including profits.[24]

Like Blue Cross, Medicare's hospital reimbursement mechanism was cost based and retrospective on a per-day-of-stay basis. Although facilitating the rapid incorporation of almost 20 million beneficiaries into the new benefit system, cost-based reimbursement also fueled utilization in an era of rapidly advancing medical technology. Because they were paid on a retrospective basis for costs incurred, hospitals had a strong incentive to use services with no incentives for efficiency.

In the decade after Medicare enactment, several amendments to the Social Security Act made significant changes. In general, amendments of the first 5 years increased the types of covered services and expanded the population of eligible persons. During the later period, amendments addressed rising concerns about the costs and quality of the program.

Many initiatives attempted to slow spiraling costs and address quality concerns. They were largely unsuccessful. In 1966 Congress enacted the Comprehensive Health Planning Act to support states in conducting local health planning to ensure adequate facilities and services and avoid duplications.[57] In 1974 the Health Planning Resources and Development Act replaced the Comprehensive Health Planning Act with health systems agencies to develop plans for local health resources based on quantified population needs. The Act also required all states to obtain approval from a state planning agency before starting any major capital project, and several states adopted certificate-of-need legislation for this purpose. Congress repealed the federal mandate in 1987, but most states still maintain some form of certificate-of-need program, focused on development of physician-owned facilities such as ambulatory surgery and diagnostic imaging centers.[58] Health systems agencies were unsuccessful in materially influencing decisions about service or technology expansion, because decisions were dominated by institutional and economic interests. Concurrent with attempts to slow cost increases through a planning approach, a number of other legislative initiatives took shape that were directly related to concerns over Medicare costs and service quality.

Professional standards review organizations, established in 1972, signaled the first federal attempt to review care provided under Medicare, Medicaid, and certain other federally funded healthcare programs.[59] Each local professional standards review organization was a not-for-profit organization composed of a group of local physicians who performed record reviews and made payment recommendations to the local Medicare intermediary. Plagued by questionable effectiveness and high administrative costs, professional standards review organizations were replaced by peer review organizations in 1982. Peer review organizations were given more specific and measurable cost and quality standards than their predecessor professional standards review organizations.[60] In 2001 peer review organizations were renamed "quality improvement organizations" as part of broad, quality improvement initiatives of the Centers for Medicare & Medicaid Services.

Both not-for-profit and investor-owned for-profit hospitals saw the opportunity for expansion offered by Medicare's guarantee of full-cost reimbursement. Between 1970 and 1980 there was a more than 200% increase in the number of hospitals involved in multihospital systems of both types.[61]

The federal budgets of 1980 and 1981 again amended the Medicare legislation, with a strong focus on reducing the number and length of hospitalizations. Amendments advocated home health services as a hospital alternative by eliminating the limit on annual number of home healthcare visits, a 3-day hospitalization requirement for home health visit coverage eligibility, and occupational therapy as a requirement for initial entitlement to home healthcare services. Budget provisions also lifted exclusion from Medicare participation of for-profit home healthcare agencies in states that did not require agency licensure.

The unsuccessful efforts at Medicare cost containment and quality control of the 1970s and 1980s culminated in Medicare's 1983 enactment of a case payment system that radically changed hospital reimbursement. The new payment system shifted hospital reimbursement from the retrospective to prospective mode. Using diagnosis-related groups (DRGs) developed for the Health Care Financing Administration, the new system provided a patient classification method to relate the type of patients a hospital treated (i.e., age, sex, gender, diagnoses) to costs.[62] The DRG payment system based hospital payments on established fees for services required to treat specific diagnoses rather than on discreet units of services. The DRGs group more than 10,000 International Classification of Disease codes into approximately 500 patient categories. Patients within each category are grouped for similar clinical conditions and expected resource use.[63] DRGs form a manageable, clinically coherent set of patient classes that relate a hospital's case mix to the resource demands and associated costs experienced by the hospital. The payment an individual hospital receives under this system is ultimately calculated using input from a variety of other data known to impact costs, such as hospital teaching status and wage data for its geographic location.

The DRG system provided incentives for the hospital to spend only what was needed to achieve optimal patient outcomes. If outcomes could be achieved at a cost lower than the preset payment, the hospital received an excess payment for those cases. If the hospital spent more to treat cases than allowed, it absorbed the excess costs. The DRG system also financially provided for cases classified as "outliers" due to complications. The DRG system did not build in allowances to the payment rate for direct medical education expenses for teaching hospitals, hospital outpatient expenses, or capital expenditures. These continued to be reimbursed on a cost basis.

The principle of case-based prospective payment soon was adopted in varying forms by numerous states and private third-party payers as their reimbursement basis. The prospective payment system raised many concerns among hospitals, healthcare providers, and consumers about its possible effects, including fears about premature hospital discharges, hospitals' questionable ability to streamline services to conform to preset payments, and the home healthcare industry's capacity to accommodate an increased caseload.

"Quicker and sicker" was the slogan popularized by the media during the first years of the prospective payment system to characterize the drive for shorter hospital stays. The media also popularized the term "patient dumping," referring to documented hospitals' transfer of patients at high risk of expensive and potentially unprofitable service needs to other hospitals.

Subsequent research on the impact of the prospective payment system demonstrated that many early concerns were unfounded and that DRGs did have a measurable impact on the overall growth of Medicare spending.[64] Extensive research also compared quality indicators before and after DRG implementation. The federal Prospective Payment Assessment Commission was established to monitor the effects of the prospective system. Studies revealed few effects on Medicare patient readmission rates attributable to the DRG system.[65] The RAND Corporation also conducted several studies of another indicator of patient care quality, in-hospital mortality rates. The studies reviewed almost 17,000 records of Medicare patients admitted to hospitals for five common diagnoses. Findings included a drop of 24% in the average length of hospital stay for these conditions and an overall improvement in mortality rates among the diagnoses studied.[65]

Concerns about patient dumping were formally addressed in the 1985 federal budget by the Emergency Medical Treatment and Labor Act of 1986, which required hospitals to treat everyone who presented in their emergency departments, regardless of ability to pay. Stiff financial penalties, as well as risk of Medicare certification loss by hospitals inappropriately transferring patients, accompanied the Emergency Medical Treatment and Labor Act provisions.[66]

Evidence indicates that the prospective payment system slowed hospital cost growth during the early years after implementation through reductions in lengths of stay, hospital personnel, and new medical technologies; however, total Medicare cost growth later reaccelerated, in part because of increased volume in outpatient spending and other factors whose impacts have not been clearly determined.[65] Concerns about the capacity of the home healthcare industry to meet anticipated increases in demand dissipated quickly. Both the not-for-profit and proprietary sectors of the industry responded by creating new or expanding existing home healthcare services as components of vertically integrated systems. In the early years of the prospective payment system, hospitals did not experience the predicted negative financial impact, and they actually posted substantial profits.[65] In fact, the federal government partially justified subsequent reductions in prospective payment on the basis that early payments were too high relative to costs.[66] It has even been suggested that the large surpluses generated by not-for-profit hospitals in the early years of prospective payment fueled hospital costs by making new surpluses available for investment.[65]

From the outset, the prospective payment system's cost-containment effectiveness was limited by its application to only inpatient hospital care for Medicare recipients. Aggressive shifting of Medicare-covered services to the outpatient setting and shifting hospital costs onto private pay patients were two major reactions that dampened the prospective payment system's cost-containment results.

Medicare Physician Reimbursement

Medicare Part B physician reimbursement was established as fee-for-service, based on prevailing fees within geographic areas. The Medicare physician payment rate increase averaged 18% annually between 1975 and 1987 and provoked legislative action.[67] Medicare first enacted a temporary price freeze for physician services.[67]

Assessments of the price freeze suggested that physicians offset the lower fees by increasing the volume of services.[67] This raised the issue of whether physicians respond to fee pressures by using more services to compensate for lower reimbursement. Concerns over absolute cost increases and overuse of costly specialty care prompted additional congressional cost-containment action.

The 1989 federal budget established a new method of Medicare physician reimbursement that became effective in 1992, using a resource-based relative value scale to replace the fee-for-service reimbursement system.[68] The resource-based relative value scale was intended to control cost growth by instituting the same payments for the same services, whether performed by a generalist or specialist physician, thereby reducing the numbers of expensive procedures and lowering the incentive for physicians to specialize. Relative value units were adjusted for geographic area variations in costs. The resource-based relative value scale continues to be used, with a committee of the AMA and national medical specialty societies recommending annual updates to the system.[68]

Balanced Budget Act of 1997

Medicare reforms enacted by the DRG prospective payment system, managed care influences, market competition, technology advances, and consumerism produced unprecedented changes in hospital and physician reimbursement, hospitals' affinity for technology, and consumer expectations of hospital care. The Medicare prospective payment system had succeeded in demonstrating that "more is not necessarily better," as lengths of stay and service intensity declined to accommodate the DRG framework, with no demonstrable negative impact on the quality of patient care. Then, in the early 1990s, the nation witnessed vigorous debates regarding the Clinton administration's National Health Security Act. Although the Act never reached a congressional vote, many months of debate

thrust national concerns about Medicare spending, lack of access to services, beneficiary costs, and provider choice into the public spotlight. Popular and political sensitivities rose against the backdrop of escalating national predictions about potential insolvency of the Hospital Insurance Trust Fund.[69]

Several trends supported the need for major changes in the Medicare system. First, Congressional Budget Office projections indicated that Medicare cost growth could not be sustained without cuts in other government programs, major increases in taxes, or larger budget deficits.[70]

Second, Medicare's fee-for-service indemnity structure was becoming rapidly outmoded, as employer-sponsored plans, Medicaid, and private insurance were rapidly embracing managed care principles.

Third, Medicare coverage left significant gaps requiring copayments and coinsurance that many beneficiaries were unable to fill with supplemental "Medi-gap" insurance policies. Although some Medicare beneficiaries were eligible for Medicaid subsidies of these expenses, subsidies created additional financial burdens for the states.

Acknowledging the president's and Congress's discord on a national health reform program, in 1995 Congress focused on slowing Medicare cost growth and achieving broader choices for Medicare beneficiaries through managed care plans as models of cost-containment and consumer satisfaction.[70]

The presidential and congressional campaigns of 1996 focused heavily on the health-care issues brought to light during debate on the National Health Security Act and consumer concerns about managed care. This political environment supported the rapid formulation and passage of the bipartisan Health Insurance Portability and Accountability Act of 1996 (HIPAA), also called the Kassenbaum-Kennedy Bill. Among its important health insurance features, HIPAA prohibited insurance companies from denying coverage due to preexisting medical conditions or denying sale of personal insurance policies to individuals who were previously covered in group plans. It also established a pilot program to enable workers to save tax-free dollars for future medical expenses through medical savings accounts.[71] Though the act accomplished important beneficial outcomes, it fell far short of addressing the pervasive problems of the overall healthcare system in general or the Medicare and Medicaid programs in particular.

The 1998 federal budget process reflected pressures to produce a balanced budget and to respond meaningfully to national health issues from both the consumer and cost-containment perspectives. The resulting Balanced Budget Act (BBA) created major new policy directions for Medicare and Medicaid and took important incremental steps toward universal coverage through an initiative to insure uninsured children through a $16 billion allocation for a new State Children's Health Insurance Program (SCHIP).[72]

The Act was characterized as containing "some of the most sweeping and significant changes to Medicare and Medicaid since their inception in 1965."[72] Overall, the BBA proposed to reduce growth in Medicare and Medicaid spending by $125.2 billion in 5 years through regulatory changes and payment changes to hospitals, physicians, post–acute care services, and health plans. It also increased premiums for Medicare Part B and required new prospective payment systems for hospital outpatient services, skilled nursing facilities, home health agencies, and rehabilitation hospitals. It also reduced allowances for medical education expenses of teaching hospitals and funded incentives to hospitals for voluntarily reducing the numbers of medical residents. As the largest Medicare spender, the BBA targeted hospitals for more than one-third of total anticipated savings. Decreased Medicare spending growth in the period 1998–2002 demonstrated the immediate impact of the BBA. After growing at an average annual rate of 11.1% for the 15 years before 1997, the average annual rate of spending growth between 1998 and 2000 dropped to 1.7%, resulting in approximately $68 billion in savings.[73]

Among the most significant policy shifts of the BBA was opening the Medicare program to private insurers through the Medicare + Choice Program, for the first time allowing financial risk sharing for the Medicare program with the private sector. The participation of private insurers was intended to increase both the impact of competitive market forces on the program and consumer awareness of alternatives to the fee-for-service system.

The BBA constituted federal commissions to carry out monitoring and recommendation functions during implementation, including the Medicare Payment Advisory Commission and an independent National Bipartisan Commission on the Future of Medicare, whose functions entailed the analyzing numerous dimensions of Medicare's financial condition and benefits design over time.[74]

Implementation of the Medicare BBA provisions experienced widespread challenges and delays. Significant changes to the Medicare and Medicaid program structure, payment methods, and amounts all drew fire from industry advocacy groups, professional organizations, and consumers. Just before several of the BBA's provisions took effect, President Clinton signed the Balanced Budget Refinement Act of 1999, providing $17.5 billion to restore cuts to industry sectors negatively impacted by the BBA and outlining later implementation schedules for many of the BBA's original mandates.[75]

The Medicare managed care enrollment initiative experienced serious challenges. Because of reduced Medicare reimbursement, costs of working with federal bureaucracy, and market shifts reducing profitability, MCOs lost their early enthusiasm for participation in the program. Plan withdrawals resulted in a decline from 6.3 million beneficiaries in 2000 to 4.6 million in 2003.[76] In response, in 2000 Congress enacted the Benefits Protection and Improvement Act that increased participating health plans' and provider payments.[77]

In 2001 the Centers for Medicare & Medicaid Services inaugurated the "Quality Initiative," encompassing every dimension of the healthcare delivery system. The Quality Initiative includes nursing homes, hospitals, home healthcare agencies, physicians, and other facilities.[78] The program collects and analyzes data to monitor conformance with standards of care and performance. In addition to the Quality Initiative, the Medicare Quality Monitoring System "processes, analyzes, interprets and disseminates health-related data to monitor the quality of care delivered to Medicare fee-for-service beneficiaries."[79] The Medicare administration also is experimenting with hospital pay-for-performance plans designed to improve quality and avoid unnecessary costs.[80]

With the goal of providing public, valid, and user-friendly information about hospital quality, in 2005 Medicare launched the website "Hospital Compare," in a collaboration with the Hospital Quality Alliance, a public–private partnership organization. Hospital Compare encompasses common conditions and criteria that assess individual hospitals' performance consistency with evidence-based practice; reporting is required for hospitals to qualify for Medicare rate updates.[81] Data from the "Hospital Consumer Assessment of Healthcare Providers and Systems" surveys has been added to the Hospital Compare information, providing patient perspectives on their hospital experience.[82]

In 2007 the Medicare administration announced that beginning in 2008 it would no longer pay for procedures resulting from hospital-acquired infections, an aggressive step in using quality standards as a basis for public reporting and payment.[83] In consultation with the Hospital Quality Forum and many other expert organizations, Medicare also identified categories of untoward hospital events, dubbed

"never happen events," for which it is investigating hospital payment reductions for resulting treatment.[84]

Medicaid and the SCHIP

In 1965 Medicaid legislation was enacted as Title XIX of the Social Security Act. Medicaid is administered by the Centers for Medicare & Medicaid Services and is a mandatory joint federal–state program in which federal and state support is shared based on the state's per capita income. Before Medicaid's implementation, healthcare services for the economically needy population were provided through a patchwork of programs sponsored by state and local governments, charitable organizations, and community hospitals.

Today, Medicaid supports healthcare and long-term care services for 47.1 million low-income Americans.[85] The program represents a major source of healthcare system funding, accounting for more than 16% of the total $1.9 trillion in personal health services spending and 41% of all spending for nursing home care in 2008.[2] The Medicaid program is the third largest source of health insurance in the United States, after employer-based programs and Medicare.

The federal government establishes broad program guidelines, but program requirements are the prerogative of state governments. Medicaid requires states to cover certain types of individuals or groups under their plans, and states may include others at their discretion. The program provides three types of coverage:

1. Health insurance for low-income families with children
2. Long-term care for older Americans and individuals with disabilities
3. Supplemental coverage for low-income Medicare beneficiaries for services not covered by Medicare, including Medicare premiums, deductibles, and coinsurance[86]

Until the enactment of Medicare Part D, the third type of coverage also paid for prescription drugs.

Medicaid federal guidelines established a mandated core of basic medical services for state programs. Included were inpatient and outpatient hospital services, physician services, diagnostic services, and nursing home care for adults. Later Medicaid amendments expanded mandated benefits to include home health care, preventive health screening services, family planning services, and assistance to recipients of Supplemental Security Income. State Medicaid programs currently must extend benefits to all pregnant women who meet federal income level guidelines and children whose family incomes fall below specified federal income guidelines. Individual states have broad discretion to include additional services in their Medicaid programs, and many have elected extended benefits beyond the core of mandated benefits.

Medicaid funding sources are distinct from those for Medicare. Medicare, which is funded from contributions of payroll taxes matched by employers, is an entitlement because individuals have contributed to their cost of coverage. Medicaid, which is funded by personal income and corporate and excise taxes, is a transfer payment representing funds transferred from more economically affluent individuals to those in need.[87]

Unlike Medicare, which reimburses providers through intermediaries such as Blue Cross, Medicaid directly reimburses service providers. Rate-setting formulas, procedures, and policies vary widely among states. Because of the variations in benefits and reimbursement policies, Medicaid has been described as "50 different programs."[87]

Throughout the 1980s as costs grew rapidly, states tested various prepaid, managed care approaches, and some implemented prospective payment systems modeled on DRG reimbursement. Several states experimented with voluntary Medicaid managed care enrollment, contracting with HMOs to provide some or all of their Medicaid benefits under federally approved demonstration projects. Through a provision of the BBA, the federal government allowed states to

mandate managed care enrollment for their Medicaid beneficiaries, and today all 50 states offer some type of Medicaid managed care plans.

In 2008, more than 70% of Medicaid beneficiaries were enrolled in managed care plans.[85] The number and proportion of Medicaid enrollees in managed care plans continue to increase as states seek ways to control costs and ensure access. All states are struggling with the burden of rising Medicaid costs. The 2008 economic recession accelerated Medicaid enrollment, spending, and growth that are expected to continue through 2010[88] (Figure 9-6).

Children's Health Insurance Program

The BBA contained a child health initiative to build on the Medicaid program by targeting uninsured children whose family income was too high to qualify for Medicaid and too low to afford private health insurance through SCHIP. SCHIP targeted enrollment of 5 million children through federal matching funds for states over the period 1998 to 2007.[89] In 1999 all 50 states were receiving federal support from BBA allocations under the SCHIP. By 2008 more than 7 million children in total had been enrolled in the program since its inception (Figure 9-7). Renamed the "Children's Health Insurance Program," the program was reauthorized in 2008 and again in 2009 with significant enhancements for the period through 2013.[89] However, in 2008, 8.1 million children—approximately 10.3% of all U.S. children—remained uninsured.[90]

Medicaid Quality Initiatives

The Centers for Medicare & Medicaid Services and State Operations has the principal responsibility for developing and carrying out Medicaid and SCHIP quality initiatives through working partnerships with the respective state's programs. The Centers for Medicare & Medicaid Services and State Operations articulates a quality strategy encompassing five key elements[91]:

1. Evidence-based care and quality measurement
2. Payment aligned with quality

3. Health information technology

4. Partnerships

5. Information dissemination, technical assistance, and sharing of best practices

The Division of Quality, Evaluation, and Health Outcomes focuses on providing technical assistance to states in their quality improvement initiatives.[92]

FUTURE PROSPECTS

A 2007 Henry J. Kaiser Family Foundation's health tracking poll on 2008 presidential election issues indicated that health care was the top domestic issue, behind only the Iraq war in voter priority for candidates' attention.[93]

The 2007 candidate, and now President Obama, campaigned with strong promises of swift, major health reform legislation to address the continuing issues of costs, quality, and access. Almost one year to the date of his inauguration as president, and after many months of acrimonious dialogue as the Senate and House constructed reform bills, in January 2010 *Modern Health Care* headlined, "Requiem for Reform," following the election of a Republican Massachusetts senator to replace the late Democratic U.S. Senator, Edward Kennedy.[94] Democrats lost their filibuster-proof Senate majority and, with it, the likelihood of passing a hoped-for comprehensive bill. Incremental alternatives remained possible, but strong partisanship suggested that outcomes would fall far short of a major overhaul of healthcare financing and the service delivery system. Passage of the Patient Protection and Affordable Care Act

| FIGURE 9-6 | Percentage Change in Total Medicaid Spending and Enrollment, 1998–2008 |

Note: Enrollment percentage changes from June to June of each year; spending growth percentage changes in state fiscal year.

Source: The Crunch Continues: Medicaid Spending, Coverage and Policy in the Midst of a Recession (#7985), The Henry J. Kaiser Family Foundation, September, 2009. This information was reprinted with permission from the Henry J. Kaiser Family Foundation. The Kaiser Family Foundation is a non-profit private operating foundation, based in Menlo Park, California, dedicated to producing and communicating the best possible analysis and information on health issues.

of 2010 recognized that America's healthcare investment is more of a moral than economic issue, as U.S. health status indicators lag behind other developed countries that spend much less and provide universal healthcare coverage.

Against the current federal backdrop, several states have continued to experiment with healthcare reform. Maine, Massachusetts, and Vermont are notable examples.[95] In 2003 Maine committed to making affordable healthcare coverage available to every citizen, to decreasing healthcare cost growth, and to enhancing care quality with a subsidized insurance product and expansions of Medicaid eligibility.[95] In 2006, Massachusetts enacted a model very close to universal coverage, using a mandate of personal responsibility to purchase health insurance combined with government subsidies to ensure affordability.[96] Since the plan's implementation, estimates are that two-thirds of pre-

viously uninsured individuals have obtained coverage.[96] Also in 2006, Vermont enacted a plan with more than 35 special initiatives targeted to increase access, contain costs, and improve quality.[97] The Vermont plan includes a new health insurance product for the uninsured that provides employer-sponsored premium assistance through employer contributions and a statewide plan for preventing and managing chronic conditions.[97]

The new healthcare reform legislation will confront policymakers with a daunting array of issues demanding creativity and courage to enact meaningful changes. Paying for required changes may be considerably easier than breaking loose from old philosophies, value systems, and politics that have brought the U.S. healthcare enterprise to its present paradoxical state of superior technology embedded in an antiquated delivery system.

| FIGURE 9-7 | Number of Children Ever Enrolled in the Children's Health Insurance Program |

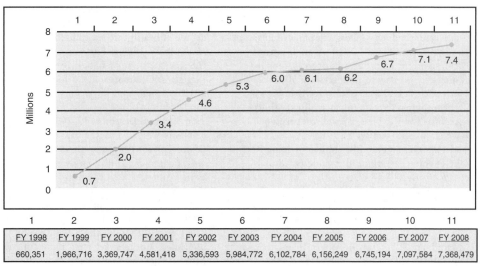

	FY 1998	FY 1999	FY 2000	FY 2001	FY 2002	FY 2003	FY 2004	FY 2005	FY 2006	FY 2007	FY 2008
	660,351	1,966,716	3,369,747	4,581,418	5,336,593	5,984,772	6,102,784	6,156,249	6,745,194	7,097,584	7,368,479

CHIP = Separate Child Health Programs and Medicaid Expansion (Title XXI)

Source: Children's Health Insurance Statistical Enrollment Data System (SEDS), January 29, 2009.

DISCUSSION QUESTIONS ─────────

1. Update the data in the chapter by using the Centers for Medicare & Medicaid Services' website to analyze national healthcare expenditures and sources of payment.

2. Using the same website, discuss the future projections for healthcare expenditures and sources of payment. What are the implications for advanced practice nursing?

3. Discuss the policy role that advanced practice nurses may assume to influence the government as a payer and provider of services.

REFERENCES ─────────────

1. Congressional Budget Office. Long-term look for health care spending: overview of the U.S. health care system. Available from http://www.cbo.gov/ftpdocs/87xx/doc8758/MainText.3.1.shtml. Accessed January 17, 2010.

2. U.S. Department of Health and Human Services, Centers for Medicare & Medicaid Services. National health expenditures tables, 2008. Available from http://www.cms.hhs.gov/nationalhealthexpenddata/downloads/tables.pdf. Accessed January 15, 2010.

3. Hartman M, Martin A, Nuccio O, et al. Health spending growth at a historic low. *Health Affairs.* 2010;29:147–152.

4. Altman S, Tompkins C, Eliat E, et al. Escalating health care spending: is it desirable or inevitable? *Health Affairs.* 2003:W1–W14. Available from http://content.healthaffairs.org/cgi/reprint/hlthaff.w3.1v1?maxtoshow=&HITS=10&hits=10&RESULTFORMAT=&fulltext=Altman+S%2C+Tompkins+C+&andorexactfulltext=and&searchid=1&FIRSTINDEX=0&resourcetype=HWCIT. Accessed January 14, 2010.

5. Anderson GF, Frogner BK. Health spending in OECD countries: obtaining value per dollar. *Health Affairs.* 2008;27:1718–1727.

6. Anderson GF, Reinhardt UE, Hussey PS, et al. It's the prices, stupid: why the United States is so different from other countries. *Health Affairs.* 2003;22:89–105.

7. Milstein A, Gilbertson E. American medical home runs. *Health Affairs.* 2009;28:1317–1318.

8. Orszag PR. Opportunities to increase efficiency in health care, June 2008. Congressional Budget Office. Available from http://www.cbo.gov/ftpdocs/93xx/doc9384/06-16-healthsummit.pdf. Accessed January 14, 2010.

9. Morris L. Combating fraud in health care: an essential component of any cost containment strategy. *Health Affairs.* 2009;28:1351–1356.

10. Chernew ME, Jacobson PD, Hofer TP, et al. Barriers to constraining health care cost growth. *Health Affairs.* 2004;23:122–128.

11. Levit K, Smith C, Cowan C, et al. Inflation spurs health spending in 2000. *Health Affairs.* 2002; 21:179.

12. U.S. Department of Health and Human Services, Administration on Aging. Profile of older Americans: 2008. Available from http://www.aoa.gov/AoARoot/Aging_Statistics/Profile/2008/index.aspx. Accessed December 14, 2009.

13. U.S. Department of Health and Human Services, Administration on Aging. Population 65 and over by age: 1900–2050. Available from http://www.aoa.gov/AoARoot/Aging_Statistics/future_growth/docs/By_Age_65_and_over.xls. Accessed December 14, 2009.

14. Coile RC Jr, Trusko BE. Healthcare 2020: challenges of the millennium. *Health Care Manage Technol.* 1999;20:37.

15. DeFrances CJ, Lucas CA, Buie VC, et al. 2006 National hospital discharge survey, July 2008. Available from http://www.cdc.gov/nchs/data/nhsr/nhsr005.pdf. Accessed December 21, 2009.

16. Smith S, Heffler S, Freeland M, et al. The next decade of health care spending: a new outlook. *Health Affairs.* 1999;18:89–90.

17. U.S. Department of Labor, Bureau of Labor Statistics. Occupational outlook handbook, 2010–2011 edition, physicians and surgeons. Available from http://www.bls.gov/oco/ocos074.htm. Accessed December 12, 2009.

18. DeNavas-Walt C, Proctor BD, Smith JC. U.S. *Census Current Population Reports, P60-236, Income, Poverty, and Health Insurance Coverage in the United States: 2008.* Washington, DC: U.S. Government Printing Office; 2009. Available from http://www.census.gov/prod/2009pubs/p60-236.pdf. Accessed January 12, 2010.

19. The Henry J. Kaiser Family Foundation. The uninsured: a primer: key facts about Americans without health insurance. Available from http://www.kff.org/uninsured/upload/7451.pdf. Accessed January 12, 2010.

20. American College of Physicians and American Society of Internal Medicine. No health insurance: it's enough to make you sick. Available from http://www/acponline.org/pressroom/applauds.htm. Accessed January 16, 2010.

21. U.S. Department of Labor, Bureau of Labor Statistics. Career guide to industries, 2010–2011, healthcare. Available from http://www.bls.gov/oco/cg/cgs035.htm. Accessed January 12, 2010.

22. Kongstvedt PR. *Essentials of Managed Health Care,* 5th ed. Sudbury, MA: Jones and Bartlett; 2007.

23. Wilson F, Neuhauser D. *Health Services in the United States,* 2nd ed. Cambridge, MA: Ballinger; 1982.

24. Stevens R. *In Sickness and in Wealth: American Hospitals in the Twentieth Century.* New York: Basic Books; 1989.

25. Conover CJ, Hall MA, Ostermann J. The impact of Blue Cross conversions on health spending and the uninsured. *Health Affairs.* 2005;24:473–482.

26. Thomasson, M. Health insurance in the United States. Available from http://eh.net/encyclopedia/article/thomasson.insurance.health.us. Accessed January 15, 2010.

27. Kongstvedt PR. *The Managed Health Care Handbook.* Gaithersburg, MD: Aspen; 1989.

28. The Henry J. Kaiser Family Foundation and Health Research and Educational Trust. Employer health benefits 2009, summary of findings. Available from http:/ehbs.kff.org/pdf/2009/7937.pdf. Accessed December 19, 2009.

29. Trespacz KL. Staff-model HMOs: don't blink or you'll miss them. *Managed Care Magazine.* Available from http://www.managedcaremag.com/archives/9907/9907.staffmodel.html. Accessed January 12, 2010.

30. Blendon RJ, Brodie M, Benson J, et al. Understanding the managed care backlash. *Health Affairs.* 1998;17:80.

31. White House Backgrounder. President Clinton releases report documenting actions federal government is taking to implement a patients' bill of rights. Available from http://www.hhs.gov/news/press/1998pres/981102.html. Accessed January 16, 2010.

32. National Conference of State Legislatures. Managed care state laws and regulations including consumer and provider protections. Available from http://www.ncsl.org/IssuesResearch/Health/ManagedCareStateLaws/tabid/14320/Default.aspx. Accessed January 16, 2010.

33. Gabel JR, Pickreign JD, Witmore HH, et al. Behind the slow growth of employer-based consumer-driven health plans. Available from http://www.hschange.com/CONTENT/900/?topic=topic01#ib1. Accessed January 15, 2010.

34. Congressional Budget Office. Projections of national health expenditures: 1997–2008, the economic and budget outlook: fiscal years 1999–2008. Available from http://www.cbo.gov/doc.cfm?index=316. Accessed January 15, 2010.

35. Levit K, Cowan C, Lazenby H, et al. Health spending in 1998: signals of change. *Health Affairs.* 2000;19:131.

36. Centers for Medicare & Medicaid Services. Health care industry market update, managed care. Available from http://www3.cms.hhs.gov/CapMarketUpdates/Downloads/hcimu11122002.pdf . Accessed January 17, 2010.

37. Chernew M, Cutler D, Keenan P, et al. University of Michigan, Economic Research Institute on the Uninsured. Increasing health insurance costs and the decline in insurance coverage. Available from http://eriu.sph.umich.edu/pdf/wp8.pdf. Accessed January 18, 2010.

38. Atlantic Information Services. Health plans, company intelligence. *Health Plan Week.* Available from http://www.aishealth.com/ManagedCare/CompanyIntel/TenLargest.html. Accessed January 21, 2010.

39. Managed Care On-line. Managed care national statistics. National managed care enrollment, 2009. Available from http://www.mcareol.com/factshts/factnati.htm. Accessed January 21, 2010.

40. Miller RH, Luft HS. HMO plan performance update: analysis of the literature, 1997–2001. *Health Affairs.* 2002;21:81.

41. Iglehart JK. The National Committee for Quality Assurance. *N Engl J Med.* 1996;335:995.

42. National Committee for Quality Assurance. Report cards. Available from http://www.ncqa.org/tabid/60/Default.aspx. Accessed January 21, 2010.

43. National Committee for Quality Assurance. Programs. Available from http://www.ncqa.org/tabid/74/Default.aspx. Accessed January 21, 2010.

44. Pawlson L, O'Kane M. Professionalism, regulation, and the market: impact on accountability for quality of care. *Health Affairs*. 2002;21:202.

45. Epstein M. The role of quality measurement in a competitive marketplace. In: Altman SH, Reinhardt UE, Eds. *Strategic Choices for a Changing Health Care System*. Chicago: Health Administration Press; 1996:217.

46. National Committee for Quality Assurance. HEDIS compliance audit program, 2010. Available from http://www.ncqa.org/tabid/205 /Default.aspx. Accessed January 21, 2010.

47. National Committee for Quality Assurance. Medicare advantage deeming program, 2009. Available from http://www.ncqa.org/tabid/102 /Default.aspx. Accessed January 21, 2010.

48. National Committee for Quality Assurance. The state of health care quality 2009. Available from http://www.ncqa.org/Portals/0/Newsroom/SOHC /SOHC_2009.pdf. Accessed January 21, 2010.

49. Fireman B, Bartlett, J, Selby J, et al. Can disease management reduce health care costs by improving quality? *Health Affairs*. 2004;23:63–64.

50. Mays GP, Au M, Claxton G. Convergence and dissonance: evolution in private sector approaches to disease management and care coordination. *Health Affairs*. 2007;20:1683–1691.

51. Moran DM. Whence and whither health insurance? A revisionist history. *Health Affairs*. 2005;24:1415–1425.

52. Health Insurance On-line. Self-funded plans. Available from http://www.online-health-insurance.com/health-insurance-resources /part2/page94.php. Accessed January 22, 2010.

53. Butler PA. ERISA update: the Supreme Court Texas decision and other recent developments. *National Academy for State Health Policy*. 2004;5. Available from http://www.statecoverage.org /node/180. Accessed January 21, 2010.

54. U.S. Congressional Budget Office. The long-term outlook for health care spending: Medicare and Medicaid: an overview. Available from http://www.cbo.gov/ftpdocs/87xx/doc8758 /AppendixA.4.1.shtml. Accessed January 19, 2010.

55. The Henry J. Kaiser Family Foundation. Medicare at a glance. Available from http://www .kff.org/medicare/upload/1066-12.pdf. Accessed January 17, 2010.

56. The Henry J. Kaiser Family Foundation. The Medicare prescription drug benefit. Available from http://www.kff.org/medicare/7044-10 .pdf. Accessed January 19, 2010.

57. American Society of Planning Officials. Reviews of government reports and public documents. *Soc Serv Rev*. 1970;44:491–492. Available from http://www.jstor.org/pss/30021773. Accessed January 24, 2010.

58. National Conference of State Legislatures. Certificate of need: state health laws and programs. Available from http://www.ncsl.org /IssuesResearch/Health/CONCertificateofNeed StateLaws/tabid/14373/Default.aspx. Accessed January 23, 2010.

59. Congressional Budget Office. Testimony on the professional standards review organizations program. Available from http://www.cbo.gov /ftpdoc.cfm?index=5226&type=0. Accessed January 23, 2010.

60. Compilation of the Social Security laws: Social Security online. Available from http://www.ssa .gov/OP_Home/ssact/title11/1154.htm. Accessed January 24, 2010.

61. Sloan FA, Vraciu RA. Investor-owned and not-for-profit hospitals: addressing some issues. *Health Affairs*. 1983;2:26. Available from http ://content.healthaffairs.org/cgi/reprint/2/2/25 .pdf. Accessed January 23, 2010.

62. Economic Expert.com. Diagnosis-related group. Available from http://www.economicexpert .com/a/Diagnosis:related:group.htm. Accessed January 23, 2010.

63. Mistichelli J. National Reference Center for Bioethics Literature. Diagnosis-related groups and the prospective payment system: forecasting social implications. Available from http://bioethics.georgetown.edu/publications /scopenotes/sn4.pdf. Accessed January 23, 2010.

64. Russell LB, Manning CL. The effect of prospective payment on Medicare expenditures. *N Engl J Med*. 1989;320:439. Available from http://content .nejm.org/cgi/content/abstract/320/7/439. Accessed January 23, 2010.

65. Thorpe KE. Health care cost containment: results and lessons from the past 20 years. In: Shortell SM, Reinhardt UE, Eds. *Improving Health Policy and Management*. Ann Arbor, MI: Health Administration Press; 1992:246.

66. Centers for Medicare & Medicaid Services. EMTALA overview. Available from http://www .cms.hhs.gov/EMTALA. Accessed January 23, 2010.

67. Kovner A. *Jonas' Health Care Delivery in the United States,* 5th ed. New York: Springer; 1995.

68. American Medical Association. The resource-based relative value scale: overview of the RBRVS. Available from http://www.ama-assn.org/ama /pub/physician-resources/solutions-managing-your-practice/coding-billing-insurance/medicare /the-resource-based-relative-value-scale /overview-of-rbrvs.shtml. Accessed January 21, 2010.

69. Board of Trustees, Federal Hospital Insurance Trust Fund. *1995 Annual Report of the Board of Trustees of the Hospital Insurance Trust Fund.* Washington, DC: U.S. Government Printing Office; 1995.

70. Reischauer RD. Medicare: beyond 2002, preparing for the baby-boomers. *Brookings Rev.* 1997;15:24.

71. U.S. Department of Labor. Health plans: portability of health coverage. Available from http ://www.dol.gov/ebsa/newsroom/fshipaa.html. Accessed January 22, 2010.

72. *The Balanced Budget Act of 1997, Public Law 105-33, Medicare and Medicaid Changes.* Washington, DC: Deloitte & Touche LLP and Deloitte & Touche Consulting Group LLC; 1997:1.

73. Medicare Payment Advisory Commission. Report to the Congress: Medicare payment policy (March 2003), chapter 1, context for Medicare spending. Available from http://www .medpac.gov/publications/congressional_reports /Mar03_Ch1.pdf. Accessed January 23, 2010.

74. National Bipartisan Commission on the Future of Medicare Task Forces. Available from http://medicare.commission.gov/medicare/task .html. Accessed January 23, 2010.

75. U.S. Department of Health and Human Services. Balanced Budget Refinement Act of 1999: highlights, November 18, 1999. Available from http://www.hhs.gov/news/pres/1999pres /1999pres/19991118b.html. Accessed January 23, 2010.

76. The Henry J. Kaiser Family Foundation. Fact sheet: Medicare, Medicare + Choice, April 2003. Available from http://www.kff.org/medicare /upload/Medicare-Choice-Fact-Sheet-Fact-Sheet.pdf. Accessed January 23, 2010.

77. Ross MN. Paying Medicare + Choice plans: the view from MedPac. *Health Affairs.* Available from http://content.healthaffairs.org/cgi/reprint /hlthaff.w1.90v1.pdf. Accessed January 23, 2010.

78. Centers for Medicare & Medicaid Services. Quality initiatives: general information. Available from http://www.cms.hhs.gov/Quality InitiativesGenInfo/01_overview.asp. Accessed January 23, 2010.

79. Centers for Medicare & Medicaid Services. About MQMS. Available from http://www.cms .hhs.gov/QualityInitiativesGenInfo/15_MQMS .asp. Accessed January 23, 2010.

80. U.S. Department of Health and Human Services, Centers for Medicare & Medicaid Services. Developing the Medicare hospital pay-for-performance plan. Available from http://www .cms.hhs.gov/MLNGenInfo/downloads/Hospital _Pay-for-Performance_plan.pdf. Accessed January 23, 2010.

81. U.S. Department of Health and Human Services, Centers for Medicare & Medicaid Services. Hospital quality compare. Available from http://www.hospitalcompare.hhs.gov/Hospital /Home2.asp?version=alternate&browser=IE% 7C6%7CWinXP&language=English&default status=0&pagelist=Home. Accessed January 24, 2010.

82. HCAHPS online. Hospital Consumer Assessment of Healthcare Providers and Systems. HC-AHPS fact sheet. Available from http://www .hcahpsonline.org/facts.aspx. Accessed January 24, 2010.

83. Pear R. Medicare won't cover hospital errors. *New York Times.* Available from http://www .nytimes.com/2007/08/19/washington/19hospital .html. Accessed January 24, 2010.

84. U.S. Department of Health and Human Services, Centers for Medicare & Medicaid Services. CMS proposes to expand quality program for hospital inpatient services in FY 2009. Available from http://www.cms.hhs.gov/apps /media/press/release.asp?Counter=3041. Accessed January 24, 2010.

85. U.S. Department of Health and Human Services, Centers for Medicare & Medicaid Services. Medicaid managed care enrollment as of June 30, 2008. Available from http://www .cms.hhs.gov/MedicaidDataSourcesGenInfo /downloads/08June30508.pdf. Accessed January 25, 2010.

86. Almanac of Policy Issues. Medicaid: an overview. Available from http://www.policyalmanac.org /health/archive/hhs_medicaid.shtml. Accessed January 25, 2010.

87. Koch AL. Financing health care services. In: Williams SJ, Torrens PK, Eds. *Introduction to Health Care Services,* 4th ed. Albany, NY: Delmar; 1993:309.

88. The Henry J. Kaiser Family Foundation. The crunch continues: Medicaid spending, coverage and policy in the midst of a recession, results from a 50-state Medicaid budget survey for state fiscal years 2009 and 2010. Available from http://www.kff.org/medicaid/upload/7985_ES .pdf. Accessed January 24, 2010.

89. U.S. Department of Health and Human Services, Centers for Medicare & Medicaid Services. Low cost health insurance for families and children. Available from http://www.cms.hhs.gov/lowcost HealthInsFamChild/. Accessed January 26, 2010.

90. The Henry J. Kaiser Family Foundation. The uninsured: a primer, October 2009. Available from http://www.kff.org/uninsured/upload /7451-05.pdf. Accessed January 25, 2010.

91. U.S. Department of Health and Human Services, Centers for Medicare & Medicaid Services. Medicaid and CHIP quality practices overview. Available from http://www.cms.hhs.gov/Medicaid CHIPQualPrac/. Accessed January 26, 2010.

92. U.S. Department of Health and Human Services, Centers for Medicare & Medicaid Services.

93. The Henry J. Kaiser Family Foundation. Health08.org. Available from http://www.kff .org/kaiserpolls/h08_pomr083007pkg.cfm. Accessed January 27, 2010.

State quality strategy tool kit for state Medicaid agencies. Available from http://www.cms .gov/MedicaidCHIPQualPrac/Downloads /qtkitwtablec.pdf. Accessed January 27, 2010.

94. Lubell J, DoBias M. Looking for a pulse. *Modern Health Care.* 2010;40:6–7, 16.

95. Lipson D, Verdier J, Quincy L, et al. Mathematica Policy Research, Inc. Leading the way? Maine's initial experience in expanding coverage through Dirigo health reforms. Available from http ://www.mathematica-mpr.com/publications /pdfs/Dirigofinalrpt.pdf. Accessed January 27, 2010.

96. The Henry J. Kaiser Family Foundation, Kaiser Commission on Medicaid and the Uninsured. Massachusetts health care reform: three years later. Available from http://www.kff.org /uninsured/upload/7777-02.pdf. Accessed January 27, 2010.

97. State of Vermont, Agency of Administration. Vermont's health care reform of 2006. Available from http://hcr.vermont.gov. Accessed January 27, 2010.

CHAPTER 10

Managing Financial Resources

Dori Taylor Sullivan

CHAPTER OBJECTIVES

1. Appreciate how the current healthcare financial environment influences practice as an advanced nurse practitioner.

2. List financial management tools and techniques essential for success as an advanced practice nurse.

3. Discuss the roles and responsibilities that advanced practice nurses have for fiscal accountability.

4. Evaluate the relationship of financial outcomes to the quality of care and service.

INTRODUCTION

The responsibilities for financial accountability will differ with each of the roles of advanced practice. Most notably, nurse managers and executives will need advanced competency to lead a department in delivering high-quality care and services within the context of the costs of delivering those services in comparison to the established resource allocation (or budget) as well as standards for best practice from others performing similar work (benchmarking). However, nurses in other roles cannot ignore or abandon responsibility

for delivering and evaluating cost-effective care. This may occur in individual interactions with clients and in developing and evaluating programs, clinical practice guidelines, and/or evidence for costs and quality patient outcomes.

This chapter begins with a brief overview of how changes in the healthcare system and environment have and will continue to influence the advanced practice nurse's financial responsibilities. The second section reviews the essential financial management tools and techniques that will position the reader for success in dealing with the money side of an operation. Once we have discussed these tools, we then discuss the major roles and responsibilities advanced practice nurses have for their areas of responsibility. Lastly, we discuss how financial outcomes relate to and must be considered in tandem with quality indicators for a realistic assessment of goal achievement.

Many nurses become anxious about accountability for running the money side of their practice. Readers of this chapter will come to recognize that a fundamental principle of leadership impact relates to the ability to direct resources to priority activities and personnel to achieve the organizational mission and goals. Thus increasing knowledge and skills with financial issues and resource allocation will assist the nurse in enacting all of the model leadership competencies. With that said, the advanced practice nurse cannot be expected to have expertise equal to those in the financial management departments. Consequently, seeking out experts for assistance in developing both operational and program budgets, and for analyzing variances and evaluating outcomes will be essential. Nevertheless, the advanced practice nurse needs to understand foundational principles and financial language to communicate needs and understand the advice he or she is given.

THE HEALTHCARE ENVIRONMENT: DECIDING WHETHER HEALTH CARE IS A RIGHT OR A PRIVILEGE

As noted earlier in this book, the United States does not have a health system but rather a fragmented approach to dealing with various illnesses. There is a general perception that special-interest groups representing the most powerful constituencies (often defined as business, the insurance industry, and the medical profession) within the healthcare field have been successful in preventing real change in the healthcare system, despite overwhelming evidence that it is not working well for many people.

Harrington and Estes (2004) reported that during the 1900s, five major initiatives were undertaken to obtain national health insurance, the most recent being the Clinton health plan in the mid-1990s. However, as the cost of health care in the United States continues to increase more rapidly than the cost of living index and concern is mounting over the dramatic increase in the number of uninsured citizens, a true reworking of the healthcare system may be on the horizon.

Geyman (2003) described six myths that he believes strongly contribute to the inability to create momentum for dramatic healthcare reform. Each of these myths is listed next, and in subsequent sections a brief explanation of the facts disputing their veracity will be provided.

- Everyone gets care anyhow.
- We do not ration care in the United States.
- The free market can resolve our problems in health care.
- The U.S. healthcare system is basically healthy, so incremental change will address its problems.
- The United States has the best healthcare system in the world.
- National health insurance is so unfeasible for political reasons that it should not be given serious consideration as a policy alternative.

Until these myths are widely recognized as untrue, there may not be sufficient momentum to fundamentally redesign and improve the current healthcare system.

EVOLUTION OF THE HEALTHCARE SYSTEM IN THE UNITED STATES

The expanding knowledge base of medicine, advancing technology, and increasing use of hospitals and other healthcare services have combined with other factors to continue the upward spiraling increases in healthcare costs. A number of changes in the financing or payment systems for health care have been introduced to try to mitigate these effects. We will provide a brief overview of the prior systems and describe newer arrangements to provide the context for why managing financial outcomes is such a critical part of the clinical leader role.

The Fee-for-Service Payment Era

The fee-for-service payment era is described as the indemnity insurance and cost-plus reimbursement environment. Hospitals worked to attract physicians who would admit their patients and provide necessary diagnostic and treatment services. Expansion in insurance coverage in the 1950s and 1960s generally paid for these services for most employed workers, while Medicare reimbursements significantly covered care for those older than age 65. Medicaid patients were a minority of patients for many institutions, and the reimbursement rates, although lower than private payers, were closer to actual costs. Little attention was devoted to care access issues by the mainstream populace, most of whom felt they could receive care whenever and wherever they required it. As late as the 1970s, relatively little attention was paid to healthcare costs by either physicians or nurses despite the urgings of administrators. Hospitals and other healthcare organizations billed charges that were reimbursed either at face value or at some percentage of the amount, referred to as a discounted fee for service.

During the 1980s, interest in traditional health maintenance organizations (HMOs) like Kaiser Permanente grew, and there was great anticipation of the ability to provide good care while reining in healthcare costs using this model. Looking back, it is clear that a failure to focus on the demographics of the early HMO enrollees (mostly healthy young families) may have led to overzealous expectations. Nonetheless, a variety of strategies to manage health care were introduced, and these concepts continue to significantly influence care and reimbursement systems.

In the late 1970s and early 1980s, concerns regarding the cost of health care were growing. Healthcare organizations and especially hospitals began embracing more traditional business approaches in considering their revenues and expenses, the efficiency of their operations, and their organizational structures. Responsibility or cost centers were seen as the location for reducing costs, leading to charging clinical leaders with understanding and managing their budgets, an often unfamiliar task.

The Advent of Prospective Payment and Diagnostic Related Groups

In 1983, a major change in reimbursement called prospective payment was adopted in the form of diagnostic related groups (DRGs). Prospective payment means that the reimbursement for a specified set of services is established before the care is provided. DRGs were originally designed as a health services research tool at Yale University; however, policymakers and regulators jumped on this opportunity to drive accountability for costs into healthcare organizations, starting with hospitals. Under the new prospective payment system, hospitals would be allotted a certain amount of reimbursement for their patients according to rates established by patients' diagnoses as categorized through DRGs. Although first applied for Medicare patients only, the use of DRGs and prospective payments was quickly embraced by private insurance companies, who also increased their use of managed care plan techniques for controlling healthcare services and costs.

Devers, Brewster, and Casalino (2004) identified another major market and policy response in addition to DRGs that increased price competition from the mid-1980s to the mid-1990s: Managed care companies started selective contracting with hospitals and other healthcare organizations to achieve the best pricing and assurance of the quality of care provided. Due to their size, managed care companies had more negotiating power than individual physicians, and this era also brought new payment arrangements related to sharing risk for high-cost patient stays that exceeded stated norms (called outliers).

These changes fueled intense scrutiny of the various services and treatments and the costs associated with them in acute care settings. Because length of stay (LOS) in the hospital is a good predictor of the amount of resources that a patient will consume, LOS became the gold standard for managing care under DRGs.

One of the interesting dialogues that also intensified under the prospective payment system focused on the issue of costs versus charges. Unlike many other businesses, healthcare organizations had little accurate knowledge of the costs of providing elements of care, and they certainly did not have good information about the costs of a typical DRG. While in some hospitals charges for care were defined as a percentage above the costs, in most cases the costs were not really known and the charges were established through a muddy process that included how much the market would bear. This consideration is important because without knowing the costs of delivering a certain service or caring for a specific patient DRG, the charges or allocated payment might be insufficient to even cover costs—which means the more a given service is provided, the faster money will be lost. Not surprisingly, hospitals became very interested in managing LOSs. In turn, an intensified focus on discharge planning and utilization review occurred and evolved toward the current views of case management. Extensive databases (public and proprietary) were created to provide comparative data for LOS and costs/charges for DRGs so performance could be assessed by each institution. Hospitals struggled to discharge patients within the suggested LOS time frames while simultaneously striving to more accurately estimate the costs of providing care. Prospective payment systems have now migrated to long-term care and home care settings, where they have touched off the same types of debates and reactions as happened in acute care.

One of the most important impacts of that change was the significant increase in patient acuity within the acute care setting; similarly, patients who were sicker with more care needs began to be seen within community settings such as home care due to the policy of earlier discharging. This phenomenon continues today and, coupled with more stringent admission criteria and migration of care services to outpatient settings, is a major factor in the dissatisfaction of many health professional groups, whose workload and intensity have also increased.

A second impact was the realization that little was known about the true costs of care for a given diagnosis, because each phase of care (triage, acute care, skilled nursing or long-term care, home care) was considered separately. Thus questions were raised as to whether costs of care increased or decreased or were just shifted to other settings when considering an episode of care rather than just hospital costs.

This recognition and the desire to better coordinate care and control costs led to the formation of integrated delivery systems through both vertical and horizontal integration strategies. An integrated delivery system (IDS) of a network may be defined as an entity that "provides or arranges to provide a coordinated continuum of services to a defined population and is willing to be held clinically and fiscally accountable for the outcomes and the health status of the population served" (Shortell, Gillies, Anderson, Erickson, & Mitchell, 1996, p. 7). Vertical integration refers to formalized relationships (ranging from agreements to ownership by a parent organization) of healthcare agencies that represent the continuum of care. For example, a hospital may have purchased or created a primary care practice, home care agency, and skilled nursing facility so that clients could receive all or most of their care with that IDS. Horizontal integration saw hospitals merge and/or be purchased with the goal of gaining efficiencies of scale as well as market clout and enhanced name recognition to promote growth and profitability. Research (Kitchener, 2004) has suggested that mergers have not been as effective a strategy as is touted and this activity has slowed to some in extent the 2000s.

Reengineering and Redesign of Healthcare Systems

The 1990s were also characterized by intense reengineering or redesign of patient care delivery systems and models. Major initiatives in cost accounting were launched in many healthcare organizations to better understand the drivers of costs and the actual costs of care for various DRGs. Knowing that in the vast majority of healthcare delivery settings the largest percentage of the budget is devoted to personnel, many of the reengineering efforts sought to decrease the overall number of professional staff by redistributing work tasks thought not to require professional knowledge to lesser-skilled and lower-paid workers. Another hallmark of this period was the decrease in management layers or levels and an increase in the span of control through loss of management positions. While processes of care delivery and support services were included and some successes achieved, the greater share of the changes were in professional roles.

Norrish and Rundall (2001) noted that hospital restructuring affects the work of registered nurses in many ways. Their summary of those impacts included:

- Nurses spending more time on administration and paperwork with less time in direct patient care—a dissatisfier for many nurses
- Contradictory findings as to whether nursing workload increased or decreased depending upon the changes made
- Less control over nursing work, with managers acquiring additional units to lead and undermining shared governance activities and structures

Nursing was perhaps the major—but not the only—discipline affected by the redesign trend. Virtually all health professions either added or increased the number of paraprofessional or support staff with the goals of better matching staff skill levels to actual workloads and, of course, trying to reduce costs. Examples in other areas include pharmacy technicians, physical and occupational therapy assistants, social work assistants, and many others.

The early 21st century finds health care still embracing a free market approach with the expectation that competition, with some regulation, will drive down the costs of care. Private insurers and government payers have adopted stringent procedures for preapproving and managing care in most settings, with virtually constant communication and oversight. However, under severe criticism from the general public, steps have been taken to soften the approaches to managing care through legislative actions. While the majority of hospitals and healthcare agencies are not-for-profit entities, an increasing number of for-profit organizations are entering the market.

The operating margin (operating profit divided by revenue as a percentage) for most hospitals has rebounded somewhat from the very low or negative margins of the 1990s, but remained very modest at 1.39% as reported by Moody's for fiscal year 2003. Physician practices, especially primary care, and home care agencies face similar situations. Nursing homes or skilled facilities in a number of states are in a true crisis. Thus the pressure related to reducing costs of care and delivering high-quality care efficiently continues to dominate most healthcare settings.

HOW IS HEALTH CARE FINANCED?

Today's healthcare industry consists of private for-profit insurance companies, HMOs, hospitals, physician groups, pharmaceutical companies, medical supply companies, and other health-related businesses (e.g., clinics, home care agencies, skilled nursing facilities). Most of the country has experienced significant consolidation of healthcare entities through the vertical and horizontal integration activities described earlier, resulting in a few larger entities. There is widespread concern that healthcare dollars have been redirected into for-profit entities of the industry, leaving those (organizations and individual professions) who provide care with fewer and fewer resources.

The major payer categories for health care in the United States remain the government, private insurers, and self-pay (often referred to as "no pay" because uninsured people account for much of this category). The term *payer mix* refers to the percentage of patients in a given healthcare organization who fall into each of these categories. With an aging population and an increasing number of uninsured people, the government (through federal and state programs) is a significant—if not the largest—payer for many healthcare organizations.

Coddington, Keen, Moore, and Clark (1990) predicted the outcomes of continuing with our market-based healthcare system, all of which have come true in the early years of the 21st century:

- More than 40 million uninsured
- Continued gaps in safety net coverage
- Double-digit health plan rate increases
- Small employers cutting coverage or even dropping health plans
- Increased co-payments and deductibles for employees
- Large rate increases for private insurers in shrinking markets
- Numerous failures of HMOs and withdrawal from the market by larger insurance companies
- Continued cost shifting in an increasingly fragmented market
- Continued inflation of healthcare costs

In 2002, $1.5 trillion was spent on health care in the United States. This amount is expected to dramatically increase to $2.5 trillion by 2011 (Heffler et al., 2004), consuming more and more of our gross national product each year.

COMPARISON OF WORLD HEALTH SYSTEM OUTCOMES: DO PEOPLE GET WHAT THEY PAY FOR?

It has been estimated that 95% of the United States' $1 trillion-plus budget is spent on medical services, with only 5% spent on health promotion and prevention (McGinnis, Williams-Russo, & Knickman, 2002). Thus it seems clear we still have an illness-oriented system.

The United States is the only country among those classified as Western industrialized nations that does not have some form of national health insurance (Geyman, 2003). While some claim that Americans do not want national health insurance, dissatisfaction with the healthcare system and the aging of the population are two major factors supporting a rise in general support for this concept. More and more often, people have direct knowledge of family or acquaintances who experienced difficulty in accessing or receiving necessary care. There are an estimated 44 million uninsured people in the United States, comprising mainly the poor and the working poor but also including increasing numbers of workers losing or unable to afford health benefits.

It is still often proclaimed that the U.S. healthcare system is the best in the world, yet virtually every health status metric—including how expensive care is—belies that claim. Starfield (2000) detailed the U.S. ranking in health status indicators from a variety of sources and concluded that the United States is not even close to being the best in the world. Some examples of health indicators showing the worst U.S. performance were low-birth-weight babies and child survival at various ages; life expectancy and age-adjusted mortality; disparities in care and outcomes across social groups; and equality of family out-of-pocket expenditures for health care. The facts demonstrate that U.S. citizens pay more for less desirable health status outcomes, with difficulties related to access and coordination of care.

IMPLICATIONS FOR ADVANCED PRACTICE NURSES

There will continue to be significant pressure to reduce overall healthcare expenditures due to rising healthcare costs as compared to normal inflation. Combined with expectations for continuous improvement and demonstration of quality outcomes, nurses can expect they will need to find ways to manage or reduce costs while maintaining or enhancing the quality of care and services.

FINANCIAL MANAGEMENT FOR ADVANCED PRACTICE NURSES

In this section, we present an overview of financial management terms and activities. While there is no expectation that readers will be financial experts, advanced practice nurses must be confident in their ability to manage the fiscal resources associated with their areas of responsibility and understand the terminology and concepts so they can talk to the finance department staff.

The Elements of Financial Management

There are four major elements to financial management: planning, controlling, organizing and directing, and decision making (Baker & Baker, 2004). Planning requires establishing goals and developing strategies for achieving those goals; developing a budget is the major activity in this element. Controlling involves assuring that the established plans or strategies are being followed, usually consisting of comparing reports of actual performance to targets. Organizing and directing relate to using resources to the best advantage. These resources may include staff, space, supply, and equipment, for example. Finally, decision making for each element involves analysis and evaluation to select the best alternatives for action.

Accounting Concepts

The field of accounting is a critical part of financial management, as it organizes information for use according to generally accepted accounting principles. Financial accounting methods are used for external reporting to third parties so that organizations may be compared across similar metrics using generally accepted accounting principles. Financial reporting is a retrospective look at what an organization has done. Managerial accounting is used within the organization to provide actionable information for planning, controlling, organizing and directing, and decision making. Industry performance metrics as well as organization-specific indicators are provided to managers as a guide for assessment and improvement of fiscal matters. In acute care hospitals, we look at metrics such as cost per equivalent discharge and hours of nursing care per patient-day translated into labor dollars. In specific areas, the indicators may relate to number of patient visits or number of procedures, calculating the revenue for those services as compared to the expenses required to provide them.

Financial management occurs within an organizational context based to some extent on the type of organization—that is, for profit or not for profit. Nonprofit organizations consist of private or government entities, neither of which pay income taxes. A common misunderstanding is that nonprofits are not allowed to make any money, when in fact they must generate more revenue than expenses to stay in business. What differs is that any margin or profit is invested back into the organization and its mission; in contrast, in a for-profit company, profits are distributed among owners and/or investors. Most healthcare organizations are nonprofit; however, there is a growing segment of for-profit businesses that own hospitals and most other types of health service delivery organizations.

Two major types of organizing structures are most frequently seen in healthcare organizations today. Traditional bureaucratic structures divide functions by type and group similar types into larger reporting structures. Each functional area or department is called a responsibility center so that financial assessments of the area may be made. The terms *profit center* and *cost center* may also be used. For example, in a health clinic there might be a primary care unit, specialty unit, pediatric unit, dental unit, and administration, human resources, and finance departments.

The type of second structure is organized by service lines or major customer groupings—for example, cancer, cardiology, and women's health. In the service line model, all of the services required by that client type are grouped so that care is coordinated and customized. Advanced practice nurses will need to understand the managerial structure as well as the financial structure and reporting for their areas, as in some cases they do not follow the same model.

Managerial Accounting and Financial Analysis

Basic Financial Terms

Revenue is defined as the value of services rendered, expressed at the facility's full established rates. The full rate for a chest X-ray might be $175, with one insurance company plan reimbursing $125 and another company only $110. Payments may be made after services are provided (fee for service or discounted fee for service) or before service is delivered, according to agreements for care. These agreements tend to establish either a predetermined, per-person payment or a negotiated amount for specified services based on the characteristics of the group to be served (Baker & Baker, 2004).

Gross revenue is the full value of services provided. *Contractual allowances* are the deductions for discounts according to the agreements in place. A deduction is also made for bad debt, or the amount of money owed that is not likely to be paid or collected. An advanced practice nurse might work with volume of activity targets such as visits or procedures or patient-days rather

than actual revenue figures, but obviously these are directly related.

The term *revenue stream* refers to how money flows into the organization or its sources of business. In the most straightforward arrangement, the expenses associated with generating that revenue are considered together to get a sense of the margin or revenue to expense ratio. The *margin* is the positive (in the black) or negative (in the red) yield after expenses are deducted from revenues.

Expenses are the costs of generating revenue, and, in complex organizations like health care, they are grouped into categories. A major distinction in expenses or costs is whether they are direct or indirect. Direct costs can be directly attributed to a responsibility center and tracked. For example, the radiology technologist and the supplies used to perform an X-ray are direct costs. Indirect costs reflect costs that are apportioned across responsibility centers to create a complete financial picture of an organization. For example, the patient billing department expenses must be supported across multiple departments as an indirect cost, but they are a necessary cost of doing business. An advanced practice nurse will be more aware of budgeted direct expenses than of indirect costs. Asking about and understanding indirect costs, however, can enhance his or her ability to plan and evaluate the costs of new programs and daily operations. Table 10-1 shows the relationship among some of these financial terms.

Another way that costs are described is based on whether they are fixed or variable. *Fixed costs* do not change when volume of activity goes up. Rent and minimum staffing requirements are two examples of fixed costs. *Variable costs* go up or down in direct relationship to changes in activity levels. Supply costs may be an example of a variable cost when each procedure uses a prepackaged tray of instruments and supplies. A *semivariable cost* changes with activity but not in direct proportion. Staffing additions are a good example of this category since there might

TABLE 10-1	Relationships Among Selected Financial Terms

Gross revenue from operations	$1,000,000
− Contractual allowances of discounts	$100,000
− Expenses (direct and indirect)	$850,000
= Net revenue	$50,000

Net revenue/gross revenue = Margin (positive or negative)

Shown as dollar value plus as a percentage of revenue

In this case, there is a positive margin of 50,000/1,000,000 = 0.05 or 5%

be a one-staff-member increase for three additional patients in a given setting but no further additions until there are five more patients.

Financial Analysis Statements

The financial status of an organization is expressed in four standard reports: the balance sheet, statement of revenue and expense, changes in fund balance/net worth, and statement of cash flows (Table 10-2). The balance sheet records what an organization owns, what it owes, and basically what it is worth (stated as the fund balance for nonprofit organizations). The assets of the organization (what it owns) are equal to its liabilities (what it owes) plus its net worth/fund balance. The balance sheet is described as a snapshot at a point in time (Baker & Baker, 2004). The statement of revenue and expense covers a period of time, such as a year, and summarizes how much revenue was generated minus the expenses used to generate the revenue, with the balance equaling the operating income. Ideally, revenues exceed expenses, leading to a positive balance or margin, often expressed as a percentage of the total operating budget. However, in health care, we sometimes see operating expenses exceeding operating revenues, leading to a negative margin. Some organizations offset this difference with investment income or transfers from other corporation entities such as a foundation.

Changes in fund balance/net worth reflect whether an organization is moving in a positive direction by increasing its value or in a negative direction by decreasing its value. An analogy would be whether an individual's personal savings account combined with the value of his or her home is a higher number this year than it was last year. If a person had to withdraw $15,000 to repair his or her home, the number may have decreased. The excess of revenues minus expenses from operations plus any gains from investment or nonoperations sources are added to the fund balance or net worth of an organization.

The statement of cash flows translates a variety of accounting elements where the cash has not yet been received along with depreciation of appropriate assets and converts them into cash flow for a designated period. While all four reports are interrelated and important, most clinical managers would focus on the first two to get a sense of the organization's overall financial condition.

The Budget Cycle

All organizations establish a fiscal year (FY), with many using calendar years. In some states, hospitals and sometimes other healthcare organizations are on standardized fiscal years for purposes of regulatory reporting and comparison. At year end, the appropriate financial and

TABLE 10-2 Leading Causes of Death and Numbers of Death (1980–2007)

Race and Cause of Death	1980	Deaths per 100,000 Standard Population	2007
All Persons			
All causes	1,989.8	All causes	2,423.7
Diseases of heart	761.1	Diseases of heart	616.1
Malignant neoplasms	416.5	Malignant neoplasms	562.9
Cerebrovascular diseases	170.2	Cerebrovascular diseases	135.9
Unintentional injuries	105.7	Chronic lower respiratory diseases	127.9
Chronic obstructive pulmonary diseases	56.1	Unintentional injuries	123.7
Pneumonia and influenza	54.6	Alzheimer's disease	74.6
Diabetes mellitus	34.8	Diabetes mellitus	71.4
Chronic liver disease and cirrhosis	30.6	Influenza and pneumonia	52.7
Atherosclerosis	29.4	Nephritis, nephrotic syndrome & nephrosis	46.4
Suicide	26.9	Septicemia	34.8
White			
All causes	1,738.6	All causes	2,074.2
Diseases of heart	683.3	Diseases of heart	531.6
Malignant neoplasms	368.2	Malignant neoplasms	483.9
Cerebrovascular diseases	148.7	Chronic lower respiratory diseases	118.1
Unintentional injuries	90.1	Cerebrovascular diseases	114.7
Chronic obstructive pulmonary diseases	52.4	Unintentional injuries	106.3
Pneumonia and influenza	48.4	Alzheimer's disease	68.9
Diabetes mellitus	28.9	Diabetes mellitus	56.4
Atherosclerosis	27.1	Influenza and pneumonia	45.9
Chronic liver disease and cirrhosis	25.2	Nephritis, nephrotic syndrome and nephrosis	36.9
Suicide	24.8	Suicide	31.3
Black			
All causes	233.1	All causes	289.6
Diseases of heart	72.9	Diseases of heart	71.2
Malignant neoplasms	45.0	Malignant neoplasms	64.0
Cerebrovascular diseases	20.1	Cerebrovascular diseases	17.1
Unintentional injuries	13.5	Unintentional injuries	13.6
Homicide	10.2	Diabetes mellitus	12.5
Certain conditions originating in the perinatal period	7.0	Homicide	8.9
Pneumonia and influenza	5.7	Nephritis, nephrotic syndrome and nephrosis	8.4
Diabetes mellitus	5.5	Chronic lower respiratory diseases	7.9
Chronic liver disease and cirrhosis	4.8	Human immunodeficiency virus (HIV) disease	6.5
Nephritis, nephrotic syndrome, and nephrosis	3.4	Septicemia	6.3

Source: Data adapted from *Health, United States, 2010*, p. 145, Centers for Disease Control and Prevention, National Center for Health Statistics.

accounting procedures are carried out to develop the final financial reports, which are usually audited by an external public accounting firm and certified as accurate in terms of meeting required standards for this type of reporting.

The budget cycle is a series of timed activities planned to arrive at an approved budget prior to the start of the next fiscal year. Depending on the size, complexity, and culture of an organization, planning for the next year's budget might start at the beginning of each fiscal year.

A critical early component of budget planning relates to forecasting and projecting the revenues and expenses for the next fiscal year. Forecasting and projecting may be led by finance executives, strategic planning directors, or other designated personnel. Environmental assessments, contractual changes, and trends in care needs or reimbursement must be analyzed and their relative impact estimated. These conclusions are then translated into what are called budget assumptions, the context for budget development. In addition, the identification of strategic priorities or organizational goals, along with the resources that will be required to accomplish them, must be factored in, whether they are organization-wide or unit-based initiatives.

Budget Development

The development of a budget requires several steps in addition to the forecasting and projections already described. First, an approach to budget development must be selected. A zero-based budget means that each year, those involved with creating the budget assume that there is a clean slate and they start building a budget without regard to the resources allocated for the current fiscal year. Zero-based budgeting can be a useful tool for realigning expenses with changing activity priorities, but it is a difficult and labor-intensive process. Most healthcare organizations use some variation of a historical budget that assumes most responsibility centers within the organization will continue to provide similar services, with adjustments made for volumes, new programs, and special projects.

In many organizations, the budget is built by each responsibility center reviewing the general budget assumptions and perhaps collaborating to develop unit-specific assumptions, if appropriate. The role of a clinical leader may involve predicting changes that would affect the unit, including volume of various services, staffing (costs and availability), equipment (needs and costs including replacement), and supplies.

In growing markets (e.g., where the population is increasing) this approach would be used more frequently since volumes and revenues are likely increasing. Using this method, the rolled-up budget (adding together all responsibility center requests) may still exceed projected revenue by millions of dollars. The budget review process usually means a process for reducing the requested allocation to try to create a balanced budget. From the perspective of the advanced practice nurse, this approach can be frustrating, as the nurse perceives he or she never gets what he or she needs or requests. It also leads to game playing and padding the budget because people know they will not get what they request, so they request more than what is needed.

More recently, some healthcare organizations in static or highly competitive markets have moved to an approach that we believe is more realistic. Similar to most household budgets, a projection of what the income is likely to be is made first, and then necessary expenses are factored in, followed by funding for whatever discretionary expenditures can be supported. Using this approach, there is little to be gained by having each responsibility center develop a new budget; rather, appropriate changes (adding or subtracting resources) are proposed based on projections and organizational goals. Adjustments are also made for salary increases, inflation of equipment costs, and other factors, usually by the finance department, after which managers may or may not review the proposed budget. While this can be frustrating, it does reflect the reality of limited resources.

An organization may also use a flexible budgeting approach that indexes or adjusts selected budget categories based on volume or other factors during the budget year. These midyear adjustments may or may not be reflected in budget reports, depending upon the budget software system capability and on the magnitude of the adjustments.

Types of Budgets

Typical budgets are organized into operating budgets and capital budgets. *Operating budgets* have two major categories: personnel and supplies/equipment. Each type of expense is named and listed on a line in the budget—thus the term *line item*. In most healthcare organizations, personnel costs are by far the largest portion of the budget, so as previously noted much effort goes into determining the necessary staffing mix, pattern, and organization. *Capital budgets* are separately created for expenditures that exceed an established dollar limit that varies across organizations. Similarly, the size of the capital budget is often determined based on what the organization believes it can afford, followed by a process for reviewing and approving capital purchases. One's ability to write a compelling justification for proposed regular and capital budget items is an important skill to acquire. Describing how a new piece of equipment will improve quality of care and decrease the professional time a service requires (and translating this information into financial terms if possible, such as a projected savings of 8 hours of professional time per week at $38 per hour for a savings of more than $15,000 per year) will be more positively received than citing that two other facilities in the area have the new equipment.

Monitoring Budget Variances

The budget variance report, as its name suggests, is a listing of each budget line item and category with the budgeted amount for the month/period and year to date, the actual amount spent for the month/period and year to date, and the difference between the two figures, or variance. The variance is often expressed as the dollar difference and the percentage the variance represents from budget. Table 10-3 shows a budget variance report for a clinical area.

The advanced practice nurse who has direct budget responsibility will be asked regularly to analyze each line item and category, determining which are tracking according to plan and which are outliers, either too high or too low. The next step is to gather the necessary information to understand why an item is over or under budget, and whether this is a good or bad thing. If things are going better than expected, there is an opportunity to learn why and maybe extend that positive impact. More often, the nurse will discover that lines are over budget, and he or she must investigate the causes. Those in a role without direct budget responsibility should recognize that this oversight occurs periodically and that each organization has different review periods.

There are three causes of budget variance for nursing: volume, efficiency, and rate variance from the budgeted amount. Volume variances are due to more or fewer patient-days or visits, efficiency variance relates to more or fewer hours per patient-day, and rate variance relates to salaries (generally the use of overtime). An explanation of the mathematics to complete this easy and very helpful analysis can be found in Finkler and Kovner (2000, p. 300).

FINANCIAL ROLES AND RESPONSIBILITIES OF ADVANCED PRACTICE NURSES

An expert in a particular area of specialization, whether with direct responsibility for managing money or with input into budgets and program development, will need the following knowledge and skills:

- Awareness of the region and the discipline's current healthcare environment, especially related to the demand for services, reimbursement mechanisms, workforce supply, and cost pressures

TABLE 10-3	Sample Budget Variance Report for a Clinical Area

| | December 2005 | | YTD | | | |
Description	Budget	Actual	Budget	Actual	Variance	Percentage
Revenue						
Gross	30,000	34,000	90,000	115,000	(25,000)	(27.7%)
Allowance	10,000	14,000	30,000	45,000	(15,000)	(50.0%)
Expenses						
Salaries	21,000	23,000	63,000	65,000	(2,000)	(0.3%)
Fringe	8,400	9,200	25,200	26,000	(800)	(0.3%)
Temporary	1,000	1,200	3,000	2,200	800	26.6%
Med supplies	5,000	4,800	15,000	12,000	3,000	20.0%
Office supplies	800	800	2,400	2,400	0	0
Telephone	400	500	1,200	1,400	(200)	(16.7%)
Copying	100	140	300	360	(60)	(20.0%)
Travel	75	65	225	210	15	.07%

Year to date (YTD) budget amounts reflect 3 months with fiscal year of October 1–September 30.

- Development of projected revenues and expenses for new and existing programs
- Monitoring and responding to budget variances
- Participating in benchmarking, either internal or external

It has been said that healthcare issues may be global but the delivery of care and solutions to those issues must be driven locally. Therefore, advanced nurse practitioners must become familiar with the dynamics within their region related to which types of services for care are in demand, what the reimbursement picture is from the major payers, what the pricing range for these services is, and which quality indicators and outcomes are expected. While the literature may provide some general direction, the most current information will come from local sources such as the hospital association and its related meeting groups, through professional networking, and from consultants.

The advanced practice nurse's role in projecting revenue and volume for preparation of an annual budget is a critical one, for it is during this process that the decisions that will affect the nurse and his or her patients for at least the next year are made. Once the nurse has a sense of the resources likely to be allocated, he or she can begin detailed planning for any changes or improvements that he or she has decided to pursue. Again, local networking along with regional or national specialty groups will likely provide the best information for program planning.

One of the most important roles a nurse manager has related to fiscal responsibility is the regular review of budget variance reports. However, whether the advanced practice nurse is a direct care provider, a manager, or in other roles, understanding the need to analyze and take action in response to budget variance reports is helpful to one's participation in the mission and vision of the organization.

TABLE 10-4	Example of a Healthcare Organization's Balanced Scorecard

Clinical outcomes and functional status of clients	Operational performance indicators
Customer satisfaction (clients, staff, physicians, payers, community)	Financial performance indicators

FINANCIAL RESULTS AND QUALITY OUTCOMES

Several authors have proposed methods for assessing overall unit or organizational performance. One of the most popular is the balanced scorecard used in general business and applied to health care (Kaplan & Norton, 1996). The balanced scorecard helps us get a true sense of how an organization or its units are performing by simultaneously considering several performance domains. The original balanced scorecard includes performance measures of finance, internal business processes, learning and growth, and the customer. Many organizations have adapted these categories, which are often displayed as quadrants of a table or circle. Table 10-4 shows a sample balanced scorecard for a healthcare organization. The point is that it will not matter much if your financial indicators are excellent if the quality outcomes and satisfaction levels of clients are poor. Similarly, if your quality is wonderful but costs more than can be supported, the organization cannot sustain success. Benchmarking can provide valuable comparison information when high-quality information with comparable organizations can be accessed.

CONCLUSION

Often understanding and managing financial resources is one of the more intimidating and challenging skills for nurses in advanced practice. Responsibilities in this area will vary according to one's role and the organizational policies and practices in the setting in which one works. However, a basic understanding of the language, processes, and justifications for cost consciousness will make the role transition to advanced practice easier.

DISCUSSION QUESTIONS

1. Identify the top two services or activities in the area in which you currently work. If you provide direct services to clients, which types of reimbursement arrangements or contracts are in place? Who are the major payers by percentage of revenue? If your area is considered an area of indirect costs, how is the support for your operation apportioned across the institution?

2. Locate the most recent balance sheet, statement of revenue and expense, and changes in fund value/net worth for your organization. Review them with a manager in nursing or finance to gain an understanding of how to read these financial statements.

3. Determine what the operating margin was for the last fiscal year. Was it positive or negative, and what does this mean?

4. Review a recent budget variance printout for your department. What were the largest variances, and do you feel confident that you understand why these variances occurred?

5. Review a balanced scorecard for the unit in which you are currently employed. Which aspects of this assessment are meeting targets, and which need improvement?

REFERENCES

Baker, J. J., & Baker, R. W. (2004). *Health care finance: Basic tools for nonfinancial managers.* Sudbury, MA: Jones and Bartlett Publishers.

Coddington, D. C., Keen, D. J., Moore, K. D., & Clark, R. L. (1990). *The crisis in health care: Costs, choices, and strategies.* San Francisco: Jossey-Bass.

Devers, K. J., Brewster, L. R., & Casalino, L. P. (2004). Changes in hospital competitive strategy: A new medical arms race? In C. Harrington & C. L. Estes (Eds.), *Health policy: Crisis and reform in the U.S. health care delivery system* (4th ed., pp. 174–183). Sudbury, MA: Jones and Bartlett Publishers.

Finkler, S. A., & Kovner, C. T. (2000). *Financial management for nurse executives and managers.* Philadelphia: W. B. Saunders.

Geyman, J. P. (2003). Myths as barriers to health care reform in the United States. *International Journal of Health Services, 33*(2), 315–329.

Harrington, C., & Estes, C. L. (2004). *Health policy: Crisis and reform in the U.S. health care delivery system* (4th ed.). Sudbury, MA: Jones and Bartlett Publishers.

Heffler, S., Smith, S., Won, G., Clemens, M. K., Keehan, S., & Zezza, M. (2004). Health spending projections for 2001–2011: The latest outlook. In C. Harrington & C. L. Estes (Eds.), *Health policy: Crisis and reform in the U.S. health care delivery system* (4th ed., pp. 250–259). Sudbury, MA: Jones and Bartlett Publishers.

Kaplan, R. S., & Norton, D. P. (1996). *Translating strategy into action: The balanced scorecard.* Boston: Harvard Business School Press.

Kitchener, M. (2004). Exploding the merger myth in U.S. health care. In C. Harrington & C. L. Estes (Eds.), *Health policy: Crisis and reform in the U.S. health care delivery system* (4th ed., pp. 162–167). Sudbury, MA: Jones and Bartlett Publishers.

McGinnis, J. M., Williams-Russo, P., & Knickman, J. R. (2002). The case for more active policy attention to health promotion. *Health Affairs, 21*(2), 78–93.

Norrish, B., & Rundall, T. (2001). Hospital restructuring and the work of registered nurses. *The Milbank Quarterly, 79*(1), 55–79.

Shortell, S. M., Gillies, R. R., Anderson, D. A., Erickson, K. M., & Mitchell, J. B. (1996). *Remaking health care in America: Building organized delivery systems.* San Francisco: Jossey-Bass.

Starfield, B. (2000). Is U.S. health really the best in the world? *Journal of the American Medical Association, 284*(4), 483–485.

CHAPTER 11

Government Regulation: Parallel and Powerful

Jacqueline M. Loversidge

CHAPTER OBJECTIVES

1. Review the history of the role of advanced practice nursing in healthcare regulation.

2. Determine the role of the state board of nursing on the regulation of advanced practice nursing.

3. Understand the methods of professional credentialing for advanced practice nurses.

4. Explore the role of professional self-regulation for the advanced practice nurse and its influence on patient safety.

5. Realize how federal regulation influences payment mechanisms for advanced practice nurses.

6. Discuss strategies that the advanced practice nurses can employ to influence regulatory changes for effective patient care delivery.

INTRODUCTION

Regulation of the U.S. healthcare delivery system and the healthcare providers who practice within the system is complex. Much of the complexity is attributable to the vastness of the industry, the manner of financing health care, and the proliferation of laws and regulations that govern practice and reimbursement in the interest of public welfare.

This chapter focuses on the major concepts of the regulation of health professionals with emphasis on advanced practice nurses (APNs). Understanding the process of licensure and credentialing and its impact on the practice of advanced practice nursing is fundamental to being a competent practitioner. Understanding the regulation of the healthcare system empowers the APN to advocate on behalf of the profession and consumers of health care.

REGULATION VERSUS LEGISLATION

The legislative process is one approach to governance. A parallel, yet equally powerful, approach is the regulatory process. Together, laws and regulations shape the way public policy is implemented. It is important for the APN to understand both processes and know how to influence each process. Major differences between the two processes are described here.

Laws are promulgated and passed by the legislative branch of government (Congress at the federal level or the state legislature for state laws) and establish the framework and authority base for the regulatory process. Once passed, laws must be implemented by administrative agencies (the executive branch) of government. Laws are written using broad language to provide for flexibility and adaptability in application of the law over time. The administrative agency charged with implementing the law adds regulations and/or rules (terms used interchangeably with the same meaning) that amplify the law and describe how the administrative agency will put the law into practice.

For example, one provision in the nurse practice act provides that a duty of the board of nursing is to examine, license, and renew the license of duly qualified individuals. The regulations amplifying that provision of law specify the criteria for eligibility, application procedures, and how and when examinations are conducted.

It is important to note that regulations may never exceed the parameters of the statute they intend to amplify. However, both statute and regulation have the force and effect of law.

The first step in establishing a new law or revising an existing law consists of the introduction of a bill by a legislator or group of legislators (sponsors) during a legislative session. The sponsor may introduce legislation to address an issue or concern of his or her constituents, or an administrative agency may seek a legislative sponsor to modify its practice act for a variety of reasons. The bill must be passed during the legislative session in which it is introduced or else it "dies" and must then be reintroduced in a subsequent session.

Legislators may amend bills at any time during the legislative process. Amendments may be made to a bill during several points of review—for example, during a subcommittee hearing, during a full committee hearing, on the floor of the House or Senate, or in a conference committee. Amendments may be favorable to the sponsor and constituency, or they may be unfavorable as a result of political maneuvering. Some amendments may change the intent of the original bill, and so there is always risk involved when bills are up for discussion and debate. For example, provisions in nurse practice acts may be changed through passage of a bill that affects another healthcare law or a statewide budget bill. It is important for the APN to monitor a bill throughout the legislative process and exert influence for positive outcomes. It is equally important for the APN to be aware of any legislation that may influence practice and the interests of healthcare consumers.

Regulations, in contrast, can be promulgated at any time during the year by an administrative agency. Some states require periodic review of regulations by the agency responsible for administering those rules in an effort to assure that rules reflect changes in the environment. The time frame for implementation of the regulation varies according to the Administrative Procedures Act (APA) of the state, but generally the regulation becomes effective within 30 to 90 days of publication of the final regulation. Regulations may be amended by the issuing agency based on public input prior to the publication of the final regulation. The administrative agency working on the regulation has discretion in determining which amendments, if any, are made; however, public comment may be very influential in determining the final outcome.

HEALTH PROFESSIONS REGULATION AND LICENSING: DEFINITIONS AND PURPOSE OF REGULATION

Regulation, as defined in *Black's Law Dictionary*, means "the act or process of controlling by rule or restriction" (Garner, 2009, p. 1398). Health professions regulation provides for ongoing monitoring and maintenance of an acceptable standard of practice for the professions in the interest of public welfare.

Regulation is needed to protect the public because of the technical complexity of the healthcare system. Diversity in educational credentialing, proliferation of types of providers, lack of public information about competency of healthcare providers, and the bundling of healthcare services all make it difficult for the public to understand and evaluate their healthcare options. The public trusts that every healthcare provider is competent to perform the duties assigned, particularly those who are licensed or registered by a state authority. Because the secondary harm that can come to an individual from an incompetent provider may be life threatening, a major role of the regulatory agency is to ensure the public safety. In addition, the regulatory process provides the public a forum to resolve complaints against healthcare providers (Sheets, 1996).

The laws (statutes) that credential and govern a profession are called *practice acts*. The practice act generally includes sections governing practice, education and credentialing, licensure and certification, disciplinary action, continuing education, the composition and scope of authority of its governing board, and its rule-making authority. Accompanying regulations (rules) specify the details related to initial licensing requirements, standards for acceptable practice, disciplinary procedures, and standards for continuing education. Some states regulate both continuing education and competence; because continuing competence is difficult to measure,

however, many states focus on the more measurable outcome of continuing education.

The regulatory process clarifies and amplifies enabling statutes and defines the methods that the governing authority will use to enforce an existing law. Regulations cannot be instituted by an administrative agency without the expressed intent of a law. Silence of the law on an issue cannot be presumed to be the will of the legislature. When there is no prior statutory authority or legislative precedent to address an issue, the legislative process must be initiated.

For example, suppose an APN petitions the board of nursing to clarify whether prescriptive authority is within the scope of practice for the APN. The board's staff refers the APN to a provision in the statute that allows the APN to "diagnose and treat" common, well-defined health problems under approved written protocols. The staff conclude that "treatment" may include prescriptive authority as an "additional act" if permitted in the approved written protocols of the nurse and physician preceptor. No specific language is found in the statute that authorizes writing prescriptions by the APN. When the medical board receives the board of nursing's opinion, an attorney general's opinion is requested. The attorney general concludes that the board of nursing may not extend the scope of practice of the APN through regulation. The expressed will of the legislature in regard to the scope of practice for the APN must be sought using the legislative process. Note that not all state boards of nursing are granted statutory authority to express formal opinions; some must rely on the express language in the practice act and regulations, the attorney general's office, or the courts.

HISTORY OF HEALTH PROFESSIONS REGULATION

At the end of the 19th century, physicians were the first healthcare providers to gain legislative recognition for their practice. The definitions of the practice of medicine are all-encompassing and include any act to diagnose or treat, or attempt to diagnose or treat, any individual with a physical injury or deformity. Herein lies the problem faced by APNs and other healthcare providers who are not physicians: how to define a scope of practice that does not overlap with this broad definition. The history of nursing regulation is characterized by efforts to accommodate this medical preemption (Safriet, 1992).

The early regulation of nurses was permissive (voluntary), providing for nurses to register with the governing board—hence the title "registered nurse." In some states, nurses were registered by the medical board prior to the establishment of a separate board of nursing. During this period, there was no competency assessment. Nurses seeking registration provided evidence of graduation from an approved nursing education program, and "good moral character" was evaluated by requiring references or endorsements from nurses registered by the board. The first board of nursing and nurse practice acts were passed in 1903 by North Carolina, followed by New York, New Jersey, and Virginia (Sheets, 1996). Boards of nursing began to establish written and practice examinations to measure competency; however, the practice acts were still permissive. Graduates of nursing-education programs not registered with the board were still permitted to practice nursing, but they were not permitted to use the title "RN."

The first mandatory licensure law was enacted by New York in 1938 (Weisenbeck & Calico, 1995). By the 1950s, mandatory licensure laws for the practice of nursing had become widespread, requiring anyone who practiced nursing to be licensed by the state board of nursing. These mandatory licensure laws protected not only the title but also the scope of practice for nurses, resulting in greater public protection.

HISTORY OF ADVANCED PRACTICE NURSING REGULATION

The 1960s set the stage for the expansion of nursing practice, as well as the practice and regulation of APNs. The birth of the federal enti-

tlement programs, Medicare and Medicaid, increased the number of individuals with access to government-subsidized health care. With a predicted shortage of primary care physicians, the first formal nurse practitioner programs were opened (Safriet, 1992).

In 1971, Idaho became the first state to legally recognize diagnosis and treatment as part of the scope of practice for the advanced practice nurse. The regulation of APNs was accomplished through joint agreement of the state board of nursing and the state board of medicine for each permissible act of diagnosis and treatment. The model of regulation established in Idaho set a precedent for subsequent models for the regulation of APNs—that is, some form of joint regulation by the board of nursing and board of medicine. The joint regulation was designed to compensate for the broad definition of the practice of medicine and is based on the determination that advanced practice nursing was a "delegated medical practice" requiring some oversight by physicians. Today, the struggle continues between nursing and medicine to define the scope of practice of the APN and to determine which regulatory board should maintain oversight.

Since 1971, virtually every state has developed some form of legal recognition of the APN. Both the American Nurses Association (ANA) and the National Council of State Boards of Nursing (NCSBN) have proposed model rules and regulations for the governing of advanced practice nursing. However, because the battles for regulation of APNs are fought in highly political state-by-state environments, there is a plethora of titles, definitions, criteria for practice, scopes of practice, reimbursement policies, and models of regulation that is difficult for policymakers to navigate and understand in today's rapidly changing healthcare delivery system.

Since 1988, *The Nurse Practitioner: The American Journal of Primary Health Care* has conducted an annual survey of each state's board of nursing and nursing organizations to gather information on the legislative status of advanced practice nursing. Significant strides have been made by many states in regard to APNs gaining sole authority for scope of practice with no requirements for direct physician supervision. As of 2010, 24 states reported that APN scope of practice is regulated solely by the board of nursing, with no statutory or regulatory requirements for physician direction, supervision, or collaboration. In 20 states, the board of nursing has sole authority for the scope of practice of APNs, but there is a requirement for physician collaboration. APNs can prescribe, including controlled substances, independent of physician involvement in 14 states; in 35 states APNs can prescribe, including controlled substances, with some degree of physician involvement (Phillips, 2010). All states now allow some form of prescriptive authority (Pearson, 2002).

METHODS OF PROFESSIONAL CREDENTIALING

Regulation of the health professions is achieved through various methods of credentialing. The method selected is determined by the state government and is based on at least two variables: (1) the potential for harm to the public if safe and acceptable standards of practice are not met, and (2) the degree of autonomy and accountability for decision making by the professional. The least restrictive form of regulation to accomplish the goal of public protection should be selected (Gross, 1984; Pew Health Professions Commission, 1994).

The term *restrictive*, as used in this context, means the degree to which the model restricts an individual who has not met the prescribed criteria in the law and received the explicit authority of the administrative agency from practicing within the scope of practice of the profession. Four methods of credentialing are used in the United States. Each of the methods is based on the regulation of the individual provider. The methods are described separately here, moving from the most restrictive to the least restrictive method of credentialing.

Licensure

A *license* is "a permission, . . . revocable, to commit some act that would otherwise be unlawful" (Garner, 2009, p. 1002). The licentiate is "one who has obtained a license or authoritative permission to exercise some function, esp. to practice a profession" (Garner, 2009, p. 1005). Licensure is the most restrictive method of credentialing and requires anyone who practices within the defined scope of practice to obtain the legal authority to do so from the appropriate administrative agency of the state.

Licensure implies competency assessment of the professional at the point of entry into the profession. A licensing examination is administered and ongoing continuing education or competency assessment by the legal authority is conducted to provide some assurance that acceptable standards of practice are met. Licensure offers the public the greatest level of protection by restricting use of the title and the scope of practice to the licensed professional who has met these rigorous criteria. Unlicensed persons cannot call themselves by the title identified in the law, and they cannot lawfully practice any portion of the scope of practice.

The administrative agency holds the licensee accountable for practicing according to the legal, ethical, and professional standards of care defined for the profession to the extent to which the laws and rules require. Disciplinary action, through an administrative disciplinary procedure that assures due process, may be taken against licensees who have violated provisions of statute or regulation. Most of the health professions are regulated by licensure because of the high degree of potential for harm to the public by individuals who are not qualified to practice the profession.

Registration

Registration is the "act of recording or enrolling" (Garner, 2009, p. 1397). Registration provides for a review of credentials to determine compliance with the criteria for entry to the profession and permits the individual to use the title "registered." Registration serves as title protection, but does not preclude individuals who are not registered from practicing within the scope of practice, as long as they do not use the title.

Registration does not necessarily imply that any competency assessment has been conducted prior to the registration. Some state laws may have provisions for removing incompetent or unethical providers from the registry or marking the registry when a complaint is lodged against a provider, but removing the person from the registry may not necessarily provide public protection because the individual may continue to practice as long as the title is not used. Some types of practitioners engage in a practice, never having been placed on a registry; an example is the lay midwife who never implies to the public that he or she is a registered nurse midwife and who does not use the title "nurse" midwife. States are required to maintain a registry of unlicensed assistive personnel who practice in long-term care facilities as a result of the Omnibus Budget Reconciliation Act of 1987.

The title "registered nurse" was formulated in the early days of nursing regulation, when the state boards registered nurses. Though nurses have been subject to licensure requirements for many years, the term *registered* has historical significance and has never been changed.

Certification

A *certificate* is "a document certifying the bearer's status or authorization to act in a specified way" (Garner, 2009, p. 255). As applied to nursing regulation, certification is a voluntary process that may involve completion of required requisite education or competency assessment, usually conducted by proprietary professional or specialty nursing organizations, denoting that the individual has achieved a level of competence in nursing practice beyond the entry-level competence measured by licensure.

Certification, like registration, is a means of title protection. *Certification* is a term that may be used by both governmental agencies and proprietary organizations. When certification is awarded by proprietary organizations, it does not have the force and effect of law. However, in some states, certification is a regulated credential; states may offer a "certificate of authority" to practice within a prescribed scope or may offer certification to assistive personnel, such as dialysis technicians. When choosing a provider, astute consumers may inquire as to whether a provider is certified as a means of assuring a level of preparedness to practice. Employers also use certification as a means of determining eligibility for certain jobs or as a requirement for promotions within the agency. Some states have enacted regulations that require an APN to be certified by a specialty nursing organization to be eligible to practice in the advanced role.

Recognition

Recognition is "confirmation that an act done by another person was authorized . . . the formal admission that a person, entity, or thing has a particular status" (Garner, 2009, p. 1385). As applied to nursing regulation, official recognition is a method of regulating APNs used by several boards of nursing that implies the board has validated and accepted credentials for the specialty area of practice. Criteria for recognition are defined in the practice act and may include requirements for certification.

PROFESSIONAL SELF-REGULATION

Self-regulation occurs within a profession through the desire of members of the profession to set standards, values, ethical frameworks, and safe-practice guidelines beyond the minimum standards defined by law. This voluntary process plays an equally significant role in the regulation of the profession, as does legal regulation. The definition of professional standards of practice and the code of ethics for the profession are examples of professional self-regulation. The members of national professional organizations set standards of practice for specialty practice and determine who can use selected titles by administering certification examinations. Continuing education require-ments, as well as documentation of practice competency, are often required for periodic re-certification. The standards are periodically re-viewed and revised to reflect current practice. Legal regulation recognizes professional stan-dards as the acceptable standard of practice when making decisions regarding what consti-tutes safe and competent care.

Even though professional organizations can develop standards, they have no legal authority to ensure compliance with said standards, as only legal regulation provides a mechanism for monitoring and enforcing compliance with standards of practice. Legal regulation and pro-fessional regulation are two sides of the same coin, working together to fulfill the profession's contract with society.

REGULATION OF ADVANCED PRACTICE NURSES

Advanced practice nursing regulation has been the focus of the Advanced Practice Task Force/Advisory Committee of the National Council of State Boards of Nursing (NCSBN) for two decades. The evolution of APN practice across the United States has resulted in a patchwork of titles, scopes of practice, and regulatory meth-ods. To bring some uniformity to the regulation of APNs and advanced practice registered nurses (APRNs), the NCSBN convened the Advanced Practice Task Force. Through the years, the task force has developed position papers for consid-eration by state boards of nursing in a quest for greater standardization and to strengthen the public protection mandate held by boards. The culmination of this work is found in the *Consensus Model for APRN Regulation: Licensure, Accreditation, Certification, & Education*. This re-port is the outcome of the work of the APRN Consensus Work Group and the National Council of State Boards of Nursing APRN Advisory Committee. It defines APRN practice, describes the APRN regulatory model, identifies the use of titles, defines specialties, describes new APRN roles and population foci, and offers strategies for implementation (APRN Joint Dia-logue Group, 2008).

National nursing certifying agencies play an important role in the professional regulation of APNs. Specialty nursing organizations develop verification examinations to measure the com-petency of nurses in an area of clinical expertise. Most boards of nursing require the APN to be certified in the clinical specialty area appropri-ate to the educational preparation to legally practice in the role. The regulatory body has the authority to accept certification examina-tions if the examination meets the criteria predetermined by the board. The board may not "surrender regulatory authority by passive ac-ceptance without evaluation of the examina-tion content, procedures and scoring process" (National Council of State Boards of Nursing, 2002). To be legally defensible for licensure pur-poses, the certification examination must meet certain psychometric standards. The founda-tional basis for regulatory sufficiency is that the examination is able to measure entry-level prac-tice; that it is based on a job analysis that de-fines job-related knowledge, skills, and abilities; and that it is developed on psychometrically sound principles of test development.

The NCSBN and the national nursing spe-cialty organizations collaborated to establish criteria that boards of nursing could use in the evaluation of certification examinations (Canavan, 1996). The Requirements for Ac-crediting Agencies and Criteria for APRN Certification Programs were developed in 1995 and updated in 2002 (National Council of State Boards of Nursing, 2002). The criteria can be lo-cated on the NCSBN website at http://www.ncsbn.org.

The national organizations that prepare cer-tification examinations for APNs include the following:

- American Academy of Nurse Practitioners
- American Association of Nurse Anesthetists Council on Certification
- American College of Nurse–Midwives Certi-fication Council

- American Nurses Credentialing Center
- National Certification Board of Pediatric Nurse Practitioners
- National Certification Corporation for the Obstetric, Gynecologic, and Neonatal Nursing Specialties

The NCSBN Advanced Practice Nursing Task Force has also sought to bring greater standardization to APN regulation in an effort to increase the mobility of APNs. In 2000, the NCSBN Delegate Assembly passed the Uniform Advanced Practice Registered Nurse Licensure/Authority to Practice Requirements. These requirements include: (1) an unencumbered RN license; (2) graduation from a graduate-level advanced practice program that is certified by a national accrediting body; (3) current certification by a national certifying body in the advanced practice specialty appropriate to educational preparation; and (4) maintenance of certification or evidence of maintenance of competence (National Council of State Boards of Nursing, 2002). Adoption of these uniform requirements by boards of nursing will enhance the ease with which APNs can become a part of the multistate regulation model. The NCSBN Model Act/Rules and Regulations were updated in August 2008 and parallel the *Consensus Model for APRN Regulation* (National Council of State Boards of Nursing, 2008).

THE STATE REGULATORY PROCESS

The 10th Amendment of the U.S. Constitution reserves all powers not specifically vested in the federal government for the states. One of these powers is the duty to protect the state's citizens (police powers). The power to regulate the professions is one way the state exercises its responsibility to protect the health, safety, and welfare of its citizens. State law provides for administrative agencies to assume the responsibility for regulation of the professions. These agencies have administrative, legislative, and judicial powers to make and enforce the laws.

Administrative agencies have sometimes been called the fourth branch of government because of their significant power in the daily execution and enforcement of the law. They are given referent authority by state and federal governments to promulgate rules and regulations, develop policies and procedures, and interpret laws to implement the agency mission.

Boards of Nursing

Each state legislature designates a board or similar authority to administer the practice act for the profession. The board's powers, duties, and composition are defined by the law. Traditionally, there are three major duties for licensing boards: (1) control entry into the profession through examination and licensure; (2) monitor and discipline licensees who violate the scope and standards of practice; and (3) monitor continuing education and/or competency of licensees to protect the public from unsafe or poor quality practice. In most states, boards of nursing have the additional duty to establish criteria for review and approval of nursing education programs that lead to licensure as a registered nurse (RN) or licensed practical nurse or licensed vocational nurse (LPN/LVN), and to set criteria for recognition of and prescriptive powers for APNs.

There are 60 boards of nursing in the United States and its territories. Each board of nursing is a member of the National Council of State Boards of Nursing. Some states have separate boards for licensing RNs and LPNs. As members of the NCSBN, the boards have the privilege of using the national licensure examination and meeting together to discuss matters of common interest (National Council of State Boards of Nursing, 2008).

Composition of the Board of Nursing

Generally, boards are composed of licensed nurses and consumer members. In most states, the governor appoints the members, although in at least one state, North Carolina, elections are conducted for the board vacancies. Nurses who are interested in serving as board members often gain appointment to those positions through the helpful endorsements of their professional associations, as well as the support of their district legislators.

Some state laws designate that nurses from specific educational and practice settings, as well as APNs, must be represented on the board of nursing. In other states, the criteria for appointment include only licensure in the profession and a residency requirement. Information on vacancies on the board of nursing can be obtained from the board office or the governor's office. Knowing the composition of the board and when vacancies occur is important to allow members of the profession to exercise political influence in gaining the desired representation on the board. Information related to serving on boards and commissions is found later in this chapter.

Board Meetings

All state government agencies function within open meeting or "sunshine" laws that permit the public to observe or participate in the discussions of the board, though boards may go into closed "executive session" when necessary; rules for executive sessions are specified in the APA and must be adhered to by the agency. The board may meet in executive session for certain reasons, including discussion of personnel matters, obtaining legal advice, contract negotiation, and disciplinary matters. Boards usually "report out" of executive session when public session resumes. All voting is a matter of public record and occurs only in open public session.

Board meetings may vary in the degree of formality. Most states' APA requires the board to post notice of meetings and the agenda in a public place, usually 30 days prior to the meeting. Sometimes the notice of meeting is published in major state newspapers. The agenda is public and available on request from the board office or from its website.

Participants in the board meeting include the board members, the board staff, and legal counsel for the board. Legal counsel advises the board in matters of law and jurisdiction. Some boards may have "staff" counsel, but many states receive advice from their representative in the state attorney general's office, known as an "assistant attorney general" (AAG). Staff or other invited guests may present reports during the meeting. Individuals may provide testimony to the board on matters of interest.

In making decisions, board members must consider several factors, including implications for the public welfare, national standards of care, impact of the decision on the state as a whole, and the legal defensibility of the decision. First and foremost, the board must act only within its legal jurisdiction. All actions of the board are a matter of public record. Most boards of nursing publish newsletters that summarize the major actions of the board during each meeting. Licensees may request to be placed on the mailing list for the newsletter if one is not automatically received.

Monitoring Competency of Nurses: Mandatory Reporting

The most critical role of the board of nursing is assuring public safety. Most nurse practice acts (NPAs) have mandatory reporting provisions that require employers to report violations of the NPA. Licensed nurses also have a moral and ethical duty to report unsafe and incompetent practice to the board of nursing. The NPA defines those acts that are considered misconduct and provides for a system of due process to investigate complaints against licensees. Procedures for filing complaints, conducting investigations, and issuing sanctions for violations are enumerated in rules and regulations of the NPA.

The licensed nurse is accountable for knowing the laws and regulations that govern the practice of nursing in the state of licensure and adhering to the legal, ethical, and professional standards of care. Some NPAs include standards of practice in the regulations. Other states may refer to professional or ethical standards established by professional associations. The employing agency also defines standards of practice through policy and procedures that must be followed by each nurse employee.

A nurse who holds a multistate license (one license that permits a nurse to practice in more than one state as long as the state is entered into a multistate compact) is held accountable for knowing and abiding by the laws of the state in which the practice occurs in addition to the home state of licensure. Multistate regulation is discussed in more detail later in this chapter. Ignorance of the law is not an excuse for misconduct.

Most boards of nursing now have the complete NPA online on their websites, as does the National Council of State Boards of Nursing (see http://www.ncsbn.org).

Instituting State Regulations

Government agencies have the authority and duty to promulgate regulations to amplify the state's statutes. As discussed earlier in this chapter, a law may provide overarching parameters, but the details of the processes required to implement the law are written into the regulations. The APA of each state specifies the process for ratifying regulations, including how the public is notified of proposed regulations and its opportunity for public comment. It is important that the APN becomes familiar with the APA to know when and how to provide comments. State processes differ: Some states have designated commissions or committees responsible for review and approval of regulations, while other states submit regulations to the general assembly or to committees of the legislature. Certain elements are common to the promulgation of regulations. These include (1) public notice that a new regulation has been proposed, or of a proposal to modify an existing regulation;

(2) opportunity to submit written comment or testimony, and in addition the opportunity to present oral testimony at a rules hearing; and (3) publication of the final regulation in a register or state bulletin.

In some states, a fiscal impact statement is required. This statement estimates the cost of compliance with the regulation. Also, in some states, the rule promulgation process requires oversight by a commission of legislators whose role it is to ensure that the regulatory agency instituting the rules does, in fact, have the authority to do so; does not exceed the scope of its rule-making authority; and does not draft rules that would conflict with its own statute or that of any related discipline. For example, in the case of nursing, legislative commissions would cross-check the statutes and rules regulating other health professions.

Monitoring State Regulations

Administrative agencies promulgate hundreds of regulations each year. Regulations that affect advanced nursing practice could be put into effect by a variety of agencies. Knowing which agencies are most likely to have the authority to put forth regulations that affect health care and professional practice, as well as monitoring the legislation and regulations proposed by those agencies, is important to protect the scope of practice of APNs.

The most obvious agencies the APN should consider tracking are the licensing boards of other health professions, such as medicine, pharmacy, counselors and therapists, and other health professionals. In this rapidly changing healthcare environment, numerous conflicts occur over scope of practice issues, definitions of practice, right to reimbursement, and requirements for supervision and collaboration.

When reviewing regulations, there are several points that are important to consider. **Exhibit 11-1** provides some key questions to consider when analyzing a regulation for its impact on nursing practice.

EXHIBIT 11-1	Questions to Ask When Analyzing Regulations

- Which agency promulgated the regulation?
- What is the source of authority (the statute that provides authority for the regulation to be promulgated)?
- What is the intent or rationale of the regulation? Is it clearly stated by the promulgating agency?
- Is the language in the regulation clear or ambiguous? Can the regulation be interpreted in different ways by different individuals? Discuss advantages of language that is clear versus ambiguous.
- Are there definitions to clarify terms?
- Are there important points that are not addressed? That is, are there omissions?
- How does the regulation affect the practice of nursing? Does it constrain or limit the practice of nursing in any way?
- Is there sufficient lead time to comply with the regulation?
- What is the fiscal impact of the regulation?

Consider the following situation and how the proposed regulations would affect the practice of the APN. Assume the board of pharmacy has drafted the following definition of the practice of pharmacy:

> The practice of pharmacy includes, but is not limited to, the interpretation, evaluation, and implementation of medical orders; the dispensing of prescription drug orders; initiating or modifying the drug therapy in accordance with written guidelines or protocols previously established and approved by a practitioner authorized to independently prescribe drugs; and the provision of patient counseling as a primary healthcare provider of pharmacy care.

If this definition was included in the pharmacy practice act requiring that anyone who "initiated or modified a drug therapy in accordance with written guidelines or protocols" must be licensed as a pharmacist by the board of pharmacy, how would this affect the practice of nursing and, especially, the APN? This is but one example of numerous definitions of scope of practice that have significant overlap with the advanced practice of nursing. A solution to this dilemma would be to negotiate for the addition of an exemption for APNs in the pharmacy practice act.

In a growing managed care market, it is also critical for APNs to be aware of regulations that mandate benefits or reimbursement policies and to lobby for inclusion of APNs. Several states have instituted open-panel legislation, known as "any willing provider" and "freedom of choice" laws. These bills mandate that any provider who is authorized to provide the services covered in an insurance plan must be recognized and reimbursed by the plan. Insurance company lobbyists, as well as business lobbyists, oppose this type of legislation. As managed care contracts are negotiated, APNs must ensure that services of the APN are given fair and equitable consideration. Other important areas include workers' compensation participation and reimbursement provisions and liability insurance laws.

APNs achieved landmark success in 1997, with grassroots lobbying efforts, to gain Medicare reimbursement for all nurse practitioners, regardless of location of practice. Prior to 1997, Medicare reimbursement for nurse practitioners was restricted to those nurse practitioners who provided services in specific geographic locations and who practiced with physician supervision.

In summary, state agencies that govern licensing and certification of healthcare facilities, administer public health services (e.g., public health, mental health, alcohol and drug abuse), and govern reimbursement, as well as the health professions licensing boards, are all agencies that could promulgate regulations that would have implications for the practice of the APN.

Serving on Boards and Commissions

One way to participate actively in the regulatory process is to seek an appointment to the state board of nursing or other board or commission that affects health policy. Active participation in the political process, especially during times of rapid change and reform, will ensure the voice of APNs is heard in setting the public policy agenda.

When seeking appointments to boards and commissions, select an agency whose mission and purposes are consistent with your interests and expertise. Because most board appointments are gubernatorial or political appointments, it is important for the APN to obtain endorsements from legislators, influential community leaders, and their professional associations.

Letters of support should document the APN's contributions to employment and community service. Delineate involvement in local, state, and national organizations. The letter from the employer should indicate a willingness to provide the time to fulfill the responsibilities of the position during the term of office. In addition, a personal letter from the APN who is seeking appointment to the governor that expresses interest in serving on the board should be offered, including the rationale for volunteering for service on the particular board or commission, evidence of a good match between one's expertise and the role of that board or commission, and expression of a clear interest in serving the public. A résumé or curriculum vitae should be attached. Letters should emphasize desire to serve over self-interest; appointment decisions should be based on how much the individual can offer the board or commission in serving the public good. This kind of public service requires a substantial time commitment; it is wise to speak to other members of the board or call the executive director or administrator of the agency to determine the extent of that commitment.

THE FEDERAL REGULATORY PROCESS

Many forces have contributed to the federal government becoming a more central figure in the regulation of the health professions. The most significant factor is the advent of the Medicare and Medicaid programs. The federal initiatives that have grown out of these programs are largely focused on cost containment (prospective payment) and consumer protection (combating fraud and abuse) (Jost, 1997; Roberts & Clyde, 1993).

With the "graying" of Americans, the cost of administering the Medicare program is skyrocketing, with predictions of bankruptcy if substantive changes are not made in either the criteria for eligibility or the methods of reimbursement. Numerous changes to the system are expected in the coming years.

One of the most significant changes occurred in July 2001 when the Centers for Medicare and Medicaid Services (CMS) was created to replace the former Health Care Financing Administration (HCFA). The reformed agency provides an increased emphasis on responsiveness to beneficiaries and providers and quality improvement. Three new business centers have been established as part of the reform: Center for Beneficiary Choices, Center for Medicare Management, and Center for Medicaid and State Operations (Centers for Medicare and Medicaid Services, 2001).

The practice of APNs has also been influenced by changes in the Medicare reimbursement policy. In 1997, legislation was passed in Congress calling for Medicare reimbursement of APNs regardless of setting; it went into effect in January 1998. These regulations provide direct reimbursement to APNs for providing Medicare Part B services that would normally be provided by a physician. These services are not restricted by site of geographic location as services have been in the past. Under this legislation, APNs can see both new and continuing patients without restriction. Reimbursement rates are set at 80% of the lesser of the actual charge or 85% of the fee schedule amount for the physician (American Academy of Nurse Practitioners, 2003). APNs must secure a Medicare provider number to be eligible for reimbursement.

The evolution of government has changed the relationship between the state and federal regulatory systems. Responsibilities once assumed by the federal government have been shifted down to the state level, such as administration of the Medicaid programs and management of the welfare program. The impetus guiding this change is that states are better equipped to make decisions about how best to assist their citizens and the sentiment against creating federal bureaucracy and increasing the tax burden. Even though states have primary authority over regulation of the health professions, federal policies also have an enormous effect on healthcare workforce regulation. All the policies related to reimbursement and quality control over the Medicare and Medicaid programs are promulgated by the U.S. Department of Health and Human Services and are administered through its financing agency, the CMS. Other federal statutes that have a regulatory impact on

healthcare providers and that the APN should be familiar with include the following:

- Clinical Laboratory Improvement Amendments of 1988 (CLIA 88)
- Occupational Safety and Health Act of 1970 (OSHA)
- Mammography Quality Standards Act of 1987 and 1992 (MQSA 87 and 92)
- Omnibus Budget Reconciliation Act of 1987 and 1990 (OBRA 87 and 90)
- Americans with Disabilities Act of 1990 (ADA)
- North American Free Trade Agreement of 1993 (NAFTA, effective date January 1, 1994)
- Telecommunications Act of 1996
- Health Insurance Portability and Accountability Act of 1996 (HIPAA)
- Patient Protection and Affordable Care Act, Public Law 111-148 (PPACA, effective date March 23, 2010)

The Veterans Administration hospitals and the Indian Health Services both are regulated by the federal government, as are the uniformed armed services. Individuals who are employed in these services must be licensed in at least one state and are subject to the laws of the state in which they are licensed and the standards of care and policies established in the federal system. The Supremacy Clause of the U.S. Constitution gives legal superiority to federal laws (Braunstein, 1995). When a federal law or regulation is enacted, it takes precedence over any state law. State laws in conflict with federal laws cannot be enforced. At times, the courts may be asked to determine the constitutionality of a law or regulation to resolve jurisdictional disputes.

The Commerce Clause of the U.S. Constitution limits the ability of states to erect barriers to interstate trade (Gobis, 1997). Courts have found that the provision of health care is interstate trade under antitrust laws, and this finding sets the stage for the federal government to preempt state licensing laws in the practice of professions across state boundaries, if it chooses to do so.

The impact of technology on the delivery of health care, such as "telehealthcare" or "telecare," allows providers to care for patients in remote environments and across the geopolitical boundaries defined by traditional state-by-state licensure. This raises the question as to whether the federal government will intercede in standardizing licensing requirements across state lines to facilitate interstate commerce, usurping the state's authority. Licensing boards are beginning to identify ways to facilitate the practice of telehealthcare, while at the same time preserving the power and right of the state to protect its citizens by regulating the professions at the state level. One innovative approach to nursing regulation, multistate regulation, is discussed later in this chapter.

The most recent of these federal initiatives is the Patient Protection and Affordable Care Act. The passing of this law in 2010 represented a national movement toward comprehensive and far-reaching national healthcare system reform. It represents the broadest revamping of health care since the Medicare and Medicaid programs were created in 1965. The provisions of the law are slated to be enacted over a 5-year period, and include requirements for consumer protection, improvement of the quality of health care, lowering of healthcare costs, increasing access to affordable care, and holding insurance companies more accountable (HealthCare.gov, 2010).

The Patient Protection and Affordable Care Act includes a number of provisions related to nursing, many of which are applicable or specific to the APN. Among these related to nursing are increased funding for a primary care workforce, grants for funding nurse-managed health centers through the Department of Health and Human Services (HHS), clarification of the funding of advanced nursing education to include accredited midwifery education, expansion of the Nurse Loan Repayment and Scholarship Programs (NLRP) to provide loan repayment for students who serve in faculty positions in accredited nursing programs for at least 2 years, and increases in the Nurse Faculty Loan Program.

Even more specifically applicable to APNs are provisions related to the inclusion of nurse practitioners and clinical nurse specialists as ACO (accountable care organization) professionals. ACOs are legally formed structures, comprising a group of providers and suppliers, to manage and coordinate care for Medicare fee-for-service beneficiaries. The law also authorizes HHS to establish a grant program for states or designated entities to establish community-based interprofessional teams to support primary care practices, increases Medicare payments for primary care practitioners, and increases reimbursement rates for certified nurse–midwives. A graduate nurse education provision would appropriate monies to establish graduate nurse education demonstration programs in Medicare. There are numerous other provisions in this law as enacted; a complete list of key provisions related to nursing may be found on the American Nurses Association website (http ://www.nursingworld.org).

However, the success of this historic legislation is threatened and the final outcome is in question.

Promulgating Federal Regulations

The federal regulatory process is a two-step process established by the federal Administrative Procedures Act. A notice of proposed rulemaking (NPR) is published in the proposed rule section of the *Federal Register*, which informs the public of the substance of the intended regulation and provides information on how the public may participate in providing comment, attending meetings, or otherwise participating in the regulatory process. The second step involves careful consideration of public comment by the agency and amendment to the regulation, if warranted. The final regulations are issued by the agency through publication in the rules and regulations section of the *Federal Register* and become effective 30 days after publication (see **Exhibit 11-2**).

EXHIBIT 11-2 The Federal Rule-Making Process

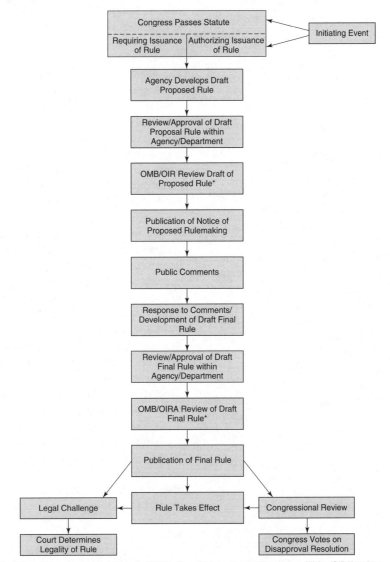

* The Office of Management and Budget's (OMB) office of Information and Regulatory Affairs (OIRA) reviews only significant rules, and does not review any rules submitted by independent regulatory agencies

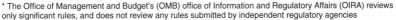

Source: Copeland, C. W. (2008, August 28). The federal rulemaking process: An overview. Congressional Research Service Report RL32240. Retrieved from http://openregs.com/docs /copeland-rulemaking-process.pdf

EMERGENCY REGULATIONS

Provisions for promulgating emergency regulations are defined at both the state and federal levels. Emergency regulations are enacted if an agency determines that the public welfare is immediately adversely affected. Emergency regulations may take effect immediately upon publication, are generally temporary, are effective for a limited time (usually 90 days, with an option to renew), and must be followed with permanent regulations that are instituted in accordance with the APA process.

LOCATING INFORMATION

The *Federal Register* is the bulletin board or newspaper of the federal government. It is published Monday through Friday, except for federal holidays, and is updated daily by 6 a.m. It contains executive orders and presidential proclamations, rules and regulations, proposed rules, notices of federal agencies and organizations, sunshine act meetings, and corrections to previous copies of the *Federal Register*. Each document in the *Federal Register* begins with a heading that includes the name of the issuing agency, the Code of Federal Regulations title, and a brief synopsis of the contents. After the heading, a preamble is published that contains the type of action, summary of action, deadline for comments, address to which the comments may be sent, a contact person, and other supplementary information (Goehlert & Martin, 1989). The *Federal Register* may be accessed online via the Governmental Printing Office (GPO) website at http://www.gpoaccess.gov /fr/index.html.

The Code of Federal Regulations (CFR) is a compilation of all final regulations issued by the executive branch agencies of the federal government. The CFR consists of 50 titles that represent broad subject areas. It is updated annually in sections; each quarter, one section of the CFR is updated according to a schedule that includes all regulations that have been passed since the prior printing. Consequently, there is never a publication that has all the regulations passed in it for the year. An index that helps in locating rules by agency name and subject headings is published and revised semiannually (Goehlert & Martin, 1989). The Code of Federal Regulations is online at the GPO website at http://www .gpoaccess.gov/cfr/index.html.

Each state government publishes similar documents that identify the proposed regulations, notices, final regulations, and emergency regulations. The publication is usually called the State Register or the State Bulletin, and the publication cycle can be obtained by calling the state legislative printing office or the state legislative information system office. Copies of these documents are usually available in the local libraries and may be available online on the state's governmental website.

The myriad of proposed regulations promulgated by agencies at the state and federal levels is so expansive that it is to the APN's advantage to belong to the appropriate professional organizations, most of which employ lobbyists whose business it is to track legislation. Specialty organization newsletters and journals, legislative subscription and monitoring services, and bulletins that summarize proposed regulations may be used to monitor these processes. Subscription services track legislation for an agency or organization and provide an abstract, including the substance of bills and regulations and the progress through the legislative or regulatory process. Both free and subscription legislative information services are available online. Examples of online services include the following:

- State Net: Information and intelligence for the 50 states and Congress, located at http ://www.statenet.com

- Thomas Legislative Information: Sponsored by the U.S. Library of Congress, located at http://thomas.loc.gov

- GPO Access: Located at http://www.gpo access.gov

- Federal Legislative Branch: Located at http ://www.USA.gov. This is the U.S. government's official web portal.

In addition, numerous private services are available and can be found by searching the Internet. Several nursing and healthcare associations also feature relevant updates and information on current legislative and public policy issues (see **Exhibit 11-3**).

PROVIDING PUBLIC COMMENT

There is a small window of opportunity for public input into the development of regulations. Most comment periods are a minimum of 30 days from the date of the publication of the proposed rule, although sometimes an NPR will provide for a longer period of time to submit comments if the agency anticipates the issue will be one of strong public interest or will be controversial in nature. It is very important that the APN is vigilant in tracking when the comment periods are set.

Public hearings may be held by an agency on a proposed rule, but are not required unless the APA establishes criteria for when a public hearing must be held by the agency. Generally, the agency is required to hold a hearing when a request is made by a specified number of individuals or agencies. Written comments received by the agency are made a part of the permanent record and must be considered by the agency's board or commission members prior to the publication of the final rule. A final rule can be challenged in the courts if the judge determines that the agency did not comply with the APA or ignored public comments.

The *Federal Register* names the individual in the agency who can be contacted to submit comments. It is best to place the comments in writing to ensure inclusion in the public record, though it is permissible to call the agency and provide comments orally if time is of the essence. Faxing comments or providing an electronic copy may also be an option if the comment period is near expiration. It is of utmost importance that the deadline posted in the *Federal Register* is met because agencies can rightfully disregard comments received after the deadline.

When providing public comment in writing, or testimony at a hearing, it is important for the APN to:

- Be specific regarding whether the regulation is supported or opposed. Give examples using brief scenarios or experiences when possible.
- Have credible data to back the position, such as statistics. Use research findings that can be explained in common language; avoid medical jargon.
- Know what the opposition is saying and respond to these concerns.
- Convey a willingness to negotiate or compromise toward mutually acceptable resolutions.
- Demonstrate concern for the public good, rather than self-interest.
- Be brief and succinct. Limit remarks to one or two pages or 5 minutes for oral testimony.

Regulatory agencies charged with public protection are more likely to address concerns that are focused on how the public may be harmed or benefit rather than concerns that seem like turf protection and professional jealousy. Demonstrate support for your position by having colleagues who represent a variety of organizations and interests submit comments. This is a powerful method to employ; it is important to demonstrate the degree of concern because the number of comments received is one way the agency measures support or nonsupport for the regulation.

STRENGTHS AND WEAKNESSES OF THE REGULATORY PROCESS

The regulatory process is much more ordered than the legislative process, in that the administrative procedures act in each state and at the federal level directs the process that must be undertaken. There is guaranteed opportunity for comment and public input, as the regulatory

| EXHIBIT 11-3 | Selected Websites of Interest |

http://www.statenet.com Legislative and regulatory reporting services from all 50 states and Congress. A subscription service that provides comprehensive and timely information on legislation.

http://thomas.loc.gov Thomas Legislative Information System. Sponsored by the U.S. Library of Congress. Summarizes bills, provides full text of bills and the Congressional Record, information on the legislative process, and U.S. government Internet resources.

http://www.ahrq.gov Agency for Healthcare Research and Quality. Provides information on healthcare research, evidence reports, clinical practice guidelines, consumer health information; hyperlinked to U.S. Department of Health and Human Services.

http://www.ctel.org Center for Telemedicine Law. Information on the latest findings in the regulation of telemedicine, proceedings of national telemedicine task force, state-by-state updates on telemedicine legislation.

http://www.nursingworld.org American Nurses Association. Access to all ANA services; access to *Online Journal of Issues in Nursing*; jointly prepared with Kent State University.

http://www.ncsbn.org National Council of State Boards of Nursing. Information on all National Council services and committee activities, access to state nurse practice acts, information on progress of multistate regulation.

http://www.hhs.gov U.S. Department of Health and Human Services. Access to all agencies within the department—that is, ACHPR, CDC, CMS, HRSA, NIH, and so forth. Includes consumer information and policy information.

http://www.hschange.com The Center for Studying Health Systems Change. A Washington, D.C.–based research organization dedicated to studying the nation's healthcare systems and the impact on the public.

http://www.nurse.org State-by-state display of advanced practice nursing organizations, links to related sites that contain legislative and regulatory information, NP Central (a comprehensive site for APN CE offerings, salary information, job opportunities).

http://www.nursingethicsnetwork.org Nursing Ethics Network. A nonprofit organization committed to the advancement of nursing ethics. Site contains ethics research findings and online inquiry.

http://www.acnpweb.org American College of Nurse Practitioners. Comprehensive site featuring latest trends and issues affecting APN practice and regulation.

http://www.aanp.org American Academy of Nurse Practitioners. Comprehensive site featuring latest trends and issues affecting APN practice and regulation.

http://www.cms.hhs.gov/hipaa Centers for Medicare and Medicaid Services. Provides latest legislative and regulatory information on reimbursement, HIPAA implementation.

http://www.hhs.gov/ocr/hipaa Office of Civil Rights. Fact sheets, sample forms, FAQs on HIPAA implementation, along with related links and educational materials.

http://www.iom.edu Institute of Medicine. Provides objective information to further science and health policy. A leading and respected authority on health issues. Access to published reports.

process has built-in delays and time constraints that slow down action. On the other hand, the regulatory process also is much more controlled by administrative agencies and can often become tedious and complex in the details of implementation. Regulations may not always be written by individuals who are knowledgeable about the substance or impact of new or revised rules, making the public input process especially important.

One power that may be provided to administrative agencies is to interpret regulations. It is especially important to be aware that existing regulations may be misinterpreted by the staff or board of an agency, resulting in a new meaning being imposed rather than the original intent of the regulation.

New interpretations to existing statutes and regulations may occur over time. For this reason, it is especially important to review opinions and/or declaratory rulings of the board, attorney general opinions, and opinions of the court. Official opinions carry the force and effect of law even though they are not promulgated according to the APA. There is a fine line between the duty to interpret existing laws and regulations and establishing new laws or standards without complying with the APA. The courts have revoked several board rulings, requiring boards to institute new regulations according to the APA. In some states, such as Ohio, official opinions interpreting statute or regulation are generated only by the attorney general's office or the courts. However, regulatory boards may offer interpretive guidelines or other documents to facilitate public understanding and compliance.

CURRENT ISSUES IN REGULATION AND LICENSURE: REGULATION IN A TRANSFORMING HEALTHCARE DELIVERY SYSTEM

The current system of regulation of healthcare professionals is based on the regulation of the individual provider and the employment set-

ting. Questions have been raised as to whether this system is the best means of public protection, or whether the system has become a means of protecting the profession and creating monopolies for services (Gross, 1984; Pew Health Professions Commission, 1994). As new healthcare occupations and professions have emerged, there has been increasing professional debate about which tasks can be accomplished by which professions. Overlapping scopes of practice have naturally emerged among nursing, medicine, pharmacy, social work, physical therapy, occupational therapy, and other licensed health professions. Overlapping scopes of practice are appropriate when competency and education to perform the acts are substantially equivalent, but restrictive practice acts have made overlapping scopes of practice a battlefield for debate—a debate with which APNs are very familiar.

The Pew Health Professions Commission (1995) published a sweeping report that began to change thinking about the existing regulatory systems. The report suggested that the current century-old regulatory system is out of sync with the nation's healthcare delivery and financing structures and in need of major reform. The web of laws and regulations created by bureaus, agencies, boards, and legal departments makes it difficult for the public and those regulated to participate in what Dower and Finocchio (1995) call an "exclusionary scheme" (p. 2). The Pew Health Professions Commission suggested that states review the regulatory process in light of the following criteria:

- Does regulation promote effective health outcomes and protect the public from harm?
- Are regulatory bodies truly accountable to the public?
- Does regulation respect consumers' rights to choose their own healthcare providers from a range of safe options?
- Does regulation encourage a flexible, rational, and cost-effective healthcare system?

- Does regulation allow effective working relationships among healthcare providers?
- Does regulation promote equity among providers of equal skill?
- Does regulation facilitate professional and geographic mobility of competent providers? (Dower & Finocchio, 1995, p. 1)

Workforce regulation has a tremendous impact on the cost and accessibility of health care. Restrictive scopes of practice limit the ability of comparably prepared providers to provide care, while employers have expanded the use of unlicensed assistive personnel (UAP) who infringe on the scope of practice defined for the licensed nurse. Boundary disputes within and across disciplines flourish—between nursing and allied health providers, allied health providers and medicine, nursing and medicine, dental hygienists and dentists, and nurses and UAPs.

The Pew Task Force on Health Care Workforce Regulation challenged the state and federal government to respond to the complex issues regarding the education and regulation of the health professions. The task force offered 10 recommendations to make the state regulatory system more responsive to the evolving healthcare system, calling for attention to standardized and understandable language, standardization of entry-to-practice requirements, assurance of initial and continuing competence of healthcare practitioners, and the redesign of professional boards, including the creation of super boards with a majority of consumer representatives. The report also called for better methods of assessing the achievement of objectives and disciplinary processes (Pew Health Professions Commission, 1995).

Since the publication of the task force's recommendations, the Institute of Medicine has issued a number of reports related to safety in healthcare systems. A part of that focus has called for licensing and certification bodies to pay greater attention to safety-related performance standards and expecta-

tions for health professionals (Kohn, Corrigan, & Donaldson, 2000).

A consensus report issued by the Robert Wood Johnson Foundation (RWJF) and the Institute of Medicine (IOM) on the future of nursing was released in October 2010. The report, *The Future of Nursing: Leading Change, Advancing Health*, provides four key messages to guide changes and remove barriers that prevent nurses from being able to function effectively in a rapidly evolving healthcare system. These messages are that (1) nurses should be enabled to practice to the full extent of their education and training; (2) nurses should be able to access higher levels of education and training in an improved educational system that allows for academic progression; (3) nurses should be full partners in the interprofessional redesign of the U.S. healthcare system; and (4) effective workforce planning and policymaking needs better data collection and information infrastructures. Eight recommendations for fundamental changes are found in the report, along with related actions for Congress, state legislatures, the Centers for Medicare and Medicaid Services, the Office of Personnel Management, and the Federal Trade Commission and Antitrust Division of the Department of Justice. The eight recommendations are as follows:

1. Remove scope-of-practice barriers
2. Expand opportunities for nurses to lead and diffuse collaborative improvement efforts
3. Implement nurse residency programs
4. Increase the proportion of nurses with a baccalaureate degree to 80% by 2020
5. Double the number of nurses with a doctorate by 2020
6. Ensure that nurses engage in lifelong learning
7. Prepare and enable nurses to lead change to advance health
8. Build an infrastructure for the collection and analysis of interprofessional healthcare workforce data (Institute of Medicine, 2010)

There is a window of opportunity to achieve significant reform in the regulation of the health professions in the 21st century. Advanced practice nurses must be open to the concept of new regulatory models that may emerge. Regulation will determine who will have access to the patient, who will serve as the gatekeeper in a managed care environment, who will be reimbursed, and who will have autonomy to practice. APNs must be visible participants throughout the political process to shape a dynamic and evolving system that is responsive to the healthcare environment and ensures consumer choice and protection.

MULTISTATE REGULATION

Technology has transformed the healthcare delivery system and is challenging the state-by-state regulatory and licensing system. Mergers, acquisitions, and buyouts of healthcare systems have produced giant conglomerates that operate across state lines, with care being coordinated by case managers who may be located in distant states. The Internet and e-mail afford patients access to hundreds of disease specialty home pages on the World Wide Web sponsored by institutions and voluntary associations. Over the past decade, a variety of telemedicine services have emerged, serving both patients and healthcare providers. United HealthCare's website, called OptumHealth (http://www.optumhealth.com) offers nursing online services. Individuals submit questions and nurses research answers and provide personalized information within 48 to 72 hours (Gobis, 1997).

Although states have done much over the years to facilitate the interstate mobility of nurses, there are still cumbersome licensure processes that make seamless transitions across geopolitical boundaries difficult or impossible. The confusion is especially prominent in the regulation of APNs. Not only are there a variety of methods used to regulate APNs, ranging from second licensure to official recognition, but titles also vary from state to state, as

do the scopes of practice and even the jurisdiction for regulation (i.e., nursing, medical, or joint boards). The NCSBN definition of Uniform Advanced Practice Registered Nurse Licensure/Authority to Practice Requirements will promote standardization of APN regulation to allow APNs to participate in multistate regulation as well as compete in a global market. Moving to a multistate regulatory system has advantages for the profession and must be carefully executed state by state to ensure that the mission of the boards to protect the public is achieved.

To that end, the NCSBN delegate assembly adopted the mutual recognition model of multistate regulation in 1997. Mutual recognition is a method of licensure in which boards voluntarily enter into an interstate compact to legally recognize the policies and processes of a licensee's home state to permit practice in the remote state without obtaining an additional license. If a violation of law occurs, the state in which the violation occurs is responsible for disciplinary action (National Council of State Boards of Nursing, 1998).

To implement the mutual recognition model of nursing regulation, each state legislature must sign the interstate compact into law. Advanced practice nurses initially were not a part of the interstate compact agreement, but with the move toward adoption of the Uniform Requirements for Licensure/Authority to Practice, APNs will be able to participate in the multistate regulation process. The APN must reside in a state that has already joined the interstate compact and subscribed to the uniform requirements. The multistate license does not, however, include prescriptive authority, which must be sought independently in the state of practice.

Given the climate in the federal government related to the business of health care and the concept that this business is interstate commerce, a number of states have quickly moved to preserve state regulation of the professions, while facilitating interstate practice. As of June

2010, 24 states are participating as "compact states" (National Council of State Boards of Nursing, 2010).

THE FUTURE OF ADVANCED PRACTICE NURSE REGULATION

Much has been written in this chapter on the problems and issues related to the regulation of APNs. However, not all of the problems associated with the full utilization and practice of the APN are external to the profession; some of the problems have been created within the profession. The proliferation of APN educational programs with numerous specialty areas that have limited scopes of practice has created much of the public confusion regarding the role and scope of practice of the APN. Multiple educational pathways to achieve APN certification and legal credentialing have further complicated the regulatory process (O'Malley, Cummings, & King, 1996). The numerous titles used for APN practice are confusing not only to the public, but also to regulatory agencies such as the Centers for Medicare and Medicaid Services that establish national reimbursement policies. Clear definitions of APN roles and titles, educational requirements, and scope of practice must become a regulatory priority.

Credentialing APNs has been a major source of debate at the national level. Should this level of provider be licensed rather than officially recognized? Should there be a core competency examination developed at the national level for APN credentialing? Do certification examinations developed by the specialty nursing organizations meet the legal defensibility of an entry-level licensure examination? Who is an APN? Should there be a minimum education requirement for use of the title? These are all questions that continue to be raised in forums between specialty nursing organizations and licensing agencies. Until the role of the APN is clearly understood by consumers and policymakers, APNs will continue to be underutilized and undervalued.

Two important issues related to the future of advanced practice nursing regulation that require monitoring by APNs include the NCSBN initiative to consider state board of nursing regulation of APNs in the future, and the related matter of the direction in which future APN education is moving, the practice doctorate.

The NCSBN 2006 draft Vision Paper, *The Future Regulation of Advanced Practice Nursing*, has been the subject of debate among advanced practice nursing organizations and the American Association of Colleges of Nursing (AACN) (American Association of Colleges of Nursing, 2006; National Council of State Boards of Nursing, 2006). The final report of the APRN Consensus Work Group and the NCSBN APRN Advisory Committee (APRN Joint Dialogue Group, 2008) was a major step in reaching a level of agreement between stakeholders in organized nursing. Major foundational requirements for licensure are described in this document, including a call for boards of nursing to be solely responsible for licensing advanced practice nurses.

Parallel to new directions in regulation of APNs is the new direction in advanced clinical nursing education. In an effort to respond to the changes in national direction for health professions education and credentialing, the AACN Board of Directors endorsed a Position Statement on the Practice Doctorate (DNP) in Nursing (American Association of Colleges of Nursing, 2004), which calls for a move in educational preparation for advanced practice nurses' to the doctorate level from the master's level by the year 2015. The AACN cites the need for change in graduate nursing education as a response to the increasing complexity of the nation's healthcare environment and points to national calls to action from the Institute of Medicine (IOM), the Joint Commission on the Accreditation of Healthcare Organizations (JCAHO; now known as The Joint Commission), and the 2005 National Institutes of Health (NIH) report calling for the development of nonresearch clinical doctorates in nursing. Two AACN task forces have been initiated to address questions related to nursing education, certification, regulation, and practice that have been raised by the development of DNP programs. As of March 2010, 120 DNP programs were currently enrolling students nationwide, and the AACN reported that 161 others were under development at U.S. nursing schools (American Association of Colleges of Nursing, 2010).

REIMBURSEMENT

Significant breakthroughs are being made in reimbursement policy for APNs, largely as a result of the formation of grassroots lobbying efforts and coalitions of APN specialty-nursing organizations. With the passage of federal legislation in 1997 allowing APNs to bill Medicare directly for services, APNs have had the opportunity to increase consumers' access to care. The managed care markets value efficiency and effectiveness in providers, so APNs are learning how to cost out services in the competitive market to win contracts and demonstrate cost-effective, quality-care outcomes to patients.

In managed care contracts where reimbursement is capitated, the amount of reimbursement is not as important as knowing whether the services can be provided for the capitated fee. Research studies are needed to document the cost of care and demonstrate nursing interventions that reduce the use of costly healthcare services over time. Studies that demonstrate the value-added activities of nursing intervention, cost–benefit analysis of interventions, and patient satisfaction with care are emerging in the literature and can be very useful in negotiating contracts for patient populations.

Understanding the business aspects of healthcare financing and creating successful practices are new roles for entrepreneurial APNs who are managing the health care for a group of clients. It is a role in which APNs are gaining more comfort and experience.

IMPACT OF THE NURSE SHORTAGE ON REGULATION AND LICENSURE

Supply and demand projections substantiate that the shortage of nurses and other healthcare providers will continue well into 2015. The factors driving this shortage include a growing aging population who will consume more healthcare services, the aging of the nursing workforce resulting in a large cohort of nurses retiring from the profession, and the inability of nursing to attract men, minorities, and young people into the profession. Even though there have been numerous initiatives at the state and federal levels to reverse this trend, the nurse shortage continues to fuel policy on work environment issues across the nation.

Several issues bear monitoring during this period of a declining nursing workforce. They include the following:

- *Delegation and supervision of unlicensed assistive personnel.* Practices for UAPs will continue to be debated and expanded as the shortage of licensed staff make it difficult to meet all the care demands of the public. Providing safe and effective care while delegating care to UAPs will place additional responsibilities on the licensed nurse.

- *Mandatory overtime legislation.* Research has shown that fatigue affects the mental acuity of an individual, leading to more errors in judgment and to medical errors that could result in harm to the patient. The Institute of Medicine has published findings that link medical errors to the number and educational level of nurses employed as well as to fatigue of the staff (Institute of Medicine, 1999). Employers have used the concept of patient abandonment to force employees to remain on duty against their will, threatening staff who leave the employment setting with patient abandonment that would result in a report to the licensing board. Laws have been passed in several states that preclude an employer from requiring staff to work beyond their scheduled assignment against their will.

■ *Staffing ratios.* In some states, nurses have organized to pass legislation to implement staffing ratios that guarantee a nurse-to-patient ratio dependent on the acuity of the patient. Staffing ratios have both positive and negative implications. Although the regulations for staffing ratios may require a set number of nurses to be employed, the minimum ratios imposed by law may be seen by the employer as the maximum number that must be employed, thereby placing a cap on hiring and negatively affecting the quality of care.

■ *Foreign nurse recruitment.* There is often an attempt to increase the recruitment of foreign-educated nurses when there is an acute nurse shortage in the United States. Legislation is often introduced during these periods of time to relax the standards for licensure and to accept competency examinations that are not equivalent to the National Council Licensure Examination (NCLEX). The nursing community must be vigilant to these attempts to lower the standards for licensure and thus prevent discrimination against U.S.-educated graduates.

■ *Proliferation of new nursing education programs.* Nationally, colleges, universities, and other accredited and legitimate public and private educational institutions are finding that the business of nursing education is becoming more attractive, and there are more qualified applicants for nursing programs then there are seats. However, proprietary organizations are also seeing nursing education as an opportunity for profit, without consideration of the infrastructure and support systems necessary to carry out a quality program. State Boards of Nursing are being challenged to strike a balance between an open marketplace and a desire to protect the stretched interests of existing programs that are struggling to maintain a cadre of qualified faculty and ensure clinical placements for their students.

Other trends and issues will surface over the next several years that may affect the regulation of nurses and APNs. It will be increasingly important to stay abreast of legislative and regulatory initiatives and to affiliate with professional organizations to preserve and protect professional standards.

CONCLUSION

Today is an era of rapid transformation in almost every aspect of life. Change is constant, and it rapidly forces adaptability and flexibility on the part of all individuals. Changes in the delivery of health care are transforming the practice and regulation of the APN. Today, the APN must develop skills to capitalize on the chaos in the healthcare system and create opportunities for the advantage of the profession rather than fear the future. One way to capitalize on the times is to become politically astute and learn to shape public policy through working with coalitions of nurses, other providers, and consumers to advocate for quality health care at an affordable cost.

Knowing how to navigate the regulatory process will give the APN the tools needed to become a confident spokesperson. Seeking and finding information on the status of issues critical to the APN, such as reimbursement, scopes of practice, and licensure issues, keeps the APN knowledgeable about how best to influence outcomes.

Participating in professional nursing organizations provides a forum for building strong coalitions and gaining power in the political process. Each APN has the ability to make a difference.

DISCUSSION QUESTIONS _____

1. Contrast the major differences in the legislative and regulatory processes.
2. Describe the major methods of credentialing. List the benefits and weaknesses of each method from the standpoint of public protection and protection of the professional scope of practice.

3. Discuss the role of professional organizations in regulating professional practice.

4. Describe an ethical dilemma that you have recently experienced. Which principles were in conflict with each other? Which principle ruled in your decision? Why?

5. Obtain a copy of a proposed or recently promulgated regulation. Using Exhibit 11-1, analyze the regulation for its impact on nursing practice.

6. Assume the board of nursing has promulgated a regulation requiring all APNs to have 20 contact hours of continuing-education credit in pharmacotherapeutics each year to maintain prescriptive authority. Write a brief (no more than two pages) testimony supporting or opposing this proposed regulation.

7. Describe the federal government's role in the regulation of health professions. Do you believe the role will increase or decrease over time? Explain your rationale.

8. Discuss the pros and cons of multistate regulation. Based on your analysis, defend a position either for or against multistate regulation.

9. Prepare written testimony for a public hearing defending or opposing the need for a second license for APNs.

10. Contrast the board of nursing and the national or state nurses association vis-à-vis mission, membership, authority, functions, and source of funding.

11. Identify a proposed regulation. Discuss the current phase of the process, identify methods of offering comments, and submit written comments to the administrative agency.

12. Download at least one resource from one of the websites listed in Exhibit 11-3 and evaluate it according to reliability of the author, last update, and appropriateness of data. Share the resources with colleagues.

13. Evaluate the board of nursing in your state using the criteria for review of regulatory agencies developed by the Pew Health Professions Commission (1995).

14. Identify the states that have implemented nurse-staffing ratios. List some of the obstacles the state has encountered in the implementation phase.

CASE STUDY 1 Regulation of Pronouncement of Death in Ohio

The profession vested with the responsibility and legal authority to pronounce death varies from state to state. In Ohio, the statutory responsibility for pronouncement of death is prescribed in Chapter 2105 of the Ohio Revised Code. This section of state law is titled "Descent and Distribution," and includes the definitions of living and death, the determination of next of kin, and the disposition of personal estates. Section 2105.34 is subtitled "Determination and Evidence of Death." This

section designates the physician as the licensee who may determine death and establishes that the criteria for the determination of death must be in accordance with section 2108.40 of the Revised Code. Death is defined in that section of state law as "either irreversible cessation of circulatory and respiratory functions *or* irreversible cessation of all functions of the brain, including the brain stem, as determined in accordance with acceptable medical standards" (emphasis

CASE STUDY 1   Regulation of Pronouncement of Death in Ohio *(continued)*

added). Mention of immunity from civil liability and criminal prosecution relative to pronouncement of death is also addressed in this section. It should be noted that this section of statute is separate from both the medical practice act and the nurse practice act.

The role of the physician in the pronouncement of death is further prescribed in Rule 4731-14-01 of the Ohio Administrative Code. This rule amplifies the Medical Practice Act and specifies that only a currently certificated physician may pronounce a person dead, though the physician may do so without personally examining the body of the deceased if a competent observer has "recited the facts of the deceased's present medical condition to the physician and the physician is satisfied that death has occurred." In this rule, licensed registered nurses and licensed practical nurses are listed, among others, as possible competent observers.

As a part of a policy course, master's-level students in a nurse practitioner track were given the option of engaging in a field experience to meet part of the requirements for the degree. Relevant criteria for the substance of the field experience included the following: (1) a researchable topic; (2) use of a scholarly approach (i.e., must use a theory or model as a foundation or framework); and (3) amenable to written and oral presentation. Several students were enthusiastic about such an opportunity and approached the course faculty, who in turn contacted her state representative. The representative encouraged this approach to learning about public policy, and willingly met with the students and two faculty members (both faculty were teaching the policy course). He brought the state nurse's association's legislative agenda with him to aid in the discussion, the goal of which was to

identify a legislative issue that would be substantively useful to nurses in Ohio.

The students, faculty, and legislator jointly decided that the restrictions requiring that the pronouncement of death be made by a physician was a timely issue. In most cases, the registered nurse is with the patient at the time of death. The requirement of physician pronouncement of death poses hardships not only on nurses who are attending to the deceased patient, but also on distraught family members who must await arrival of the physician. In many facilities, the attending physician may be the one required to make the decision; in facilities such as long-term care, there may be a substantial delay between the actual time of death and the arrival of the physician. Modification of the statute to permit registered nurses to pronounce death would be of great benefit to Ohio nurses, their clients, families, and significant others.

Once the legislative issue was identified, the students proceeded to the research phase of the project. The legislator and faculty members served as resources and guides, suggesting that students first determine whether this change had been made in other states. Students found that nurses had been granted authority to pronounce death in 22 other states. From that list, they conducted a telephone survey of nurses who had been intimately involved in the legislative change in 5 of those 22 states. The telephone interviews revealed that the bulk of the opposition experienced during the process came from organized medicine (e.g., state medical associations).

The next step was to work with stakeholders to identify major issues. The majority of stakeholders were supportive, and included the state nurses association and organizations representing hospice and long-term care. The state medical association indicated that it would not oppose language permitting nurses to pronounce death, although it did indicate it would not support language allowing nurses to sign the death certificate. Nurses who researched this issue were told by those who worked on legislation in other states that physicians were reimbursed for signing a death certificate but not for pronouncing death.

A bill was drafted and introduced into the Ohio House of Representatives by the faculty members' representative. The state medical association remained neutral during introduction. The bill was assigned to the House Health Committee. While it was in committee, the state medical association sought to amend the bill by eliminating the nurses' authority to pronounce death in acute care facilities, by adding language describing requirements for documentation of death, and by defining what it would mean to notify the physician of death in a "timely manner." The bill spent the better part of the General Assembly in Committee, but passed out of committee. At this time, other politically charged advanced nurse practice issues were pressing in the legislature, such as removing barriers to prescribing Schedule II drugs. Whether those issues were a distraction from this bill or whether the bill garnered support from more legislators, the bill moved successfully out of the House. The bill then became stuck in a "lame duck" session, meaning that November elections had occurred and the political party of the governor's office and the General Assembly changed; the current legislators would no longer hold a majority and the probability of many bills awaiting passage was unlikely. The current legislative leadership announced that there would be no lame duck

session and the pronouncement bill died in session without ever getting to the Senate.

The bill's sponsor left the legislature to take a position in his home district. The House bill lost momentum without his influence in the Senate when the new Senate leadership did not seem interested in picking up the bill.

Whether or not nurses will eventually be given legislative authority to pronounce death will be dependent on whether a sponsor can be found and is willing to reintroduce the issue in the next General Assembly, the level of energy that organized nursing is willing to spend on this particular issue, and the positions of various stakeholders relative to the bill's support or opposition. At this juncture, registered nurses in Ohio continue to be limited to the same role they have always played in the pronouncement of death—that of a competent observer.

1. Identify ways to increase the likelihood for the legislation to pass in this General Assembly or the next.
2. Determine a complete list of possible stakeholders. Which groups may be interested in this change in regulation besides the state nurses association, state medical association, hospice association, hospital association, and long-term care?
3. Discuss the notion of "incremental legislation," noting the changes that were made to the language while the bill was in the House Health Committee.
4. Who do you think could carry on the work started by students after they graduate? What do you think students learned from this field experience?
5. Whom would you choose to spearhead this bill? For what reasons?

CASE STUDY 2 Changes in Regulations

Advanced practice nurses may find themselves in teaching roles. Schools of nursing often employ APNs to teach advanced practice students, or may be asked to teach assessment skills at the undergraduate level. APNs engaged in teaching roles must have an understanding of the regulations affecting nursing education in addition to those affecting general and advanced nursing practice. This case focuses on changes in education rules in one state, although the process could easily be applied to changes in any regulations affecting nursing.

In most states, education regulations devote a section to the supervision of nurse students by qualified faculty and instructional personnel, and also speak to the leadership of the nursing program by qualified administrators (e.g., chairs, deans, or directors). In one state, a long-standing regulation accounted for the occasional absence of the program administrator in the case of illness or other personal reason. The regulation read that if the program administrator was absent for a period of 30 or more business days, a qualified interim administrator would need to be named, and the board of nursing notified. This regulation, in effect, protected the integrity of the nursing programs by assuring continuity of program leadership.

During a revision of all of the education regulation, which, in that state, is required every five years, the rule was redrafted so that the period of time was extended to 90 days from 30 days, and it is believed that this was an effort to make the rule more "generous." However, additional language in the same regulation was added so that the scope of the rule expanded from the coverage of short absences, lasting a month or more, to include the vacating of the position by the administrator—that is, resignation. In addition, the word "interim" was deleted. In effect, a nursing program would have to replace the ad-

ministrator within a 90-day period. In most cases, this time frame is inadequate to conduct a search and hire a qualified person to fill the position. It is not uncommon for chair or dean searches to take up to a year in most colleges and universities.

A group of nursing education program leaders in the state discussed the impact of the regulation change as it was stated in draft form. The board of nursing held an open public hearing as a part of the rule-making process; the group sent a representative to give both oral and written testimony. The board of nursing heard the testimony, and as a result had a more complete understanding of the meaning of the rule change to nursing education programs. The board of nursing redrafted the regulation; the revised draft still included both absences and vacancies, but also included language that required the designation of a qualified registered nurse to replace the program administrator *or* to serve as an interim program administrator.

Keeping in mind that it is imperative for nursing programs to comply with all board of nursing rules to maintain their approval status, consider the following questions:

1. If the draft language had not been changed, what would have been the effect on nursing programs if an administrator resigned unexpectedly?
2. What is the impact of the word "or" in the revised language?
3. Identify ways that APNs can stay abreast of potential changes in relevant nursing or related regulations.
4. Discuss the value of involvement with nursing organizations as a means to have an impact on changes in regulations. That is, how might a regulatory agency weigh the testimony of an individual versus the testimony of an organization representative?

REFERENCES

American Academy of Nurse Practitioners. (2003). Medicare reimbursement fact sheet. Retrieved from http://www.aanp.org/NR/rdonlyres/D498CAF2-7BE6-4D89-A588-9DBC9CBD901A/0/Medicare ReimbursementFactsheet.pdf

American Association of Colleges of Nursing. (2004). AACN position statement on the practice doctorate in nursing. Retrieved from http://www.aacn.nche.edu/DNP/DNPPositionStatement.htm

American Association of Colleges of Nursing. (2006). Nursing organizations respond to NCSBN's draft 2006 APRN vision paper. Retrieved from http://www.aacn.nche.edu/Education/ncsbnvision.htm

American Association of Colleges of Nursing. (2010). Doctor of nursing practice (DNP). Retrieved from http://www.aacn.nche.edu/Media/FactSheets/dnp.htm

APRN Joint Dialogue Group. (2008). Consensus model for APRN regulation: Licensure, accreditation, certification & education. Retrieved from https://www.ncsbn.org/170.htm

Braunstein, M. (1995). Homecare in cyberspace. *Computer Talk for Homecare Providers,* 5–12.

Canavan, K. (1996). Credentialing agencies agree on outside review. *American Nurse, 28*(5), 6.

Centers for Medicare and Medicaid Services. (2001, June 14). Fact sheet: The new Centers for Medicare and Medicaid services. Retrieved from http://www.hhs.gov/news/press/2001pres/20010614a.html

Copeland, C. W. (2008, August 28). The federal rulemaking process: An overview. Congressional Research Service Report RL32240. Retrieved from http://openregs.com/docs/copeland-rulemaking-process.pdf

Dower, C., & Finocchio, L. (1995). Health care workforce regulation: Making the necessary changes for a transforming health care system. *State Health Workforce Reforms, 4,* 1–2.

Garner, B. A. (2009). *Black's law dictionary* (9th ed.). St Paul, MN: West.

Gobis, L. J. (1997). Licensing and liability: Crossing the borders with telemedicine. *Caring, 16*(7), 18–24.

Goehlert, R. U., & Martin, F. S. (1989). *Federal administrative law. Congress and law making: Researching the legislative process* (2nd ed.). Santa Barbara, CA: ABC-CLIO.

Gross, S. (1984). *Of foxes and hen houses.* Westport, CT: Quorum.

HealthCare.gov. (2010). About the law: Patient Protection and Affordable Healthcare Act. Retrieved from http://www.healthcare.gov/law/about/Index.htm

Institute of Medicine. (1999). To err is human: Building a safer health system. (Report of the IOM). Retrieved from http://www.iom.edu/CMS/8089/5575.aspx

Institute of Medicine. (2010). The future of nursing: Leading change, advancing health. Retrieved from http://www.iom.edu/~/media/Files/Report%20Files/2010/The-Future-of-Nursing/Future%20of%20Nursing%202010%20Recommendations.pdf

Jost, T. S. (1997). *Regulation of the health professions.* Chicago: Health Administration Press.

Kohn, L. T., Corrigan, J. M., & Donaldson, M. S. (Eds.). (2000). *To err is human: Building a safer health care system.* Institute of Medicine of the National Academies. Washington, DC: National Academies Press.

National Council of State Boards of Nursing. (1998, April). *Multi state regulation task force communiqué.* Chicago: Author.

National Council of State Boards of Nursing. (2002). Regulation of advanced nursing practice position paper. Retrieved from https://www.ncsbn.org/1993_Position_Paper_on_the_Regulation_of_Advanced_Nursing_Practice.pdf

National Council of State Boards of Nursing. (2006). Draft—Vision paper: The future regulation of advanced practice nursing. Retrieved from https://www.ncsbn.org/Draft_APRN_Vision_Paper.pdf

National Council of State Boards of Nursing. (2008). APRN model act/rules and regulations. Retrieved from https://www.ncsbn.org/170.htm

National Council of State Boards of Nursing. (2008). Contact a board of nursing. Retrieved from https://www.ncsbn.org/515.htm

National Council of State Boards of Nursing. (2010). Map of NLC states. Retrieved from http://www.ncsbn.org/nlc

O'Malley, J., Cummings, S., & King, C. S. (1996). The politics of advanced practice. *Nursing Administration Quarterly, 20*(3), 62–69.

Pearson, L. J. (2002). Fourteenth annual legislative update. *Nurse Practitioner, 27*(1), 10–52.

Pew Health Professions Commission. (1994). *State strategies for health care workforce reform.* San Francisco: UCSF Center for the Health Professions.

Pew Health Professions Commission. (1995). *Report of task force on health care workforce regulation* (executive summary). San Francisco: UCSF Center for the Health Professions.

Phillips, S. J. (2010). 22nd annual legislative update. *Nurse Practitioner, 35*(1), 24–47.

Roberts, M. J., & Clyde, A. T. (1993). *Your money or your life: The health care crisis explained.* New York: Doubleday.

Safriet, B. J. (1992). Health care dollars and regulatory sense: The role of advanced practice nursing. *Yale Journal of Regulation, 9,* 2.

Sheets, V. (1996). *Public protection or professional self-preservation.* NCSBN Monograph, 3.

Weisenbeck, S. M., & Calico, P. A. (1995). *Issues and trends in nursing* (2nd ed.). St. Louis, MO: Mosby.

CHAPTER 12

Advanced Practice Nurses and Public Policy, Naturally

Jeri A. Milstead

CHAPTER OBJECTIVES

1. Identify the scope of health policy and the role of advanced practice nurse as change agent to influence health outcomes.

2. Discuss trends in nursing education and clinical practice that will inform health policy at the local, state and national levels.

3. Describe the concepts in the paradigms known as "sick care" vs. "health care" and its impact on health care reform.

4. Analyze current demographic and socioeconomic variables that affect access to health care in the United States.

5. Differentiate between the terms public policy, entity and process.

6. Explore strategies for helping advanced practice nurses to integrate legislative skills into their practices in order to change health policy.

INTRODUCTION

This chapter addresses the policy process as a broad range of decision points, strategies, activities, and outcomes that involve elected and appointed government officials and their staffs, bureaucratic agencies, private citizens, and interest groups. The process is dynamic, convoluted, and ongoing, not static, linear, or concise. The idea of "messy" may be uncomfortable to nurses who are known to expect action immediately, but participating in the political arena requires patience, tact, diplomacy, and persistence. Knowledgeable nurses in advanced practice must demonstrate their commitment to action by being a part of relevant decisions that will ensure the delivery of quality health care by appropriate providers in a cost-effective manner.

So why would anyone suggest that working at the policy level is "natural" to our profession? Some nurses are experienced in their political activity. They have served as chairs of legislative committees for professional organizations, worked as campaign managers for elected officials, or presented testimony at congressional or state hearings; a few actually have run for office. Still, there is a perception that "legislation" and "policy" are interchangeable, and that perception misses a lot of what policy is about.

Nursing as a practice profession is based on theory and evidence. For many years, that practice has been interpreted as direct, hands-on care of individuals. Although this still is true, the profession has matured to the point where the provision of expert, direct care is not enough. Nurses of the third millennium can stand tall in their multiple roles of provider of care, educator, administrator, consultant, researcher, political activist, and policymaker. The question of how much a nurse in advanced practice can or should take on may be raised. The Information Age continues to present new knowledge exponentially. Nurses have added more and more tasks that seem important to a professional nurse and are essential for the provision of safe care to the client. Is political activism necessary? All health professionals are expected to do more with fewer resources. Realistically, how much can a specialist do?

Drucker (1995), in addressing the need for more general-practitioner physicians rather than specialists, redefined the generalist of today as one who puts multiple specialties together rapidly. Nursing can benefit from that thought. In Drucker's definition, the advanced practice nurse (APN) must be a multidimensional generalist/specialist. This means that the APN combines knowledge and skills from a variety of fields or subspecialties effectively to design the new paradigm of healthcare delivery. It also means that the APN must demonstrate competence in the multiple roles in which he or she operates. To function effectively in the role of political activist, the APN must realize the scope of the whole policy process, and the process is much broader than how a bill becomes a law.

It is natural for nurses to talk with bureaucrats, agency staff, legislators, and others in public service about what nurses do, what nurses need, and the extent of their cost-effectiveness and long-term impact on health care in this country. For too long, nurses talked only to one another. Each knew his or her value, and each told great stories; they "preached to the choir" of other nurses instead of sharing their wisdom with those who could help change the healthcare system for the better. We finally are listening to those who have espoused interprofessional collaboration, and we are realizing that, together with our colleagues in medicine, psychology, pharmacy, allied health, and other professions, we can join forces and make a stronger presence in determining policy. In the end, the patient is the winner.

Today's nurses, especially those in advanced practice who have a solid foundation of focused education and experience, know how to market themselves and their talents and know how to harness their irritations and direct them toward positive resolution. Nurses are embracing the whole range of options available in the various parts of the policy process. They are initiating opportunities to sustain ongoing, meaningful dialogues with those who represent the districts and states and those who administer public programs. Nurses are becoming indispensable to elected and appointed officials, and they are demonstrating leadership by becoming those officials and by participating with others in planning and decision making.

The advanced practice nurse of the third millennium is technically competent; uses critical thinking and decision models; possesses vision that is shared with colleagues, consumers, and policymakers; and functions in a vast array of roles. One of these roles is policy analyst. Although Florence Nightingale demonstrated great political influence in the 19th century (Nightingale, 1859), this aspect of the nurse's role was slow to become integrated into the scope of practice of the advanced practice nurse. In reality, policy and politics represent a natural domain for nurses.

We are on the brink of an opportunity for the full integration into practice of the impending major changes in the delivery of care in the United States. Nurses have prepared for these changes by initiating new nurse education programs, expanding the number of master's and doctoral programs, and focusing on issues important to patients such as the just and equitable delivery of health care.

CHANGES IN NURSING EDUCATION AND PRACTICE

Education and practice reflect or direct alterations in the delivery of health care. A 2008 survey of registered nurses (Health Resources and Services Administration, 2008) reported that there were 3,063,162 registered nurses in the United States, 84.8% of whom were working in nursing. Projections indicate that the long-standing nurse shortage will become worse as baby boomers retire. This group of consumers grew up in a time of abundance and will expect an abundance of health services when they leave the workforce. Nurse education programs recognize the opportunity to expand program enrollment but are faced with a dearth of qualified faculty and appropriate clinical space.

Nurse educators and administrators are using technology to enhance and supplement the learning process. Patient simulators are models that can mimic healthcare problems in a laboratory. These models are very sophisticated and expensive, and can be programmed to mirror a heart attack, congestive heart failure, or any number of health conditions and emergencies. For best effect, students work in teams

with colleagues from nursing, medicine, physical therapy, emergency medical technology, medical residents, and others. The lab approach can ease the need for clinical experience because of the focused approach and because a scenario can be analyzed and replayed for different outcomes. Boards of nursing are concerned about how much simulation is appropriate, but it is clear that simulation is an asset to learning. Another benefit of simulation is the experience of working with a team. Interprofessional education is fairly new in most educational programs, although the concept has been discussed for many years. The use of simulators may be a way to implement the idea of interprofessional collaboration.

Online education has also become a major force in the United States. Whether described as *distance learning, electronic education,* or another similar term, most nurse education programs use at least some form of teaching that is not face-to-face (F2F) in a single classroom. Distance learning was pioneered as "television courses" in the 1960s, in which a group of students met together at a location remote from the customary classroom and were taught by a faculty member in the primary classroom. Today's e-learning affords opportunities to learn in a flexible, "anytime" schedule that is not grounded in geography or time. The sophistication of software systems provides students and faculty with a wide range of presentations.

Telehealth, an outgrowth of e-learning and advanced diagnostic technology, allows patients and providers access to each other's domain without concerns about transportation, time lost from work, childcare during visits, and other major reasons why patients do not make or keep appointments. This sophisticated technology first was tested by military personnel and found to be an effective method for training and for practice. Currently, a physician in Washington, D.C., is testing the use of an Internet-ready cell phone to track disease compliance (Neergaard, 2010). Ethical issues, cost of equipment, and the learning curve of the provider and patient will dictate how much telehealth the public will embrace.

Although the profession has not solved the "entry" problem, there are efforts to move closer to requiring a bachelor of science in nursing (BSN) degree as the beginning point for professional nursing. Aiken, Clarke, Cheung, Sloan, and Silber (2003) report that hospitals with higher proportions of baccalaureate-prepared nurses demonstrate decreased patient morbidity and mortality. More than 90 nurse generalist and specialty organizations are on record as supporting the BSN as an entry point to professional nursing. Some states are moving legislation or regulation to require that graduates of hospital diploma and associate degree programs obtain a BSN within 10 years of graduation to be relicensed as registered nurses (RNs). Academic institutions have created programs to expand the number of graduates.

Accelerated nurse education programs, recalling similar programs during World War II, have been developed at the bachelor's and master's degree levels. These programs were created to accept applicants with college degrees in fields other than nursing and provide the student with opportunities to graduate with degrees in nursing in an abbreviated time period; graduates are eligible to sit for the National Council Licensing Exam (NCLEX-RN) to become registered nurses. These popular programs provide new avenues that address the nurse shortage.

A new education model at the master's level was created by the American Association of Colleges of Nursing (AACN), the national organization of deans and directors of baccalaureate and higher-degree nurse programs. During meetings of leaders of AACN, the American Organization of Nurse Executives, and other employers of nurses, AACN asked: Are educational institutions providing appropriate professionals for the workforce? The answer was that the nurses of today and the future should be educated to manage a population of patients/clients (such as a group of diabetics or those with congestive heart failure) both in a hospital setting and after discharge and should be able to make changes at a microsystem (i.e., unit) level. The clinical nurse leader (CNL) master's level program was proposed in 2003 to address those recommendations. In 2011, there were more than 100 CNL programs, whose graduates can sit for a national certification exam that provides credibility to employers (Commission on Nurse Certification, 2011).

At about the same time as the CNL program was initiated, much work had been accomplished in moving APNs toward doctoral education as an entry point. The rationale for this position included granting a degree appropriate to the knowledge base and credit hours required in APN programs and placing the advanced practitioner on a level with other health professionals. Note that a physician (MD), dentist (DDS), physical therapist (DPT), occupational therapist (OTD), and audiologist (AuD) require a practice doctorate. In 2004, AACN members voted to establish a doctor of nursing practice (DNP) degree and to require that all APN education be offered through DNP programs by 2015 (American Association of Colleges of Nursing [AACN], 2010a). The DNP will be an expert in patient care and will design, administer, and evaluate the delivery of complex health care in new organizational arrangements. Areas of concentration are offered in direct care, informatics, executive administration, and health policy. Although some nurse educators still debate AACN's decision (Cronenwett et al., 2011), more than 153 DNP programs currently exist. A concern that DNP programs might siphon students from PhD programs has proved unfounded (AACN, 2011).

The CNL and DNP also reflect a change in how health care is provided. Certified CNLs work at the unit micro level (not the health systems macro level) and provide direct care to groups of patients, which includes teaching with the goal of self-management of their own health problems. Patients learn to notice early indicators of changes in their conditions so that they may seek help before serious symptoms arise, with the goal being to keep patients as healthy as possible and to reduce hospital readmissions. The DNP provides care at the systems level; that is, this provider is alert to problems in the healthcare organization and can seek solutions through policy changes. DNPs develop relationships within and outside the healthcare network in order to facilitate transformation.

Perhaps the greatest potential for change in the education of nurses will be the effect of the report from the Institute of Medicine (IOM) of the National Academies, *The Future of Nursing: Leading Change, Advancing Health* (Institute of Medicine [IOM], 2010). Under the aegis of the IOM and funded by the Robert Wood Johnson Foundation (RWJF), the report recognizes that nurses (the largest healthcare workforce in the United States) must be an integral part of a healthcare team. The report provided four key messages:

- Nurses should practice to the full extent of their education and training.
- Nurses should achieve higher levels of education and training through an improved education system that promotes seamless academic progression.
- Nurses should be full partners with physicians and other healthcare professionals in redesigning health care in the United States.
- Effective workforce planning and policy making require better data collection and an improved information infrastructure (IOM, 2010, pp. 1–3).

How the messages will be received by the intended audiences—"policy makers; national, state, and local government leaders; payers; and healthcare researchers, executives, and professionals—including nurses and other—as well as [by] licensing bodies, educational institutions, philanthropic organizations, and consumer advocacy organizations" (IOM, 2010, p. 4)—can have a seismic impact on nursing education, practice, administration, and research. Removing barriers to practice, expanding leadership

opportunities, doubling the number of nurses with doctorates, and greatly increasing bachelor's degrees to 80% of the workforce will require money, commitment, energy, and creativity. As Donna Shalala, chair of the committee that initiated the report, noted at the 2010 annual meeting of the American Academy of Nursing, this report is the most important report on nursing in the past century.

It is now up to nurses to use the report to advance health care so that both patients and professionals will benefit. Nurses must not only reform nurse education and practice, but also provide leadership in gathering other healthcare professionals (practitioners and educators) together to begin paradigm-changing discussions to reform the entire system. The new system will focus on sick care, prevention of disease/disability, and health promotion. Research will continue to produce breakthroughs in medical science. Research on outcomes of treatment will become essential. **Exhibit 12-1** compares the old paradigm of sick care and the new paradigm of health care.

There has been talk for decades about reforming the U.S. healthcare system. In the 1990s, President Bill Clinton established a group that made major recommendations, but the constant pressure of special-interest groups, such as pharmaceutical and insurance companies that protected their own interests, delayed and ultimately derailed any serious attempt at overhauling this huge system. During the George W. Bush administration, defense was the number one issue on the agenda and health care was not a priority.

Today's policymakers seem to be more polarized than at any time in recent history; choices often are dichotomous or mutually exclusive, and rulings follow a strict party line. Compromise can be perceived as losing power, and power seems to be revered over common sense or the common good. Splinter groups or loose arrangements of radical thinkers have appeared on the political scene and are challenging the traditional two- or three-party system.

| EXHIBIT 12-1 | Comparison of Old Sick Care Paradigm with New Healthcare Paradigm |

Old Paradigm	New Paradigm
Hospital-based acute care	Short-term hospital, outpatient surgery, mobile/satellite clinics, telehealth/telemedicine
Physician in charge	Team approach
Nurse as subordinate	Nurse as full team member
Physician as primary decision maker	Relevant professionals and patient make treatment decisions
Segmented care focused on separate body parts/systems	Seamless, coordinated, holistic care
Primary care physician and specialist separated	Patient-centered home health
Paper records; some electronic health records (EHRs)	EHR systems that generate data used for change
Fee-for-service	Mix of reimbursement packages
Hierarchical organizations	Value-based organizations
Positivist, linear thinking	Complexity science: patterns noted in chaos, networks essential, quantum principles

A long-time congressperson told this author that she has never seen this much bitterness and antagonism in her 30-plus years of elected office. Nurses will have to be especially sensitive to the political positions of all policymakers when working in this arena. Communications techniques learned in basic baccalaureate and graduate programs will enable the nurse to transcend some of the pressures encountered in working through the political process.

The healthcare system in the United States is on the brink of huge changes. Many health problems are the result of lifestyles that do not support health. Obesity, hypertension, and cardiovascular illnesses are only three such conditions that are mentioned frequently. To promote a healthy population, we are in the early phases of a move toward prevention of illness and disability and promotion of healthy living. Many people know how to live a healthy life, but just as many do not actually engage in healthy practices. Healthcare professionals are changing the way they assess, diagnose, counsel, and treat patients.

People are living longer and are encountering many chronic problems. Who would have thought five years ago that cancer today would be considered a chronic disease? Surgery has made great strides, especially as minimally invasive methods and robotics have been perfected. Genetics has opened up a whole discipline that incorporates gene splicing and manipulation, genetic testing and counseling, and many other approaches to what have been considered irreversible or inevitable conditions. The use of prosthetics in many forms and for many body parts is maturing into a fast-growing business, especially with the recovery and return of military personnel from wars. Body parts grown in laboratories from stem cells taken from a recipient will reduce the probability of autorejection. Ethical questions are integral to policy arguments, especially as appropriations are examined with a critical eye toward costs.

Federal reform has mandated programs and policies that will demand action that is different from what is available today. The Patient Protection and Affordable Care Act of 2010 (commonly known as the Affordable Care Act [ACA]) is a federal law that will transform how, where, and by whom health care is provided. Whether the programs envisioned in the law will succeed (i.e., meet the needs of the populace and be politically acceptable) will be played out through federal and state legislatures, presidential influence, and judicial decisions. In 2011, for example, bills were introduced to seriously amend and terminate the law. Nurses and nurse organizations will be strong voices in the debates that will have lasting influence on health care in this country.

Hospitals are concerned with staffing the workforce with nurses and other healthcare providers. Staffing levels have become a huge issue, with two opposing camps: one supports actual numbers of nurses per patient or per unit and the other supports principles of staffing rather than actual numbers. The California Nurses Association (CNA), originally a state affiliate of the American Nurses Association, broke from ANA mainly over staffing issues. The CNA (the group kept the name), under the umbrella of the National Nurses Organizing Committee (NNOC), became politically active in several states as those states considered their requirements to establish legal, specific, numerical nurse-to-patient ratios. ANA, in contrast, established "principles of staffing" that required including patient acuity, diagnosis, type of nursing unit, and other considerations rather than specific numbers. Buerhaus (2008, 2009) presents data and thoughtful discussion to support the need for nurses as the primary workforce in the United States.

Most care providers recognize the problems inherent in offering care to the uninsured and underinsured. The disparity in care seen in low socioeconomic groups and vulnerable populations (e.g., children, the elderly) and groups with specific health concerns (e.g., diabetics, smokers) presents enormous challenges. Nurses have proffered solutions that have not been taken seriously by major policy players.

For some policymakers, these trends make it seem as if nurses are trying to expand the scope of their practice. This perception often reflects the reality that policymakers do not know what nurses do or appreciate the actual dimensions of their roles. The nurse of today and the future is "not your mother's nurse," to paraphrase an automobile commercial. Haas's (1964) early study of nurses clarified that their role had four dimensions: task, authority or power, deference or prestige, and affect or feelings. Each of those dimensions has changed drastically over the past 10 years. Nurses simply want to practice at the level of their education and within legal and professional definitions.

Expanding the boundaries of historical nursing takes skill in negotiation, diplomacy, assertiveness, expert communication, and leadership. Sometimes physician and nurse colleagues are threatened by these behaviors, and it takes persistence and certainty of purpose to proceed. Nurses must speak out as articulate, knowledgeable, caring professionals who contribute to the whole health agenda and who advocate for their patients and the community.

The American Academy of Nursing (AAN), a prestigious organization of approximately 1500 select nurse leaders, created a Raise the Voice campaign that "provides a platform to inform policymakers, the media, health providers and consumers about nurse-driven activities and solutions for an ailing health care system" (American Academy of Nursing, 2010, p. 1). This program, funded by a grant from the Robert Wood Johnson Foundation, cites "Edge Runners"—nurses who are leading the way to healthcare reform by creating models of care that "demonstrate significant clinical and financial outcomes" (p. 2). AAN members are committed to transforming the healthcare system from the "current hospital-based, acuity-oriented, physician-dependent paradigm towards a patient-centered, convenient, helpful, and affordable system" (p. 1).

A major influence in how health care is delivered is occurring as more and more people use social media. Patients bring articles about diseases and conditions to their healthcare providers. Providers surf the Internet and other computer networks in search of accurate information. The expansion of knowledge and the rapidity with which it can be disseminated has grown exponentially in ways that were not possible even five years ago. A unique resource, *The Nurse's Social Media Advantage* (Fraser, 2011), explains social media and, more importantly, discusses the necessity for nurses to understand how to use media resources to practice effectively in a fast-changing world.

DEVELOPING A MORE SOPHISTICATED POLITICAL ROLE FOR NURSES

There has been a major shift in the roles that nurses assume. In addition to clinical experts, nurses are entrepreneurs, decision makers, and political activists. The nurse's role must be examined to determine if there is a power differential, what the unwritten rules are that acknowledge deference, and how both actors exhibit or control feelings. Many nurses realize that to control practice and move the profession of nursing forward as a major player in the healthcare arena, nurses have to be involved in the legal decisions about the health and welfare of the public—decisions that often are made in the governmental arena.

For many nurses, political activism used to mean letting someone else get involved. Today's nurse "tunes in" to bills that reflect a particular passion (e.g., driving and texting), disease entity (e.g., diabetes), or population (e.g., childhood obesity). Although this activity indicates a greater involvement in the political process, it still misses a broader comprehension of the whole policymaking process that provides many opportunities for nurse input before and after legislation occurs.

Nurses who are serious about political activity realize that the key to establishing contacts with legislators and agency directors is through ongoing relationships with elected and appointed officials and their staffs. By developing credibility with those active in the political process and demonstrating integrity and moral purpose as client advocates, nurses are becoming players in the complex process of policymaking.

Nurses have learned that by using nursing knowledge and skill they could gain the confidence of government actors. Communications skills that were learned in basic skills classes or in psychiatric nursing classes are critical in listening to the discussion of larger health issues and in being able to present nursing's agenda. Personal stories gained from professional nurses' experience anchor altruistic conversations with legislators and their staffs in an important emotional link toward policy design. Nurses' vast network of clinical experts produces nurses in direct care who provide persuasive, articulate arguments with people "on the Hill" during appropriations committee hearings and informal meetings.

Nurses participate in formal, short-term internship programs with elected officials and in bureaucratic agencies. Most of the programs were created by nurse organizations that were convinced of the importance of political involvement. The interns and fellows learn how to handle constituent concerns, how to write legislation, how to argue with opponents yet remain colleagues, and how to maneuver through the bureaucracy. They carry the message of the necessity of the political process to the larger profession, although the rank and file still are not active in this role.

As nurses move into advanced practice and advanced practice demands master's and doctoral degree preparation, the role of the nurse in the policy process has become clearer. Through the influence of nurses with their legislators, clinical nurse specialists, certified nurse–midwives, certified registered nurse anesthetists, and certified nurse practitioners are named in several pieces of federal legislation as duly authorized providers of health care. The process has been slow; however, the deliberate way of including more nurse groups over time demonstrates that "getting a foot in the door" is an effective method of instituting change in the seemingly slow processes of government. Some groups of nurses do not understand the political implications of incrementalism (the process of making changes gradually) and want all nurse groups named as providers at one time. They do not understand that most legislators do not have any idea what registered nurses do. Those nurse lobbyists who worked directly with legislators and their staff in early efforts bore the brunt of discontent within the profession and worked diligently and purposefully to provide a unified front on the Hill and to expand the definition of provider at every opportunity. The designation of advanced practice nurses as providers was an entry to federal reimbursement for some nursing services, representing a major move toward improved client and family access and health care. Advanced practice nurses became acutely aware of the critical importance of the role of political activist. Not only did APNs need the basic knowledge, but they also understood the necessity of practicing the role, developing contacts, working with professional organizations, writing fact sheets, testifying at hearings, and maintaining the momentum and persistence to move an idea forward.

However, many nurses still focus their political efforts and skills on the legislative process. They understand the comprehensiveness of the policy process, the much broader process that precedes and follows legislation. For APNs to integrate the policy role into the character of expert nurse, they must recognize the many opportunities for action. APNs cannot afford to "do their own thing"—that is, only provide direct patient care. They cannot ignore the political aspects of any issue. Nurses who have fought the battles for recognition as professionals, for acknowledgment of autonomy, and for formal acceptance of clinical expertise worthy of payment for services have enabled APNs today to provide reimbursable, quality services to this nation's residents.

The American Association of Colleges of Nursing continues to emphasize the importance of understanding and becoming involved in policy formation, and the organization and financing of health care for the registered nurse and the APN through documents on essential components of baccalaureate, master's, and doctoral education in nursing. Content essential at the undergraduate level includes "policy development . . . legislation and regulatory processes . . . social policy/public policy . . . and political activism and professional organizations" (AACN, 2008a, p. 21). Content at the master's level for all students, regardless of their specialty or functional area, includes "policy, organization, and finance of health care" (AACN, 2008b, p. 6). Required content for doctoral students in advanced practice includes behaviors to "critically analyze . . . demonstrate leadership . . . inform policy makers . . . educate others . . . advocate for the profession" (AACN, 2006, p. 13).

Today's nurses have a much clearer understanding of what constitutes nursing and how nurses must integrate political processes into their practices to further the decisions made by policymakers. Nurses continue to focus on the individual, family, community, and special populations in the provision of care to the sick and infirm and on the activities that surround health promotion and the prevention of disease and disability. Advanced practice nurses have a foundation in expert clinical practice and can translate that knowledge into understandable language for elected and appointed officials as the officials respond to problems that are beyond the scale or impact of individual healthcare providers. As nurses continue to refine the art and science of nursing, forces external to the profession compel the nursing community to consider another aspect—the business of nursing—that is paradoxical to the long history of altruism.

21ST-CENTURY ORGANIZATIONS

The whole economic basis of capitalism—that is, the manufacturing system—had become rapidly outdated by the beginning of the 21st century. The new paradigm for organizations in the 21st century began with changes within one's head with a move to a perspective that is outside the usual way of thinking. What work is done, where it is done, how it is done, and what it costs are mundane questions that demand creative answers.

Complexity science acknowledges patterns in chaos, complex adaptive systems, and principles of self-organization and has great applicability to nursing (Curtin, 2010; Lindberg, Nash, & Lindberg, 2008). "The quantum concept of a matrix or field . . . that connects everything together" (Curtin, 2011) informs us that nurses are focused masses of energy who direct their behaviors and actions with patients in an intentional way towards accomplishing healthy states. The nurse–patient (or nurse–provider) relationship is not incidental or haphazard, but fully cognizant of purpose (Curtin, 2010; Husted & Husted, 2008).

Quantum thinking also is crucial to the effectiveness of an organization in the 21st century (Porter-O'Grady & Malloch, 2011). Partnerships are valued over competition, and the old rules of business that rewarded power and ownership have given way to accountability and shared risk. Transforming the old systems into the new systems does not mean merely automating processes or restructuring the organizational chart. Transformation involves a radical, cross-functional, futuristic change in the way people think. Long-term planning is balanced with strategic planning, and vertical work relationships are replaced with networks and webs of people and knowledge. All workers at all levels share a commitment to the organization and an accountability to define and produce quality work. Rhoades, Covery, and Shepherdson (2011) are "convinced that positive, people-centered cultural values lead to higher performance" (p. 1). All workers share responsibility for self-governance, from which both the organization and the worker benefit (Porter-O'Grady, Hawkins, & Parker, 1997). Control is replaced by leadership. The new leader does not use policing techniques of supervision, but enables and empowers colleagues through vision, trust, and respect (Bennis & Nanus, 1985; Kouzes & Posner, 2007; Porter-O'Grady & Wilson, 1995). Encouragement, appreciation, and personal recognition are celebrated together in an effective organization (Kouzes & Posner, 1999).

WHAT IS PUBLIC POLICY?

What do the changes in education, practice, and organizations have to do with policymaking, especially in the public arena? A brief overview of the entire policy process will clarify what policy is and how influencing government policies has become crucial to the profession of nursing.

In this chapter, *policy* is an overarching term used to define both an entity and a process. The purpose of *public policy* is to direct problems to government and secure government's response, while *politics* is the use of influence to direct the responses toward goals. Although there has been much discussion about the boundaries and domain of government and the extent of difference between the public and private sectors, that debate is beyond the scope of this chapter.

The definition of public policy is important because it clarifies common misconceptions about what constitutes policy. In this book, the terms *public policy* and *policy* are interchangeable. The process of creating policy can be focused in many arenas and most of these are interwoven. For example, environmental policy deals with health issues such as hazardous material, particulate matter in the air or water, and safety standards in the workplace. Education policy, more than tangentially, is related to health—just ask school nurses. Regulations define who can administer medication to students; state laws dictate which type of sex education can be taught. Defense policy is related to health policy when developing, investigating, or testing biological and chemical weapons. Health policy directly addresses health problems and is the specific focus of this book.

POLICY AS AN ENTITY

As an entity, policy is seen in many forms as the "standing decisions" of an organization (Eulau & Prewitt, 1973, p. 495). As formal documented directives of an organization, official government policies reflect the beliefs of the administration in power and provide direction for the philosophy and mission of government organizations. Specific policies usually serve as the "shoulds" and "thou shalts" of agencies. Some policies, known as position statements, report the opinions of organizations about issues that members believe are important. For example, state boards of nursing (government agencies created by legislatures to protect the public through the regulation of nursing practice) publish advisory opinions on what constitutes competent and safe nursing practice.

Agency policies can be broad and general, such as those that describe the relationship of an agency to other governmental groups. Procedure manuals in government hospitals that detail steps in performing certain nursing tasks are examples of the results of policy directives, but are not considered policies. Policies serve as guidelines for employee behavior within an institution. Although policies and procedures often are used interchangeably, policies are considered broader and reflect the values of the administration.

Laws are types of policy entities. As legal directives for public and private behavior, laws serve to define action that reflects the will of society—or at least a segment of society. Laws are made at the international, federal, state, and local levels and have the impact of primary place in guiding conduct. Lawmaking usually is the purview of the legislative branch of government in the United States, although presidential vetoes, executive orders, and judicial interpretations of laws have the force of law.

Judicial interpretation is noted in three ways. First, courts may interpret the meaning of laws that are written broadly or with some vagueness, although laws often are written deliberately with language that addresses broad situations. Agencies that implement the laws then write regulations that are more specific and that guide the implementation. However, courts may be asked to determine questions in which the law is unclear or controversial (Williams & Torrens, 1988). For example, the 1973 Rehabilitation Act prohibited discrimination against handicapped persons by any program that received federal assistance. Although this may have seemed fair and reasonable at the outset, courts were asked to adjudicate questions of how much accommodation is "fair" (Wilson, 1989).

Second, courts can determine how some laws are applied. Courts are idealized as being above the political activity that surrounds the legislature. They also are considered beyond the influence of politically active interest groups. The court system, especially the federal court system, has been called upon to resolve conflicts between levels of government (state and federal) and between laws enacted by the legislature and their interpretation by powerful interest groups. For example, courts may determine who is eligible or who is excluded from participation in a program. In this way, special-interest groups that sue to be included in a program can receive "durable protection" from favorable court decisions (Feldstein, 1988, p. 32).

Third, courts can declare the laws made by Congress or the states unconstitutional, thereby nullifying the statutes entirely (Litman & Robins, 1991). Courts also interpret the Constitution, sometimes by restricting what the government (not private enterprise) may do (Wilson, 1989).

Regulations are another type of policy initiative. Although they often are included in discussions of laws, regulations are different. Once a law is enacted by the legislative branch, the executive branch of government is charged with administrative responsibility for implementing the law. The executive branch consists of the president and all of the bureaucratic agencies, commissions, and departments that carry out the work for the public benefit. Agencies in the government formulate regulations that achieve the intent of the statute. On the whole, laws are written in general terms, and regulations are written more specifically to guide the interpretation, administration, and enforcement of the law. The Administrative Procedures Act (APA) was created to provide opportunity for citizen review and input throughout the process of developing regulations. The APA ensures a structure and process that is published and open, in the spirit of the founding fathers, so that the average constituent can participate in the process of public decision making.

All of these entities evolve over time and are accomplished through the efforts of a variety of actors or players. Although commonly used, the terms *position statement, resolution, goal, objective, program, procedure, law*, and *regulation* really are not interchangeable with the word *policy*. Rather, they are the formal expressions of policy decisions. For the purposes of understanding just what policy is, nurses must grasp policy as a process.

POLICY AS A PROCESS

In viewing policy as a guide to government action, nurses can study the process of policy-making over time. Milio (1989) presents four major stages in which decisions are made that translate to government policies: (1) agenda setting, (2) legislation and regulation, (3) implementation, and (4) evaluation. Agenda setting is concerned with identifying a societal problem and bringing it to the attention of government. Legislation and regulation are formal responses to a problem. Implementation is the execution of policies or programs toward the achievement of goals. Evaluation is the appraisal of policy performance or program outcomes.

In each stage, formal and informal relationships are developed among actors both within and outside of government. Actors can be individuals, such as a legislator, a bureaucrat, or a citizen, but they also can be institutions, such as the presidency, the courts, political parties, or special-interest groups. A series of activities occurs that brings a problem to government, which results in direct action by the government to address the problem. Governmental responses are political; that is, the decisions about who gets what, when, and how are made within a framework of power and influence, negotiation, and bargaining (Lasswell, 1958).

Although one can explain each of the stages of the policy process and explore them for areas in which nurses can provide influence, one must recognize that the policy process is not necessarily sequential or logical. The definition of a problem, which usually occurs in the agenda-setting phase, may change during legislation. Program design may be altered significantly during implementation. Evaluation of a policy or program (often considered the last phase of the process) may propel onto the national agenda (often considered the first phase of the process) a problem that differs from the original. However, for the purpose of organizing one's thoughts and conceptualizing the policy process, the policy process is examined from the linear perspective of stages.

Even before the process itself can be studied, nurses must understand why it is so important to be knowledgeable about the components and the functions of the process and how this public arena has become an integral part of the practice of advanced nursing.

WHY NURSES AND PUBLIC POLICY?

Registered professional nurses have studied the basics of how a bill becomes a law in their baccalaureate programs. An extension of the focus on legislation usually is provided in graduate schools. However, most nurses (and most nurse educators) do not have a clear understanding of the total policy process. To focus on legislation misses a whole range of governmental and political activities—activities in which professional nurses should have a central place.

Nurses and nursing are at the center of issues of tremendous and long-lasting impact, such as access to providers, quality of care, and reasonable cost. Issues crucial to the profession are being decided, such as who is eligible for government reimbursement for services and what is the appropriate scope of practice of registered nurses in advanced practice. If nurses wait until legislation is being voted on before they become involved, it is too late to affect decisions.

Nurses have learned the legislative process. They have written letters and made visits to their legislators. Now nurses must move forward and apply the knowledge of the whole policy process by speaking out to a variety of appropriate governmental actors and institutions so that nurses can move issues onto the national agenda, lobby Congress with alternative solutions, and provide nursing expertise as policies and programs are being designed. In addition, nurses must be the watchdogs as programs are implemented so that target groups are served and services are appropriate. Nurses should be experts at program evaluation and continuing feedback to ensure that old problems are being addressed, new problems are being identified, and appropriate solutions are being considered.

The opportunities for nurse input throughout the policy process are unlimited and certainly not confined narrowly to the legislative process. Nurses are articulate experts who can address both the rational shaping of policy and the emotional aspects of the process. Nurses cannot afford to limit their actions to monitoring bills; they must seize the initiative and use their considerable collective and individual influence to ensure the health, welfare, and protection of the public and healthcare professionals.

AN OVERVIEW OF THE POLICY PROCESS

Although other sources address specific components of the policy process in depth and from a theoretical perspective, advanced practice nurses also need an overview of the total process so that they do not get stuck on legislation. Many useful articles and books have been written about policy in general and even about specific policies, but few have addressed the scope of the policy process or defined the components. The elements of agenda setting (including problem definition), government response (legislation, regulation, or programs), and policy and program implementation and evaluation are distinct entities, but are connected as parts of a whole tapestry in the process of public decision making.

Agenda Setting

Getting a healthcare problem to the attention of government can be a tremendous first step in getting relief. The actual mechanism of defining a healthcare problem is a major political issue. APNs have the capacity and opportunity to identify and frame problems from multiple sources.

The choice of a clinical problem on which to focus one's energy is a major decision. A nurse may be working in a specialized area and may see a need for more research or alternatives to existing treatment options; for example, those who work with patients and families with breast cancer already may have a passion for issues critical to this area. Other topics receiving attention include diabetes, obesity, AIDS, early detection and treatment of prostate cancer, child and parent abuse, cardiac problems in women, and empowering caregivers (Hash & Cramer, 2003; Pierce & Steiner, 2003).

Professional problems that are especially critical to nurses in advanced practice include reducing barriers to autonomy and reimbursement for nursing services. Workplace issues include advocacy for workplace safety and management strategies for training and redeploying nurses as work sites change. Related social problems that affect nurses include the increase of street violence and bioterrorism. A plethora of problems and "irritations" can arouse the passion of a nurse in advanced practice.

APNs must come to understand the concepts of windows of opportunity, policy entrepreneurs, and political elites. "Sound bites" and "word bites" are tools that are used to gain the attention of viewers and readers and serve as a shortcut or an abbreviated version of a statement. Originally created as off-hand remarks, these oral and written snippets have become planned tactics. For example, a nurse who speaks at a press conference or who delivers a message to a politician should have a written message that includes bulleted sound or word bites that underscore the message and that emphasize the important points. These brief, focused points can serve as references for the media or a politician as they consider the message later.

Government Response

The government response to public problems often emanates from the legislative branch and usually comes in three forms: (1) laws, (2) rules and regulations, and (3) programs. Because only senators and representatives can introduce legislation (not even the president can bring a bill to the floor of either house), these elected officials command respect and attention.

The work of legislation is not clear-cut or linear. Informal communication and influence are the coin of the realm when trying to construct a program or law from the often vague wishes of disparate groups. The committee structure of both houses is a powerful method of accomplishing the work of government. Conference committees are known as the "Third House of Congress" (*How Our Laws Are Made*, 1990) because of their power to force compromise and bring about new legislation. APNs must appreciate the difference between the authorization and appropriations processes and seek influence in both arenas.

Becoming involved directly with legislators and their staffs has been a training ground for many APNs. Supporting or opposing passage of a bill often has served as the first contact with the political process for many nurses, but this place often has been the stopping point for many nurses because they were unaware of other avenues of involvement, such as the follow-up process of regulations and rulemaking.

Lowi (1969) notes that administrative rulemaking is often an effort to bring about order in environments that are unstable and full of conflict. Some regulations codify precedent; others break new ground and address issues not previously explicated. An example of the latter is the Federal Trade Commission's (FTC) Trade Regulation Rules. In 1964, the FTC, whose mission is to protect the consumer and enforce antitrust legislation, wrote regulations requiring health warnings on cigarette packages. The tobacco industry reacted so fiercely that Congress quickly passed a law that nullified the regulations and replaced them with less stringent ones (West, 1982). Decades passed before no-smoking rules actually were mandated in public places. Other ways to sanction agencies whose rules are viewed as too restrictive are to reduce budget allocations and increase the number of adjudications or trial-like reviews. Advanced practice nurses must become knowledgeable about the regulatory process so that they can spot opportunities to contribute or intervene prior to final rulemaking ("The Regulatory Process," 1992).

Programs are concrete manifestations of solutions to problems. Program design often is a joint effort of legislative intent, budgetary expediency, and political feasibility. There are many opportunities for nurses in advanced practice to become involved in the design phase of a program. Selecting an agency to administer the program, choosing the goals, and selecting the tools that will ensure eligibility and participation are all decisions in which the APN should offer input.

Policy and Program Implementation

It is important that APNs keep reminding their colleagues that the phases of the policy process are not linear and that policy activities are fluid and move within and among the phases in dynamic processes. The implementation phase includes those activities in which legislative mandates are carried out, most often through programmatic means. The implementation stage also includes a planning ingredient. Problems occur in program planning if technological expertise is not available. This is particularly important to nurses, who are experts in the delivery of health care in the broadest sense.

If government officials do not know qualified, appropriate experts, decisions about program planning and design often are determined by legislators, bureaucrats, or staff who know little or nothing about the problem or the solutions. As excellent problem solvers, APNs have many opportunities to offer ideas and solutions. One strategy is to employ second-order change to reframe situations and recommend pragmatic alternatives to implementers (de Chesnay, 1983; Watzlawick, Weakland, & Fisch, 1974). Bowen (1982) uses probability theory to demonstrate how program success could be improved. She suggests putting several clearance points (instances where major decisions are made) together so that they could be negotiated as a package deal. She also advocates beginning the bargaining process with alternatives that have the greatest chance for success and using that success as a foundation for building more successes, a strategy she refers to as a "band-wagon approach" (p. 10). In the past, nurses have done the opposite: focused on failure and perceived lack of nursing power. APNs have begun to note successes in the political arena and are building a new level of success and es-

teem. The nurse in advanced practice today uses the strategies of packaging, success begets success, and persistence in a deliberate way so that nurses can increase their effective impact in the implementation of social programs.

Although nurses most often work toward positive impact, they have found that opposition to an unsound program can have a paradoxical positive effect. Although not in the public arena, an example of phenomenal success in the judicious use of opposition occurred when the professional body of nursing rose up as one against the American Medical Association's 1986 proposal to create a new type of low-level healthcare worker called a registered care technician. The power emerged as more than 40 nurse organizations stood together in opposition to an ill-conceived proposal that would have placed patients in jeopardy and created dead-end jobs.

Policy and Program Evaluation

For nurses who have worked beyond the nursing process through the process of clinical reasoning (Pesut & Herman, 1999), evaluation seems to be a logical component of the policy process. Evaluation is the systematic application of methods of social research to public policies and programs. Evaluation is conducted "to benefit the human condition to improve profit, to amass influence and power, or to achieve other goals" (Rossi & Freeman, 1995, p. 6). Evaluation research is a powerful tool for defending viable programs, for altering structures and processes to strengthen programs, and for providing rationale for program failure. Goggin, Bowman, Lester, and O'Toole (1990) propose that researchers investigate program implementation within an analytical framework rather than a descriptive one. They argue that a "third generation" of research established within a sound theory would strengthen the body of knowledge of the policy process. APNs can contribute to both the theory and the method of evaluation.

Evaluation should be started early and continued throughout a program. An unconscionable example of a program that should have been stopped even before it was begun is the Tuskegee "experiment." From 1932 to 1972, a group of African Americans was used as a control group and denied antibiotic treatment for syphilis, even after treatment was known to be successful (Thomas & Quinn, 1991). Beyond evaluation research, this study clearly points out the moral and ethical concerns that are mandated when researchers work with human beings. Should a study or program be started at all? At what point should it be stopped? What is involved in "informed consent"? If a program involves experimental therapy, what are the methods for presenting subjects with relevant data so that participation preferences are clear (Bell, Raiffa, & Tversky, 1988)? These kinds of questions should be considered automatically by today's researchers, but it is the responsibility of APNs as consumer agents to ask the questions if they have not been asked or if there is any doubt about the answers.

A BRIGHT FUTURE

The multiple roles of the APN—provider of direct care, researcher, consultant, educator, administrator, consumer advocate, and political activist—reflect the changing and expanding character of the professional nurse. Today is the future; nurse action today sets the direction for what health care becomes for coming generations. As true professionals with a societal mandate and a comprehensive body of knowledge, nurses function as visionaries who are grounded in education, research, and experience. APNs serve as the link between human responses to actual and potential health problems and the solutions that may be addressed in the government arena.

Full integration of the policy process becomes evident when professional nurses discern early the social implications of health problems, seize the opportunity to inform public officials with

whom the nurses have credible relationships, provide objective data and subjective personal stories that help translate big problems down to a level of understanding, propose alternative solutions that acknowledge reality, and participate in the evaluation process to determine the effectiveness and efficiency of the outcomes.

EDUCATING OUR POLITICAL SELVES

Nurses in advanced practice must be politically active. Basic content in undergraduate nursing programs must be reexamined in light of the needs of the profession. Educators must do more than plant the seeds of interest and excitement in baccalaureate students; they must model activism by talking about the bills they are supporting or opposing, by organizing students to assist in election campaigns, and by demanding not only that students write letters to officials but also that they mail them and provide follow-up.

Educators can develop games in which students maneuver through a virtual bureaucracy to move a health problem onto the agenda. Brainstorming techniques can lead students to discover innovative alternative solutions. Baccalaureate students can analyze policy tools to discover how and when to use them. Teachers of research methods and processes can use political scenarios to point out how to phrase clinical questions so that legislators will pay attention. Program effectiveness can be studied in research and clinical courses. The theoretical components taught in class and followed by practical application through participation in political and legislative committees in professional organizations must serve as "basic training" for the registered nurse.

Graduate education must demand demonstrated knowledge and application of more extensive and sophisticated political processes. All graduate program faculty should serve as models for political activism. The atmosphere in master's and doctoral programs should heighten the awareness of students who are potential leaders.

Faculty can motivate students by displaying posters that announce political events and by including students in discussions of nursing issues framed in a policy context. Students who spot educators at rallies and other political and policy occasions are learning by example, so faculty should advertise their experiences as delegates to political and professional conventions. A few faculty can serve as mentors for students who need to move from informal to sustained, formal contact with policymakers and who have a policy track in their career trajectories. Both faculty and students should consider actual experience in government offices as a means of learning the nitty-gritty of how government functions and of demonstrating their own leadership capabilities.

If students hesitate and seem passive about involvement, educators must help these nurses determine where their passions lie, which may help students focus on where they might start. Often the novice can be enticed by centering on a clinical problem. Every nurse cannot assume responsibility for all of the profession's problems or work on every healthcare issue. Issues can be at the practice level or the systems level (e.g., funding for nurse education or nurse-led research). Each nurse must choose the issue on which to invest energy, time, and other resources. Nurses can make a difference in the new healthcare system.

STRENGTHENING ORGANIZED NURSING

The most productive and efficient way to act together is through a strong professional organization. Just as organizations in general have restructured and reengineered for more efficient operation, so will the professional associations. APNs have a knowledge base that includes an understanding of how organizations develop and change. This theoretical knowledge must serve as a foundation for leadership in directing new organizational structures that are responsive to members and other important bodies. National leaders must talk with state and local leaders as new configurations are conceived. States must confer among themselves to share innovations and knowledge about what works and what does not.

Issues such as the role of collective bargaining units within the total organizational structure, the position of individual membership vis-à-vis state membership, the political role of a specialized-interest group (nurses) in creating public policy, and the issue of international influence in nursing and health care require wisdom and leadership that APNs must exert as the American Nurses Association addresses its place as a major voice of this country's nurses. The National League for Nursing (NLN) will exert leadership as nurse education programs move toward baccalaureate programs. Accrediting agencies (e.g., Commission for Credentialing in Nursing Education and the NLN Accrediting Commission) must continue to be visionary and flexible in developing criteria and processes for accreditation. Boards of nursing must not become trapped in the slowness with which government bureaucracy can be mired, but must be on the forefront of developing regulations that protect the public and allow nurses to work at their top capacity.

Issues inherent in multistate licensure are being debated today, and the outcome will reflect the extent to which nurses will use concepts of telehealth in their practices. Because APNs already are eligible for Medicare reimbursement for telehealth services that are provided in specified rural areas (Burtt, 1997), these nurses are rich resources and must be included in reasoned discussions on this issue. State boards of nursing in every state and jurisdiction face issues of appropriate methods of recognizing advanced nursing practice, the role of the government agency in regulating nursing and other professions, and the analysis of educationally sound and legally defensible examinations for candidates.

Nurses who have been reluctant to become political cannot afford to ignore their obligations any longer. Each nurse counts and, collectively, nursing is a major actor in the effort to ensure the country's healthy future. Nurses have expanded their conception of what nursing is and how it is practiced to include active political participation. A nurse must choose the governmental level on which to focus: federal, regional, state, or local. The process is similar at each level: Identify the problem and become part of the solution.

Advanced practice nurses understand the scope of service delivery, continuity of care, appropriate mix of caregivers, and the expertise that can be provided by multidisciplinary teams. By being at the forefront of understanding, nurses have a moral and ethical mandate to lead the public-policy process. Dynamic political action is as much a part of the advanced practice of nursing as is expert direct care.

WORKING WITH THE POLITICAL SYSTEM

By now, many APNs have developed contacts with legislators, appointed officials, and their staffs. A new group that holds great potential for nurse interaction is the Senate Nursing Caucus (AACN, 2010b). Established in March 2010, this group will provide a forum for educating senators on issues important to nurses, as well as for hearing concerns of the senators. Four senators established the caucus: Jeff Merkley (Democrat–Oregon), Mike Johanns (Republican–Nebraska), Barbara Mikulski (Democrat–Maryland), and Olympia Snowe (Republican–Maine). The Senate Nursing Caucus follows the lead of the Congressional Nursing Caucus in the U.S. House of Representatives, begun in 2003 by Representatives Lois Capps (Democrat–California) and Ed Whitfield (Republican–Kentucky) (American Nurses Association, 2003). Members hold briefings on the nurse shortage, patient and nurse safety issues, preparedness for bioterrorism, and other relevant and pertinent issues and concerns.

APNs must stay alert to issues and be assertive in bringing problems to the attention of policymakers. It is important to bring success stories to legislators and officials—they need to hear what good nurses do and how well they practice. Sharing positive information will keep the image of nurses in an affirmative and constructive picture. Legislators must run for office (and members of the U.S. House of Representatives do so every 2 years), so media coverage with an APN who is pursuing noteworthy accomplishments is usually welcomed eagerly.

Nurses absolutely must "get their act together" and work toward presenting a unified voice on issues that affect the public health and the nursing profession. Whatever their differences in the past—anger from entry-into-practice arguments that have dragged on for more than half a century; disparagement and animosity among those with varied levels of education; cerebral and pragmatic concerns about gaps between education and practice, practice and administration, or administration and education—nurses must put these kinds of divisive, emotional issues behind them if they expect to be taken seriously as professionals by elected and appointed public officials and policymakers.

Nurses cannot afford to stop arguing critical issues internally, but they must learn how to argue heatedly among themselves—and then go to lunch together. Nurses can learn lessons from television shows such as *Meet the Press, This Week, The O'Reilly Factor,* and *The McLaughlin Group* about how to challenge, contest, dispute, contend, and debate issues passionately, then shake hands and respect the opponent's position. Passionate issues must not polarize the profession any longer and, more important, must not stand in the way of a unified voice to the public.

CONCLUSION

Nurses in advanced practice must have expert knowledge and skill in change, conflict resolution, assertiveness, communication, negotiation, and group process to function appropriately in the policy arena. Professional autonomy and collaborative interdependence are possible within a political system in which consumers can choose access to quality health care that is provided by competent practitioners at a reasonable cost. Nurses in advanced practice have a strong, persistent voice in designing such a healthcare system for today and for the future.

The policy process is much broader and more comprehensive than the legislative process. Although individual components can be identified for analytical study, the policy process is fluid, nonlinear, and dynamic. There are many opportunities for nurses in advanced practice to participate throughout the policy process. The question is not whether nurses should become involved in the political system, but to what extent. In the whole policy arena, nurses must be involved with every aspect. Knowing all of the components and issues that must be addressed in each phase, the nurse in advanced practice finds many opportunities for providing expert advice. APNs can use the policy process, individual components, and models as a framework to analyze issues and participate in alternative solutions.

Nursing has a rich history. The professional nurse's values of altruism, respect, integrity, and accountability to consumers remain strong. In some ways, the evolution of nursing roles has come full circle, from the political influence recognized and exercised by Nightingale to the influence of current nurse leaders with elected and appointed public officials. The APN of the 21st century practices with a solid political heritage and a mandate for consistent and powerful involvement in the entire policy process.

DISCUSSION QUESTIONS

1. Read Nightingale's *Notes on Nursing* and other historical sources of the mid-1800s and discuss how Nightingale's personal and family influence moved her agenda for the Crimea and for nursing education, and how this has implications for the future.

2. Discuss implications of the "BSN in 10" movement in relation to your own education. Research opportunities for BSNs and for APNs. Dream about positions that might not be available today.

3. Compare the definition of nursing according to Nightingale, Henderson, the ANA, and your own state nurse practice act. What are the differences in a legal definition versus a professional definition? What are the similarities? What did definitions include or not include that reflected the state of nursing at the time? Construct a definition of nursing for today and for 10 years from now.

4. Discuss the role of research in nursing. What has been the focus over the past century? What is the pattern of nursing research vis-à-vis topic, methodology, and relevance? To what extent do you think nursing research has had an impact on nursing care? Cite examples.

5. Trace the amount of federal funding for nursing research. Do not limit your search to federal health-related agencies; that is, investigate departments (e.g., Commerce, Environment, Transportation), military services, and the Veterans Administration. Which funding opportunities exist for nurse scientists?

6. Read books and articles about the changing paradigm in healthcare delivery systems. Discuss the change in nursing as an occupation and nursing as a profession. What does this mean in today's transformational paradigm?

7. Consider a thesis, graduate project, or dissertation on a specific topic (e.g., clinical problems, healthcare issues) using the policy process as a framework.

8. Identify policies within public agencies and discuss how they were developed. Interview members of an agency policy committee to discover how policies are changed.

9. Have faculty and students bring to class official governmental policies. Which governmental agency is responsible for developing the policy? For enforcing the policy? How has the policy changed over time? What are the consequences of not complying with the policy?

10. Identify nurses who are elected officials at the local, state, or national level. Interview these officials to determine how the nurses were elected, what their objectives are, and to what extent they use their nurse knowledge in their official capacities. Ask the officials if they tapped into nurse groups during their campaigns. If so, what did the nurses contribute? If not, why?

11. Discuss the major components of the policy process and discuss the fluidity of the process. Point out how players move among the components in a nonlinear way.

12. Using Exhibit 12-1 as a framework, construct a healthcare organization in which access is provided and quality care is assured. What are the barriers to this type of paradigm?

13. Develop an assessment tool by which students can determine their own level of knowledge and involvement in the policy process. Reminder: Stretch your thinking beyond legislative activity.

14. Watch television programs in which participants discuss national and international issues, then analyze the verbal and nonverbal communication patterns, pro-and-con arguments, and other methods of discussion. Discuss your analysis within the framework of gender differences in communication and utility in the political arena.

15. Construct a list of ways in which nurses can become more knowledgeable about the policy process. Choose at least three activities in which you will participate. Develop a tool for evaluating the activity and your knowledge and involvement.

16. Select at least one problem or irritation in a clinical area and brainstorm with other APNs or graduate students on how to approach a solution. Discuss funding sources; be creative.

17. Attend a meeting of the state board of nursing, the district or state nurses association, or a professional convention. Identify issues discussed, resources used, communication techniques, and rules observed. Evaluate the usefulness of the session to your practice.

18. Discuss which skills (e.g., task, interpersonal) and attitudes are required for the nurse in the new paradigm. Who is best prepared to teach these skills, and what teaching techniques should be used? How will they be evaluated? Develop a worksheet to facilitate planning.

19. Discuss at least five strategies for helping nurses integrate these skills into their practices.

REFERENCES

Aiken, L. H., Clarke, S. R., Cheung, R. B., Sloan, D. M., & Silber, J. H. (2003). Hospital nurse staffing and patient mortality, nurse burnout, and job dissatisfaction. *Journal of the American Medical Association, 290*(12), 1617–1623.

American Academy of Nursing. (2010). Raise the voice. Retrieved from http://www.aannet.org /i4a/pages/Index.cfm?pageid=3301

American Association of Colleges of Nursing. (2006). *Essentials of doctoral education for advanced nursing practice.* Washington, DC: Author.

American Association of Colleges of Nursing. (2008a). *Essentials of baccalaureate education for professional nursing practice.* Washington, DC: Author.

American Association of Colleges of Nursing. (2008b). *Essentials of master's education for advanced practice nursing*. Washington, DC: Author.

American Association of Colleges of Nursing. (2010a). Fact sheet: The doctor of nursing practice. Retrieved from http://www.aacn.nche.edu/media/FactSheets/dnp.htm

American Association of Colleges of Nursing. (2010b). Senate nursing caucus. Retrieved from http://www.aacn.nche.edu/Government/SenNursingCaucus.htm

American Association of Colleges of Nursing. (2011). Press release: Despite educational challenges facing schools of nursing, new AACN data confirm sizable growth in doctoral nursing programs. Retrieved from http://www.aacn.nche.edu/media/NewsReleases/2011/enrollsurge.html

American Nurses Association. (2003, March 19). American Nurses Association commends Reps. Capps, Whitfield for forming congressional nursing caucus. Retrieved from http://www.nursingworld.org/_pressrel/2003/pr0319.htm

Bell, D. E., Raiffa, H., & Tversky, A. (1988). *Decision making*. Cambridge, UK: Cambridge University Press.

Bennis, W., & Nanus, B. (1985). *Leaders*. New York: Harper and Row.

Bowen, E. (1982). The Pressman-Wildavsky paradox: Four addenda on why models based on probability theory can predict implementation success and suggest useful tactical advice for implementers. *Journal of Public Policy, 2*(1), 1–22.

Buerhaus, P. (2008). The future of the nursing workforce in the United States: Data, trends, and implications. *Journal of the American Medical Association, 300*(16), 1950.

Buerhaus, P. I. (2009). Messages for thought leaders and health policy makers. *Nursing Economic$, 2*(2), 125–127.

Burtt, K. (1997). Nurses use telehealth to address rural health care needs, prevent hospitalizations. *The American Nurse, 29*(6), 21.

Commission on Nurse Certification. (2011). History of CNL certification. Retrieved from http://www.aacn.nche.edu/CNC/pdf/history.pdf

Cronenwett, L., Dracup, K., Grey, M., McCauley, L., Meleis, A., & Salman, M. (2011). The doctor of nursing practice: A national workforce perspective. *Nursing Outlook, 59*(1), 9–17.

Curtin, L. (2010). Quantum nursing. *American Nurse Today, 5*(9), 47–48.

Curtin, L. (2011). Quantum nursing II: Our field of influence. *American Nurse Today, 6*(1), 56.

de Chesnay, M. (1983). The creation and dissolution of paradoxes in nursing practice. *Topics in Clinical Nursing, 5*(3), 71–80.

Drucker, P. F. (1995). The age of social transformation. *Quality Digest*, 36–39.

Eulau, H., & Prewitt, K. (1973). *Labyrinths of democracy*. Indianapolis, IN: Bobbs-Merrill.

Feldstein, P. J. (1988). *The politics of health legislation*. Ann Arbor, MI: Health Administration Press.

Fraser, R. (2011). *The nurse's social media advantage*. Indianapolis, IN: Sigma Theta Tau International.

Goggin, M. L., Bowman, A. O'M., Lester, J. P., & O'Toole, L. J., Jr. (1990). *Implementation theory and practice: Toward a third generation*. New York: HarperCollins.

Haas, J. E. (1964). *Role conception and group consensus* (Research Monograph No. 17). Columbus, OH: The Ohio State University, Bureau of Business Research.

Hash, K. M., & Cramer, E. P. (2003). Empowering gay and lesbian caregivers and uncovering their unique experiences through the use of qualitative methods. *Journal of Gay and Lesbian Social Services, 15*(1/2), 47–64.

Health Resources and Services Administration. (2008). The RN population: Findings from the 2008 national sample survey of registered nurses. Retrieved from http://bhpr.hrsa.gov/healthworkforce/_rnsurveys/rnsurveyinitial2008.pdf

How our laws are made. (1990). (House Document 101–139). Washington, DC: U.S. Government Printing Office.

Husted, J., & Husted, G. L. (2008). *Bioethical decision making in nursing and health care: A symphonological approach* (4th ed.). New York, NY: Springer.

Institute of Medicine. (2010). *The future of nursing: Leading change, advancing health*. Washington, DC: Author.

Kouzes, J., & Posner, B. (2007). *The leadership challenge* (4th ed.). San Francisco, CA: Jossey-Bass.

Kouzes, J., & Posner, B. (1999). *Encouraging the heart: A leader's guide to rewarding and recognizing others*. San Francisco, CA: Jossey-Bass.

Lasswell, H. D. (1958). *Politics: Who gets what, when, how*. New York: Meridian Books.

Lindberg, C., Nash, S., & Lindberg, C. (2008). *On the edge: Nursing in the age of complexity*. Medford, NJ: Plexus Press.

Litman, T. J., & Robins, L. S. (1991). *Health politics and policy* (2nd ed.). Albany, NY: Delmar.

Lowi, T. (1969). *The end of liberalism*. New York: Norton.

Milio, N. (1989). Developing nursing leadership in health policy. *Journal of Professional Nursing, 5*(6), 315.

Neergaard, L. (2010, July 26). Cell phone doctoring. *The Columbus Dispatch.* Retrieved from http://www.dispatch.com/content/stories/business/2010/07/26/cell-phone-doctoring.html

Nightingale, F. (1859). *Notes on nursing.* Cambridge, UK: Cambridge University Press.

Patient Protection and Affordable Care Act of 2010. (2010). Pub. L. No. 111-148, 124 Stat. 119.

Pesut, D., & Herman, J. (1999). *Clinical reasoning: The art and science of critical and creative thinking* (2nd ed.). Albany, NY: Delmar Learning.

Pierce, L., & Steiner, V. (2003). The male caregiving experience: Three case studies. *Stroke, 34*(1), 315.

Porter-O'Grady, T., Hawkins, M. A., & Parker, M. L. (1997). *Whole-systems shared governance: Architecture for integration.* Gaithersburg, MD: Aspen.

Porter-O'Grady, T., & Malloch, K. (2011). *Quantum leadership: Advancing innovation, transforming health care* (3rd ed.). Sudbury, MA: Jones & Bartlett Learning.

Porter-O'Grady, T., & Wilson, C. K. (1995). *The leadership revolution in health care: Altering systems, changing behaviors.* Gaithersburg, MD: Aspen.

The regulatory process. (1992, December 4). *Capitol Update, 10*(23), 1.

Rhoades, A., Covery, S. R., & Shepherdson, N. (2011). *Building values: Creating an equitable culture that outperforms the competition.* San Francisco, CA: Jossey-Bass.

Rossi, P. H., & Freeman, H. E. (1995). *Evaluation: A systematic approach* (5th ed.). Beverly Hills, CA: Sage.

Thomas, S. B., & Quinn, S. C. (1991). The Tuskegee syphilis study, 1932 to 1972: Implications for HIV education and AIDS risk reduction education programs in the black community. *American Journal of Public Health, 8*(11), 1498-1505.

Watzlawick, R., Weakland, C. E., & Fisch, R. (1974). *Change.* New York: W. W. Norton.

West, W. F. (1982, September/October). The politics of administrative rulemaking. *Public Administration Review,* 420-426.

Williams, S. J., & Torrens, P. R. (Eds.). (1988). *Introduction to health services* (3rd ed.). Albany, NY: Delmar.

Wilson, J. Q. (1989). *American government institutions and policies* (4th ed.). Lexington, MA: D. C. Heath.

Quality, Safety, and Information Systems for Advanced Practice

With specialized knowledge and practical application of that knowledge to influence patient outcomes, nurses in advanced practice have the fiduciary responsibility not only to provide and/or manage quality care, but also to take leadership roles within the practice setting to promote a culture of quality. As described in Part 2, quality is one of the major components of the healthcare triad, along with cost and access. In Part 3, we consider quality issues and the intersection of quality and information technology.

There are many definitions of quality and many perspectives on what healthcare quality means. Consumers, providers, payers, and regulators may all have differing viewpoints about what healthcare quality is and how it should be measured and reported. However, with the national, healthcare industry, and societal interest in the costs of health care and the outcomes of that care, the Institute of Medicine's def-inition (IOM, 2001) of quality is a well-accepted one and the one used for this book. This agency defines healthcare quality as "The degree to which health services for individuals and populations increase the likelihood of desired health outcomes and are consistent with current professional knowledge."

Further, in its report titled *Crossing the Quality Chasm,* the IOM (2001) has described six quality aims for health care. Specifically, health care should be

1. Safe
2. Effective
3. Patient centered
4. Timely
5. Efficient
6. Equitable

These characteristics of quality should be foremost in mind as readers study Part 3.

Patient safety is one of the top—if not *the* top—current quality issues politically and professionally. Nevertheless, it is essential to think broadly about healthcare quality, going beyond just safety, and to keep foremost in one's thinking all of the aforementioned characteristics of quality.

With the recent emphasis on patient safety as a result of the 2000 IOM report, *To Err Is Human,* a concerted, ongoing effort focused on assessing and improving patient safety has been a major driver in health care. In this report, the IOM documented the serious and pervasive nature of the United States' overall patient safety problem, concluding that more than 98,000 deaths per year occurred due to medical error, and stating that the U.S. healthcare system had a severe problem.

In 2008, the Robert Wood Johnson Foundation (RWJF) and the IOM realized the need to assess and transform the nursing profession. Their 2-year initiative resulted in the 2010 IOM Consensus Report entitled *The Future of Nursing: Leading Change and Advancing Health.* Through extensive dialogue, the committee developed four goals linked to policy, safety and education:

1. Nurses should practice to the full extent of their education and training.
2. Nurses should achieve higher levels of education and training through an improved education system that promotes seamless academic progression.
3. Nurses should be full partners, with physicians and other healthcare professionals, in redesigning health care in the United States.
4. Effective workforce planning and policy making require better data collection and information infrastructure.

With the passage of the 2010 Affordable Care Act and the national recognition that nurses work on the front lines of patient care, collaborative efforts will be made to ensure that the U.S. healthcare system provides seamless, affordable, quality care that is accessible to all and leads to improved health outcomes.

In Chapter 13, Sullivan introduces the work of the IOM regarding patient safety and outlines principles of quality improvement (QI). She traces the history of quality initiatives in health care from quality to assessment to today's performance improvement. Along the way, this author reviews tools and techniques for improving quality and performance. This chapter is both informative, providing analysis of quality programs and health care, and practical, offering strategies for measuring quality and forming quality teams.

The last three chapters in Part 3 are dedicated to the use of information technology and electronic health records—factors that are transforming the U.S. healthcare environment into a more technologically sophisticated field. In Chapter 14, Godin first describes the basic components of information technology and security issues that arise from computerized medical records. Although these information systems have multiple uses—from financial reporting and analysis to documentation of care—perhaps the most important facet for the advanced nurse practitioner is the ability to use clinical systems to analyze patient outcomes and improve quality.

In Chapter 15, Barey discusses the implications of adoption of the electronic health record (EHR). This trend is being driven by legislation—specifically, the passage of the American Recovery and Reinvestment Act of 2009 (ARRA), including the HITECH Act, which offers incentives to health organizations and providers to become "meaningful users" of EHRs. The eight components of an EHR are reviewed: (1) health information and data; (2) results management; (3) order entry management; (4) decision support; (5) electronic communication and connectivity; (6) patient support; (7) administrative processes; and (8) reporting and population health management (IOM, 2003).

Chapter 16 explores clinical documentation, confidentiality and privacy concerns, and interface terminologies. Specific information and clinical application features that are useful to advanced practice nurses in a variety of settings are highlighted as part of this discussion.

REFERENCES

Institute of Medicine. (2000). *To err is human: Building a safety health system.* Washington, DC: Author.

Institute of Medicine. (2001). *Crossing the quality chasm: The IOM health care quality initiative.* Washington, DC: Author.

Institute of Medicine. (2010). *The future of nursing: Leading change and advancing health.* Washington, DC: Author.

CHAPTER 13

Healthcare Quality

Dori Taylor Sullivan

CHAPTER OBJECTIVES

1. Trace the history of quality and performance improvement approaches in healthcare organizations.

2. List the major principles of quality and performance improvement.

3. Discuss the role that the management of information and information technology play in achieving the best results from improvement efforts.

4. Relate the concept of evidence-based practice to quality improvement in general and the role of the advanced nurse practitioner.

5. List the significant accrediting and regulatory bodies influencing quality measurement in health care and discuss their focus.

INTRODUCTION

In this chapter, quality improvement is presented along with ways to build a culture of quality. The advanced nurse practitioner plays a major role in identifying priorities for improvement, establishing and maintaining quality standards, participating in data collection activities for regulatory and accreditation purposes, and assuring that improvements are evaluated for safety, efficacy, and effectiveness. As a role model, the advanced nurse practitioner can play a key role in creating a quality of culture or a commitment to continuous improvement in the organization.

This chapter provides an overview of the evolution of performance improvement in health care followed by the major principles of quality and performance improvement common to all the major approaches. Regardless of the specific quality improvement program that an organization has selected or developed, most of the principles will be applicable. For example, the commitment to data-driven decisions for improvement is universal. While the initial focus of performance improvement was on administrative processes, the practice rapidly spread to clinical systems and outcomes; so we discuss this as a special case of performance improvement.

The chapter suggests how evidence-based practice is related to performance improvement and particularly the impact of the quality of available data to inform identification of best practices. Finally, the chapter presents a summary of what the major regulatory and accreditation agencies are requiring related to quality improvement, patient safety, and outcomes of care.

INTRODUCTION OF CONTINUOUS QUALITY IMPROVEMENT TO HEALTH CARE

Sometime around 1980, the concept of *quality assurance* (QA) began to be popular in clinical settings in acute care hospitals. Early QA efforts were mostly a counting activity and, while carried out with the best intentions, tended to focus on aspects of care that were relatively easy to count rather than processes or outcomes of most interest to practitioners. These early QA activities received a lukewarm reception from most disciplines and were met with relative disdain from physicians. As is often noted by measurement experts, it seems that the things that are easy to measure are relatively unimportant, while those things that would really make a difference are difficult to measure and interpret. The fact that the focus of QA tended to be determined and imposed by a central authority was another strike against these early efforts. The result was general compliance with the mandates but little enthusiasm and limited use of the findings.

The Quality Movement and Its Translation into Health Care

During the 1980s, the work of Deming (1986) was noticed by healthcare leaders. Deming is considered the ultimate guru of *total quality management* (TQM), based on his work rebuilding the manufacturing businesses of war-torn Japan beginning around 1950. Deming promoted what he termed constancy of purpose and systematic analysis, with measurement of process steps in relation to capacity or outcomes. The TQM approach incorporated the view, as the name implies, that the entire organization must be committed to quality and improvement to achieve the best results—and to promote joy in work.

The staggering success of these improved Japanese businesses was first recognized by some industries in the United States, including manufacturing; slowly other sectors took note. Health care was a natural extension given the concerns about quality and cost of care that were beginning to accelerate. Soon after gaining popularity in health care, the quality improvement movement was translated into public and higher education. While some were quick to label quality improvement as a fad, it has flourished in health care and education and has become a business standard for success.

Besides Deming, other experts quickly gained national prominence. New and existing consulting firms created or added quality and performance improvement consulting and education services to assist the many healthcare organizations eager to introduce these powerful methods. Juran (1988) and Joiner (1994) are two other widely recognized experts in quality improvement, both of whom lead international consulting firms devoted to quality management principles, culture, and techniques. Today the field encompasses hundreds of trademarked approaches to quality, making it impossible to cover them all. We can, however, identify and discuss the most important principles of quality and performance improvement.

Language of Quality Improvement

First, a word about the jargon of *quality improvement* (QI). Over time, different terms became popular and then faded away as newer terms were embraced. The relatively early TQM was somewhat displaced by *continuous quality improvement* (CQI) and then by *performance improvement* (PI). Although there are distinctions made by the originators of these and other terms, for our purposes we will use quality and performance improvement to describe a comprehensive and formal system of principles, methods, and techniques to systematically measure and improve processes and outcomes. Also, how quality is defined differs somewhat among various approaches; however, virtually all definitions of quality include meeting or exceeding customer needs, decreasing variation, and minimizing or eliminating defects or errors from products or services.

Quality improvement may focus on enhancing existing processes or designing quality processes. When existing processes are believed to be incapable of yielding the desired results, redesign or reengineering of a process is undertaken. Hammer and Champy (1993) explained reengineering as the "fundamental rethinking and radical redesign of processes to achieve dramatic improvements in critical, contemporary measures of performance, such as cost, quality, service, and speed" (p. 22). While there are clearly differences in improving versus redesigning a work process, we will use the term "quality improvement" (QI) to describe all such efforts.

Principles of Quality and Performance Improvement

Scholtes (1988) aptly notes that many elements of quality leadership have "appeared separately in fads that swept through business schools and organizations (pp. 1–10)," such that many are unfamiliar with a comprehensive approach to performance improvement that has been termed "a new way of doing business." The principles shown in Table 13-1 and described in the following pages, as presented by Scholtes about the Joiner model, may be worded differently in various approaches, but their meaning is the same.

Customer Focus

The customer is the center of quality efforts as an organization strives to meet or exceed customer goals and provide value. Quality approaches recognize external customers (the users of products or services) and internal customers (those within the organization that receive goods or services from other departments).

The translation of QI principles into health care requires that we think about the term "customer" a bit differently. In a strict business sense, customers are the ones who pay for the service or product they receive. The case in health care is more complex, because much of the cost of health care is borne by third parties, including employers, insurance companies, and the government, as opposed to clients themselves. Also, frequently the goals and desires of clients are in conflict with those of the payers. Some have referred to the client as the ultimate customer, so as not to confuse where our primary obligation

TABLE 13-1	Principles of Quality Leadership

1. Customer focus
2. Obsession with quality
3. Recognizing the structure in work
4. Freedom through control
5. Unity of purpose
6. Looking for faults in systems
7. Teamwork
8. Continued education and training

Source: Scholtes, 1988, pp. 1–11.

lies. That said, most healthcare organizations and their clinical managers typically try to identify and balance the needs of these major customers, which sometimes are conflicting.

A related principle in this customer focus is to measure, not assume or guess about, what customers need and want. This focus on data and information recurs in many of the quality principles.

Obsession with Quality

Everyone in an organization must be obsessed with quality! This principle may be best defined by the phrase "building a culture of quality," where the norm becomes the relentless pursuit of quality products and services through efficient and effective methods of execution. Building a culture of quality requires attention to staff education, clear communication of goals and expectations, provision of necessary resources, organizational systems that are efficient and effective, and alignment of performance and rewards systems.

Recognizing the Structure in Work

All work consists of processes that are structured, not random. The structure and processes must be studied, measured, analyzed, and improved systematically to achieve the best results. Quality improvement includes specific tools and techniques to quantify and understand work, providing the data needed to create improvements.

To best understand the structure of work, management and staff must work together since each brings valuable information to the activity. We must appreciate that the people directly involved in the work have the best information about how that work is performed—and how it could be done better. In addition, the focus on work rather than individual performance engages staff in a positive way. This approach fundamentally changes the relationship between staff and management and fosters trust, respect, and empathy. One should

recognize these as elements of transformation leadership.

Freedom Through Control

Quality improvement embraces the idea of quality control and reducing variation to produce regular desired results. Standardizing processes and ensuring that everyone uses those standards should make work processes more efficient and effective. The increase in productivity should allow for more freedom to develop new ideas for the business, enhance service to the customer, and improve skills in key areas. For example, in a clinical service area, if the scheduling procedure for clients is a refined and effective process, the scheduler or receptionist should not have to spend as much time on the telephone or negotiating with patients or providers, freeing up time for other important activities.

Unity of Purpose

Unity of purpose speaks to a clear and widely understood vision for the organization that unites or aligns all who work there. It is the vision that guides quality improvement efforts and provides criteria for decision making and problem solving when issues or opportunities arise. In a truly patient-centered healthcare organization, we would expect to see tangible efforts to promote comfort, safety, and timeliness.

During a recent visit to an ambulatory surgery facility, the following actions were noted. A sign in the reception area asked patients to come up to the desk if they had been waiting longer than 15 minutes to be called for registration. Upon changing into a hospital gown, patients were provided with two warmed bath blankets. While awaiting surgery, patients were asked if they wanted fresh warmed blankets, and blankets were also wrapped around a family member who was chilled. No one in that organization raised questions about the cost of providing this service, as patient satisfaction data clearly supported how much this amenity was valued, both for its physical comfort and communication of caring at a stressful time.

Looking for Faults in Systems

The QI philosophy and culture specifies aggressive continuous improvements of all work systems. The most important factor underlying this principle is accepting that systems rather than individual people are responsible for 80% to 85% of the results achieved (claims made by Deming and Juran, and supported by the Pareto principle, or 80/20 rule). Loosely translated, the Pareto principle says that 80% of the poor results or troubles come from 20% of the problems. Or, as some managers like to say, 20% of their staff causes 80% of the problems!

Realistically, we cannot work on all systems at the same time, so a way to identify priorities for improvement is essential. This is usually done through the collection of performance data on critical indicators across the organization (sometimes called a dashboard report or report card). In addition, departments create function-specific performance indicators that reflect improvement foci for specific areas. There needs to be some alignment or relationship between organization-wide goals and focus and those of the departments, since it is at the point of service within the departments that quality happens or doesn't happen. An example of this alignment might be an organizational commitment to improving turnaround time. For radiology, this might mean the reading of reports. In the lab, the measure would be time until test results are available. In the rehabilitation department, it might relate to readying special rooms or equipment between clients so there would be decreased waiting time and more appointments possible during a day.

Teamwork

There are few, if any, important work tasks that people do completely by themselves. Thus we rely on others who play a part in supplying us with the products and services (including infor-

mation) that we need to do our jobs well—or who need to work collaboratively with us to achieve the desired results. Teamwork differs from individuals or groups in that teams are defined by having members who are committed to working toward a common goal or vision. The best team results are achieved when there is a diversity of ideas and relevant skills on the team that represent the important aspects of the work to be improved.

Continued Education and Training

An ongoing commitment to education and training across the organization is critical to keeping the culture of quality alive and thriving. There are always new techniques and ideas to be shared and enhanced skills for obtaining, managing, measuring, analyzing, and using information for improvement. Furthermore, education tends to make staff feel valued and important while enhancing their skills in a concrete way.

TOOLS AND TECHNIQUES FOR IMPROVING QUALITY AND PERFORMANCE

Improving quality and performance in any organization requires attention to three major areas: leadership, skills for gathering and using information related to work analysis, and the people factor. The Joiner triangle (Scholtes, Joiner, & Streibel, 2003, p. xxi) in Figure 13-1 shows the relationship of these elements where quality leadership and the scientific approach represent the skills and tools for work analysis and improvement and all one team represents the people factor. Teamwork is at the heart of most QI efforts because teamwork reflects how work is typically accomplished and because more brainpower with different perspectives usually develops better solutions. We next present an overview of each of these areas so that you can consider the implications for your role as an advanced nurse practitioner.

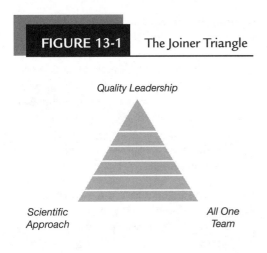

FIGURE 13-1 The Joiner Triangle

Quality Leadership

Scientific Approach *All One Team*

Source: In Scholtes, P., Joiner, B., Streibel, B. (2003). *The TEAM Handbook* (3rd ed.). Madison, WI, Oriel Inc., p. xxi.

Leadership for Quality

The role of leaders in an organization endeavoring to create a culture of quality and continuous improvement cannot be underestimated. Any serious initiative to create a quality organization must be sincerely embraced at the senior levels of the organization as well as by nurse managers and advanced nurse practitioners and be constantly reinforced through actions and reward structures, or what has been called "walking the talk." Staff are experts at identifying inconsistencies in leader behavior, and they use any incongruence to decide whether to believe and invest in what is being proffered.

Scholtes (1988) identified six steps needed for quality leadership and a continuous improvement culture. First, senior leadership must first commit to a rigorous education program for their team; this program must address all three elements of the triangle. Second, they should define the organizational culture characteristics and values that they wish to develop that are consistent with continuous improvement. Third, senior leaders should develop a multiyear improvement strategy (2 years is recommended) so that a pathway is clearly defined.

The fourth step is a plan for educating the entire workforce, usually done in phases for logistical and cost reasons. This is a significant undertaking that, when well done, yields powerful results by introducing a new way of thinking about work improvement and relationships. Fifth, a formal network of support and guidance (often defined as access to quality facilitators with advanced knowledge of QI techniques) should be established and communicated. Sixth, the specific improvement projects should be identified and initiated.

As an advanced nurse practitioner, you will be called on to be a formal and/or informal leader for quality improvement initiatives. Knowing the process of quality improvement can assist you to be more effective in this role.

Using the Scientific Method

In simple terms the scientific method can be used to test our assertions. More precisely, the scientific method is a set of orderly, systematic, controlled procedures for acquiring dependable, empirical—typically quantitative—information about a topic or question (Polit & Beck, 2004). This method involves four steps after identifying a question or, in our case, a work process, to focus on: assessment and data collection, problem identification, interventions, and evaluation (Table 13-2).

Some commonly used tools for data collection, analysis, and problem identification have evolved from the quality movement: traditional statistical control processes (mostly from manufacturing) and the discipline of management engineering. For our purposes, we describe only the most frequently used tools so that readers can get a feel for this skill set. Our purpose is to introduce readers to the tools. Readers can build their knowledge base by searching the Internet and/or working with a quality improvement department. Readers' charge is to determine the specific quality approach, methods, and tools used in their own organization so that their knowledge and skill development target those specific areas.

TABLE 13-2	Steps in the Scientific Method

1. Assessment and data collection
2. Problem identification
3. Selection of interventions or solutions
4. Evaluation of results

Flowcharts

A flowchart is a diagram that uses standardized symbols to create a paper picture of steps and decisions that make up a work process. There are several variations of flowcharting but each serves the purpose of defining the detail and order of a process. Flowcharts may be developed as a team activity, or individuals may be assigned to create a flowchart based on their understanding of the work process. There are often conflicting opinions about process flowcharts, so one of the major purposes they serve is to develop a common view of an existing or proposed process, a first step in reducing variation.

Pie Charts and Pareto Charts

Most people are familiar with pie charts, which display the percentage of categories or responses using the wedges of a circle that look like slices of pie. The size of the wedge reflects the frequency or size of that category. Similarly, Pareto charts use the same information as a pie chart but depict the categories or responses in a bar graph that orders the named categories from highest to lowest in terms of frequency or impact. The purpose of the Pareto chart is to determine whether in each case the rule holds true—that is, whether 20% of the categories will explain 80% of the problems.

Cause and Effect (Fishbone) Diagrams

Fishbone diagrams are used to categorize and analyze possible problem causes related to a desired or problematic effect or outcome. The shape of the diagram resembles a fish with

bones—hence the name. The fishbone diagram is a picture of lists with increasing amounts of detail as more "bones" are added to the descriptions of possible causative factors. As with flowcharts, cause and effect diagrams may be developed by the team or by individual/small group efforts and then compared.

Operational Definitions

Operational definitions specify a concept or element and how it will be measured. For example, a definition of good turnaround time for a pathology report could be more precisely stated as a typed, signed, final report delivered to the ordering physician within 72 hours of receipt of the specimen. Without precise definitions of effects or outcomes, it becomes difficult to measure the impact of various work process steps or issues.

Run Charts (Time Plots) and Control Charts

A run chart or time plot depicts a series of observations or measures of a work process over time. The purpose of seeing variations over time is to look for patterns that could lead to understanding causes of variation or diminished performance so that effective improvement strategies can be created. Recall that one of the first steps in QI is decreasing variation; the run chart shows the amount of variation over time. For example, suppose the clinical manager of an emergency clinic wishes to see the number of patient visits by day of week so that he can develop a better staffing plan. A 2-week run chart shows that visits are much higher on Thursdays, Fridays, and Saturdays. The next step might be to analyze time of day of visits for those days on a second run chart.

A control chart is a run chart with boundaries for expected variation drawn into the display. The values for these boundaries are calculated from statistical control formulas that a quality expert could assist in determining. Variation within the boundaries is referred to as common cause or normal variation. Points of variation outside the boundaries are termed special cause and require further investigation.

Checksheets

Checksheets are forms developed to facilitate collection of observed data about a work process step or element. Checksheets should be as simple as possible with the goal of showing patterns or amounts easily. As an example, consider the case of a courier service that provides service to a freestanding nutrition center. The center might develop a checksheet to document whether the courier is on time and how many items he is delivering. These data could be used to decrease the service and reduce costs or to investigate an improved method of accomplishing this activity.

Gap Analysis

A gap analysis is used to assess the nature and amount of difference between the current state and the desired state of designated characteristics or outcomes. The best gap analyses incorporate measurement data to support the description of the current state and definition of the desired future. For instance, if a goal is to have active participation in shared governance of a department, one could count the number of staff participating on councils.

Root Cause Analysis

Root cause analysis is a formalized investigation and problem-solving approach focused on understanding the underlying causes of an event as opposed to focusing on symptoms of a problem. Root cause analysis seeks to determine what happened, how it happened, and why it happened, with the overall goal of making recommendations for prevention of future events. The four steps in root cause analysis are data collection, causal factor charting, identification of root causes, and generation of recommendations and implementation of changes (Rooney & Vanden Heuvel, 2004). A root cause summary table may be used to summarize the findings and recommendations of the analysis.

The People Factor and Teams

Each of us has probably experienced an unproductive or uncomfortable group meeting, where differing opinions and dialogue did not result in a consensus or decision. Consensus may be defined as an idea or proposal that all team members can positively support, even though it may not be their personal first choice or preference. Achieving consensus is generally preferred to majority rules voting or an authoritarian decision because it promotes better solutions and improved team relationships as well as buy-in from members.

Team Communication and Decisions

Using structured communication and decision-making tools improves team functioning and outcomes. The tools and techniques described here are designed to promote efficient presentation of ideas and opinions after which agreements can be developed for how to proceed.

Brainstorming

Brainstorming is a technique that enables a group to generate and list many ideas within a short time period. It also promotes relatively equal participation, assuring that talkative members do not monopolize the discussion.

Participants contribute one item in order with no comments about the ideas allowed. People may pass if they have nothing to add during that round, and the session is stopped by time or lack of additional ideas. The group then clarifies their understanding of each idea and may combine similar items. The next steps are for the group to agree on criteria for evaluating these ideas or how to reduce the list to the best ideas to make it manageable.

Multivoting

Multivoting allots a certain number of votes to each participant that each uses for his or her most preferred items from a brainstorming or other list. Multivoting reduces the list of ideas by retaining only those items with a higher number of votes. It is often used following a brainstorming session to focus the team on one or more items. After combining similar items, the remaining items are numbered. Each member is given a specified number of votes. Items with the lowest vote totals are eliminated and another multivoting session may be conducted; this process can be repeated as many times as needed.

Nominal Group Technique

This technique is a more formalized approach to determine priorities from a list generated by participants. It combines elements of brainstorming, as participants write down their ideas independently in response to a question or topic. A master list of the ideas is compiled on a flip chart. Each participant is then asked to assign a rating or number of points to a specified number of the ideas presented. This technique is helpful for relatively new teams or controversial topics.

Affinity Diagrams

Creating an affinity diagram is an action strategy to develop categories or see how numerous elements might be related based on perceptions of a group. Each member is instructed to write down three to five responses to a question, writing each response on a separate sticky note. The individual notes are then posted on a large wall by all participants. Participants are instructed to group the sticky notes together as best makes sense to them without speaking to others. Each individual can move the sticky notes into whatever configuration he or she prefers, but the next person can come along and undo it. After a period of time the group tends to arrive at a good enough solution. The clusters of notes depict a number of broad categories or themes that emerge. This activity can promote enhanced understanding of underlying causes of issues.

Lessons Learned for Promoting QI Team Effectiveness

In addition to the structured QI tools just discussed, consideration must be given to how to structure team activities for the best outcomes, acknowledging that individuals have needs and motivations that may detract from team effectiveness. As a culture of quality develops in a unit or organization, the norm is to question and improve everything and defensiveness decreases. However, to promote optimal team functioning and outcomes, attention must be given to establishing a clear charge, selecting the team members, and assigning roles. These recommendations apply whether the team is from one unit or comprised of several departments across the organization, so it is important to make the appropriate adjustments depending upon the type of team.

Team Charge

Most organizations create a formal mechanism for deciding upon improvement priorities relying on appropriate performance data and quality indicators. Once the decision is made that a cross-functional team (composed of staff from multiple departments or areas) should be convened to address an improvement opportunity, a formal charge to the team is prepared. This charge should include the specific nature of the improvement opportunity and the desired outcomes, timelines, resources available, team members, and any other parameters or assumptions the team needs to accomplish its charge. A team charge is similar to a team charter, differing only in how much detail is fleshed out by the person or group creating the team.

Selection of Members

The selection of team members is crucial to team success. Individuals who have process owner status, meaning that they have primary responsibility for this work, must be included both for their knowledge and to promote buy-in for recommended improvements. If one wants to establish a team on one's unit to improve the response time of the night shift and there is a night charge person, it is essential to have the charge person on the team. Staff who actually perform the work and are closest to the provision of services should also be team members. Those who supply information, products, or services (suppliers) as well as internal and possibly external customers should also be represented, either as team members or through invitations to join certain meetings. The size of a QI team varies among organizations and projects, but most experts seem to agree that between seven and nine members is the best number for team effectiveness.

Team Roles

There are six basic roles in a QI team: team leader or chair, team member, recorder, timekeeper, facilitator or quality adviser, and executive champion. Depending on the size of the team, some of these roles may be combined or even rotated; whatever the plan, the team needs to ensure that all the functions are assigned and carried out.

Team Leader

The team leader is formally in charge of the team's efforts, including meeting schedules and agendas, between-meeting assignments, maintenance of the formal team records, and communication with others regarding the team's work (unless this is specifically assigned to a team member for specific requests). The team leader role may be performed by cochairs if desired. The team leader works closely with the facilitator for guidance and feedback on team performance and next steps. Whenever possible, the next meeting's agenda and between-meeting assignments should be reviewed and documented near the end of the meeting.

Team Member

Team members accept responsibility for sharing their ideas and information, preparing for meetings, completing between-meeting assignments, committing to continued learning, and contributing to overall team effectiveness.

Recorder

It is highly recommended that the team's work be captured on flip charts or smart boards so that all members can see and assist with what is being recorded. In addition, this method of recording eliminates the need to spend time writing minutes after the meeting, as meeting documentation can be typed from the recording sheets. Any reports or charts prepared may also be attached and distributed to foster the team's work progress. The recorder function may be assigned to a specific team member or, more often, it is rotated among members.

Timekeeper

As the name suggests, this team role is responsible for helping the team manage its time. Agendas should include suggested time allocations for each agenda item and/or the team should discuss how to best use the available time at each meeting. The timekeeper notifies the team when the allocated time has elapsed, at which point the team can decide to stop the discussion or agree to continue for an amount of time.

Facilitator

The facilitator or quality adviser may be from the quality or education department or it could be a colleague who has received in-depth quality training. The facilitator has three main responsibilities. First and foremost, the facilitator works with the team leader to plan out the team's work and consider which QI tools or methods might be most helpful at different stages of the project. Second, the facilitator attends team meetings to observe and make recommendations to the team about its level of effectiveness and its enhancement. Many facilitators take 5 minutes at the end of each meeting to elicit members' perceptions of what went well and facilitated work versus what could be done better for the next time. Third, the facilitator is an expert in QI and provides formal or just-in-time training as needed to foster team progress.

Champion

Each QI team should have a senior leader appointed as the executive champion of the team's project. For unit teams, the advanced nurse practitioner would be identified as the champion.

Frequently, the team leader and the facilitator encounter issues or barriers that require assistance or advice from senior administration. And while the champion does not attend all team meetings, that person does establish regular communication, and this provides information to show that the team is on track to meet the improvement goals. Table 13-3 provides a summary of QI tools and techniques, and Table 13-4 lists the team decision methods.

Ground Rules

Ground rules (or rules of engagement) evolve from team discussions about how members wish to behave with one another to promote member satisfaction and team success. Ground rules often include expectations related to prompt attendance, participation, interruptions (pagers and phones), decision making, conversational courtesies (such as no interrupting when others are speaking), and confidentiality agreements when appropriate. Once ground rules are established through consensus, it is easier to hold members accountable for compliance.

WHAT MAKES QUALITY IMPROVEMENT SUCCESSFUL?

The traditionalist QI approaches developed by Deming, Juran, and Joiner, among others, remain the method of choice in numerous healthcare organizations. Others have opted to follow two newer models: General Electric's (GE) Six Sigma and Work Out (GE, n.d.) and Studer Group's Pillars of Excellence (Studer Group, n.d.). The Six Sigma and Pillars of Excellence approaches have been adopted by growing numbers of healthcare organizations. These approaches, while evolutionary in terms of QI, retain the core principles presented earlier in this chapter.

Many QI approaches have led to spectacular organizational successes. The major factors in this success may be summarized into three themes. First is the commitment of leadership to the fundamental principles of quality, improvement, measurement, empowerment, and involvement. Leaders must visibly, powerfully, and continuously talk and walk the talk! Second, a clear and consistent model for QI should be selected and refined for use in an organization; this would also be used at the unit level. The QI field is cluttered with jargon and people become easily frustrated if the language changes all the time. Staff want to master QI skills, and that is more difficult to do without a clear model, terms, and processes. Third, there must be an investment in building a quality infrastructure to provide the human and material resources required for QI success. An advanced nurse practitioner needs to assure that staff teams have sufficient resources and direction for success. Members of a staff may also be

TABLE 13-3	Summary of QI Tools and Techniques

QI Tools	QI Techniques
Flowchart	Brainstorming
Pie chart/Pareto chart	Multivoting
Cause and effect (fishbone) diagram	Nominal group technique
Operational definitions	Affinity diagrams
Run and control charts	Structured discussion
Checksheets	
Root cause analysis	

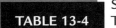

TABLE 13-4	Summary of QI Team Concepts

Team charge (opportunity, outcomes, timelines, resources, assumptions)

Selection of members

Size of team

Team roles (leader, member, recorder, timekeeper, facilitator, executive champion)

Ground rules

asked to develop additional QI skills to support efforts throughout the organization.

Benchmarking is a term denoting the use of information from other organizations to use as a comparison or benchmark in evaluating an organization's performance. Benchmarking may be a relatively informal, collegial process or, more often, an extensive and detailed project. The utility of benchmarking data is enhanced when there are common operational definitions for key data elements and metrics for reporting. It also works better when the organizations, or at least the specific area or work process being benchmarked, share important characteristics.

Recently the emphasis in benchmarking has been on best or better practices. For example, if a hospital is trying to reduce length of stay for patients having total knee replacements, it should access information from a hospital having the lowest lengths of stay and excellent quality outcomes. This comparison yields two helpful things. It provides a reality-based sense of the possible in the current environment, and it allows for learning about how the length of stay reduction is achieved.

Many healthcare organizations belong to proprietary benchmarking service companies or groups and can regularly access performance data in areas of interest such as patient satisfaction. These comparisons may also facilitate the

identification of organizational or departmental improvement priorities if there is a major difference in efficiency and/or effectiveness of the care or services under study.

Benchmarking is discussed in more detail in the section on accrediting and regulatory agencies' quality initiatives. We now turn our attention to the special case of clinical improvement and the related concept of evidence-based practice.

CLINICAL-PROCESS IMPROVEMENT AND EVIDENCE-BASED PRACTICE

The successes in administrative and support processes using QI skills led to transferring this approach to clinical processes and outcomes. While QI was largely driven by administrators at the beginning, physician leaders and other clinicians recognized the opportunities that a structured approach to improvement provided. Further, given the long tradition of a research-based approach to care, a renewed interest in using research evidence to guide care decisions and protocols developed. The term *evidence-based medicine* or *evidence-based practice* was coined and reflects this renewed emphasis by medicine, nursing, and other health disciplines. We also note how advances in information technology have accelerated and supported clinical improvement and evidence-based practice.

Clinical-Process Improvement

Clinical-process redesign or improvement means "the effective design of the continuum of care to satisfy customers, improve patient outcomes, maximize efficiencies, and improve the organizational climate" (Strongwater & Pelote, 1996, p. ix). The specific outcomes of general interest specified by these authors include clinical outcomes, functional outcomes (physical, social, and quality of life), patient satisfaction, and organizational climate (staff satisfaction and readiness to change), along with cost and utilization indicators.

As individual healthcare organizations identified clinical-process improvement as a major strategic goal, entities that support hospitals and other agencies developed clinical-improvement programs and resources to assist their constituencies. For example VHA, Inc., a national membership organization for community hospital systems, and the University Healthsystems Consortium (UHC), a member organization for academic medical center hospitals and systems, each created divisions for clinical improvement. VHA, Inc., and UHC added physicians, nurses, and other quality experts to their staffs to provide consultation and other resources to support their members' efforts. The development of comparative databases for benchmarking and creating peer relationships for learning and improvement blossomed during the 1990s, and entire conferences were regularly held to advance this area.

At about the same time, the Agency for Healthcare Research and Quality (AHRQ) came into being and began assimilating research to issue practice guidelines with the expectation of improving patient outcomes. The stated mission of AHRQ is to improve the quality, safety, efficiency, and effectiveness of health care for all Americans (AHRQ, n.d.). The AHRQ develops consensus around evidence-based best practices for priority healthcare concerns like pain, incontinence, and others. This brings us to evidence-based practice.

Evidence-Based Practice

Evidence-based practice (EBP) is the integration of best research evidence with clinical expertise and patient values to deliver optimal care (Sackett, Straus, Richardson, Rosenberg, & Haynes, 2000). *Best research* means clinically relevant, patient-centered research studies. *Clinical expertise* refers to the role of clinical skills and experience as well as unique patient presentations. The inclusion of *patient values* reflects the need to individualize care to meet individual preferences, needs, and concerns to best serve that patient. These authors further assert that to carry out EBP there must be sufficient research published on the specific topic of interest, the health practitioner must have skills in accessing and critically analyzing research, and the practice must allow for implementing changes based on the evidence. Table 13-5 summarizes a five-step process for EBP.

The evaluation of evidence is often done using a system for grading or leveling the quality of the evidence according to accepted research standards. There are several systems for

---

TABLE 13-5	Summary of EBP and the Five-Step Process

Evidence-based practice (EBP) is the integration of best research evidence with clinical expertise and patient values to optimize clinical outcomes and quality of life (Sackett, Straus, Richardson, Rosenberg, & Haynes, 2000, p. 1).

1. Formulate a question arising from patient clinical problems based on current knowledge and practice.

2. Search for and access relevant evidence or research.

3. Evaluate the evidence using established criteria for scientific merit.

4. Choose interventions or changes in practice, justifying the selection with the most valid evidence for the patient population to which it will be applied.

5. Implement the change(s) and evaluate the results.

grading evidence with one example being the following three-grade system:

- Level I or A: a multisite randomized clinical trial or several single-site randomized studies
- Level II or B: a quasi-experimental study
- Level III or C: a correlational or descriptive study

While EBP in health care is not totally new, the emphasis and widespread commitment to its use, facilitated by exploding and more readily available evidence, continues to grow and has become the standard of care. Another factor contributing to EBP is the time pressure experienced by most healthcare providers. Instead of having to go to a library, clinicians can use their PDAs or a computer with Internet access to quickly locate current research data and critical reviews on a particular topic. There are also evidence-based clinical guidelines available for purchase to guide practice in the field.

Recognizing that patient outcomes result from the efforts of numerous disciplines, the most effective EBP models combine the interventions of the involved disciplines for various patient conditions, although each discipline retains responsibility for assessing its own professional practice. For further information about and examples of current evidence-based improvement initiatives, refer to the websites for the Institute for Healthcare Improvement (www.ihi.org) and ZYNX (www.zynx.com).

Despite its popularity, some barriers to EBP have been identified, most commonly accessibility of research findings, anticipated benefits of using research, organizational support to use research, and support from others (Retsas, 2000). Healthcare organizations need to find ways to foster the culture of quality and support systems to make EBP a way of life to provide the best and most cost-effective care. Advanced nurse practitioners will be expected to use research knowledge and skills to promote safe, high-quality care. Those who have not already done so should consider taking a formal or continuing education course to enhance their competence in this area.

Managing Information and Information Technology

The evolution of computerization and information technology (IT) in health care is a complex and interesting topic. For our purposes, we comment on the critical role of IT and some of the issues and decisions that will critically affect our ability to improve quality and enhance efficiency using IT advances. We expect that all readers have some experience with IT systems in their organizations, whether it be for managing staffing or supplies, scheduling visits or procedures, tracking records, entering medical orders, or using electronic medical records.

One of the major issues in health care is the jigsaw puzzle approach to computerization in most healthcare organizations. For a variety of reasons, different departments or functions were automated at different times, after which more comprehensive software systems became available. Decisions related to interfacing abilities (getting the systems to talk to one another and share information) versus extinction of the original system in favor of wider benefits are quite common. Comprehensive software systems can now be purchased for many healthcare setting needs related to client medical records, tracking, services, payments, and outcomes; financial matters; staff and patient scheduling; and many others.

Automation tends to improve information access, communication, and documentation; decrease redundancy of data entry; facilitate the use of data for research and QI; and promote easier compliance with regulatory requirements. The initial and ongoing costs of these systems along with information security can be significant challenges. Another challenge is data integrity—that is, verifying that the data in the system are accurately coded, entered, and available. While many healthcare organizations are making progress in implementing a fully automated medical record, most are still working at this process.

Leapfrog Group is a conglomerate of non-healthcare *Fortune* 500 company leaders committed to modernizing the current healthcare system (Milstein, 2000). This increasingly influential group has identified three evidence-based initiatives it believes will dramatically improve outcomes: (1) computerized physician order entry (CPOE), (2) evidence-based hospital referrals (EHR), and (3) intensive care unit physician staffing (IPS) (Hudon, 2003, p. 233). We discuss the first two, as they directly relate to subsequent content.

Implementation of a CPOE system addresses several components of medical errors related to medications, namely the legibility of orders, completeness of information, and the ability to use a clinical decision support system (CDSS) to cross-check for dangerous drug interactions or contraindications. Although evidence clearly supports improved quality and financial outcomes related to CPOE, the initial expenses are substantial. These statements could apply to many software systems available to healthcare agencies. Another factor is that most would agree that computerization often does not save professional time but does improve the quality and availability of data.

The EHR recommendation supports that consumers should have access to quality and outcome data for specific conditions and procedures so that they can make informed choices regarding where to seek care. We address this in more detail in the section on regulatory and accrediting quality initiatives.

Advanced nurse practitioners will need to be involved in the implementation of systems that include their areas or serve their areas specifically. Also, it is generally recommended that representative advanced nurse practitioners and the staff on the front line participate in the selection of software systems to provide the end-user perspective. Thus enhancing knowledge of information technology systems and ca-pabilities will lead to better use of information for evidence-based practice and quality, financial, and other purposes.

ACCREDITATION AND REGULATORY FOCUS ON QUALITY

The major accreditation and regulatory entities in health care have taken significant steps to promote quality and safety in the delivery of health care. Although many of the efforts focused on hospitals, they noted that other settings would likely have similar issues. Recommendations for assessing other settings (such as nursing homes, ambulatory care, and home care) to identify differences and effective solutions were frequently encouraged. In this section, we review some of the major changes and recent requirements that focus on improving the quality of care and patient safety with attention to cost-effectiveness and service utilization—changes that have significant impact on advanced nurse practitioners in most settings.

Joint Commission Performance Improvement and Safety Standards

The Joint Commission, formerly known as the Joint Commission on the Accreditation of Health Care Organizations (JCAHO), provides voluntary accreditation services to hospitals, home-care agencies, ambulatory care, long-term care, behavioral health, laboratories, and office-based surgery, among others. The Joint Commission should be lauded for an early effort to require contemporary QI activities of its accredited facilities. As early as 1987, JCAHO's Agenda for Change called for demonstration of systematic QI efforts, including closing the loop by evaluating the impact of improvement strategies. At the same time, JCAHO began development of performance measures that evolved into the ORYX initiative, a requirement for benchmarking clinical outcomes of selected conditions.

Since 1999, The Joint Commission has met with stakeholder groups to develop a set of hospital core measures. Three initial major diagnoses were selected for testing after extensive pilot testing, feedback from pilot hospitals, and information derived from the Centers for Medicare & Medicaid Services (CMS) of the U.S. Department of Health and Human Services (HHS): acute myocardial infarction (AMI, nine measures), heart failure (HF, four measures), and community-acquired pneumonia (CAP, five measures). A fourth area, pregnancy and related conditions (PR), was added later, as was the measure for surgical infection prevention (SIP). Additional measures are under development with the stated intent to stay consistent with CMS goals and initiatives.

Two other Joint Commission requirements deserve mention in the context of quality and safety. The Joint Commission calls for a patient safety plan that reflects a comprehensive approach for reporting, analyzing, and preventing medical errors through a variety of actions. Specific attention is given to sentinel events, defined as "an unexpected occurrence involving death or serious physical or psychological injury, or the risk thereof" (www .jcipatientsafety.org). In an assessment of 2,966 hospital sentinel events reported between 1995 and 2004, JCAHO listed the top five root causes of sentinel events from all categories as communication, orientation and training, patient assessment, staffing, and availability of information.

For our purposes and because of the role hospitals play in the current system, we have used the Joint Commission accreditation of hospitals as an exemplar to illustrate how quality and safety requirements have evolved. Advanced nurse practitioners should become knowledgeable of the Joint Commission or other accreditation agency standards for their areas, many of which have headed in similar directions. The next section summarizes reports from the Institute of Medicine (IOM) and highlights the information that drove some of these changes.

IOM Reports

Three reports among the many issued by the IOM of the National Academies fueled the focus on measuring and reporting quality and safety in health care. Each of these reports is briefly presented with the major recommendations.

The first of the three reports, *To Err Is Human* (IOM, 2000), garnered major headlines with its finding that as many as 98,000 deaths each year in the United States were due to medical errors. This number surpasses the number of deaths from motor vehicle accidents, breast cancer, and AIDS. It was also reported that the cost of one category of these errors, preventable adverse drug reactions, was about $2 billion. The goal of the report was to break what was called the "cycle of inaction" and improve the quality and safety of the delivery of health care in the United States. A four-tiered set of recommendations was made:

1. A national focus to create leadership, resources, tools, and protocols to increase the knowledge base on healthcare safety.

2. Identification and learning from errors with mandatory reporting of events.

3. Raising standards and expectations for improving safety among oversight organizations, purchasers of care, and professional groups.

4. Creation of safer systems in healthcare organizations leading to safe practice at the level where care is delivered—the ultimate goal of all the recommendations.

The next pivotal IOM report, *Crossing the Quality Chasm* (IOM, 2001), called for fundamental changes to the healthcare system to increase the benefits of care while decreasing harm. It acknowledged that the current system does not make the best use of resources due to the impact of errors and overuse. The report also stated that the system is plagued by outmoded systems of work and called for public and private purchasers of care, healthcare organizations, clinicians, and patients to work together to redesign healthcare processes. Six aims for redesign of the healthcare system were established, indicating the new system should be safe, effective, patient centered, timely, efficient, and equitable. The IOM also suggested that HHS take a role in identifying priority conditions and fostering research and improvements in care delivery based on this knowledge. Finally, the report listed 10 principles to guide the redesign of the healthcare system:

1. Care should be based on continuous healing relationships.
2. Care should be customized based on patient needs and values.
3. Patients should have control with shared decision making.
4. There should be shared knowledge and a free flow of information.
5. Evidence-based decision making should be evident.
6. Safety should be designed in as a system priority.
7. There should be transparency to promote informed decision making.
8. The system should anticipate patient needs, not just respond.
9. There should be a continued decrease in waste within the system.
10. There needs to be cooperation among clinicians.

In its 2004 report, *Keeping Patients Safe: Transforming the Work Environment of Nurses,* the IOM was asked by AHRQ to conduct a study with two aims: (1) identify key aspects of the work environment for nurses that were likely to have an impact on patient safety, and (2) recommend potential improvements in nurses' work conditions that would likely increase patient safety. This report emphasized the critical role that nurses play in patient safety and confirmed that the evidence supported the contention that aspects of nurses' work environments were

threats to patient safety. The IOM specifically noted the impact of reengineering or redesign in health care as detrimental by decreasing nurses' trust in administration and diminishing the voice of nurses in patient care at multiple levels. *Keeping Patients Safe* contains a wealth of detailed research evidence about many aspects of work environments and is worth reading in its entirety. Although the report targets nurses, many of the principles and recommendations can be applied to other healthcare providers. The report identified transformational leadership and evidence-based practice for management as two important concepts for improving work environments.

Specific recommendations were made in the following areas:

- Nurse staffing ratios and practices
- National data reporting of staffing
- Increased resources for knowledge and skill development from orientation through length of tenure
- Support for interdisciplinary activities that promote collaboration
- Limits on hours worked
- Design of work environments and care processes with a recommendation to first focus on medication administration and hand washing
- Creating an overall culture of safety within healthcare organizations

The later IOM reports built upon the work of the prior reports and had substantial impact on the healthcare system and professional communities. The imprint of the IOM report recommendations can be seen in later health initiatives.

CMS Initiatives

In November 2001, HHS and CMS announced a quality initiative designed to measure and report on healthcare quality for consumer use with the support of Medicare's quality improvement organizations. The CMS launched the Hospital Quality Initiative in 2003, which aimed to define and standardize hospital data for collection, data transmission requirements, and performance measures. A 10-measure starter set focused on acute myocardial infarction (AMI), heart failure (HF), and pneumonia (PNE). Another 12 measures are under discussion under the auspices of the Hospital Quality Alliance (CMS, 2004).

Building on the Hospital Quality Initiative and work related to nursing home quality, pilot testing of improved measures for nursing home quality occurred in 2002 and 2003. It was reported that about 3 million elderly and disabled Americans received care in approximately 17,000 Medicare and Medicaid certified nursing homes in 2001. As of January 2004, the CMS Nursing Home Quality Initiative listed 14 quality measures on its Nursing Home Compare website for comparison in the areas of delirium, pain (acute and chronic), pressure sores, decline in activities of daily living, bedfast, worsening anxiety or depression, incontinence, indwelling catheters, mobility decline, physical restraints, urinary tract infections, and weight loss. New initiatives in the creation of staffing quality measures and background checks for employees are under development.

The CMS Home Health Quality Initiative was launched in 2003 to assess and report on quality measures for the significant number of individuals receiving home care services. About 3.5 million elderly and disabled Americans received care from nearly 7,000 Medicare certified home health agencies in 2001 (CMS, 2003). The home care quality indicators rely heavily on data provided from the Outcomes and Assessment Information Set (OASIS) introduced in the late 1990s to fulfill provisions of the Balanced Budget Act (BBA) of 1997 related to prospective payment for Medicare patients. The OASIS assessment purports to include core items of a comprehensive assessment for an adult home care patient and provide data for

purposes of outcome-based quality improvement. The National Quality Foundation (NQF) is working with CMS on additional measures that are likely to include improvements related to ambulation, bathing, transferring, managing oral medications, pain interfering with activity, dyspnea, urinary incontinence, acute care hospitalization, discharge to community, and emergent care.

In the ambulatory care domain, CMS is again working with the NQF to endorse a set of standards, building on work initiated by the CMS and the American Medical Association's Physician Consortium for Performance Improvement, which is part of the National Committee for Quality Assurance. The standards are expected to address asthma and respiratory illness, depression and behavioral health, bone conditions such as osteoporosis, arthritis, diabetes, heart disease, hypertension, prenatal care, and prevention/immunization/screening activities (CMS, n.d.).

Additional quality measures for other healthcare settings may be found in the Joint Commission and CMS standards as well as in other accrediting and regulatory bodies' published information. Advanced nurse practitioners should access these other quality standards relevant to their areas. We have presented an array of current activities to underscore the wide and intensive efforts under way to measure and report quality, since it is a major responsibility of healthcare leaders.

Medicare Pay for Performance Initiatives

CMS is developing and implementing a set of pay for performance initiatives to support QI in the care of Medicare beneficiaries. CMS is focusing first on hospitals, physicians, and physician groups, to be followed by home health and dialysis. As part of a demonstration project, incentive payments will be made to hospitals that demonstrate high quality based on data from 34 quality measures relating to five clinical conditions. A similar demonstration project began in selected physician practices across the country in spring 2005. More information about other pay for performance proposals can be accessed on the CMS website.

CONCLUSION

In summary, there is increasing evidence that the healthcare system is fragmented, unacceptably unsafe, and costly. The mounting evidence and public attention have led to unprecedented cooperation among major accrediting, regulatory, and professional groups to address this evolving crisis in health care. As you consider the information just presented, please reflect on the congruencies among the priority areas identified by major agencies like The Joint Commission, AHRQ, and CMS. Today, evidence-based management and decision making are identifying clearer priorities for healthcare improvement. In addition, there is a comprehensive effort to include all settings where health care is delivered, which is especially important considering the shift of services outside of hospitals in recent years.

With advanced knowledge and skills, advanced nurse practitioners must be on the cutting edge in assimilating and acting on quality and performance standards driven by external forces (primarily accrediting and regulatory agencies) and internal mandates (health system corporate entities and organization-wide goals). Success in this area calls for balancing scientific or data-driven changes for improvement with the human side of the equation, recognizing that it takes time for people to embrace change. The creation of a culture of quality can enhance the staff's ability to positively improve care, control costs, and accelerate the pace of change that is needed.

An advanced nurse practitioner will need to hone his or her skills and commitment to mastering the skills of QI so that he or she can serve as a resource and role model to nursing staff. He or she will also be called upon to have an up-to-date knowledge of the current and expected quality measures that relate to clinical expertise and the area in which he or she is employed. The detailed planning for compliance with quality reporting depends heavily upon information management and technology, both system-wide applications and unit-based software systems.

While all these changes in QI and public reporting can feel a bit overwhelming, they are introducing a new era of excitement by refocusing health providers on our mission through outcomes-based QI and enhancing the care delivered to clients. The systematic use of evidence to support or redefine how to best provide care is energizing and supports interdisciplinary collaboration. This focus on quality care and outcomes is assisting healthcare organizations to reinvent themselves and cut through the status quo system (or existing system) that no longer serves us or our patients well.

DISCUSSION QUESTIONS

1. What is the culture of your organization as it relates to QI?

2. Describe and name the overall approach to QI that is used in your organization. What is the nature of your participation in QI?

3. What are the most significant external quality standards or measures for your area(s), and from which accrediting or regulatory bodies are they derived?

4. Identify a current quality concern or improvement opportunity within your scope of responsibility and then consider if there is evidence to support considering a change.

REFERENCES

AHRQ (Agency for Healthcare Research and Quality). (n.d.). Mission statement. Retrieved May 10, 2005, from http://www.ahrq.gov/about/profile.htm

CMS (Centers for Medicare & Medicaid Services). (2003, March 21). Home health quality initiative overview. Retrieved from http://www.cms.hhs.gov /quality/

CMS (Centers for Medicare & Medicaid Services). (2004, January). Nursing home quality initiative. Retrieved from http://www.cms.hhs.gov/quality/

CMS (Centers for Medicare & Medicaid Services). (2004, November 22). Building on the foundation: Hospital measures for public reporting, CMS fact sheet. Retrieved from http://www.cms .hhs.gov/quality/

Deming, W. E. (1986). *Out of the crisis.* Cambridge, MA: MIT Center for Advanced Engineering Study.

GE (General Electric). (n.d.). Six Sigma. Retrieved May 5, 2005, from http://www.ge.com/sixsigma /keyelements.html

Hammer, M., & Champy, J. (1993). *Reengineering the corporation: A manifesto for business revolution.* New York: HarperCollins.

Hudon, S. (2003). Leapfrog standards: Implications for nursing practice. *Nursing Economics, 21*(5), 233–236.

IOM (Institute of Medicine). (2000). *To err is human: Building a safer health system.* Washington, DC: National Academy Press.

IOM (Institute of Medicine). (2001). *Crossing the quality chasm: A new health system for the 21st century.* Washington, DC: National Academy Press.

IOM (Institute of Medicine). (2004). *Keeping patients safe: Transforming the work environment of nurses.* Washington, DC: National Academy Press.

Joiner, B. L. (1994). *Fourth-generation management: The new business consciousness.* New York: McGraw-Hill.

Juran, J. M. (1988). *Juran on planning for quality.* New York: The Free Press.

Milstein, A. (2000). Statement on behalf of the business roundtable. Retrieved May 16, 2005, from http://www.brtable.org/document.cfm/372

Polit, D., & Beck, C. T. (2004). *Nursing research: Principles and methods* (7th ed.). Philadelphia: Williams & Wilkins.

Retsas, A. (2000). Barriers to using research evidence in nursing practice. *Journal of Advanced Nursing, 31*(3), 599–606.

Rooney, J. J., & Vanden Heuvel, L. N. (2004, July). Root cause analysis for beginners. *Quality Progress,* 45–53.

Sackett, D. L., Straus, S. E., Richardson, W. S., Rosenberg, W., & Haynes, R. B. (2000). *Evidence-based medicine: How to practice and teach EBM* (2nd ed.). Edinburgh: Churchill Livingstone.

Scholtes, P., Joiner, B., & Streibel, B. (2003). *The TEAM handbook* (3rd ed.). Madison, WI: Oriel Inc.

Strongwater, S. L., & Pelote, V. (1996). *Clinical process redesign: A facilitator's guide.* Gaithersburg, MD: Aspen.

Studer Group. (n.d.). Health care flywheel. Retrieved May 15, 2005, from http://www.studergroup.com /$spindb.query.2flywheel.studview

CHAPTER 14

Information Technology for Advanced Nursing Practice

Michelle Godin

CHAPTER OBJECTIVES

1. Understand basic computer concepts and components.

2. Appreciate security issues that have evolved as a result of the introduction of technology in health care.

3. Discuss the implications of the Health Insurance Portability and Accountability Act for advanced practice nursing.

4. Discuss the use of information systems for the storage and retrieval of data for individual clients and for populations.

5. Discuss the use of technology for initiating a line of inquiry into a comprehensive database so as to improve patient outcomes.

INTRODUCTION

The use of information technology in today's health care is inescapable. More and more healthcare organizations and provider practices are computerizing patient data for easy retrieval and data analysis. It is essential for advanced nurse practitioners to be knowledgeable about information technology and how it can best be utilized in their daily practice not only for the care of the individual patient but also to evaluate quality, safety, and costs of care.

This chapter begins with the basic computer concepts of the hardware and software components. It then discusses the concept of information privacy and confidentiality. With the advent of technology, controls over the access to patient data became an all-important national concern.

The enactment of the Health Insurance Portability and Accountability Act (HIPAA) created rules to govern the access and release of health information. The chapter ends with information on specific categories of computer applications with which nurses in advanced practice should be the most familiar.

BASIC COMPUTER CONCEPTS

There are two major components with any computer system: the hardware and the software. The hardware component is defined as the physical component of the system. The software component is defined as the elements responsible for the operation of the system and the performance of specific tasks.

Hardware

The hardware of the computer systems is made up of four separate elements. The first element is the central processing unit (CPU). The CPU decides where and when to send information. It functions with the internal clock, which sets the speed. The clock speed of a computer will be identified by its megahertz. Many of the computers today have speeds in gigahertz (1 gigahertz is equal to 1,000 megahertz). The speed to process information is identified by bytes, but you will probably see information listed as KB, or kilobytes, which is 1,000 bytes.

The CPU is where the "brains" and the computer memory reside. There are three types of memory: random access memory, read-only memory, and cache. Random access memory (RAM) is the primary working memory of the computer. Think of it as a scratch pad to do the current work. The data is temporarily stored in this area and is deleted from the system when the computer is shut off. The read-only memory (ROM) is the section where there is permanent storage of information. This section is where the actual programs and instructions for the computer are stored. Cache is a special memory that allows for rapid access to information based on what information is used repeatedly.

Input devices are the second element of the hardware components. The computer system needs a means to receive the data. There are a variety of devices currently available: keyboards, light pens, mice, touch screens, bar code readers, microphones, scanners, cameras, and biometrics scans (retinal or fingerprint). The variety of devices allows for the input of information to be performed under different circumstances. A light pen, touch screen, and bar code reader have an advantage over a keyboard at a patient's bedside, while a mouse or keyboard work better at the nursing station when one is putting in physician orders. When deciding on the type of input device, it is important to assess not only the type of data being entered but the environment in which the entry is occurring.

The third element of the hardware component is the output. The reason for entering data into a computer system is the ability to store, analyze, and retrieve it. The main output device is the screen display. The screens have advanced greatly over time. Depending upon the data to be displayed, the screen size can range from a few inches for handheld devices, such as personal digital assistants (PDAs), to 20 inches for desktop monitors that display patient tracking information. The decision on the type of display is usually dependent upon the type of data being displayed. For instance, clinical documentation with large volumes of data are difficult to display on small handheld screens but can be viewed with greater ease on larger desktop monitors. Some applications will make recommendations on screen size to maximize the functionality of the application.

Printers, which display the collected data in a printed form, are also considered output devices. Most organizations today use either laser or inkjet printers and many of them print in both black-and-white and color. The advent of the multifunctional device has also brought a new output device into the healthcare setting. These devices allow for not only the printing of information but the copying, scanning, or faxing of the information as well. The decision on which type of printer to select is usually based on the primary output requirements. The use of color printing can be based on financial constraints since the current cost of color toner for the printer is significantly higher than the black toner.

The last element of the hardware is the storage devices. Disks, tapes, flash or jump drives, CDs, and DVDs are all different types of storage devices. These devices can serve as both input and output devices. The purpose is to retain information in a storage space separate from the main computer memory. This allows for portability and backup capability of the data.

Software

There are two categories of software utilized by computer systems. The first category is the operating system. This category of software is responsible for handling the tasks that make the computer work, such as figuring out which keys were pressed and in which order, sending messages to printers, and identifying errors and problems. DOS, GUI, UNIX, and Linux are some of the terms referring to types of operating systems.

The larger category of software is the applications. These are the individual programs developed to perform specific functions. Most computers will have as basic features a word processing product (for typing documents and memos) and a spreadsheet product (for calculating numbers and analyzing data). Depending upon the job requirements of the user, a computer may also have a presentation product (used to create slides and posters) and a database management product (for categorizing and analyzing large amounts of data).

SECURITY CONSIDERATIONS

When using any type of computer in a healthcare setting, there are two levels of security to protect patient information. The first type is the physical security of the device(s) which possess a dilemma. Workstations should be positioned in such a way to protect them from unauthorized access while at the same time ensuring that they are visible. However, safety concerns must be balanced with the need to avoid interruptions of staff when using the computer, along with the need to avoid placing the computers in direct view of unauthorized users. A computer in a staff lounge or locker room might be great for staff to access their hospital e-mail, but it should not have software that would allow access to patient information. Mobile devices should be stored in locked areas when not in use to prevent theft as well as unauthorized access.

The second type of security is password security. To protect access to data and information, multiple layers of passwords are essential. The more sensitive the data is, the more layers that should be required to access the data. Application passwords grant a user access to a specific application. For example, advanced nurse practitioners might need access to a certain program to document patient care, but the housekeeping staff would have no reason for access to that application. The next layer of the password security is location. In this layer, the user's access to the application is limited by the department or location of the device. As with the previous example, while all nurses have access to document, only those nurses who work on the psychiatric unit will be able to access and document those particular patient records. The last layer of security is based on the job requirement. Access to an application is given but only to the specific sections of the application that are necessary for the user to perform his or her job. An example of this is a nurse's aide, whose job requires him or her to document vital signs. He or she is given access to document that particular element of the patients' care, but will not be able to access any other part of the patient record.

The use of all the layers of security allows an organization to maintain the integrity of the patient information and protect the privacy and confidentiality of the data. The main focus of the security is to give access to individuals based on what their job requirements are and only what they need to perform that job efficiently and effectively.

INFORMATION PRIVACY AND CONFIDENTIALITY ISSUES

The Health Insurance Portability and Accountability Act (HIPAA) was enacted by the U.S. Congress in 1996. It comprises two titles or sections. Title I addresses the issue of healthcare access, portability, and renewability. The focus of this section is on the rules governing an individual's ability to obtain healthcare coverage. Table 14-1 outlines the details.

Title II addresses preventing healthcare fraud and abuse. The second title is of particular importance to healthcare organizations and their employees, including the advanced nurse practitioner. It is broken down into five sections: privacy rule, transactions and code set rule, security rule, unique identifiers rule, and the enforcement rule. The privacy rule became effective on April 14, 2003, and established the regulations for the use and disclosure of protected health information (PHI). PHI is any information about health status, provision of health care, or payment for health care that can be linked to an individual. It requires reasonable effort to disclose only the minimum amount of information and the use of reason-

able steps to ensure the confidentiality of communication with others. This rule also requires organizations to appoint a privacy officer and a person responsible for receiving complaints and to train all members of the workforce in the proper care of PHI.

The transactions and code set rule became effective on October 6, 2004, and requires that all medical providers who file claims electronically use HIPAA standard codes to be paid. These codes were developed to force a standardization of the data stream from each organization to the insurance companies.

The security rule was implemented on April 21, 2005, and complements the privacy rule by outlining three types of security safeguards necessary for compliance. The administrative safeguards are policies and procedures designed to show how an organization will comply with the act. Physical safeguards work to control physical access to protect against the inappropriate access to protected data. Technical safeguards allow for the control of access to computer systems and protect communications containing PHI transmitted electronically. Table 14-2 lists some of the specific controls that an organization must have in place to comply with this specific rule.

The enforcement rule went into effect on March 16, 2006, and set a monetary penalty for violating the HIPAA rules. The last rule is the establishment of unique identifiers. This rule

---

TABLE 14-1   HIPAA Title I Highlights

- Regulates the availability and breadth of group and individual health insurance plans.
- Prohibits any group health plan from creating eligibility rules or assess premiums for individuals in the plan based on health status, medical history, genetic information, or disability.
- Limits restrictions that a group health plan can place on benefits for preexisting conditions.
- Forbids individual health plans from denying coverage or imposing preexisting condition exclusions on individuals who have at least 18 months of creditable group coverage under any group, state, or federal health plans at the time they seek individual insurance.

TABLE 14-2	HIPAA Security Rule Control Safeguards

Administrative Safeguards

■ Designation of a privacy officer.

■ Indication of classes of employees who have access to PHI (must be restricted on a need-to-know basis).

■ Demonstrate ongoing training and education.

■ Document the process involved in auditing records. Audits should be conducted both on a routine basis and when an event occurs.

Physical Safeguards

■ Oversight of addition and removal of hardware and software from the network.

■ Equipment with PHI should be monitored.

■ Hardware and software must be limited to properly authorized individuals.

■ Workstations should be removed from high-traffic areas and monitor screens should not be in direct view of the public.

Technical Safeguards

■ Encryption software must be used to protect information.

■ Measures must be taken to ensure that data is not altered in an unauthorized manner.

---

went into effect on May 23, 2007, and established a unique national provider identifier (NPI) for every healthcare provider who files healthcare forms. Every healthcare organization and provider must possess an NPI number when submitting claims.

The enactment of HIPAA has forced each and every healthcare entity to review and reassess its controls over who has access to information. The auditing of patient records is not limited to who accessed a specific patient record. It goes to the level of whether or not an individual had reason to access the individual record and which specific information was accessed.

HOSPITAL INFORMATION SYSTEMS

Computers have been around since the 1930s, but it was not until the 1950s that hospitals began to utilize the technology. Not surpris-

ing, financial and statistical calculations were the first applications to be utilized within the hospital setting. Patient charges, payroll, inventory control, and patient statistics (birth and death rates) were more easily and rapidly calculated utilizing the computer than by manual methods. The first hospital computer was developed in the late 1960s to address clinical applications and was very unsuccessful. Hardware and software were expensive and inflexible, and the input devices were expensive and unreliable.

A hospital information system (HIS) refers to computer systems that support patient care. There are two categories of systems within a hospital setting: clinical systems, which allow the organization to provide, monitor, and evaluate patient care; and administrative systems, which allow the organization to monitor the quality of care as well as the revenue and expenditures related to the delivery of care.

Clinical Systems

Nursing Information Systems

A nursing information system (NIS) is one of the major types of clinical systems. This type of system allows for the assessment of the patient and the documentation of the care and teaching delivered. There are two approaches to documentation.

The first is menu-driven screens that present content in prearranged categories that allow the practitioner to select the most applicable items. The categories are designed around the nursing process from admission through to discharge based on the nursing diagnosis. Most are modeled after the paper forms currently in use.

The second approach is to utilize care protocols. In this type of documentation, a specific protocol is selected based on the admission diagnosis. The protocol lists the elements of care to be initiated and monitored during each patient day. The documentation is related to the ability of the patient to achieve the established daily protocol goals.

There are many advantages to an NIS, but there are also some disadvantages, as can be seen in Table 14-3.

Clinical Information Processing Systems

Another major type of clinical system is the clinical information processing system. These systems are responsible for recording and storing patient data from a variety of clinical settings. Many departments have specific systems that facilitate their own unique activities (e.g., medical records, operating room, emergency department, home care). Other systems cross departments to assist in the delivery of patient care. The specific systems of order entry, patient monitoring, radiology, laboratory, and pharmacy systems will be reviewed in more detail.

TABLE 14-3　Advantages and Disadvantages in Utilizing a Nursing Information System

Advantages

- Increased observation due to forced recall.
- Increased accuracy and reliability of observations. If done in real time, no need to write on paper and then transcribe. No time to forget.
- Legibility with less time required to read and interpret accurately.
- Decrease time in writing notes.
- Available for statistical analysis. Elements already coded and can be selected.
- Teaching tool to guide observations. Can develop specific elements to help the staff with what they need to look for.
- Errors and omissions are decreased or eliminated with protocol followed.

Disadvantages

- Charting may be longer due to need for review of content prior to selection.
- Wording may not match the user's language. Standard dictionaries are not readily available.
- Pre-established content and need to make sure protocols are individualized for patients with comorbidities.

The beginning point of these systems is the order entry process. Orders are entered into a computer system, which processes the orders and sends information to specific departments requesting services. The receiving departments, through requisitions, process the order and perform a test or deliver a service.

Order Entry

There are two methods of order entry. One is simple data entry by selecting items from menus. The other method is to utilize sets of orders based on clinical guidelines or best practices. This type of order entry can be quicker depending upon the amount of flexibility in completing individual orders. Many orders sets will have multiple orders covering items such as antibiotics or pain medication to allow the practitioner to individualize the type and dose of drug most appropriate for a specific patient. The order sets can also include directions for other departments such as holding meals when a specific radiology exam is ordered and having the pharmacy send the preparations for tests.

An advantage of an order entry system is the rapid initiation of orders. Orders are entered and transmitted, and the receiving department will be notified of the request for services in real time. Additionally, as the orders are entered, the system can prompt for prerequisite pieces of information that must be entered before an order can be initiated. An example would be the requirement for the medical reason for an exam on a radiology order before the order is sent to radiology to be performed, thereby documenting the medical necessity. This assures that important pieces of data regarding the patient are recorded and communicated.

As a response to ongoing patient safety issues, the trend in today's healthcare environment is for physician order entry. This type of order processing requires the physician to input the orders directly into the computer system, thereby eliminating any transcription errors. With this method there is an additional advantage in the ability of an order entry system to provide the physician with alerts regarding such factors as allergies and medication interactions. These alerts warn a physician of a potential problem and offer options for the physician to change the orders before they are carried out.

Patient Monitoring

Patient monitoring systems include all types of devices that automatically collect data regarding the patient condition. Cardiac monitors, IV pumps, pulse oximeters, and blood pressure cuffs are some examples of these devices. The advantage of this type of system is the ability to quickly detect a deviation in a patient's condition and alert the appropriate personnel, freeing up clinicians from watching the monitors and focusing on the patient.

Radiology

A radiology imaging system allows for the processing of an exam from the scheduling of exams to the storage of images. Most systems today provide for the images using digital technology rather than film. Providers can be sitting at any desktop anywhere and view the images on the monitor. This allows for rapid turnaround in the treatment of injuries especially during the evening and night hours. On-call physicians can view images from their homes to immediately begin initiating treatment plans.

Laboratory

A laboratory information system allows for the processing of lab specimens. These systems receive the request from the order entry system and provide the results to the clinicians. Many of these systems report the results directly into an HIS. Within the HIS, a patient's data can be readily viewed and trended over time and can be viewed from any computer. Inherent in the system is avoidance of duplication of tests within predetermined time frames and alerts for results outside established parameters (both high and low). These alerts can be tied directly to many communication tools such as PDAs to immediately alert clinicians of potential problems and allow for rapid treatment.

Pharmacy

The ability to track the ordering, dispensing and administration of drugs is at the heart of a pharmacy information system. Beginning with the ordering of the pharmaceuticals, the pharmacy systems have been extremely beneficial to assist in the delivery of quality care. The primary advantage of these systems is the prevention of medication errors. Once orders are entered into the system, the orders are reviewed and verified by pharmacists. The orders are checked against the patient's allergy profile, a drug interaction profile, and available laboratory results to assure that any foreseeable problems from the drugs will be avoided. Medication dispensing devices both within the pharmacy and on the nursing units create a system where the proper drug is selected. In the pharmacy, the robotic system selects the drug based on the order and delivers it to the nursing unit. On the nursing unit, the nurse selects the drug from the dispensing device by selecting the correct patient and drug. The device then opens only the drawer where the drug is contained. This allows for accurate record keeping of administration of medications and can keep the pharmacy aware of drug levels in the devices.

Administrative Systems

Administrative systems assist the organization in supporting the patient care process and can be used to monitor patient outcomes so as to improve quality and safety. Table 14-4 lists a variety of systems that are considered administrative systems.

A specific type of administrative system used in most healthcare organizations is a staffing and scheduling system. This system allows for the efficient and effective scheduling of both patients and staff. Patient scheduling systems

---

TABLE 14-4 Categories of Administrative Information Systems and Their Uses

System

- Human resources
- Payroll
- Risk management
- Quality management
- Financial systems
- Material management

Uses

- Track applicants and employee information regarding work status, credentials, and performance evaluation
- Time and attendance with salary data for proper accounting of pay
- Occurrence and incident tracking for a variety of issues involving patients and employees
- Review of patient outcome data to help identify trends and make performance improvements
- Includes accounting and contract management for reimbursement
- Manages the charging and inventory of supplies for the organization

---

allow the organization to schedule appointments for services that maximize the equipment and the staff in the best possible manner. Staff scheduling systems perform a similar function. Staff scheduling systems have two components: a scheduling component and a staffing component. The scheduling component develops a plan for when the staff will be working. Most schedules are developed 4–6 weeks in advance, balancing employee days on and off with requests for vacation and holiday. The staffing component uses a patient volume indicator (visits, patient days, acuity, or hours per patient day) to determine what the required staff needs for a department.

Decision support systems are specialized administrative systems that bring together all the data that has been collected in the clinical systems as well as the administrative systems. The data can then be used by administrators or clinicians to help in the decision-making process by identifying trends, developing models for future endeavors, and demonstrating the financial position of projects.

The ability to utilize a decision support system requires the capability to query the database effectively. The first step in the query is to get the question right. Which specific data elements are necessary? The ability to identify the exact elements that are needed is crucial. Time can be wasted on running and rerunning database queries if the elements are not correct. Another question to be asked is, In which database are the elements located? If the elements are not in the same database, additional querying skills might be required to achieve the right elements.

EDUCATIONAL APPLICATIONS

There is an additional computer application that can be useful for any professional—applications developed specifically for educational functions. The use of computers and the Internet have changed the face of education and training forever. Many individuals use the Internet daily, seeking information that now can come from anywhere in the world. The use of educational applications, either on a computer or through the Internet, allows individuals to gain knowledge at their own pace and at a time that is convenient for the individuals.

Educational applications have three main uses: to provide education, to evaluate education, and to determine the competency.

Provide Education

Education applications provide education in a variety of methods, including the following:

- Drills and practice sessions: The computer serves as a supplement for the teacher. The main concepts and new material are presented by the teacher while the computer allows the student to practice.
- Tutorial: This method provides certain original portions of the content. It relies on coaching the student through a situation in sequences in which the student can discover the correct answers.
- Simulation and gaming: This is used when a student has received the basic information about a topic and then uses the information with the computer to gain a deeper understanding. This method enables the student to explore situations that might be too expensive, dangerous, or time consuming in real life, in which the ramifications of wrong answers can endanger or hurt patients.

Evaluate Education

Using the computer to evaluate education allows the instructor or student to determine whether the content of educational lessons has been learned. The programs are geared to the specific tasks, abilities, and progress of the student. The systems have the ability to provide feedback and reinforcement to the student regarding their performance. For the instructors, reports from the system can be used to assess the progress of the student and where there are potential areas that need improvement.

Determine Competency

The last step in the educational process is to determine competency in the subject matter. The Nursing Competency Licensing Exam (NCLEX) is a perfect example of that process in action. Graduate nurses take a computerized exam in which the computer determines if they have reached a level of knowledge to allow a professional license to be issued.

One of the advantages of an educational computer system is that the applications can be used for both staff and patients. They can be used to orient new staff and train staff and patients on the functionality of new equipment. Because the applications are programmable, they can be adapted for any skill level and in any language that is required. This is of great benefit for patients who may have limited medical background and would like to review information privately and at a time of their own convenience.

There is another advantage, which is the effect the applications have on teaching itself. Educational applications have helped shift the emphasis from the teacher and teaching to the learner and learning. Students can be independent and supplement their learning with additional methods that are more suited to their learning style.

Instructors also benefit since they are able to allow the educational applications to provide content better suited to the computer simulation and focus on the students. Some educational applications have also assisted in teaching content where there is no faculty staff that possesses expertise in the content. These same applications can also assist in presenting specific disease situations in which there is a lack of clinical exposure.

CONCLUSION

This chapter presented a look into the growing and ever-changing world of information technology. Every day one hears about a new device or application that has been developed. Each practitioner must evaluate that information and determine what is usable in their practice to maintain good quality patient outcomes.

DISCUSSION QUESTIONS

1. Describe the hardware components that you currently use in practice. Based on this chapter, what do you see as the strengths and weaknesses of this system?

2. Describe the software components that you currently use in practice. Based on this chapter, what do you see as the strengths and weaknesses of this system?

3. What security issues have you faced in your practice and/or what opportunities for improvement exist in your current system?

4. How will HIPAA affect your role as an advanced practice nurse? How does this differ for each of the various advanced nursing practice roles?

5. Consider a current clinical issue or concern in your practice. What information do you need to better understand the scope of the issue? Is there data stored in the system that would help you understand the issue? If so, how can you retrieve it? If not, what new data would you need to enter the system?

CHAPTER 15

The Electronic Health Record and Clinical Informatics

Emily B. Barey

CHAPTER OBJECTIVES

1. Describe the common components of an electronic health record.

2. Assess the benefits of implementing an electronic health record.

3. Explore the ownership of an electronic health record.

4. Evaluate the flexibility of the electronic health record in meeting the needs of clinicians and patients.

INTRODUCTION

The significance of electronic health records (EHRs) to nursing cannot be underestimated. Although EHRs on the surface suggest a simple automation of clinical documentation, in fact their implications are broad, ranging from the means by which care is delivered to the types of interactions nurses have with patients, to the use of technology in the research surrounding EHRs that will inform the nursing practice of tomorrow. A basic knowledge of EHRs and nursing informatics is now considered by many to be an entry-level nursing competency. As stated by participants in the Technology Informatics Guiding Education Reform (TIGER, 2006) summit on evidence and informatics transforming nursing, "the nation is working full-speed to realize the 10-year goal of Electronic Health Records for its citizens" (p. 1). Nurses must become active participants in this effort to capture healthcare information, generate knowledge, and enhance patient care. "This is a critical juncture for nurses, who comprise 55% of the healthcare workforce, number more than 3 million, and who must become more aware and involved at every level of the Informatics Revolution" (TIGER, p. 1). Although EHR standards are evolving and barriers to adoption remain, the collective work has a positive momentum that can only benefit clinician and patient alike.

This trend has been underscored by the passage of the Health Information Technology for Economic and Clinical Health Act of 2009 (HITECH). It is essential that this competency be developed so that nurses can participate fully in the changing world of healthcare information technology.

This chapter has four goals. The first is to describe the common components of an EHR. The second and third are to review the benefits of implementing an EHR and to provide an overview of successful ownership of an EHR, including nursing's role in promoting the safe adoption of the use of an EHR in day-to-day practice. The fourth goal is to discuss the flexibility of an EHR in meeting the needs of both clinicians and patients, including an introduction to interoperability.

SETTING THE STAGE

The U.S. healthcare system faces an enormous challenge in trying to improve the quality of care and simultaneously control costs. EHRs have been proposed as one solution to achieve this goal (Institute of Medicine [IOM], 2001). In January 2004, President George W. Bush raised the profile of EHRs in his State of the Union address by outlining a plan to ensure that most Americans have an EHR by 2014. He stated that "by computerizing health records we can avoid dangerous medical mistakes, reduce costs, and improve care" (Bush, 2004). This proclamation generated an increased demand for understanding EHRs and ways to promote their adoption, but relatively few healthcare organizations were motivated to pursue more rapid adoption of EHRs. The Healthcare Information and Management Systems Society (HIMSS) has been tracking EHR adoption since 2005 through its "Stage 7"

Award and reports that most of the country's healthcare organizations are in Stage 0–3, reflecting only the basic components of laboratory, radiology, and pharmacy ancillaries installed; a clinical data repository including a controlled medical vocabulary; and simple nursing documentation and clinical decision support available (HIMSS, 2010b).

Since then, President Barack Obama's administration has passed the American Recovery and Reinvestment Act of 2009 (ARRA), including the HITECH Act to specifically incentivize health organizations and providers to become "meaningful users" of EHRs. These incentives will come in the form of increased reimbursement rates from the Centers for Medicaid and Medicare Services (CMS) and ultimately will result in a payment penalty to the healthcare organization if adoption of an EHR is not obtained by January 2015. The final rule was published by the Department of Health and Human Services (DHHS) in July 2010 for the first phase of implementation, and more details are expected to be completed for the second and third phases in 2011 and 2012, leading up to the 2015 deadline (DHHS, 2010).

COMPONENTS
Overview

Before the ARRA, there were several definitions of EHRs, each with its own terminology and developed with a different audience in mind. These sources included the federal government (Certification Commission for Healthcare Information Technology, 2007), the IOM (2003), the HIMSS (2007), and the National Institutes of Health (Robert Wood Johnson [RWJ], 2006). Under ARRA, there is now an explicit requirement for providers and hospitals to use a certified EHR that meets a set of standard functional definitions to be eligible for the increased reimbursement incentive. DHHS has granted two organizations the authority to accredit EHRs: The Drummond Group and the Certification Commission for Healthcare Information Technology. These bodies are authorized to test and certify EHR vendors against the standards and test procedures developed by the National Institute of Standards and Technology (NIST) and endorsed by the Office of the National Coordinator for Health Information Technology for EHRs.

The NIST test procedure includes 45 certification criteria ranging from the basic ability to record patient demographics, document vital signs, and maintain an up-to-date problem list, to more complex functions, such as electronic exchange of clinical information and patient summary records (NIST, 2010). **Box 15-1** lists the 45 certification criteria outlined by NIST.

Despite ARRA, the IOM definition also remains a valid reference point. This definition is useful because it has distilled all the possible features of an EHR into eight essential components with an emphasis on functions that promote patient safety, a universal denominator that everyone in health care can accept. The eight components include (1) health information and data, (2) results management, (3) order entry management, (4) decision support, (5) electronic communication and connectivity, (6) patient support, (7) administrative processes, and (8) reporting and population health management (IOM, 2003). Each is described in more detail here, and with the exception of EHR infrastructure functions, such as security and privacy management, controlled medical vocabularies, and interoperability standards, the 45 NIST standards easily map into the IOM categories.

Health Information and Data

Health information and data comprise the patient data required to make sound clinical decisions including demographics, medical and nursing diagnoses, medication lists, allergies, and test results (IOM, 2003).

Results Management

Results management is the ability to manage results of all types electronically, including laboratory and radiology procedure reports, both current and historical (IOM, 2003).

Order Entry Management

Order entry management is the ability of a clinician to enter medication and other care orders, including laboratory, microbiology, pathology, radiology, nursing, supply orders, ancillary services, and consultations directly into a computer (IOM, 2003).

Decision Support

Decision support is the computer reminders and alerts issued in an attempt to improve the diagnosis and care of a patient, including screening for correct drug selection and dosing, medication interactions with other medications, preventive health reminders in such areas as vaccinations, health risk screening and detection, and clinical guidelines for patient disease treatment (IOM, 2003).

Electronic Communication and Connectivity

Electronic communication and connectivity is the online communication among healthcare team members, their care partners, and patients including e-mail, Web messaging, and an integrated health record within and across settings, institutions, and telemedicine (IOM, 2003).

Patient Support

Patient support is the patient education and self-monitoring tools, including interactive computer-based patient education, home telemonitoring, and telehealth systems (IOM, 2003).

Administrative Processes

Administrative processes are the electronic scheduling, billing, and claims management systems, including electronic scheduling for inpatient and outpatient visits and procedures, electronic insurance eligibility validation, claim authorization and prior approval, identification of possible research study participants, and drug recall support (IOM, 2003).

BOX 15-1	NIST Certification Criteria for Electronic Health Records

Criterion Number	Certification Criteria
§170.302(a)	Drug–drug, drug–allergy interaction checks
§170.302(b)	Drug formulary checks
§170.302(c)	Maintain up-to-date problem list
§170.302(d)	Maintain active medication list
§170.302(e)	Maintain active medication allergy list
§170.302(f)(1)	Vital signs
§170.302(f)(2)	Calculate body mass index
§170.302(f)(3)	Plot and display growth charts
§170.302(g)	Smoking status
§170.302(h)	Incorporate laboratory test results
§170.302(i)	Generate patient lists
§170.302(j)	Medication reconciliation
§170.302(k)	Submission to immunization registries
§170.302(l)	Public health surveillance
§170.302(m)	Patient specific education resources
§170.302(n)	Automated measure calculation
§170.302(o)	Access control
§170.302(p)	Emergency access
§170.302(q)	Automatic log-off
§170.302(r)	Audit log
§170.302(s)	Integrity
§170.302(t)	Authentication
§170.302(u)	General encryption
§170.302(v)	Encryption when exchanging electronic health information
§170.302(w)	Accounting of disclosures (optional)
§170.304(a)	Computerized provider order entry
§170.304(b)	Electronic prescribing
§170.304(c)	Record demographics
§170.304(d)	Patient reminders
§170.304(e)	Clinical decision support
§170.304(f)	Electronic copy of health information
§170.304(g)	Timely access
§170.304(h)	Clinical summaries

BOX 15-1	NIST Certification Criteria for Electronic Health Records *(continued)*

§170.304(i)	Exchange clinical information and patient summary record
§170.304(j)	Calculate and submit clinical quality measures
§170.306(a)	Computerized provider order entry
§170.306(b)	Record demographics
§170.306(c)	Clinical decision support
§170.306(d)(1)	Electronic copy of health information
§170.306(d)(2)	Electronic copy of health information

Note: For discharge summary

§170.306(e)	Electronic copy of discharge instructions
§170.306(f)	Exchange clinical information and patient summary record
§170.306(g)	Reportable lab results
§170.306(h)	Advance directives
§170.306(i)	Calculate and submit clinical quality measures

Source: National Institute of Standards and Technology (NIST). (2010). Meaningful use test measures: Approved test procedures. Retrieved from http://healthcare.nist.gov/use_testing/finalized_requirements.html

Reporting and Population Health Management

Reporting and population health management are the data collection tools to support public and private reporting requirements including data represented in a standardized terminology and machine-readable format (IOM, 2003).

NIST's criteria do not provide an exhaustive list of all possible features and functions of an EHR. Different vendor EHR systems may combine different components in their offerings, and often a single set of EHR components does not meet the needs of all clinicians and patient populations. For example, a pediatric setting may demand functions for immunization management, growth tracking, and more robust order entry features to include weight-based dosing (Spooner & The Council on Clinical Information Technology, 2007). These types of features may not be provided by all EHR sys-

tems, and it is important to consider EHR certification as a minimum standard.

ADVANTAGES

There are mixed reviews of the advantages of an EHR. Much has been written about the potential promise of reduced cost, improved quality, and outcomes, but very few of these gains have been substantiated except anecdotally (Sidorov, 2006). Possible methods to estimate EHR benefits include using vendor-supplied data that have been retrieved from their customer systems, synthesizing and applying studies of overall EHR value, creating logical engineering models of EHR value, summarizing focused studies of elements of EHR value, and conducting and applying information from site visits (Thompson, Osheroff, Classen, & Sittig, 2007). However, the time and effort involved completing this work is exacerbated by the fact that historically there was no standard by which to measure adoption or expected benefits (RWJ, 2006; Thompson et al.). With the advent of ARRA there are now 25 meaningful use objectives for eligible providers and 24 meaningful use objectives for eligible hospitals (CMS, 2010a). In addition, the final rule calls for providers to report on three required clinical quality measures and three additional quality measures of their choice from a list of 44 possible measures (CMS, 2010b). Eligible hospitals must report on 15 clinical quality measures. Although these objectives and measures will provide a universal benchmark for moving forward in terms of EHR benefits, for most healthcare organizations these outcomes alone will not provide sufficient return on investment to warrant the capital investment that must be made to implement an EHR, and additional benefits will continue to be sought.

The four most common benefits are (1) an increased delivery of guideline-based care, (2) an enhanced capacity to perform surveillance and monitoring for disease conditions, (3) a reduction in medication errors, and (4) a decreased use of care (Chaudhry et al., 2006). These findings were echoed by two similar literature reviews. The first focused on the use of informatics systems for chronic illness and found that the processes of care most positively impacted were guideline adherence; visit frequency (i.e., a decrease in emergency department visits); provider documentation; patient treatment adherence; and screening and testing (Dorr et al., 2007).

The second review was a cost–benefit analysis of health information technology completed by the Agency for Healthcare Research and Quality that studied the value of an EHR in the ambulatory care and pediatric settings, including its overall economic value. The Agency for Healthcare Research and Quality highlighted the common findings already described and also noted that most of the data available for review came from six leading healthcare organizations in the United States, underscoring the challenge of generalizing these results to the broader healthcare industry (Shekelle, Morton, & Keeler, 2006). As noted previously by the HIMSS Stage 7 Awards, the challenge to generalize results persists in the hospital arena and elsewhere, with fewer than 1% of U.S. hospitals or eight leading organizations providing most of the experience with a comprehensive EHR to date (HIMSS, 2010d). Finally, all three literature reviews cited here indicated that a limited number of hypothesis-testing studies have been carried out, and even fewer that reported cost data.

The descriptive studies, however, do have value and should not be hastily dismissed. Although not as rigorous in their design, they do describe the advantages of an EHR well and often include useful implementation recommendations learned from practical experience. According to these types of reviews, EHR advantages include simple benefits, such as no longer having to interpret poor handwriting and handwritten orders, reduced turnaround time for laboratory results in an emergency department, and decreased time to administration of the first dose of antibiotics in an inpatient nursing unit (Husk & Waxman, 2004; Smith et al., 2004).

In the ambulatory care setting, evidence of improved management of cardiac-related risk factors in patients with diabetes and effective patient notification of medication recalls have been demonstrated (Jain et al., 2005; Reed & Bernard, 2005). Two other unique advantages that have great potential are the ability to use the EHR and decision support functions to identify patients who qualify for research studies or who qualify for prescription drug benefits offered by pharmaceutical companies at safety-net clinics and hospitals (Embi et al., 2005; Poprock, 2005).

The HIMSS Davies Award may be the best resource for combined quantitative and qualitative results of successful EHR implementation. The Davies Award recognizes healthcare organizations that have achieved both excellence in implementation and value from health information technology (HIMSS, 2010a). One recent winner demonstrated a significant avoidance of medication errors because of barcode scanning alerts, a \$3 million decrease in medical records expenses as a result of going paperless, and a 5% reduction of duplicate laboratory orders by using computerized provider order entry alerting (HIMSS, 2010c). Another recent winner also noted a 13% decrease in adverse drug reactions through the use of computerized physician order entry, and a decrease in methicillin-resistant *Staphylococcus aureus* nosocomial infections from 9.8 per 10,000 discharges to 6.4 per 10,000 discharges in less than a year using the EHR flagging function that made clinicians immediately aware that contact precautions were required for methicillin-resistant *S. aureus*–positive patients (HIMSS, 2009). At both organizations, qualitative and quantitative evidence of high end-user adoption and satisfaction with use of the EHR was noted as well.

Without an EHR system, any of these benefits would be very difficult and costly to accomplish. Thus, despite limited standards and published studies, there is enough evidence to warrant pursuing widespread implementation of the EHR (Halamka, 2006) and certainly enough as discussed here to warrant further study of the use and benefit of EHRs.

OWNERSHIP

The implementation of an EHR has the potential to affect every member of a healthcare organization. The process of becoming a successful owner of an EHR has multiple steps and requires integrating the EHR into both the organization's day-to-day operations and long-term vision, and into the clinician's day-to-day practice. All members of the healthcare organization—from the executive level to the clinician at the point of care—must feel a sense of ownership to make the implementation successful for themselves, their colleagues, and their patients. Successful ownership of an EHR may be defined in part by the level of clinician adoption of the tool, and this section reviews key steps and strategies for the selection, implementation

and evaluation, and optimization of an EHR in pursuit of that goal.

Historically, many systems were developed locally by the information technology department of a healthcare organization. It was not unusual for software developers to be employed by the organization to write needed systems and interfaces between them. As commercial offerings were introduced and matured, it became less and less common to see homegrown or locally developed systems. As a result, the first step of ownership is typically a vendor selection process for a commercially available EHR.

During this step, it is important to survey the organization's level of interest, identify possible barriers to participation, document desired functions of an EHR, and assess the willingness to fund the implementation (Holbrook, Keshavjee, Troyan, Pray, & Ford, 2003). Although clinicians should drive the project, the assessment should also include the needs and readiness of the executive leadership, information technology, and project management teams. It is essential that leadership understands that this type of project is as much about redesigning clinical work as it is about technically automating it, and that they agree to accept accountability for its success (Goddard, 2000). In addition, this preacquisition phase should concentrate on understanding the current state of the health information technology industry to identify appropriate questions and the next steps in the selection process (American Organization of Nurse Executives, 2006). These first steps begin to identify any organizational risks that might threaten a successful implementation and pave the way for initiating a change management process to educate the organization about the future state of delivering health care with an EHR system.

The second step of the selection process is to select a system based on the organization's current and predicted needs. It is common during this phase to see a demonstration of several vendors' EHR products. Based on the completed needs assessment, the organization should establish key evaluation criteria to compare the different vendors and products. These criteria should include both subjective and objective items that cover such topics as common clinical workflows, decision support, reporting, usability, technical build requirements, and maintenance of the system. Providing the vendor with these guidelines will ensure that the process meets the organization's needs; however, it is also essential to let the vendor demonstrate a proposed future state from its own perspective. This process is critical to ensuring that the vendor's vision and the organization's vision are well aligned. It also helps spark additional dialogue about the possible future state of clinical work at the organization and the change required in obtaining it. Such demonstrations not only provide the ability to compare and contrast the features and functions of different systems, but also are a good way to engage the organization's members in being a part of this strategic decision.

Implementation planning should occur concurrently with the selection process, particularly the assessment of the scope of the work, initial sequencing of the EHR components to be implemented, and resources required. However, it begins in earnest once a vendor and product have been selected. In addition to further refining the implementation plan, participants in the planning process must identify key metrics by which to measure the EHR's success. An organization may realize numerous benefits from implementing an EHR. The organization should choose metrics that match its overall strategy and goals in the coming years and may include expected improvements in financial, quality, and clinical outcomes. Commonly used metrics include reducing the number of duplicate laboratory tests through duplicate orders alerting, reducing the number of adverse drug events through the use of barcode medication administration, meaningful use objectives and measures, and those EHR advantages mentioned previously. To be sure that the benefits

are realized, it is important to avoid choosing so many that they become meaningless or unobtainable, to carefully and practically define those that are chosen, to measure before and after the implementation, and to assign accountability to a member of the organization to ensure the work is completed.

End-user adoption of the EHR is also essential to realizing its benefits. Clinicians must be engaged to use the EHR successfully in their practice and daily workflows so that data may be captured to drive the decision support that underlies so many of the advantages and metrics described. To promote adoption, a change management plan must be developed in conjunction with the EHR implementation plan. The most effective change management plans offer end users several exposures to the system and relevant workflows in advance of its use, and continue through the go-live and post-live time periods. Successful pre-live strategies include end users' involvement as subject-matter experts to validate the EHR workflow design and content build, hosting end-user usability testing sessions, shadowing end users in their current daily work in parallel with the new system, and formal training activities. The goal of these pre-live activities is not only to ensure that the EHR implementation will meet end-user needs but also to assess the impact of the new EHR on current workflow and process. The larger the impact, the more change management is required above and beyond system training. For example, simulation laboratory experiences may be offered to ensure a more thorough dress rehearsal for a significant workflow change, executive leadership may need to convey their support and expectations of clinicians about a new way of working, and generally more anticipatory guidance is required to communicate to those impacted.

Training may be delivered via a variety of media, and often a combination of approaches works best, including classroom time, electronic learning, independent exercises, and peer-to-peer support "at the elbow." Training must be workflow based and reflect real clinical processes. Training must also be planned and budgeted for through the post-live period to ensure that competency with the system is assessed at go-live and that any necessary retraining or reinforcements are made in the 30 to 60 days post-live. This not only promotes the reliability and safe use of the system as it was designed, but also can have a positive impact on end users' morale, giving them the sense that they are being supported beyond the initial go-live period and have an opportunity to move from basic skills to advanced proficiency with the system.

Finally, the implementation plan should account for the long-term optimization of the EHR. This step is commonly overlooked and often results in benefits falling short of expectations because the resources are not available to realize them permanently. It also often means the difference between end users of EHRs merely surviving the change as opposed to becoming savvy about how to adopt the EHR as another powerful clinical tool, akin to the stethoscope. Optimization activities of the EHR should be considered a routine part of the organization's operations, should be resourced accordingly, and should emphasize the continued involvement of clinician users to identify ways that the EHR can enable meeting the overall mission of the organization. Many organizations start an implementation of an EHR with the goal of transforming their care delivery and operations. Rather than simply automating a previously manual or fragmented process, transformation often includes improving the process to realize better patient care outcomes or added efficiency. Although some transformation is experienced with the initial use of the system, most of this work is done post-implementation and is reliant on widespread clinician adoption of the EHR. As such, it makes optimization a critical component to successful ownership of an EHR. **Box 15-2** reviews the barriers to, and methods for, successful acceptance of EHRs.

FLEXIBILITY AND EXPANDABILITY

Health care is as unique as the patients themselves. It is delivered in a variety of settings, for a variety of reasons over the course of a patient's lifetime. In addition, patients rarely receive all their care from one healthcare organization, and choice is a cornerstone of the American healthcare system. An EHR must be flexible and expandable to meet the needs of patients and caregivers in all these settings, despite the challenges.

At a very basic level, there is as yet no EHR system available that can provide all functions for all specialties to a degree that all clinicians would successfully adopt. A good example is oncology. Most systems do not yet provide the advanced ordering features required for complex treatment planning. An oncologist could use a general system, but he or she would not find as many benefits without additional features for chemotherapy ordering, lifetime cumulative dose tracking, or the ability to adjust a treatment-day schedule and have a new schedule be recalculated for the remaining days of the plan.

Further, most healthcare organizations do not yet have the capacity to implement and maintain systems in all care areas. As one physician stated, "implementing an EMR is a complex and difficult multidisciplinary effort that will stretch an organization's skills and capacity for change" (Chin, 2004, p. 47). These two conditions are improving every day at both vendor and healthcare organizations alike, and were recently fueled by ARRA incentives (see **Box 15-3**).

ARRA has also set the expectation that despite the number of settings in which a patient may receive care, there is a minimum set of data from those records that must flow or "interoperate" between each setting and the unique EHR systems used. Today, interoperability exists through what is called a continuity of care document. This data set includes patient demographics, medication, allergy, and problem lists, among others, and the continuity of care document formatting and exchange is required to be

BOX 15-2	Resistance to Implementation *Julie A. Kenney and Ida Androwich*

For an implementation to be successful, a few things need to happen. The informatics nurse specialist (INS) needs to understand and use change management theory to ensure that the implementation of the new EHR system will be successful. It is a well-known fact that nurses can make or break a system implementation. Indeed, a nursing staff that is involved early in the implementation process has been found to be a major determinant in a successful implementation.

Assessing nursing attitudes and concerns early in the process can aid the INS in determining the best way to proceed with staff education and implementation rollout. Nurses may feel that the implementation that should be making their job easier is actually making it more challenging (Trossman, 2005). Nurses who feel that the system has been forced onto them will very likely be highly resistant to the change. This is why it is imperative that nurses be involved in the design, development, and implementation of the EHR. Nurses who have been involved in the implementation process will ensure that the product meets the needs of the staff, which will result in high end-user satisfaction (McLane, 2005).

Another challenge facing those wishing to implement an EHR is that writing is nearly automatic for most, but using a computer is not. This barrier to us can be overcome by ensuring that data entry and system navigation make for a system that is user friendly (Walsh, 2004). Voice data entry is an easy way to enter data into the system and may be a way for those who are not comfortable with computers to still use the system effectively (Walsh). Another way for staff to improve the chance that staff will accept the new EHR is to ensure that they have had adequate training prior to the implementation as well as ensure continued support and education after the implementation. The implementation of a new EHR system requires the staff to make significant changes to how they work and how they handle patient information. The INS who is familiar with change management and the NI process should have an integral role in the redesign of workflow processes in order to ensure a smooth transition from a paper record to an electronic record.

Many excellent EHR systems that have been installed fail due to poor implementation planning. It is imperative that nurses are employed in the information systems (IS) department (Trossman, 2005).

References

McLane, S. (2005). Designing an EMR planning process based on staff attitudes toward and opinions about computers in healthcare. *CIN: Computers, Informatics, Nursing, 23*(2), 85–92.

Trossman, S. (2005). Bold new world: Technology should ease nurses' jobs, not create a greater work load. *American Journal of Nursing, 105*(5), 75–77.

Walsh, S. (2004). The clinician's perspective on electronic health records and how they can affect patient care. *BMJ: British Medical Journal, 328*(7449), 1184–1187.

BOX 15-3	Cloudy EHRs

A paradigm shift from healthcare facility-owned machine-based computing to offsite, vendor-owned cloud computing, Web browser–based login accessible data, and software and hardware could link systems together and reduce costs. Hospitals with shrinking budgets and extreme IT needs are exploring the successes in this area achieved in other industries, such as Amazon's S3. As providers strive to implement potent EHRs, they are looking for the cloud-based models that offer the necessary functionality without having to assume the burden associated with all of the hardware, software, application, and storage issues. However, in the face of the HITECH Act and its associated penalties, how can we overcome the challenges to realize the benefits? There are advantages and disadvantages of cloud computing. Notably, while they explore this new paradigm, healthcare providers must relinquish control as they continue to strive to maintain security. The vendors, which are responsible for developing and maintaining this new environment, are also facing challenges brought on by the legislature and healthcare providers. As the vendors and healthcare providers work together to improve the implementation and adoption of the cloud-based EHR, the sky is the limit!

supported by EHR vendors and healthcare organizations seeking ARRA meaningful use incentives. Despite this positive step forward, financial and patient privacy hurdles must still be overcome to achieve an expansive EHR. Most health care is delivered by small community practices and hospitals, many of which do not have the financial or technical resources to implement an EHR. DHHS recently loosened regulations so that physicians may now be able to receive healthcare information technology software, hardware, and implementation services from hospitals to alleviate the cost burden on individual providers and foster adoption of the EHR.

Finally, patient privacy is a pivotal issue to determine how far and how easy it will be to share data across healthcare organizations. In addition to the Health Insurance Portability and Accountability Act privacy rules, many states have regulations in place related to patient confidentiality. The recent experience of the state of Minnesota foreshadows what all states will soon be facing. In 2007, Governor Tim Pawlenty announced the creation of the Minnesota Health Information Exchange (State of Minnesota, 2007). Although the intentions of the exchange were to promote patient safety and increase healthcare efficiency across the state, it raised significant concerns about security and privacy. New questions arose about the definition of when and how patient consent is required to exchange data electronically, and older paper-based processes needed to be updated to support real-time electronic exchange (Minnesota Department of Health, 2007). For health exchanges such as these to reach their full potential, the public must be able to trust that their privacy will be protected, or else the healthcare industry risks that patients may not share a full medical history, or worse yet, may not seek care, effectively making the exchange useless.

THE FUTURE

Despite the challenges, the future of EHRs is an exciting one for patient and clinician alike. Benefits may be realized by stand-alone EHRs as described here, but the most significant transformation will come as interoperability is realized between systems. As the former national information technology coordinator in the DHHS, David Brailer, notes the potential of interoperability:

> For the first time, clinicians everywhere can have a longitudinal medical record with full information about each patient. Consumers will have better information about their health status since personal health records and similar access strategies can be feasible in an interoperable world. Consumers can move more easily between and among clinicians without fear of their information being lost. Payers can benefit from the economic efficiencies, fewer errors, and reduced duplication that arises from interoperability. Healthcare information exchange and interoperability (HIEI) also underlies meaningful public health reporting, bioterrorism surveillance, quality monitoring, and advances in clinical trials. In short, there is little that most people want from health care for which HIEI isn't a prerequisite. (Brailer, 2005, p. W 5-20)

The future also holds tremendous potential for EHR features and functions that will include not only more sophisticated decision support and clinical reporting capacity, but also improved biomedical device integration, ease of use and intuitiveness, and access through more hardware platforms.

Implementations of EHRs will also become more commonplace in the near future with ARRA putting pressure on healthcare organizations to move more quickly toward their adoption. More organizations adopting EHRs will facilitate broader dissemination of implementation best practices, with the hope of further shortening the time to taking advantage of advanced EHR features.

SUMMARY

It is an important time for health care and technology. EHRs have come to the forefront and will remain central to shaping the future of health care. In an ideal world, all nurses—from entry level to executives—will have a basic com-

petency in nursing informatics to participate fully in shaping the future use of technology in the practice at a national level and wherever care is delivered. Such initiatives as TIGER are imperative for adoption and ultimately more visibility of nursing in the later phases of the ARRA meaningful use standards, which are still being defined.

DISCUSSION QUESTIONS

1. What are the implications for nursing education as the EHR becomes the standard for caring for patients?

2. What are the ethical considerations related to interoperability and a shared EHR?

REFERENCES

American Organization of Nurse Executives. (2006, September). Defining the role of the nurse executive in technology acquisition and implementation. Washington, DC: Author. Retrieved from http://www.aone.org/aone/pdf/Guiding%20Principles%20for%20Acquisition%20and%20Implementation%20of%20Information%20Technology.pdf

Brailer, D. J. (2005, January). Interoperability: The key to the future healthcare system. *Health Affairs—Web Exclusive*, W 5-19–W 5-21. Available from http://content.healthaffairs.org/cgi/reprint/hlthaff.w5.19v1

Bush, G. W. (2004). State of the Union address. Retrieved from http://www.whitehouse.gov/news/releases/2004/01/20040120-7.html

Centers for Medicare and Medicaid Services. (2010a). EHR incentive programs: Meaningful use. Retrieved from https://www.cms.gov/EHRIncentivePrograms/35_Meaningful_Use.asp

Centers for Medicare and Medicaid Services. (2010b). Quality measures: Electronic specifications. Retrieved from http://www.cms.gov/QualityMeasures/03_ElectronicSpecifications.asp#TopOfPage

Certification Commission for Healthcare Information Technology. (2007). Certification commission announces new work group members. Retrieved from http://www.cchit.org/about/news/releases/Certification-Commission-Announces-New-Work-Group-Members.asp

Chaudhry, B., Wang, J., Wu, S., Maglione, M., Mojica, W., Roth, E., Morton, S., & Shekelle, P. (2006).

Systematic review: Impact of health information technology on quality, efficiency, and costs of medical care. *Annals of Internal Medicine, 144*(10), E-12–E-22.

Chin, H. L. (2004). The reality of EMR implementation: Lessons from the field. *The Permanente Journal, 8*(4), 43–48.

Department of Health and Human Services. (2007). HIT certification: Background. Retrieved from http://www.dhhs.gov/healthit/certification/background

Department of Health and Human Services. (2010). Medicare and Medicaid programs: Electronic health record incentive program. Retrieved from http://www.ofr.gov/OFRUpload/OFRData/2010-17202 _PI.pdf

Dorr, D., Bonner, L. M., Cohen, A. N., Shoai, R. S., Perrin, R., Chaney, E., & Young, A. (2007). Informatics systems to promote improved care for chronic illness: A literature review. *Journal of the American Medical Informatics Association, 14*(2), 156–163.

Embi, P. J., Jain, A., Clark, J., Bizjack, S., Hornung, R., & Harris, C. M. (2005). Effect of a clinical trial alert system on physician participation in trial recruitment. *Archives of Internal Medicine, 165,* 2272–2277.

Goddard, B. L. (2000). Termination of a contract to implement an enterprise electronic medical record system. *Journal of American Medical Informatics Association, 7,* 564–568.

Halamka, J. D. (2006, May). Health information technology: Shall we wait for the evidence? [Letter to the editor]. *Annals of Internal Medicine, 144*(10), 775–776.

Healthcare Information and Management Systems Society (HIMSS). (2007). Electronic health record. Retrieved from http://www.himss.org/ASP/topics_ehr.asp

Healthcare Information and Management Systems Society (HIMSS). (2009). HIMSS Davies Organizational Award Application: MultiCare. Retrieved from http://www.himss.org/davies/docs/2009_RecipientApplications/MultiCareConnect HIMSSDaviesManuscript.pdf

Healthcare Information and Management Systems Society (HIMSS). (2010a). *HIMSS Davies Organizational Award Application: Sentara.* Forthcoming.

Healthcare Information and Management Systems Society (HIMSS). (2010b). EMR Adoption Model. Retrieved from http://www.himssanalytics.org/hc_providers/stage7Award.asp

Healthcare Information and Management Systems Society (HIMSS). (2010c). Recipient list. Retrieved from http://www.himssanalytics.org/hc_providers/stage7Hospitals.asp

Healthcare Information and Management Systems Society (HIMSS). (2010d). Davies Award. Retrieved from http://www.himss.org/davies/

Holbrook, A., Keshavjee, K., Troyan, S., Pray, M., & Ford, P. T. (2003). Applying methodology to electronic medical record selection. *International Journal of Medical Informatics, 71,* 43–50.

Husk, G., & Waxman, D. A. (2004). Using data from hospital information systems to improve emergency care. *Academic Emergency Medicine, 11*(11), 1237–1244.

Institute of Medicine. (2001). *Crossing the quality chasm: A new health system for the 21st century.* Washington, DC: National Academies Press.

Institute of Medicine. (2003). *Key capabilities of an electronic health record system: Letter report.* Washington, DC: National Academies Press.

Jain, A., Atreja, A., Harris, C. M., Lehmann, M., Burns, J., & Young, J. (2005). Responding to the rofecoxib withdrawal crisis: A new model for notifying patients at risk and their healthcare providers. *Annals of Internal Medicine, 142*(3), 182–186.

Minnesota Department of Health. (2007, June). *Minnesota Health Records Act—HF 1078 fact sheet.* Minneapolis, MN: Author. Retrieved from http://www.health.state.mn.us/e-health/mpsp/hra factsheet2007.pdf

National Institutes of Health. (April, 2006). *Electronic health records overview.* McLean, Virginia: The MITRE Corporation.

National Institute of Standards and Technology. (2010). Meaningful use test measures: Approved test procedures. Retrieved from http://healthcare.nist.gov/use_testing/finalized_requirements.html

Poprock, B. (2005, September). *Using Epic's alternative medications reminder to reduce prescription costs and encourage assistance programs for indigent patients.* Presented at the Epic Systems Corporation user group meeting, Madison, WI.

Reed, H. L., & Bernard, E. (2005). Reductions in diabetic cardiovascular risk by community primary care providers. *International Journal of Circumpolar Health, 64*(1), 26–37.

Robert Wood Johnson Foundation. (2006). Health information technology in the United States: The information base for progress. Retrieved from http://www.rwjf.org/programareas/resources/product.jsp?id=15895&pid=1142&gsa=1

Shekelle, P. G., Morton, S. C., & Keeler, E. B. (2006). *Costs and benefits of health information technology. Evidence report/technology assessment, No. 132* [Prepared by the Southern California Evidence-based Practice Center under Contract No. 290-02-0003]. Agency for Healthcare Research and Quality Publication No. 06-E006. Rockville, MD: Agency for Healthcare Research and Quality.

Sidorov, J. (2006). It ain't necessarily so: The electronic health record and the unlikely prospect of reducing healthcare costs. *Health Affairs, 25*(4), 1079–1085.

Smith, T., Semerdjian, N., King, P., DeMartin, B., Levi, S., Reynolds, K., Ryan, J., & Dowd, J. (2004). *Nicolas E. Davies Award of Excellence: Transforming healthcare with a patient-centric electronic health record system.* Evanston, IL: Evanston Northwestern Healthcare. Retrieved from http://www.himss.org/content/files/davies2004_evanston.pdf

Spooner, S. A., & The Council on Clinical Information Technology. (2007). Special requirements of electronic health record systems in pediatrics. *Pediatrics, 119,* 631–637.

State of Minnesota, Office of the Governor. (2007). New public–private partnership to improve patient care, safety and efficiency. Retrieved from http://www.governor.state.mn.us/mediacenter/press releases/2007/PROD008303.html

Technology Informatics Guiding Education Reform. (2006). Evidence and informatics transforming nursing. Retrieved from http://www.amia.org/inside/releases/2006/tiger_press%20release_amia.pdf

Thompson, D. I., Osheroff, J., Classen, D., Sittig, D. F. (2007). A review of methods to estimate the benefits of electronic medical records in hospitals and the need for a national database. *Journal of Healthcare Information Management, 21*(1), 62–68.

CHAPTER 16

IOM Core Competency: Utilize Informatics

Marion J. Ball

CHAPTER OBJECTIVES

1. Discuss the Institute of Medicine competency: Utilize informatics.

2. Describe informatics and its relationship to nursing.

3. Explain the purpose of documentation and key issues related to informatics and documentation.

4. Identify informatics tools used in healthcare delivery.

5. Describe telehealth and its relationship to healthcare delivery and nursing.

6. Examine the impact of the use of biomedical equipment on nursing care.

7. Compare and contrast high-touch care with high-tech care.

INTRODUCTION

Nursing professionals are the foot soldiers of the healthcare delivery system and, therefore, must be well equipped to carry out the best possible care for their patients. Having a solid understanding of the use of technological enabling tools is essential to be able to give the best possible patient care. The Technology Informatics Guiding Education Reform (TIGER; http://www.tigersummit.com) initiative is working on bringing the most essential skills for the profession to the table. This initiative addresses eight areas:

1. Standards and interoperability
2. Healthcare IT national agenda/healthcare IT policy
3. Informatics competencies
4. Education and faculty development
5. Staff development/continuing education
6. Usability/clinical application design
7. Virtual demonstration center
8. Leadership development

In fighting the battle of disease and suffering, nurses are the ones who can win the battle if they are well prepared. This means a good grasp of informatics is an essential ingredient. Thus this chapter focuses on one of the Institute of Medicine's (IOM) healthcare profession core competencies: utilize informatics. Informatics/information technology (IT) is an important topic in all areas of life today; with the explosion of technology there are many opportunities for communication and sharing of knowledge. The impact of informatics on nursing care is explored in this chapter. Other issues that need to be addressed are documentation, confidentiality and privacy of information, and telehealth. This chapter also includes content about biomedical equipment, an expanding area in healthcare technology that impacts nurses and nursing care. Some of this equipment also uses IT. Nurses today cannot avoid technology, whether it is used for communication or for care provision. The chapter concludes with discussion of the concern about high-touch care versus high-tech care: How do they relate? This is an important issue for nurses to consider. **Figure 16-1** identifies key elements in this chapter.

THE IOM COMPETENCY: UTILIZE INFORMATICS

The IOM description of its fifth healthcare profession core competency is as follows: "communicate, manage knowledge, mitigate error, and support decision making using information technology" (IOM, 2003, p. 4). Informatics is more than just understanding what IT is; it also includes how that technology is used to

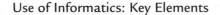

FIGURE 16-1   Use of Informatics: Key Elements

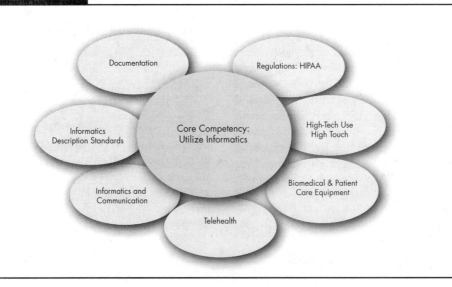

prevent errors and improve care. From the initial use of computers to management of financial records to the current use of informatics, there has been a major move toward IT application in care. Some examples are greater use of informatics to find evidence to implement evidence-based practice; use of informatics in research; greater consumer access to information via the Internet; and more specific clinical applications, such as reminder and decision systems, telehealth, teleradiology, online prescribing, and use of email for provider–provider communication and patient–provider communication. Additional details and examples are discussed later in this chapter. The IOM concludes that every healthcare professional should meet the following informatics competencies (2003, p. 63):

- Employ word processing, presentation, and data analysis software
- Search, retrieve, manage, and make decisions using electronic data from internal information databases and external online databases and the Internet
- Communicate using email, instant messaging, email lists, and file transfers
- Understand security protections such as access control, data security, and data encryption, and directly address ethical and legal issues related to the use of IT in practice
- Enhance education and access to reliable health information for patients

A position statement from the Healthcare Information and Management Systems Society addressed the IOM report *The Future of Nursing* from the perspective of informatics (2011). The following recommendations were made and align with the IOM report on the key points of leadership, education, and practice:

- Partner with nurse executives to lead technology changes that advance health and the delivery of health care.
- Support the development of informatics departments.

- Foster the evolution of the chief nursing informatics (NI) officer role.
- Transform nursing education to include informatics competencies and demonstrable behaviors at all levels of academic preparation.
- Promote the continuing education of all levels of nursing, particularly in the areas of electronic health records (EHRs) and health IT.
- Ensure that data, information, knowledge, and wisdom form the basis of 21st-century nursing practice by incorporating informatics competencies into practice standards in all healthcare settings.
- Facilitate the collection and analysis of interprofessional healthcare workforce data by ensuring data can be collected from existing IT systems.

The statement also indicates that nurses play a critical role in healthcare informatics and need to continue to do so.

> Nurses are key leaders in developing the infrastructure for effective and efficient health information technology that transforms the delivery of care. Nurse informaticists play a crucial role in advocating both for patients and fellow nurses who are often the key stakeholders and recipients of these evolving solutions. Nursing informatics professionals are the liaisons to successful interactions with technology in healthcare. (Healthcare Information and Management Systems Society, 2011)

INFORMATICS

Informatics is complex, and the fact that it is changing daily makes it even harder to keep current. Healthcare delivery has been strongly influenced by the changes in informatics, but what is informatics?

Definitions and Description

Informatics has opened doors to many innovative methods of communication with patients and among providers, individuals, and healthcare organizations (HCOs) of all types. It often saves time, but can lead to information overload.

Physicians are using email to communicate with patients (e.g., sending appointment reminders, sharing lab results, and answering questions). The Web has provided opportunities to build communities of people with common chronic diseases to help them with disease management. HCOs have developed websites to share information about their organizations with the public (a marketing tool for services). In addition, these websites provide HCOs with an effective method for internal communication; staff can access some parts of the sites with special passwords. Informatics is also used to evaluate the performance of the HCO and individual healthcare providers. IT has a major impact on quality improvement; today, it is much easier to collect, store, and analyze large amounts of data that in the past were collected by hand. Insurers rely heavily on informatics to provide insurance coverage, manage data, and analyze performance, which has a direct impact on whether care is covered for reimbursement. Informatics has allowed governments at all levels—local, state, national, and international—to collect and use data for policy decision making and evaluation.

Informatics has its own language and is a highly specialized area. Nurses do not have to be informatics experts, but they do need to understand the basics. Some terms have become so common that the majority of people know what they are (such as Internet and email). Some terms that are useful to know are listed next.

- Clinical data repository: A physical or logical compendium of patient data pertaining to health; an "information warehouse" that stores data longitudinally and in multiple forms, such as text, voice, and images (American Nurses Association [ANA], 2008).
- Clinical decision support systems: Computer applications designed to facilitate human decision making. Decision support systems are typically rule based. These systems use a knowledge base and a set of rules to analyze data and information and provide recommendations (ANA, 2008).

- Clinical information system: A clinical information system supports the acquisition, storage, manipulation, and distribution of clinical information throughout an HCO, with a focus on electronic communication. This system uses IT that is applied at the point of clinical care. Typical clinical information system components are electronic medical records (EMRs), clinical data repositories, decision support programs (such as application of clinical guidelines and drug interaction checking), handheld devices for collecting data and viewing reference material, imaging modalities, and communication tools such as electronic messaging systems.
- Coding system: A set of agreed-on symbols (frequently numeric or alphanumeric) that are attached to concept representation or terms to allow exchange of concept representations or terms with regard to their form or meaning. Examples are the Perioperative Nursing Data Set and the Clinical Care Classification System (ANA, 2008).
- Computer literacy: The knowledge and skills required to use basic computer applications and computer technology.
- Data: Discrete entities that are described objectively without interpretation.
- Data analysis software: Computer software that can analyze data.
- Data bank: A large store of information; it may include several databases.
- Database: A collection of interrelated data that are organized according to a scheme to serve one or more applications. The data are stored so that several programs can use data without concern for data structures or organization. An example is the National Database of Nursing Quality Indicators (ANA, 2008).
- Data mining: Locating and identifying unknown patterns and relationships within data.

- Email list: A list of email addresses that can be used to send one email message to many addresses at one time.

- Encryption: To change information into a code, usually for security reasons, to limit access.

- Information: Data that have been interpreted, organized, or structured.

- Information literacy: The ability to recognize when information is needed and to locate, evaluate, and effectively use that information (ANA, 2008).

- Knowledge: Information that is synthesized so that relationships are identified and formalized (ANA, 2008).

- Minimum data set: The minimum categories of data with uniform definitions and categories; they concern a specific aspect or dimension of the healthcare system that meets the basic needs of multiple data users. An example is the Nursing Minimum Data Set (ANA, 2008).

- Nomenclature: A system of designations (terms) that is elaborated according to pre-established rules. Examples include System-atized Nomenclature of Medicine—Clinical Terms International, and the International Classification for Nursing Practice (ANA, 2008).

- Security protections (access control, data security, and data encryption): Methods used to ensure that information is not read or taken by unauthorized persons.

- Software: Computer programs and applications.

- Standardized language: A collection of terms with definitions for use in informational systems databases. A standardized language enables comparisons to be made because the same term is used to denote the same condition. Standardized language is necessary for documentation in EHRs (ANA, 2008).

- Wisdom: The appropriate use of knowledge to solve human problems; understanding when and how to apply knowledge (ANA, 2008).

Nursing Standards: Scope and Standards of Nursing Informatics

Nursing informatics (NI) is a specialty that integrates nursing science, computer science, and information science to manage and communicate data, information, knowledge, and wisdom in nursing practice. NI supports consumers, patients, nurses, and other providers in their decision making in all roles and settings. This support is accomplished through the use of information structures, information processes, and IT. The goal of NI is to improve the health of populations, communities, families, and individuals by optimizing information management and communication (ANA, 2008, p. 1).

This specialty area has expanded, and all nurses need to understand basic IT concepts and their application to nursing practice. Undergraduate nursing programs often include IT in the curriculum, sometimes as a course on informatics, although not all programs include this content. This is now a problem because of the emphasis on informatics as a healthcare professions core competency. Some schools of nursing offer master's degrees in NI.

Three major concepts related to information are important to understand (Englebardt & Nelson, 2002):

1. Data are discrete entities that are described objectively without interpretation.

2. Information is defined as data that are interpreted, organized, or structured.

3. Knowledge is information that is synthesized so that relationships are identified and formalized.

The flow from data to wisdom can be described as data naming, collecting, and organizing following this pattern: (1) information—organizing and interpreting; (2) knowledge—interpreting, integrating, and understanding; and (3) wisdom—understanding, applying, and applying with compassion. **Figure 16-2** illustrates this flow.

"Wisdom is defined as the appropriate use of knowledge to manage and solve human problems. It is knowing when and how to apply knowledge to deal with complex problems or specific human needs" (Nelson & Joos, 1989, p. 6). "While knowledge focuses on what is known, wisdom focuses on the appropriate application of that knowledge. For example, a knowledge base may include several options for managing an anxious family, while wisdom would help decide which option is most appropriate for a specific family" (ANA, 2008, p. 5).

Nurses first need to understand the importance of data collection and data analysis and then how to apply data and knowledge—leading to wisdom. Data are important to the delivery of nursing care. In hospitals, data can be used to evaluate outcomes, identify problems for a specific group of patients, and assist in making plans for change to improve care. In the community, aggregated data are often collected to better understand the health issues in a population or community and to formulate a plan of action.

Certification in Informatics Nursing

Nurses who practice in the area of informatics can be certified if they meet the eligibility criteria and complete the certification examination satisfactorily. The following were the application eligibility criteria required for the informatics certification exam sponsored by the American Nurses Credentialing Center for 2008–2009 (ANA, 2007). The nurse must:

- Hold a current, active registered nurse license within a state or territory of the United States or the professional, legally recognized equivalent in another country
- Have practiced the equivalent of 2 years full time as a registered nurse
- Hold a baccalaureate or higher degree in nursing or a baccalaureate degree in a relevant field
- Have completed 30 hours of continuing education in informatics within the last 3 years
- Meet one of the following practice hour requirements:
  a. The nurse must have practiced a minimum of 2,000 hours in NI within the last 3 years.
  b. The nurse must have practiced a minimum of 1,000 hours in NI in the last 3 years and must have completed a minimum of 12 semester hours of academic credit in informatics courses that are a part of a graduate-level NI program.
  c. The nurse must have completed a graduate program in NI containing a minimum of 200 hours of faculty-supervised practicum in informatics.

FIGURE 16-2 From Data to Wisdom

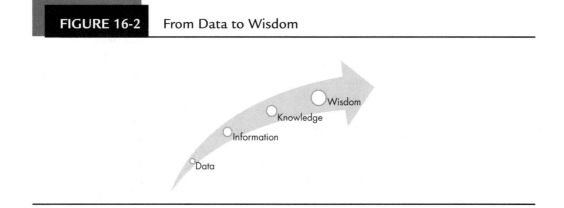

These are not simple criteria; they take time to meet, and they provide a good overview of the need for expertise in this area. All criteria must be met before a nurse can apply to take the certification examination.

The informatics nurse is involved in activities that focus on the methods and technologies of information handling in nursing. Informatics nursing practice includes the development, support, and evaluation of applications, tools, processes, and structures that help nurses to manage data in direct care of patients and also in nursing education and research. The work of an informatics nurse can involve any and all aspects of information systems, including theory formulation, design, development, marketing, selection, testing, implementation, training, maintenance, evaluation, and enhancement. "Informatics nurses are engaged in clinical practice, education, consultation, research, administration, and pure informatics" (ANA, 2007, p. 1). It is clear that a nurse who wants to function in this specialty area must have excellent computer skills, understand the practice needs for information, and know how best to apply IT to nursing practice. The nurse must also be able to work collaboratively in interprofessional teams and demonstrate leadership. By speaking for the needs of the practicing nurse, the informatics nurse represents all nurses in practice—clinical, education, and research—as applies to the specific situation.

Informatics: Impact on Care

The IOM recommendations indicate that informatics can lead to safe, quality care, and it can. However, applying informatics is not perfect.

> There is a perception that technology will lead to fewer errors than strategies that focus on staff performance; however, technology may in some circumstances lead to more errors. This is particularly true when the technology fails to take into account end users, increases in staff time, replicates an already bad process or is implemented with insufficient training. The best approach is not always clear, and most approaches have advantages and disadvantages. (Finkelman & Kenner, 2009, p. 55)

Nurses need to take an active role in the development of IT for patient care and not wait to be asked to participate. When an HCO is choosing a system for an EMR, nurses need to be involved to ensure that the system meets nursing care documentation requirements and that relevant data can be collected to assist nurses in providing and improving care. Nurses may serve in key IT roles to guide development and implementation, and these nurses may have special training or education in informatics. Nurses may also serve as resources in identifying needs and testing systems to ensure that the systems are nurse user friendly. Many nurses who provide feedback about systems do not have special IT training; they review the system to determine if it is user friendly for nurses who have limited informatics knowledge and help to determine if the system meets documentation needs and standards. All nurses need be skilled in managing and communicating information, and they are primarily concerned with the content of that information.

Coordination of care is very important, of course. One of the barriers to seamless coordination is the lack of interoperable computerized records (Bodenheimer, 2008). In 2007, only 34.8% of physician offices used computerized records; this percentage represented a major increase from the 2005 rate of 23.9%, and 49.8% of the hospitals had adopted the EMR, with more adding such systems each year. Data for 2009 (U.S. Department of Health and Human Services, 2011) indicate that 41% of office-based physicians and 81% of hospitals planned on taking advantage of the federal incentive payments for adoption and meaningful use of certified EHR technology. To improve information sharing and coordination of care, ideally these rates should be 100%, but this is a costly, complex change to implement (National Center for Health Statistics, 2010). The federal incentive program can make a significant difference in adoption of this critical healthcare informatics technology. Today, information can rarely be shared among multiple systems, which is a shortcoming that needs to be resolved. For example, there should be ability to share current information among healthcare providers in private practice and clinics and the hospitals when it is needed.

Innovative methods to improve coordination that focus on informatics have been developed. One method is to use electronic referral, or e-referral. This process allows a healthcare provider to send an email to another provider, such as a specialist, with information about the patient and to ask for consultation. In many situations, it eliminates the need to see the patient. The specialist reviews such information as lab reports, surgical reports, and so on, and can share his or her opinion with the healthcare provider. It is critical that this type of service be reimbursed, or it will not be used. Health Insurance Portability and Accountability Act (HIPAA) requirements must also be considered to ensure patient privacy. Timely information flow from the hospital to posthospital care should improve patient coordination. Not having this stream of information is a major drawback; even though the technology to improve it is available, it is not freely used.

Implications for Nursing Education and Nursing Research

Informatics is important not only for practice, but also for nursing education and nursing research. There is greater and greater use of IT in nursing education. The increased use of online courses throughout the nursing curriculum, at both the undergraduate and graduate levels, has revolutionized nursing education. It has required that faculty consider more interactive learning methods. Informatics also impacts simulation, allowing faculty to create complex learning scenarios that use the computer and computerized equipment. As students personally use more technology, they expect greater use of IT in education. Such tools as iPods, personal digital assistants (PDAs), and mobile phones, and Internet tools such as Facebook

and MySpace provide instant information and can be very interactive. These methods can be used to increase student–faculty communication and have the potential to provide different methods for student–faculty supervision in the clinical area. This is particularly true in areas such as community health, when students visit multiple sites and faculty move from site to site to see students.

Nursing research uses informatics in data collection and analysis; it saves time and improves the quality of data collection and analysis.

> The capacity for a mega-repository of clinical and research findings will allow for a richer science derived from multiple perspectives. Nurses have the responsibility to initiate practice-based inquiry, participate in clinical nursing research, and use nursing research to enhance patients' well-being and contribute to the body of nursing knowledge. (Appleton, 1998, as cited in Richards, 2001, p. 10)

This quote is not a recent one, but the message is the same today, though we have yet to really reach this status.

DOCUMENTATION

Over time, nursing documentation has increased in terms of its relevance to nurses and to other healthcare professionals, thus increasing its impact on patient care and patient outcomes.

> Clear, accurate, and accessible documentation is an essential element of safe, quality, evidence-based nursing practice. Nurses practice across settings at position levels from the bedside to the administrative office; the registered nurse (RN) and the advanced practice registered nurse (APRN) are responsible and accountable for the nursing documentation that is used throughout an organization. This may include either documentation on nursing care that is provided by nurses—whether RN, APRN, or nursing assistive personnel—that can be used by other non-nurse members of the health care team or the administrative records that are created by the nurse and used across organization settings. (ANA, 2010, p. 3)

According to the ANA (2010), nursing documentation is used for the following purposes:

- Communicate within the healthcare team
- Communicate with other professionals
- Verify credentialing—to monitor performance
- Provide legal support
- Learn about regulation and legislation—to provide data for audits and monitoring
- Receive reimbursement—determine services for reimbursement
- Do research—data for studies
- Conduct quality process and performance improvement

The format and content of nursing documentation have also changed. It is a professional responsibility to document planning, actual care provided, and outcomes. Care coordination and continuity are supported by documentation. With many different staff caring for patients around the clock, it is critical that there be a clear communication mechanism, and this mechanism is documentation. Verbal communication is important, but a written document must be available. Staff can refer to documentation when other care providers are not available. Documentation serves as a record of the patient's care; it provides data for reimbursement and regarding quality improvement and staff performance; and it supports interprofessional teamwork. Through documentation, outcomes and evaluation of patient care are made clear.

The medical record is a legal document, and as such, there are rules that must be followed. Once documentation has been created, changes to it must be accompanied by a note indicating who made the change(s) and when (date and time). Only certain staff can document; they must note the date and time on the documentation and include their name and credentials. If there are questions about care or a legal action, such as a malpractice suit, the medical record is the most important evidence. Medical records need to be saved. A nurse can say that he

or she provided certain care, but if it was not documented, then it is as if it did not occur.

Iyer and Camp (1999, p. 5), listed the following standard critical concerns that pertain to documentation:

- The medical record reflects the nursing process.
- The medical record describes the patient's ongoing status from shift to shift (inpatient care) or from patient visit to patient visit (ambulatory care).
- The plan of care and medical record complement each other.
- The documentation system is designed to facilitate retrieval of information for quality improvement activities and for research.
- The documentation system supports the staffing mix and acuity levels in the current healthcare environment.

The following guidelines (Iyer & Camp, 1999) continue to be important for all who document:

- Do not include opinion, but rather objective information in documentation. The nurse does not make subjective comments (e.g., comments about the patient being uncooperative, lazy, impolite, and so on). Nurses document only what they have done and objective data. A nurse would not document another staff member's actions. Supervision of care can be documented.
- Write neatly and legibly. Many HCOs now use computerized documentation, though not all HCOs have moved to an EMR system. If a computerized system is used, typos may be a problem. Other issues arise in electronic systems that use a checklist for a particular section of the EMR but do not allow for narrative notes. Nurses and others may be frustrated when they cannot add a narrative note.
- Use correct spelling, grammar, and medical terminology.

- Use authorized abbreviations. Using unapproved abbreviations can increase risk of errors.

- Use graphic records to record specified patient data, such as vital signs and medication administration.

- Record the patient's name on every page (for hard copy medical records); this should be part of the EMR.

- Follow HCO rules about verbal and telephone orders.

- Transcribe orders carefully; double-check and ask questions if not clear. In computerized systems, orders do not need to be transcribed; however, this does not mean that there is no risk of an error in an order. All orders need careful review, and if they are not clear, they may require follow-up.

- Document omitted care.

- Document medications and outcomes.

- Document patient noncompliance and reason(s).

- Document allergies, and use this information to prevent errors and complications.

- Document sites of injections.

- Record all information about intravenous therapy and blood administration.

- Report abnormal laboratory results.

- Document as soon as possible after care is delivered. If documentation is done late, note this in the record. The nurse should not leave blank areas to come back to for later documentation.

- When quoting, use quotation marks and note who made the statement.

- When documentation is corrected because of a mistake, follow the HCO policies regarding corrections as per a hard copy record or electronic record. Medical records are never rewritten.

- Document patient status change.

- When contacting the physician, document the time, date, name of physician, reason for the call, content, physician response, and steps taken after the call. This note should not include subjective analysis of the response, such as that the physician was rude.

The Joint Commission does not provide details as to what must be in a medical record (or the term used by the Joint Commission, *record of care/treatment, and services*), but it does provide some guidelines that are required for accreditation (Clark, 2011; Joint Commission, 2011):

- The following content noted by the Joint Commission needs to be included: the patient's name, address, and date of birth; name of any legally authorized representative; assessment; diagnosis; clinician notes and actions; signatures and countersignatures as required; dates; details of procedures performed; laboratory reports; medications administered; and treatment plans. This does not mean that other data cannot be included, and frequently there are other data. This is the minimum requirement.

- Records should be clear and understandable.

- Records must create a system of communication and an audit trail.

- Storage of documents must be secure and reasonable. For example, the system would consider who has access to records and prevent casual viewing by nonstaff. All Medicare storage rules must be followed.

- The HIPAA must be followed.

This list applies to hospital medical records. The content is somewhat different for other types of settings, such as ambulatory care, long-term care, and home care, although some information would be the same. Nurses are not involved in documenting in all these categories because other staff members also have documentation responsibilities.

In 2010, the standard for record of care/ treatment and services was one of the top 10 noncompliant standards (Clark, 2011). The three areas where hospitals often did not meet compliance were:

1. Complete and accurate medical record.
2. Verbal orders received and recorded by qualified staff
3. Patient assessed and reassessed per defined time frame

Nurses are involved in all three aspects of these documentation standards.

A NEED: STANDARDIZED TERMINOLOGY

Health care has expanded in multiple directions and includes the services of many different healthcare providers. Communication among the providers is not easy. Certainly, there are issues regarding willingness to communicate, lack of time to communicate, and so on, but a critical problem is the lack of a common professional language. For those entering health care, such as nursing students, this is probably a surprising comment. Each healthcare professional area has its own language; there are common medical terms, but each has a specific language that is often not known or understood by other healthcare professionals.

"Creating a common language is no small task. Developing and adhering to distinct profession-specific terms may be a manifestation of professionals' desire to preserve identity, status or control" (IOM, 2003, p. 123). This problem affects all the core competencies and the ability to develop educational experiences that meet the competencies across healthcare professions, such as nursing, medicine, pharmacy, and allied health. It does not just relate to informatics; however, because informatics is dependent on language, the issue of shared language is even more important. The IOM recommends that an interprofessional group created by the Department of Health and Human Services develop a common language across health

disciplines "on a core set of competencies that includes patient-centered care, interprofessional teams, evidence-based practice, quality improvement, and informatics" (IOM, 2003, p. 124). Accomplishing this requires that healthcare professionals are willing to actively work together to achieve this goal. Once this is accomplished, the next major step is getting different healthcare professionals to accept a universal language. This will require compromises.

The data element sets and terminologies are foundational to standardization of nursing documentation and verbal communication that will lead to a reduction in errors and an increase in the quality and continuity of care. It is through standardization of nurse documentation and communication of a patient's care that the many nurses caring for a patient develop a shared understanding of that care. Moreover, the process generates the nursing data needed to develop increasingly more sophisticated decision support tools in the electronic record and to identify and disseminate best nursing practices (ANA, 2006).

These statements are an example of why developing and accepting a universal language is difficult but necessary. The statements are nursing focused. How to move from this approach and blend with others, such as medicine, is the challenge.

Systems and Terminologies: Informatics Complexity

Informatics is not as simple as email and Internet. There are many database systems, terms, and other factors that make this a complex area. The following provides examples to illustrate informatics complexity.

Examples of Systematic Collection of Nursing Care Data or Data Element Sets

■ *Nursing Minimum Data Set:* This data set describes patient problems across healthcare settings, different populations, geographic areas, and time. These clinical data also assist in identifying nursing diagnoses, nursing interventions, and nurse-sensitive patient outcomes. The Nursing Minimum Data Set is also useful in assessing resources used in the provision of nursing care. The goal is the ability to link data between HCOs and providers. Data can also be used for research and healthcare policy.

■ *Nursing Management Minimum Data Set:* This data set focuses on nursing administrative data elements in all types of settings.

Interface Terminologies

■ *Clinical Care Classification:* The clinical classifications software for the *International Classification of Diseases, 10th revision, Clinical Modification* (ICD-10-CM) is a diagnosis and procedure categorization scheme that can be used in many types of projects that analyze data on diagnoses and procedures. The software is based on ICD-10-CM, a uniform and standardized coding system. The ICD-10-CM includes more than 13,600 diagnosis codes and 3,700 procedure codes (Centers for Disease Control and Prevention, 2011). Clinical care classification focuses on home care and includes diagnoses, interventions, and outcomes.

■ *International Classification of Nursing Practice:* This classification system is a unified nursing language system that applies to all types of nursing care. It is a compositional terminology for nursing practice that facilitates the development of and the cross-mapping among local terms and existing terminologies. It includes nursing diagnoses, nursing interventions, and nursing outcomes (International Council of Nurses, 2008).

■ *North American Nursing Diagnosis Association, Nursing Intervention Classification, and Nursing Outcome Classification:* The North American Nursing Diagnosis Association (NANDA) focuses on nursing diagnoses, Nursing Intervention Classification (NIC) on nursing interventions, and Nursing Outcome Classification (NOC) on nursing outcomes. The NANDA, NIC, and NOC terminology is frequently used by both nursing students and faculty.

■ *Omaha System:* The Omaha system is a comprehensive, standardized taxonomy designed to improve practice, documentation, and information management. It includes three components: the problem classification scheme, the intervention scheme, and the problem rating scale for outcomes. When the three components are used together, the Omaha system offers a way to link clinical data to demographic, financial, administrative, and staffing data (Omaha System, 2011). The Omaha system is used in home health care, community health, and public health services.

■ *Perioperative Nursing Data Set:* The Perioperative Nursing Data Set is a standardized nursing vocabulary that addresses the perioperative patient experience from preadmission until discharge, including nursing diagnoses, interventions, and outcomes. The Perioperative Nursing Data Set was developed by a specialty organization, the members of the Association of periOperative Registered Nurses, which has been recognized by the ANA as a data set useful for perioperative nursing practice (Association of periOperative Registered Nurses, 2008).

Examples of Multiprofessional Terminologies

■ *ABC Codes:* ABC coding solutions manage care, claims, and outcomes related to alternative medicine, nursing, and other integrative healthcare practices. ABC codes, paired with ABC terminology, currently describe more than 4,300 unique instances of care and services and/or supply items specific to the practice of alternative medicine, nursing, and other integrative healthcare practitioners. The codes fill the gaps left by the existing standard HIPAA code sets and provide for comprehensive and seamless coding (ABC Coding Solutions, 2011). This data coding system applies to nursing and other healthcare services and focuses on interventions.

■ *Logical Observation Identifiers Names and Codes:* This is a clinical terminology classification used for laboratory test orders and results. It is one system designated for use in U.S. federal government systems for the electronic exchange of clinical health information (National Library of Medicine, 2008a). This system can be used to collect data about assessments and outcomes for nursing and other healthcare services.

■ *The Current Procedural Terminology:* This is a code used for reimbursement (Larkin, 2008).

■ *Systematized Nomenclature of Medicine—Clinical Terms:* This is a comprehensive clinical terminology. It is one of several designated standards for use in U.S. federal government systems for the electronic exchange of clinical health information (National Library of Medicine, 2008b). This system is applicable to nursing and other healthcare services and focuses on diagnoses, interventions, and outcomes.

With the increased use of technology for documentation, nursing has been more concerned about two issues (Schwiran & Thede, 2011):

1. How to differentiate nursing's contributions to patient care from those of medicine

2. How to incorporate descriptions of nursing care into the health record in a manner that is commensurate with its importance to patients' welfare

In a study conducted by Schwiran and Thede (2011), the researchers examined nurses' knowledge of and experience with standardized nursing technologies. The results indicate that most nurses do not have much knowledge of or experience with standardized nursing technologies such as the examples provided here, and even knowledge of and use of Nursing Interventions

Classification, Nursing Outcomes Classification, and North American Nursing Diagnosis Association are not strong. Given that there is increased use of informatics, this lack of knowledge will affect nurses' ability to participate actively in informatics.

Informatics: Types and Methods

For informatics to be effective, three concerns must be addressed.

First, the HCO must have effective and easily accessible IT support services. Staff must be able to pick up the telephone and get this support. Failure of the information system has major implications for patient care, so backup systems are critical.

The second critical concern is staff training. This requires resources—financial resources, trainers, and time. Staff need time to attend training, and there must be recognition that it takes time for staff to learn how to use the system.

Incorporation of informatics with any of the methods described next (and others that are not included in this chapter) is a major change in care delivery. Change is stressful for staff, and it needs to be planned, representing the third concern. Too much change at one time can increase staff stress, impact the success of using more informatics in the future, decrease staff motivation to participate, and increase the risk of errors that might impact patient outcomes. It is not difficult to find nurses who will complain about a hospital's attempt to increase the use of informatics, particularly if it has been badly planned. Often, in these complaints, staff note that the system selected was not effective and that they had no part in the process.

Equipment and software can be very costly, and decisions regarding these are critical. Time must be taken to evaluate equipment and software to make sure they meet the needs and demands of the organization and users such as nurses. Examples of current activities in this area are automated dispensing of medications and bar coding; computerized monitoring of adverse events; the use of electronic medical/ health records, provider order entry systems, clinical decision support systems, PDAs, and computer-based and reminder systems; accessing patient records at the point of care; prescribing via the Internet; and using nurse call systems, voice mail, the telephone for advice and other services, online support groups for patients and families, the Internet or virtual appointments, and smartphones. These possibilities are discussed next.

Automated Dispensing of Medications and Bar Coding

Pharmacies in all types of HCOs are using or moving toward using automatic medication dispensing systems with bar coding. These systems select the medication based on the order and prepare it in single doses for the patient. The bar code is on the packaged dose. This code can then be compared with the bar code on the patient's identification band using a handheld device. This system can decrease errors, and it supports all five rights of medication administration:

1. Right drug
2. Right patient
3. Right amount
4. Right route
5. Right time

Bar coding can also be used to collect data about prescribed and administered drugs. Data can then be used for quality improvement and for research. Bar coding systems are expensive to install and maintain, but they can make a difference in reducing errors.

Computerized Monitoring of Adverse Events

Computerized systems that monitor adverse events assist in identifying and monitoring adverse events. Developing and using a database of these events facilitates analysis of data and

the development of interventions to decrease adverse events.

Electronic Medical/Health Records

The EMR/EHR is slowly replacing the written medical record for an individual patient while he or she receives care within a specific healthcare system. A second type of electronic system is the personal health record (PHR). The PHR is less common than the EMR, but there is much hope that it will become standard in the future. The PHR is a computer-based health record for which data are collected over the long term—for a lifetime. With the patient's permission, the healthcare provider can access this record easily to obtain information. To reach this point, there must be agreement on a minimum data set—that is, uniform definitions of data (i.e., standardized language) that would enable all healthcare providers to understand and use the information. There is still much to be done to make this a reality in every HCO, including clinics and medical offices, but the technology is available.

The EMR is a record of the patient's history and assessment, orders, laboratory results, description of medical tests and procedures, and documentation of care provided and outcomes. Care plans are included. Information can be easily input, searched, and reviewed, and reports can be printed. Data can be stored for the long term, which is harder to do with written records requiring storage space, which then may not be easy to find. In addition, written records can be less readable over time. The hard copy record is also not always easy to access in a hospital unit. If one person is using the record, others cannot use it. With the EMR, this is not a problem as long as staff can access the computerized record system. The EMR systems do require security and backup saving systems.

The following is a summary by Iyer and Camp (1999, pp. 129–130) of the advantages for using EMRs:

- Legible records
- Readily available records

- Improved nursing productivity
- Reduction in record tampering
- Support of the nursing process in the system
- Reduction of redundant documentation
- Clinical prompts, reminders, and warnings
- Categorized nursing notes
- Automatically printed reports
- Documentation according to standards of care
- Improved knowledge of outcomes
- Availability of data
- Prevention of medication errors
- Facilitation of cost-defining efforts
- Printed discharge information

EMR documentation may take place at the unit workstation, at a hallway computer station, at the bedside in the hospital, or in an examining room in a clinic. Bedside systems are better; they are easy to access when the nurse or other healthcare professional needs information, and point-of-care documentation is enhanced.

The ANA believes that the public has a right to expect that health data and healthcare information will be centered on patient safety and improved outcomes throughout all segments of the healthcare system, and that healthcare-related data and information will be accurately and efficiently collected, recorded, protected, stored, utilized, analyzed, and reported. Principles of privacy, confidentiality, and security cannot be compromised as the industry creates and implements interoperable and integrated healthcare information technology systems and solutions to convert from paper-based media for documentation and healthcare records to the newer format of EHRs, including individual PHR products. The ANA strongly supports efforts to further refine the concept and requirements of the patient-centric EHR, including the creation of standards-based electronic health records and supporting infrastructures that promote efficient and effective interprofessional and patient communications and decision making wherever care is provided.

Similar attention must be paid to the secondary uses of data and information to generate knowledge that leads to improved and effective decision tools. All stakeholders, including nurses and patients, must be integral participants in the design, development, implementation, and evaluation phases of the electronic health record. This effort requires the attention and action of nurses, the professional and specialty nursing organizations, and the nursing profession to ensure the EHRs are designed to facilitate and support critical thinking and decision making, such as in the nursing process, and the associated documentation activities. It is the ANA's position that the registered nurse must also be involved in the product selection, design, development, implementation, evaluation and improvement of information systems and electronic patient care devices used in patient care setting (ANA, 2009).

In July 2010, the Office of the National Coordinator for Health Information Technology and the Centers for Medicare and Medicaid Services issued new rules in identifying criteria that hospitals and eligible providers must meet to be considered meaningful users of health IT (U.S. Department of Health and Human Services, 2010). Hospitals and eligible providers are not able to receive federal funding related to the EMR initiative unless they meet these requirements, which is a significant amount of funding. There are five purposes for establishing these rules:

1. To improve quality, safety, efficiency, and reduce health disparities
2. To engage patients and their families (through electronic communication)
3. To improve care coordination
4. To ensure adequate privacy and security protection for personal health information
5. To improve the health of the population as well as public health—through data collection and analysis of data

All of these purposes are in line with the IOM Quality Chasm reports.

Provider Order Entry System

The provider order entry system has also been called a professional order entry system (POES), but this terminology is changing to include all healthcare professionals who might write profession-specific orders, such as nursing orders. Such a system is included in the EMR, though it can be a stand-alone system. When this kind of system is in place, the healthcare provider inputs orders into the system rather than writing them. One clear advantage is legibility; written orders are often very difficult to read because handwriting varies, which has led to many errors. It takes time to transcribe written physician orders into a form in which the orders can be used. During this process, risk of transcription errors is increased. Typing orders into a computer can also lead to typos, although this is less of a problem.

Clinical decision support systems can be incorporated into the professional order entry system. This combination enhances the professional order entry system and can lead to improved care and a decrease in errors.

Clinical Decision Support Systems

The advent of this type of system is leading to major changes in healthcare delivery. Clinical decision support systems provide immediate information that can influence clinical decisions. Some of the systems actually intervene when an error is about to be made. For example, suppose an order for a medication is put into a patient's EMR; the computerized system might indicate that the patient is allergic to that medication and signal this fact by immediately sending an alert, stopping the order. The nurse can also get alerts that the patient is at risk for falls or decubiti. In the past, nurses depended on textbooks or journals that the unit might have to find information, and information searches were often not done effectively. Easy electronic access to current information eliminates many problems related to obtaining information when needed. This, too, can improve the quality of care. Evidence-based

practice relies heavily on access to evidence-based practice literature, which is most easily accessible via the Internet and databases.

There still needs to be more research done to fully understand the impact of clinical decision support systems on patient outcomes. A study published in 2011 indicates that there was no consistent association between use of such systems and quality of care in a study that included 3 billion patient visits (Romano & Stafford, 2011). Only one of 20 indicators—diet counseling for high-risk adults—demonstrated significantly better performance when a clinical decision support system was used. Earlier studies showed that use of clinical decision support systems improved outcomes. Criticism of this study questions whether its results were influenced by the following factors: (1) Clinical decision support systems rules may have been different in systems studied; (2) this study focused on medication management, whereas earlier studies were broader; and (3) this study looked at the outcome of a single visit rather than cumulative effect. Clearly, more research is needed to better determine the effectiveness of using clinical decision support systems.

Use of Personal Digital Assistants

PDAs have become popular with the general public. Many mobile telephones now have PDA capability, such as access to the Internet and storage of information. These handheld devices can hold a significant amount of information, serve as a calendar, keep contact information, and are an effective method for transmission of information. Nurses who use PDAs carry information with them and can look up side effects of a medication or any other type of medical information to help them as they provide care. In some cases, the nurse can access EMRs to get to patient information through the PDA. Some textbooks can now be uploaded into PDAs, such as pharmacology and clinical laboratory resources. This is very useful information for the nurse to have available when needed, because it is accessible in seconds at the point of care. Nurses who work outside a structured setting, such as in public health or in home care, find this type of system very useful for support information and for documentation needs (patient information, visit data, and so on); however, they must be very careful to comply with HIPAA regulations.

Computer-Based Reminder Systems

These systems are used to communicate with patients via email to remind them of appointments and screenings and to discuss other health issues. In the future, this method will most likely take the place of telephone calls to remind patients of appointments. Such a system also must maintain HIPAA compliance. For example, who will have access to the computer and email? Only the patient should have access to the information unless the patient wants the information to be shared.

Access to Patient Records at the Point of Care

Many hospitals are moving toward providing access to the patient records either in the patient's room or in the hallway via computers. In the future, more nurses will carry small laptops that allow access to the EMR when needed. This reduces time spent returning to the workstation to get information. Documentation can be completed as soon as care is provided, which reduces errors and improves quality because all care providers know when care has been provided. Point-of-care access decreases the chance that something may be forgotten, documented incorrectly, or not documented at all. In addition, it saves nurses time and eliminates the need to delay documentation. For example, without this type of access, nurses may document at certain times during the shift such as midmorning or near the end of a shift—an approach that can lead to errors, incomplete data in the record if the nurse forgets information, and situations in which other providers need current patient information that has not yet been documented.

Internet Prescriptions

There has been rapid growth in access to prescriptions via the Internet. The medications are then mailed to the patient. The consumer does have to be careful and check the legitimacy of the source to prevent errors.

Nurse Call Systems

Nurse call systems are a form of informatics that are very important in communication within a healthcare system. They allow for improved and efficient communication and are a great improvement over the old method of yelling out for a staff member. There are many types of nurse call systems, such as pagers, light signals, buzzers, methods that allow patients to talk directly to nurses through a direct audio system that the nurse can easily access, mobile telephones, miniature label microphones, and locator badges. The goal is to get a message to the right person as soon as possible and maintain privacy and confidentiality. This can improve care, reduce errors, and make staff more efficient, preventing the unnecessary work of trying to obtain and share information.

Voice Mail

Computer-based messaging systems are found in all healthcare settings today so that staff can leave and receive voice messages. Staff and patients can use these systems, often reducing the need for callbacks. Complicated systems can annoy consumers, and there is an impersonal quality to this form of communication, though it is part of everyday life today. One has to be very careful about leaving voice mails. Clearly, others can listen to messages, and this can lead to a HIPAA violation.

Telephone for Advice and Other Services

Patient advice systems are used mostly by insurers and managed care. Nurses use their assessment skills and provide advice to patients who call in with questions. Typically, insurers develop standard protocols that the nurses use for common questions, but nurses must still use professional judgment when providing advice. This type of service should not become "cookbook" care in which there is no consideration of assessment and individual patient needs. Assessment is the key to successful telephone nursing so as to identify the interventions required that may or may not be found in the guidelines. Some physician offices have telephone advice services that are manned by a physician in the practice or by a nurse. Pediatric practices are the most common type of practice using this system. Patient advice systems via telephone require clear documentation policies and guidelines that include content related to whom is called, when, and for what reason, and the required assessment data and interventions. Telephone advice systems are typically used to answer questions, remind patients of appointments or follow-up needs, and to check in on how a patient is doing.

Hospitals are also using the telephone to begin the admission process for patients with scheduled admissions. Patients are called before the admission date, asked questions related to required admission information, and told what to expect on admission. Pretesting may be scheduled prior to admission. This saves the hospital time and is more cost-effective, and pretesting can be more convenient for the patient. This method can also identify problems that may impact the needed patient care so that they can be addressed early on.

Online Support Groups for Patients and Families

Online support groups can focus on any problem or disease. Patients and their families can use chat rooms, email, and websites for information sharing. Consumers gain information, education about their health and health needs, and support from others with similar problems. A healthcare provider may or may not be involved. Privacy issues must be discussed with participants and the risk of lack of privacy.

Internet or Virtual Appointment

Use of the Internet as a means of increasing accessibility to a physician or advanced practice nurse is growing. Members of younger generations, as well as some senior citizens, are using the Internet to gain advice from health professionals. Portable family histories can be maintained in this fashion and passed on to a new primary care provider. Those patients and families who have limited resources—financial, transportation, or insurance—can more affordably receive medical advice in this format. It also keeps some employees from missing work to take a child or other family member to an appointment. Many of these sites link into cellular devices to send an alert of high importance to whoever is on call for virtual hours. This ensures that high-priority questions and advice get to the health professional quickly (Larkin, 2008). These types of services will most likely increase in the future.

Smartphones

Smartphones are also used in healthcare. These phones give providers access to information, Internet, email, and text messaging, and, of course, telephone access. Security and privacy are of concern and must be considered when smartphones are used.

THE FUTURE OF INFORMATICS AND MEDICAL TECHNOLOGY

The future is likely to see major expansion in the use of technology. Some of the possible technological approaches are already being used in some areas. One area that is growing is the use of embodied conversation agents to provide reinforcement of discharge teaching, particularly when there is low health literacy (Paasche-Orlow, 2010). Cutting-edge technology is sometimes hard to believe. Some of the possibilities are discussed next.

Nanotechnology

Nanotechnology—microscopic technology on the order of one billionth of a meter—will likely impact the diagnosis and treatment of many diseases and conditions (Gordon, Lutz, Boninger, & Cooper, 2007). Some of the pending technologies are highlighted here:

- Sensing patients' internal drug levels with miniature medical diagnostic tools that circulate in their bloodstreams.
- Chemotherapy delivered directly to a tumor site, reducing systemic side effects.
- New monitoring devices for the home: a talking pill bottle that lets patients push a button to hear prescription information; bathroom counters that announce whether it is safe to mix two medications; a shower with built-in scales to calculate body mass index; measuring devices in the bathroom to track urine frequency and output and upload these data to a system or care manager; noninvasive blood glucose monitors to eliminate sticks; and sensors to compute blood sugar levels using a multiwavelength reflective dispersion photometer.

Wearable Computing

A computer can be worn, much as eyeglasses or clothing is worn, and interactions with the user can be based on the context of the situation (ANA, 2008). With heads-up displays, embedded sensors in fabrics, unobtrusive input devices, personal wireless local area networks, and a host of other context sensing and communication tools, wearable computers can act as intelligent assistants or data collection and analysis devices. Many of these devices are available now using smart fabrics. These wearable computer and remote monitoring systems are intertwined with the user's activity so that the technology becomes transparent. Sensors and devices can gather data during the patient's daily routine, providing healthcare providers or researchers with periodic or continuous data on the person's health while he or she is at work, at school, exercising, or sleeping, rather than the current snapshot captured during a typical hospital or clinic visit. A few applications for wearable computing include sudden infant death syndrome monitoring for infants; ambulatory cardiac and respiratory monitoring; monitoring of ventilation during exercise; monitoring the activity level of poststroke patients; monitoring patterns of breathing in asthma; assessment of stress in individuals; arrhythmia detection and control of selected cardiac conditions; and daily activity monitors (Offray Specialty Narrow Fabrics, 2007).

HIPAA: ENSURING CONFIDENTIALITY

The 1996 Health Insurance Portability and Accountability Act (HIPAA) has had a major impact on healthcare delivery systems and how they communicate. Privacy and confidentiality have long been issues in health care, of course. Because HIPAA focuses on the issue of information and confidentiality, it applies to IT. The law also requires data security and electronic transaction standards. This law was necessary because with the growth of information sharing, it became increasingly evident that the transactions and systems were not ensuring privacy and confidentiality—key elements that had long been part of the healthcare delivery system.

Privacy is the right of a person to have personal information kept private. In the healthcare setting, this issue relates to professional ethics. Privacy considerations even apply to family members unless the adult patient specifically communicates that it is acceptable for family members to be given information; such permission cannot be assumed. The law requires that only necessary information be shared among providers, including insurers. Patients may also access their medical records. Information cannot be openly shared—for example, discussing patient information in public places, calling a patient's place of work or home and leaving a message that reveals information about health or health services, and so on, must not be done. Carrying documents outside an HCO with patient identifier information is prohibited;

this has implications for students who may take notes or have written assignments that include this information. How information is carried in PDAs or laptops is also of concern. The new technology has been moving so fast that these critical issues have not been addressed effectively.

The law requires that staff know the key elements of HIPAA and apply them. As a result, HCOs and healthcare profession schools, such as nursing programs, are required to provide information and training about HIPAA. There are large fines if the law is broken. Patients are informed about HIPAA when they enter the health system; they are given written information and asked to sign documents to indicate that they have been informed. Ensuring that the requirements are met must be incorporated into IT, which has become a major method for communicating health information.

TELEHEALTH: A GROWING INTERVENTION

Telehealth, or telemedicine, is the use of telecommunications equipment and communications networks for transferring healthcare information between participants at different locations. Telehealth applies telecommunication and computer technologies to the broad spectrum of public health and medicine. This technology offers opportunities to provide care when face-to-face interaction is impossible (such as in home care, in school-based care, and in rural areas) and can be used in a variety of settings and situations as long as the equipment is available. Two-way interactive video is the most effective telehealth method.

> Telenursing refers to the use of telecommunications technology in nursing to enhance patient care. It involves the use of electromagnetic channels (e.g., wire, radio and optical) to transmit voice, data and video communications signals. It is also defined as distance communications, using electrical or optical transmissions, between humans and/or computers. (Skiba, 1998, p. 40)

Issues that arise with telehealth are the cost of equipment and its use; training for staff and for patients if they need to actively use equipment; limited or no insurance coverage for telehealth services; the need for clear policies, procedures, and protocols; privacy and confidentiality of information; and regulatory issues (e.g., a nurse who is located and licensed in one state providing telenursing for a patient in another state where the nurse is not licensed). Telehealth also has implications for international health care because it provides a method for connecting expertise to patients who may need care that is not accessible in their home country.

INTERNET

Nurses use the Internet to obtain information and for communication through email. Patients/consumers also use the Internet more and more. It can be an excellent source for all types of information, including health and medical information. When the Internet is used as a source of health information, it is important that nurses assess the websites, because they are not all of the same quality. A nurse needs to consider the following factors when evaluating a website:

■ The source or sponsor of the website; the most reliable sites are sponsored by the government, academic institutions, healthcare professional organizations, and HCOs.

■ The current status of the information: When was it posted or revised?

■ Accessibility of the information on the site: Can one find what one needs?

■ References provided for content when appropriate.

Examples of other biomedical and patient care technologies include the following.

Remote Telemetry Monitoring

Remote telemetry monitoring is technology that informs staff when a patient's condition has changed. The patient is on a monitor, and signals are sent to staff through a page system. Staff are informed of the patient's identity, heart rate, and readout of rhythm without being right next to the patient.

Robotics

The use of robotics in patient care will expand (ANA, 2008). Robots have been used for many years to deliver supplies to patient care areas. Robotics enables remote surgeries and virtual reality surgical procedures. Hand-assist devices help patients regain strength after a stroke ("Robotic Brace," 2007). Robots are providing a remote presence to allow physicians to virtually examine patients by manipulating remote cameras ("Telemedicine Pioneer Helps Physicians," 2007). They are being used for microscopic, minimally invasive surgical procedures. One example is the da Vinci surgical system, which helps surgeons perform such procedures as mitral valve repairs, hysterectomies, and prostate surgeries (da Vinci Surgery, 2008). In the future, robots may also be used in direct patient care—for instance, to help lift morbidly obese patients.

Genetics and Genomics

Advances in mapping the human genome (genetics), understanding individual DNA, and examining the impact of external factors such as the environment (genomics) will have a dramatic impact on patient care (ANA, 2008). Such data, especially once they are integrated into EMRs or PHRs, will lead to advances in customized patient care and medications targeted to individual responses to medications. Care and medication can be precisely customized to patients based on their unique DNA profile and how they have responded to medications and other interventions in the past; this will dramatically change how patients are managed for specific diseases and conditions and extend into the prevention of some diseases. The inherent complexity of customized patient care will demand computerized clinical decision support. Predictive disease models based on patients' DNA profiles will emerge as clinicians

better understand DNA mapping. These advances have implications for a new model of care and for the informatics nurse's participation in the development of genomic IT solutions. More than ever, patients will need to be partners in this development as part of patient-centered care. Nurses are beginning to collaborate more with bioengineers and informatics experts to develop new products, participate in research using these products, and help to develop implementation and evaluation plans to use with these products.

HIGH-TOUCH CARE VERSUS HIGH-TECH CARE

High-touch care is what most people go into nursing for, but nursing is much more than this today. This chapter has described the increasing influence of technology on all segments of health care. This influence will not decrease in the future, but rather increase. Nurses do need to understand and know how to use technology that is applied to their practice areas. They need to be involved in the development of this technology when possible, and they must be involved in the implementation of the technology. But there are concerns. When we talk through machines, do we lose information and the personal relationship? How can this be prevented so that we are not disconnected from our patients? How can we ensure that the information we are getting is correct and complete? Are people able to communicate fully through some of these other means? It is clear that over time, the public has become increasingly comfortable with informatics, which they are using more and more in their everyday lives. As nursing uses informatics, nurses need to keep in mind the potential for isolation and the need for effective communication, and they must not forget the need for touch and face-to-face communication.

The future will include many more new uses of technology, and change is ongoing. For example, the eICU (e-intensive care unit) is used to monitor patients from afar to improve patient outcomes (Kowalczyk, 2007). This system allows intensivists at a remote monitoring center to view patients' vital statistics, electrocardiograms, ventilators, and X-ray and lab results. The eICU includes two-way conference video capability so that patients and staff can interact when required. Such a system is attached to four hospitals in Iowa and their ICUs, for example. This type of system has advantages: Experts can be located in one place and then consult with multiple locations and staff. This is particularly useful in providing expert medical care for residents in rural and remote areas. There is no reason that this type of system would be limited to physician consultation; it could be used for nurses. For example, a nurse clinical specialist could view data and consult on patient care with nurses in various ICUs. The potential is there for increased access to information and expertise. The other side of this innovation is the effect on the touch side of care when the provider is not actually in the room with the patient. It is not clear how this might impact care because these types of systems are very new.

CONCLUSION

This chapter has explored the current and future in the world of healthcare informatics and some aspects of biotechnology. There is much more to this subject than use of email, and the chapter has identified many diverse examples. The core competency to utilize informatics is critical. If graduates of the healthcare profession schools cannot understand and use informatics, the safety and quality of the care provided will be impacted. Communication, coordination, documentation, and care provision (including monitoring and decision making) are linked to informatics. However, each nurse must not get so involved in informatics and technology that the patient as a person is lost—the patient–nurse relationship is an important component of patient-centered care.

DISCUSSION QUESTIONS

1. What is informatics, and why is it important in health care and nursing?

2. Describe the certification requirements for an informatics nurse and the role.

3. Describe four examples of healthcare informatics and implications for nursing.

4. Why is documentation important?

5. Explain how the EMR and PHR can increase quality of care and decrease errors. Provide examples.

6. Discuss issues related to confidentiality and informatics.

7. Divide into small teams. Identify an HCO in your local community and try to find out how it uses informatics. You can focus on the entire organization or select a department or a unit. Are there any future plans to increase the use of informatics?

8. In a team of classmates, develop six questions to ask a nurse who works in a hospital that uses an EMR. Each student on the team will then interview one registered nurse. After the interviews, combine your data and analyze the results.

9. Speak to a registered nurse who works in staff development/education in an HCO. Discuss the training that staff members receive for using informatics.

10. If you have used an EMR in clinical practice, what was it like for you? If you have not yet done this, interview a senior student and ask about the experience.

11. Which biomedical equipment have you used or seen used? How does the use of this equipment impact care?

12. What is your opinion of the potential conflict between high-touch care and high-tech care? Discuss with your team.

CASE STUDY

A 6-year-old has come to the attention of the child welfare department as a possible victim of sexual abuse. The child lives in a very rural part of a western state. Rather than have the child travel a distance to experts, she was taken to the nearest clinic staffed by sexual assault nurse examiners and a knowledgeable pediatrician skilled in sexual abuse examinations. At the time of the examination, pictures were taken of the child's body, including the genital area. These pictures are crucial if charges are filed. To ensure that an accurate diagnosis is made, local experts wish to have a second opinion because the results of the physical examination were not believed to be completely definitive. The experts for the second opinion were linked via the Internet and Internet videoconferencing equipment so that the two teams could talk and view de-identified (because the information was going across unsecure Internet channels) photos.

Within 15 minutes, it was determined that the hymen was intact and no penetration had occurred. Other markers indicated that there was evidence of child abuse, but none that supported a claim of sexual assault. This case used an EMR, digitized photos, and Internet consultation to arrive at a diagnosis that had both medical and legal implications.

Case Questions

1. Discuss the impact of the use of these methods in the case on the nurse–patient relationship and on patient confidentiality including HIPAA requirements.
2. How else might this technology be used?
3. What is your opinion of the human, caring part of the care process in relation to this case description?

RESOURCES

Alliance for Nursing Informatics: http://www.alliance
ni.org/

American Nursing Informatics Association: http
://www.ania-caring.org/mc/page.do?sitePageId=
101757&orgId=car

American Telemedicine Association: http://www
.atmeda.org/

Ending the Document Game: http://endingthe
documentgame.gov/ medicationRecord.html

Healthcare Information and Management Systems
Society: http://www.himss.org/asp/topics_nursing
Informatics.asp

Technology Informatics Guiding Educational Reform (TIGER Initiative): http://www.tigersummit
.com/About_Us.html

REFERENCES

ABC Coding Solutions. (2011). ABC coding. Retrieved from http://www.abccodes.com/ali/abc
_codes/

American Nurses Association (ANA). (2006). Nursing practice information infrastructure: Glossary. Retrieved from http://www.nursingworld.org/npii
/glossary.htm

American Nurses Association (ANA). (2007). Informatics nurse certification exam. Retrieved from http://www.nursecredentialing.org/Nurse
Specialties/Informatics.aspx

American Nurses Association (ANA). (2008). *Nursing informatics: Scope and standards of practice*. Washington, DC: Author.

American Nurses Association (ANA). (2009). Electronic health record (Position statement).

Silver Spring, MD: Author. Retrieved from http ://www.nursingworld.org/MainMenuCategories /HealthcareandPolicyIssues/ANAPosition Statements/practice.aspx

American Nurses Association (ANA). (2010). *ANA's principles for nursing documentation.* Silver Spring, MD: Author.

Appleton, C. (1998). Nursing research: Moving into the clinical setting. *Nursing Management, 29*(6), 43–45.

Association of periOperative Registered Nurses. (2008). Perioperative data set. Retrieved from http ://www.aorn.org/PracticeResources/PNDSAnd StandardizedPerioperativeRecord/

Bodenheimer, T. (2008). Coordinating care: A perilous journey through the healthcare system. *New England Journal of Medicine, 358,* 1065–1071.

Centers for Disease Control and Prevention (CDC). (2011). *International Classification of Diseases (ICD-10).* Retrieved from http://www.cdc.gov/nchs/icd /icd10.htm

Clark, S. (2011). Medical record documentation makes top 10 non-compliance list for first half of 2010. *HIM Connection.* Retrieved from http://www .hcpro.com/CCP-258429-237/Medical-record-documentation-makes-Joint-Commission-top-10-noncompliance-list-for-first-half-of-2010.html

da Vinci Surgery. (2008). Surgery enabled by da Vinci®. Retrieved from http://www.davinci surgery.com/davinci-surgery/

Englebardt, S., & Nelson, R. (2002). *Healthcare informatics: An interdisciplinary approach.* St. Louis, MO: Mosby-Year Book.

Finkelman, A., & Kenner, C. (2009). *Teaching IOM.* Silver Spring, MD: American Nurses Association.

Gordon, A., Lutz, G., Boninger, M., & Cooper, R. (2007). Introduction to nanotechnology: Potential applications in physical medicine and rehabilitation. *American Journal of Physical Medicine and Rehabilitation, 86,* 225–241.

Healthcare Information and Management Systems Society. (2011, June 17). Position statement on transforming nursing practice through technology and informatics. Retrieved from http://www .himss.org/ASP/index.asp

Institute of Medicine (IOM). (2003). *Health professions education.* Washington, DC: National Academies Press.

International Council of Nurses (ICN). (2008). International Classification for Nursing Practice

(ICNP). Retrieved from http://www.icn.ch/icnp _def.htm

Iyer, P., & Camp, N. (1999). *Nursing documentation.* St. Louis, MO: Mosby.

The Joint Commission (JC). (2011). *Comprehensive accreditation manual for hospitals.* Chicago, IL: Author.

Kowalczyk, L. (November 19, 2007). Teletreatment: Monitoring from afar, "eICUs" fill the gap. Retrieved from http://www.boston.com/business /globe/articles/2007/11/19/tele_treatment/

Larkin, H. (2008). Your future chief of staff? *H&HN: Hospitals & Healthcare Networks, 82*(3), 30–34.

National Center for Health Statistics. (2010). More physicians switch to electronic medical record. Retrieved from http://nchspressroom.wordpress .com/2010/04/02/more-physicians-switch-to-electronic-medical-record-use/

National Library of Medicine (NLM). (2008a). Logical observation identifiers names and codes. Retrieved from http://www.nlm.nih.gov/research /umls/loinc_main.html

National Library of Medicine (NLM). (2008b). Unified medical language system: SNOMED clinical terms. Retrieved from http://www.nlm.nih .gov/research/umls/Snomed/snomed_main .html

Nelson, R., & Joos, I. (1989, Fall). On language in nursing: From data to wisdom. *PLN Vision,* p. 6.

Offray Specialty Narrow Fabrics. (2007). Smart textiles. Retrieved from http://www.osnf .com/p_ smart.html

Omaha System. (2011). The Omaha System: Solving the clinical data-information puzzle. Retrieved from http://www.omahasystem.org/

Paasche-Orlow, M. K. (2010). Usability of conversational agents by patients with inadequate health literacy: Evidence from two clinical trials. *Journal of Health Communication, 15*(Suppl. 2, special issue), *Health Literacy Research: Current Status and Future Directions,* 197–210.

Richards, J. (2001). Nursing in a digital age. *Nursing Economics, 19*(1), 6–10, 34.

Robotic brace aids stroke recovery. (2007). Retrieved from *Science Daily* website: http://www.science daily.com/releases/2007/03/070321105223.htm

Romano, M., & Stafford, R. (2011). Electronic health records and clinical decision support systems: Impact on national ambulatory care quality. *Archives of Internal Medicine, 171,* 897–903.

Schwiran, P., & Thede, L. (2011). Informatics: The standardized nursing terminologies: A national survey of nurses' experiences and attitudes. *Online Journal of Issues in Nursing, 16*(2). Retrieved from http://www.nursingworld.org/MainMenu Categories/ANAMarketplace/ANAPeriodicals /OJIN/TableofContents/Vol-16-2011/No2-May-2011/Standardized-Nursing-Terminologies.aspx

Skiba, D. J. (1998). Health-oriented telecommunications. In M. J. Ball, K. J. Hannah, S. K. Newbold, & J. V. Douglas (Eds.), *Nursing informatics: Where caring and technology meet* (pp. 40–53). New York, NY: Springer.

Telemedicine pioneer helps physicians on the move stay close to patients. (2007). Retrieved from Cisco Systems website: http://www.cisco.com/en/US /solutions/collateral/ns339/ns636/ns418/ns554 /net_customer_profile0900aecd804073a3.pdf

U.S. Department of Health and Human Services. (2010). Meaningful use. Retrieved from http ://www.hhs.gov/news/imagelibrary/video /2010-07-13_press.html

U.S. Department of Health and Human Services. (2011). Surveys show significant proportions of hospitals and doctors already plan to adopt electronic health records and qualify for federal incentive payments. Retrieved from http://www.hhs .gov/news/press/2011pres/01/20110113a.html

Theoretical Foundations, Research, and Evidence-Based Practice

The chapters included in Part 4 are not intended to be a summary of major nursing theories or research methods, but rather provide a foundation for understanding, critiquing, evaluating, and using theory and research for advanced practice. Theory can provide a framework that encompasses what nurses know, do, and think, and it can guide the advanced practice nurse to know what to ask, what to observe, what to focus on, and what to think about (Chinn & Kramer, 1995).

The terminology and definitions surrounding theory can be confusing for the novice advanced practice nurse to fully understand. Further, scholars of nursing theory do not always agree on the definitions, leading to a lack of clarity in this field of study. As way of introduction to Part 4, the generally agreed-upon definitions of terms that provide the foundation for the chapters in this part are presented here.

What is *theory*? As with many concepts, a variety of definitions for this term have been proposed, which typically share a common set of characteristics. For our purposes, theories are organized systems that describe, explain, predict, or prescribe phenomenon. They are composed of *concepts* (constructs or variables) and *propositions* (hypotheses) that specify the relationships among the concepts. Further theories are substantiated by and derived from established evidence and can be repeatedly confirmed by observation and testing.

Four types of theories are derived from the preceding definition:

1. *Descriptive theories* describe concepts of a discipline.
2. *Explanatory theories* explain how the concepts relate to one another.
3. *Predictive theories* predict the relationships between the concepts of a phenomenon

and predict under which conditions it will occur.

4. *Prescriptive theories* prescribe interventions and the consequences of interventions.

Additionally, four levels of theory can be placed on a continuum ranging from very abstract and broad (metatheory) to very specific and narrow (practice theories):

1. *Metatheory* is the most abstract and cannot be easily tested. There are no theories labeled as such in nursing. The most commonly cited examples of metatheory are the big bang and evolution.

2. *Grand theories* define broad perspectives for nursing practice and are less abstract than metatheory. As such they can be tested. Some of the more well-known nursing theories classified as grand theory are those proposed by Nightingale, Parse, Leininger, Benner, and Henderson. There are many more, however, and a search of the Internet can lead to a long list of nursing grand theories.

3. *Middle-range (midrange) theories* are moderately abstract and have a limited number of concepts. They can be tested directly. Midrange theories can predict and prescribe nursing interventions and patient outcomes. Many new midrange nursing theories have been proposed over the last two decades. They are often used for both nursing research and practice. Some examples include theories of uncertainty, comfort, pain, social support, and quality of life. A search of the Internet can reveal many nursing middle-range theories useful to the advanced practice nurse.

4. *Practice theory* traces the outline for practice. Objectives are set and actions are set to meet the objectives.

Another important fundamental understanding of nursing theory is needed before reading the chapters in Part 4. In 1984, Fawcett presented a seminal paper on the metaparadigms of nursing. It is now widely accepted, but not universally, that the metaparadigms for nursing theory are as fourfold:

■ Nursing

■ Health

■ Person

■ Environment

Theory, practice, research, and evidence-based practice (EBP) are intimately intertwined. Theory informs practice, just as practice informs theory. Research is used to test the theory, but at the same time can be used to develop and refine theory. As nursing goes forward as a discipline, and as consumers and policymakers demand effective, cost-conscious, evidence-based practice, we must understand theory and research and use them to guide practice, while simultaneously analyzing and critiquing our practice to generate new theories that can be tested by research.

In the first chapter in Part 4 (Chapter 17), Kenney provides a foundation to appreciate the value and relevance of theory from nursing and other disciplines and application to practice. In Chapter 18, Gortner and Sultz discuss knowledge development in nursing; Chapter 19, Sultz and Young provide a historical overview of nursing research and highlight the role the Agency for Healthcare Policy and Research (AHCPR) has played in the development of clinical practice guidelines. Future trends related to nursing research, including population research, EBP, and outcomes research, are reviewed. Current opportunities and goals of the National Institute of Nursing Research (NINR) are outlined, with a focus on health promotion, chronic disease management. and reproductive health. It is essential for advanced practice nurses to have a solid foundation in the utilization of EBP guidelines to incorporate research findings into clinical decision making.

In Chapter 20, Houser gives a broad overview of the five elements necessary in the EBP process: (1) formulating an appropriate question, (2) performing an efficient literature search, (3) critically appraising the best available evidence, (4) applying the best evidence to clinical practice, and (5) assessing outcomes of care. Clinical scenarios and strategies to overcome barriers to EBP utilization are illustrated.

In the last chapter in Part 4 (Chapter 21), Tymkow eloquently compares and contrasts clinical scholarship and EBP and the role of the doctor of nursing practice (DNP) to this end. The AACN DNP essentials document further defines the skills, tools, and methods necessary to implement and support clinical scholarship and EBP as the following: (1) translating re-search in practice, (2) quality improvement and patient-centered care, (3) evaluation of practice, (4) research methods and technology, (5) participation in collaborative research, and (6) disseminating findings from evidence-based practice.

The AACN recommends separate course work in research and an informal survey of doctor of nursing practice and master of science in nursing curricula demonstrates that most often research is done in separate courses in advanced nurse practice programs. Thus it is not the intention of this book to explicate the research process and methods in detail, but rather to put the need for health research and nursing research into a broader context so the reader can appreciate how research improves practice and informs decision making.

CHAPTER 17

Theory-Based Advanced Nursing Practice

Janet W. Kenney

CHAPTER OBJECTIVES

1. Describe the value and relevance of theory-based nursing for advanced practice nurses.

2. Discuss issues for applying theories in nursing practice.

3. Discuss the structure of nursing knowledge and the transformative process for theory-based practice.

4. Explain the relationship between theory and critical thinking.

5. Discuss the process for selecting and applying appropriate nursing, family, and other disciplines' models and theories to advanced nursing practice.

INTRODUCTION

All professional disciplines are based on their unique knowledge, which is expressed in models and theories that are applied in practice. The focus of nursing knowledge is on humans' health experiences within the context of their environment and the nurse–client relationship. Theory-based nursing practice is the application of various models, theories, and principles from nursing science and the biological, behavioral, medical, and sociocultural disciplines to clinical nursing practice. Conceptual models and theories provide a broad knowledge base to assist nurses in understanding and interpreting the client's complex health situation and in planning nursing actions to achieve desired client outcomes. "Explicit use of conceptual models of nursing and nursing theories to guide nursing practice is the hallmark of professional nursing" (Fawcett, 1997, p. 212); it distinguishes nursing as an autonomous health profession.

This chapter describes the value and relevance of theory-based nursing for advanced practice nurses and discusses some underlying concerns about applying theories in nursing practice. The structure of nursing knowledge and the transformative process for theory-based practice are explained, along with the importance of critical thinking. An overview of various models and theories of nursing, family, and other disciplines is provided. Finally, the process for selecting and applying appropriate models and theories in nursing practice is thoroughly described.

RELEVANCE OF THEORY-BASED PRACTICE IN NURSING

The value of theory-based nursing practice is well documented in numerous books and journal articles. Although many articles illustrate the application of a nursing model or theory to clients with a specific health problem, Alligood (1997b) reviewed the nursing literature and found that about 68% of the articles reflect a medical approach to nursing. She also noted that most nurses described their practice in terms of a specialty area, types of care or health problems, and nursing interventions.

All nurses use knowledge they acquired during their formal education and clinical experience to guide their practice. Some nurse practitioners consistently use models and theories to guide their practice, but most nurses are unaware of existing theories and models or do not know how to apply them. Many nurses are not aware of what knowledge they use or where they learned it; thus their implicit knowledge tends to be fragmented, diffused, incomplete, and greatly influenced by the medical model (Fawcett, 1997). Although graduate nurse practitioner students learn about nursing models

and theories, their education often emphasizes application of medical knowledge as the base for their nursing practice. In essence, the use of medical knowledge and policies of healthcare delivery systems has replaced nursing knowledge and influenced some nurses to become "junior doctors," instead of "senior nurses" (Meleis, 1993).

Theories and models from nursing and behavioral disciplines are used by advanced practice nurses to provide effective, high-quality nursing care. Many nurses believe that use of nursing theories would improve the quality of nursing care but that they do not have sufficient information about them or the opportunity to use them (McKenna, 1997b). According to Meleis (1997), theories improve quality of care by clearly defining the boundaries and goals of nursing assessment, diagnosis, and interventions and by providing continuity and congruency of care. Theory also contributes to more efficient and effective nursing practice and enhances nurses' professional autonomy and accountability. Aggleton and Chalmers (1986) claim that providing nursing care without a theory base is like "practicing in the dark." Kenney (1996) reported that professional nurses can effectively use theories and models from nursing and behavioral disciplines to:

- Collect, organize, and classify client data
- Understand, analyze, and interpret clients' health situations
- Guide formulation of nursing diagnoses
- Plan, implement, and evaluate nursing care
- Explain nursing actions and interactions with clients
- Describe, explain, and sometimes predict clients' responses
- Demonstrate responsibility and accountability for nursing actions
- Achieve desired outcomes for clients

The healthcare revolution requires that nurses demonstrate efficient, cost-effective, high-quality care within organized delivery systems. "Nursing theory-based practice offers an alternative to the dehumanizing, fragmented, and paternalistic approaches that plague current delivery systems" (Smith, 1994, p. 7). With changes in the current third-party reimbursement systems, nurses will be paid for effective theory-based practice that enhances clients' health and their quality of life. To accomplish this, nurse practitioners must use critical thinking skills combined with theory-based knowledge and clinical expertise to achieve desired client outcomes.

ISSUES RELATED TO THEORY-BASED NURSING PRACTICE

In recent years, the enthusiasm for using nursing models and theories in practice has waned due to criticisms about the theory–practice gap and the lack of relevance to clinical practice. Also, there are philosophical concerns about whether only nursing models should guide practice and whether models and theories of nursing and other disciplines may be integrated in practice. This section discusses some of these issues.

The theory–practice gap refers to the lack of use or inability of nurses to use nursing and other theories in clinical practice. McKenna (1997b) claims that theories are not being used in a systematic way to guide nursing practice, although using theories may improve the quality of care. He believes nurses do not use nursing theories because they do not know about them, understand them, believe in them, or know how to apply them, or because they are not allowed to use them. Professional nursing practice more often reflects the medical or organizational model of care than application of relevant nursing models or theories.

According to Rogers (1989, p. 114), "Nursing knowledge . . . is often seen as being unscientific, intuitive, and highly subjective." Some nurses believe that conceptual models and theories are too abstract to apply in nursing practice; they do not provide sufficient information to guide nursing judgments, are subject to different interpretations, are incomplete, and lack

adequate testing and refinement (Field, 1987; Firlet, 1985). Others argue that some nursing theories were never meant to be directly applied in nursing practice but were intentionally kept abstract to stimulate thinking, provide new insights, and develop creative ways of viewing nursing (McKenna, 1997b).

As a practice discipline, nursing models and theories should be useful in practice, or their value is questionable. When models and theories are logical and consistent with other validated theories, they may provide the rationale and consequences of nursing actions and lead to predictable client outcomes. Numerous articles and chapters describe application of various models to clinical nursing practice. However, rigorous research studies on how nursing models and theories contribute to desirable nursing actions and client outcomes are lacking.

Another issue is whether only nursing models and theories are appropriate for the discipline, as nursing is an applied science. Most professional nurses are familiar with theories from other disciplines, such as systems theory, family theories, developmental theories, and others; in clinical practice, nurses often combine their nursing and medical knowledge with theories from other disciplines. Some nurse scholars argue that nursing practice must be based on nursing models and theories, as they are consistent with nursing's view of human science and provide the structure for explaining nursing's unique contribution to health care (Cody, 1996; Mitchell, 1992). Because nursing models or theories represent the theorist's unique beliefs about persons, health, and nursing and guide how nurses interact with clients, McKenna (1997b) believes that an eclectic approach, combining theories from nursing and other disciplines, may compromise nursing theories if the concepts are removed from their original context and interwoven with other theories.

In contrast, Meleis (1997) argues that because nurses study other disciplines, nursing theory tends to reflect a broad range of perspectives and premises. Many nursing theorists have incorporated or borrowed theories from other disciplines and then transmuted them to fit within the context of nursing so that their nursing theories comprise shared knowledge used in a distinctive way (Timpson, 1996).

A related issue is whether professional nurses should consistently use only one nursing model or use various models and theories from nursing and other disciplines in their practice. Most professions, like nursing, have multiple theories that represent divergent and unique perspectives about the phenomena of concern to their practice. Within nursing, conceptual models and theories range from broad conceptual models, or grand theories, to specific practice theories. There are advantages and disadvantages to using one or more theories in clinical practice. Depending on the nurse's knowledge and clinical practice area, some nursing models and theories may be more appropriate than others. However, some would argue that use of just one nursing theory limits the nurse's assessment to only those things addressed by the theory, and the nurse may be forced to fit the client situation to the theory.

Others believe that nurses should consider a variety of nursing theories and select the model or theory that best fits the client's health problems. The majority of early nursing theories were based on traditional scientific methods and reflect a reductionistic perspective of humans as passive beings, consisting of elementary parts that respond to external stimuli in a linear, causal, and predictive way (Benner & Wrubel, 1989). Nursing models based on this perspective ultimately dehumanize individuals into disparate parts and systems and lead to fragmented, nonholistic nursing care (Aggleton & Chalmers, 1986). More contemporary nursing models view humans as continuously changing during reciprocal interactions with their environment; thus individual reactions to nursing care are not predictable, nor can they be controlled. However, these newer nursing models are more abstract than earlier models and

are less likely to offer specific guidelines for nursing actions. Professional nurses are expected to develop unique, creative nursing actions suitable for each client's health problem and lifestyle, and theories from other disciplines may be integrated to complement and strengthen some limitations in both early and contemporary nursing models.

Cody (1996) contends that eclecticism, or selecting the best theory from other sources, is not necessarily wrong, but constantly borrowing theories from other disciplines does not contribute to the science of nursing or differentiate nursing from other professions. He believes that nursing practice ought to reflect a coherent, nursing theoretical base to guide practice in specific ways and contribute to the quality of care.

Since professional nurses provide health care for a variety of clients, each of whom is unique, yet some of whom may have similar health concerns, nurses must use a broad knowledge base from nursing and other disciplines to select and apply relevant models and/or theories that are congruent with the client's situation. Health care, based on appropriate nursing models and theories, that integrates appropriate family, behavioral, and developmental theories, is most likely to achieve desired client health outcomes.

STRUCTURE OF NURSING KNOWLEDGE AND PERSPECTIVE TRANSFORMATION

Advanced practice nurses must first understand the structure of nursing knowledge and the process of transforming nursing models and theories into useful perspectives prior to implementing theory-based practice. Fawcett (1995) described the structural hierarchy of nursing knowledge or nursing science. Nursing's metaparadigm, which includes the major concepts of person, health, environment, and nursing, provides the foundation from which nursing philosophies, conceptual models, and theories are derived. Each nurse theorist developed unique definitions of her major concepts, based on her education, practice, and personal philosophy (values, beliefs, and assumptions) about humans, health, nursing, and environment. The theorist's philosophy also influenced her conceptual model, which describes how the concepts are linked; the model explains the relationships among client–health–nursing situations (Sorrentino, 1991). Conceptual nursing models are usually called "grand theories" because they are broad and abstract and may not provide specific directions for nursing actions. Some nurse theorists have developed midrange or practice theories from their models, which describe specific relationships among the concepts and suggest hypotheses to be tested.

According to Rogers (1989), an individual's personal meaning perspective or conceptual model provides a frame of reference or lens that influences how one perceives, thinks, and behaves in the world, yet most people are not aware of how their perspective influences and affects their view of themselves, others, and their world because underlying beliefs are held in the unconscious mind. In practice, nurses' perceptions, thoughts, feelings, and actions are guided by their personal framework or perspective of nursing, which provides a cognitive structure based on their assumptions, beliefs, and values about nursing (Fawcett, 1995). Many nurses unconsciously use a medical or institutional model as their perspective for organizing care. The prevalent values of such models or perspectives are efficiency, standardized care, rules, and regulations, such as "critical care pathways" (Rogers, 1989). As nurses become aware of the differences between the present and potential possibilities of nursing practice, they experience a cognitive dissonance or discomfort from an awareness of what is versus what could be (Rogers, 1989). Thus, only when nurses experience cognitive dissonance in practice will they change their frame of reference and use nursing models and theories.

For professional nurses to apply conceptual nursing models and theories, a dramatic change, or perspective transformation, must occur (Fawcett, 1995; Rogers, 1989). Perspective transformation is the process of moving from one frame of reference or perspective to another when unresolved dilemmas arise and create dissonance in one's current perspective (Mezirow, 1979). It is a process of critical reflection and analysis of other explanations or perspectives that might resolve the dilemma and explain or guide one's understanding and actions. This process involves gradually acquiring a new perspective that leads to fundamental changes in the way nurses experience, interpret, and understand their world and their relationships with others (Fawcett, 1995).

Fawcett (1995) describes nine phases leading to perspective transformation. Initially, the prevailing stability of the current nursing practice is disrupted when use of a nursing conceptual model or theory-based practice is introduced. Dissonance occurs as nurses consider their own perspective for practice and the challenge of changing to a new conceptual model or theory. Some nurses identify discrepancies between their current practice and how the new model or theory could affect their practice. Confusion may follow as nurses struggle to learn about the model or theory and how to apply it in practice. Nurses often feel anxious, angry, and unable to think during these phases and may grieve the loss of familiar perspectives of nursing. Their former perspective no longer seems useful, yet they have not internalized the new model or theory well enough to use it effectively. While dwelling with uncertainty, nurses acknowledge that their confusion is not due to personal inadequacy, and as their anxiety diminishes, they begin to critically examine former practice methods and explore the possibilities of implementing a new model or theory (Fawcett, 1995; Rogers, 1989).

With the discovery that a new model or theory is coherent and meaningful, synthesis occurs.

As ways to apply the new model become clearer, new insights assist nurses to understand the usefulness of the conceptual model or theory in nursing practice (Fawcett, 1995). Resolution occurs as nurses become comfortable using the new model; they may feel a sense of empowerment and view their practice differently. Gradually, nurses consciously change their practice during reconceptualization; they shift from their former patterns to new ways of thinking and acting within the new model or theory. The final phase, return to stability, occurs when nursing practice is clearly based on the new nursing model or theory. Acceptance of a new perspective or paradigm, along with the corresponding assumptions, values, and beliefs, concludes the transformation process.

Models and theories from nursing and other disciplines provide the cognitive structures that guide professional nursing practice. This body of knowledge helps nurses explain what they know and the rationale for their nursing actions that facilitate the client's health (Fawcett, 1997). Theory-based nursing practice depends on the depth of nurses' knowledge of models and theories and their understanding about how to apply them in practice (Alligood, 1997a). Nursing models and theories represent ideal, logical, unique perspectives or maps of the person and health. They provide a structure and systematic approach to examine clients' situations, identify relevant information, interpret data for nursing diagnoses, and plan effective nursing care through critical thinking, reasoning, and decision making (Alligood, 1997a; Mayberry, 1991; Timpson, 1996).

Nurses must use critical thinking skills to apply models and theories to their clients' health concerns. Paul and Nosich's (1991) definition of critical thinking, which follows, is a commonly accepted one:

> Critical thinking is the intellectually disciplined process of actively and skillfully conceptualizing, applying, analyzing, synthesizing, or evaluating information gathered from, or generated by, observation, experience, reflection, reasoning, or communication, as a guide to belief and action. (p. 4)

According to Cradock (1996), it is not what they know that makes nurses advanced practitioners, but rather how they use what they know. Advanced practice nurses must make expert clinical decisions based on reflection, complex reasoning, and critical thinking to apply theoretically based knowledge to diverse client situations (Spiracino, 1991). Critical thinking combines ideas from both models and theories with clinical experience and provides the structure for unique, creative nursing practice with each client (Alligood, 1997a; Field, 1987; Mayberry, 1991; Sorrentino, 1991). Several nurse authors believe that nursing theories will become the stimuli for reflection and critical thinking, leading to realms for creative expressions in nursing practice (Chinn, 1997; Marks-Moran & Rose, 1997). Theory-based nursing and critical thinking are the foundations of advanced nursing practice (Mitchell, 1992). Specific critical thinking skills for each component of the nursing process are identified in **Table 17-1**.

MODELS AND THEORIES APPLICABLE IN ADVANCED NURSING PRACTICE

Theory-based nursing practice is the creative application of various models, theories, and principles from nursing, medical, behavioral, and humanistic sciences. Models and theories from relevant disciplines provide the knowledge base to understand various aspects of the client's health concerns and guide appropriate nursing management. In advanced nursing practice, the client may be an individual, families, or an aggregate, such as a community or special population. Knowledge of relevant models and theories from nursing and other disciplines enables the nurse to select those that best fit each client. This section provides a brief overview of some nursing, family, community, and other models and theories that may be relevant and useful to nurse practitioners.

TABLE 17-1	Application of Critical Thinking Skills to the Nursing Process

Components and Definitions	Critical Thinking Skills and Activities
Assessment An ongoing process of data collection to determine the client's strengths and health concerns	Collect relevant client data by observation, examination, interview and history, and reviewing the records Distinguish relevant data from irrelevant Distinguish important data from unimportant Validate data with others
Diagnosis The analysis/synthesis of data to identify patterns and compare with norms and models A clear, concise statement of the client's health status and concerns appropriate for nursing intervention	Organize and categorize data into patterns Identify data gaps Recognize patterns and relationships in data Compare patterns with norms and theories Examine own assumptions regarding client's situation Make inferences and judgments of client's health concerns Define the health concern and validate with the client and health team members Describe actual and potential concerns and the etiology of each diagnosis Propose alternative explanations of concerns
Planning Determination of how to assist the client in resolving concerns related to restoration, maintenance, or promotion of health	Identify priority of client's concerns Determine client's desired health outcomes Select appropriate nursing interventions by generalizing principles and theories Transfer knowledge from other sciences Design plan of care with scientific rationale
Implementation Carrying out the plan of care by the client and nurse	Apply knowledge to perform interventions Compare baseline data with changing status Test hypotheses of nursing interventions Update and revise the care plan Collaborate with health team members
Evaluation A systematic, continuous process of comparing the client's response with the desired health outcomes	Compare client's responses with desired health outcomes Use criterion-based tools to evaluate Determine the client's level of progress Revise the plan of care

Nursing Models and Theories

Numerous nursing models and theories have been reported in the literature since the 1950s. Some well-known nurse theorists' works are cited; readers are encouraged to seek other sources for more information about their models and theories. The early nurse theorists' conceptual models focused on individual clients and described nursing goals and activities. Peplau's interpersonal model described a goal-directed, nurse–client interpersonal process to promote the client's personality and living. Orlando's model explained a deliberative nursing approach to understand nurse–patient relationships and the communication process. Hall's core–care–cure model expanded and clarified nursing actions to promote clients' health. Levine's model identified four principles of human conservation to guide nursing activities.

More contemporary nursing theories have been published since 1970, when Rogers introduced her science of unitary man. She described mutually evolving relationships between humans and their environment that are expressed as changing energy fields, patterns, and organization. Orem's self-care model identified requisites for an individual's self-care and specific nursing systems to deliver care according to the client's self-care needs. King designed a systems model that included the individual, family, and society, then developed her theory of goal attainment, which described nurse–patient transactions to achieve the client's goals. Roy's adaptation model identified three types of stimuli that affect a patient's four modes of functioning. She described how the nurse identifies maladaptive behaviors and alters stimuli to enhance the client's adaptation. Paterson and Zderad developed a model of humanistic nursing. Leininger's transcultural nursing model explained differences between universal and cultural-specific views of health and healing, and how nurses can provide culturally congruent health care. According to Watson, nursing is the art and science of human care; nurses engage in transpersonal caring transactions to assist persons to achieve mind–body–soul harmony. Johnson's behavioral systems model focused on nurturing, protecting, and stimulating the individual's seven subsystems to maintain balance and stability. Neuman designed a complex healthcare systems model that identified different types of stressors and levels of defense; nursing actions were based on three levels of prevention. Parse developed a man–living–health theory in which nurses assist individuals to explore their past, present, and future life experiences and illuminate possible lifestyle choices to enhance their health and lives. Newman's theory of health as expanding consciousness considers disease as part of health, and explores time and rhythm pattern recognition with changes in life and health.

Family Models

Although most nursing models were originally designed to focus on individual clients, a few are applicable to families. King views the family as a social system or group of interacting individuals and family health as dynamic life experiences. Roy views the family as part of the client's immediate social environment, whereas Neuman's concept of family comprises harmonious relationships among family members. These nurse theorists focused on the individual client, with the family seen as context. If the family is viewed as the client, the nurse must decide what the model should focus on—family development, interactions and stress, family systems, structure and function, or a combination of these models, such as the Calgary family model.

Family development models are based on the premise that the life cycle of families follows a common sequence of events from marriage through child rearing, retirement, and bereavement. Most are based on the typical nuclear two-parent family and emphasize the stages and adult's responsibilities to accomplish desired goals. Duvall's (1977) model is well known. Stevenson (1977), a nurse theorist, also designed a family model.

Family interactional models view family members as a unit of interacting personalities within a dynamic life process. These models focus on how members' perceptions and interpretations of themselves and other family members determine their behaviors and actions. Also, these models consider how members' roles affect their interaction with others. Satir's family interaction model is an example. Family stress and coping models, based on the work of Lazarus and Folkman, were developed by Moos and Billings (1982) to identify how the family appraised the situation, dealt with their problems, and handled the resulting emotions. McCubbin and McCubbin (1993) designed the double ABCX model, which examines family life stressors and resources, along with changes that affect their adaptation to health problems and their ability to manage family crises. Curran's (1985) healthy family model identified characteristics of healthy families and common stressors affecting families.

Family systems models view the whole family as greater than and different from the sum of its parts or members. These models focus on the family with a hierarchy of subsystems (mother-father, parent-child) and supersystems in the community (social, occupational, recreational, and religious networks) that interact with the family system. Olson, Russell, and Sprenkle's (1983) model identifies 16 types of family systems based on the premise that a balance must be maintained in family cohesion, so that members do not become too enmeshed or too distant, and on adaptability, wherein too much change creates chaos and too little change leads to rigidity. Communication between family members is the third dimension. The Beavers system model (Beavers & Voeller, 1983) examines the structure, flexibility, and competence of a family and its members. Centripetal families enjoy close family relationships, while centrifugal families seek satisfaction outside the family.

Family structural-functional models view the family as a social system composed of nuclear and extended family members, along with their social–communicative interactions to achieve family functions. According to Friedman (1992), the structural components include family composition, values, communication patterns, members' roles, and the power structure. Functional components of this model include physical necessities and care; economic, affective, and reproductive behaviors; socialization and placement of family members; and family coping abilities. The structural and functional components are interrelated, and each part is affected by changes in other parts.

A model that combines many of the aforementioned models is the Calgary family model, developed by Wright and Leahey (1994). The major components include the internal and external family structure, similar to Friedman's (1992) model, along with family context, such as race, ethnicity, social class, religion, and environment. Family functions are viewed as instrumental or daily living activities, and expressive activities, including communication (emotional, verbal, and behavioral), problem solving, roles, influences, beliefs, and alliances or coalitions. Family developmental stages and tasks, similar to Duvall's (1977), are also part of this comprehensive model.

Any family model may be combined with and complement a nursing model because nursing practice may involve individual clients or families. Nurses with knowledge of various family models are more likely to select the most appropriate and relevant one to meet the family's health concerns.

Community Models

Many community models are useful to nurses, but they differ according to whether community is considered a target population or aggregate or a geographic area. McKay and Segall (1983) described an aggregate model, in which the focus is on a group of individuals who share common characteristics, but who may not interact with one another. Shamansky and Pesznecker (1981) identified three interdependent factors that constitute a geographical community: (1) persons who reside in an area; (2) space and time, which include the community's history and environmental features; and (3) purpose factors that explain functional processes such as government policies, educational services, and forms of communication. The community-as-client model, designed by Anderson, McFarlane, and Helton (1986), combines both the aggregate and geographical community. It addresses the following eight subsystems of the aggregate in the community: physical environment, education, safety and transportation, politics and government, health and social services, communication, economics, and recreation. A community nursing process model was developed by Goeppinger, Lassiter, and Wilcox (1982). It examines the following eight processes in a community: commitment of members, awareness of others' views, articulation of community needs, effective communication within and among members, conflict containment and accommodation, participation in organizations, management of relations with the larger society, and mechanisms to facilitate participant interactions and decision making. Knowledge of several community models facilitates selection of the most appropriate one.

Other Useful Models and Theories

Nurses and theorists in other disciplines have developed many relevant models and theories that are useful in advanced nursing practice. Some of these models include Maslow's hierarchy of needs, Erikson's stages of development, Piaget's cognitive development of children, Pender's (1987) health promotion/disease prevention model, and Loveland-Cherry's (1989) family health promotion model. In addition, numerous theories of stress, crises, coping, grief, bereavement, death, and dying have been developed in the psychology and behavioral disciplines. Nurses have transformed some of these theories to encompass a health–illness context. Nurses who are cognizant of a variety

of nursing, family, community, and behavioral models and theories are more likely to select the best fitting model for their clients.

SELECTION OF RELEVANT MODELS AND THEORIES

This section provides an overview of several nurse scholars' criteria and guidelines for selecting models and theories. Meleis (1997) identified six criteria to guide selection of suitable models and theories for practice. McKenna (1997a) described seven selection criteria based on a review of the literature. Kim (1994) constructed a framework for practice theories with four dimensions to consider in selecting nursing models and theories. Fawcett and associates (1992) suggested that nurses consider three questions to determine the best fit between the client's health concerns and various models and theories. Relevant criteria from these scholars' work were integrated with the author's prior work to delineate five guidelines for selecting appropriate models and theories (Christensen & Kenney, 1996).

Meleis (1997) wrote that selecting models and theories for nursing practice is both a subjective and objective process. She identified the following six criteria for nurses to consider in the selection process:

1. Personal—the nurse's comfort with the theory and congruency with the nurse's own philosophical views of life
2. Mentor—the model or theory learned from a nurse mentor or educator
3. Theorist—their reputation in the discipline and degree of recognition
4. Literature—support the amount of literature available about the theory and the theory's significance for one's specialty
5. Sociopolitical congruency—the model or theory's acceptability within the nurse's workplace and whether major structural or practice changes are required

6. Utility—the ease in which nurses can understand and apply the model or theory in practice settings

McKenna (1997a) reviewed the literature and identified the following seven criteria for selecting models and theories:

1. The type of client—The client's needs should direct the choice because the theory provides guidelines to achieve the client's goals.
2. Healthcare setting—The type of clinical setting and nursing practice are contextual factors that affect selection of theories.
3. Parsimony/simplicity—Simple and realistic theories are more likely to be understood and applied in practice.
4. Understandability—Nurses must understand a theory if they expect to use it.
5. Origins of the theory—The credibility, prior use, and testing of the theory should be considered.
6. Paradigms as a basis for choice—Nurses must decide between the totality or simultaneity paradigm, as each provides a different view of clients and nursing actions.
7. Personal values and beliefs—The theory must be congruent with the nurse's own views about humans, health, and nursing.

In her article on practice theories, Kim (1994) defined two dimensions of theories, which include four sets of practice theories relevant to selecting models and theories. One dimension is the target, which addresses both the philosophy of care for the person and the philosophy of therapy for the client's problems. The other dimension is the nurse-agent, which includes two phases—deliberation and enactment. The four sets of practice theories serve to guide nurses in choosing theories that will (1) explain the patient's problems and ideas about therapy for the problems; (2) provide ideas about how the nurse should approach the patient, such as through communication, caring,

or empowerment; (3) explain how to make decisions about appropriate nursing actions for the patient; and (4) explain what happens during enactment of nursing actions. Kim proposed that a science of nursing practice could be developed from this framework.

Fawcett and associates (1992) identified questions to guide nurses' selection of appropriate theories and models. The nurse must understand the differences among various models and theories in nursing and other disciplines to answer these questions. The following three questions will help the nurse identify the most appropriate model:

1. Does the theory or model address the client's problems and health concerns?
2. Are the nursing interventions suggested by the model consistent with the client's expectations for nursing care?
3. Are the goals of nursing actions, based on the model or theory, congruent with the client's desired health outcomes?

These questions help nurses decide which models and theories will assist them to organize the data into patterns, identify other health concerns, and determine congruency of the client's and nurse's view of nursing and health.

The first step toward theory-based nursing practice is the conscious decision to use theories in practice (Fawcett, 1997). The second step is recognizing that use of conceptual nursing models and theories requires a major change in how the nurse thinks about and interacts with clients to alleviate their health concerns. This change, referred to earlier as a perspective transformation, occurs gradually as the nurse discards one framework of practice and learns another perspective. Adopting and applying new models and theories in practice depends on nurses having knowledge of various models and theories and understanding how these models and theories relate to each other (Alligood, 1997a).

GUIDELINES FOR SELECTING MODELS AND THEORIES FOR NURSING PRACTICE

After deciding to implement theory-based nursing practice, the author believes that each nurse must engage in the five steps described here:

1. Consider personal values and beliefs about nursing, clients, health, and environment. Each nurse has a personal frame of reference or perspective of nursing practice, based on his or her conscious or unconscious assumptions, beliefs, and values about nursing. One's perspective of nursing provides a cognitive structure that guides one's perceptions, thoughts, feelings, and nursing actions (Fawcett, 1995). Clarifying one's own values and beliefs about clients, health, and nursing practice is necessary before a perspective transformation can occur.

2. Examine the underlying assumptions, values, and beliefs of various nursing models, and how the major concepts are defined. After clarifying one's own values and beliefs, the nurse examines the definitions of major concepts in various models and theories to determine whether they are congruent with one's own beliefs (Alligood, 1997a). Nursing models and theories are based on different values and beliefs about the nature of the client's behaviors and abilities, definitions of health and environment, and the appropriate nursing actions to facilitate clients' health. Each nursing model and theory provides a unique view for specific nursing practice. Some nursing models reflect a totality paradigm and view humans as having separate biological, social, psychological, and spiritual parts that respond to environmental stimuli or change, such that the nurse's role is to facilitate adaptation or equilibrium to maintain health. Other nursing models reflect a simultaneity paradigm and propose that humans are intelligent beings, capable of making informed decisions about their lives, and that they continuously engage in a dynamic, mutual interaction with their environment. In this paradigm, the nurse's role is to guide clients in choosing lifestyles and/or therapies that are acceptable to them and facilitate their growth and life–health process.

3. Identify several models that are congruent with one's own values and beliefs about nursing, clients, and health. Each nurse must consider whether the theorist's underlying values are congruent with the nurse's own personal values and beliefs about clients, health, and nursing because the theorist's values guide the nurse's critical thinking and reasoning processes (Alligood, 1997a). Models and theories reflect the theorist's views about people and nursing. They directly affect how nurses approach their clients, which information they gather, how that information is processed, which nursing activities are appropriate, and which client outcomes are expected based on the model. For example, some traditional nursing models define the person as a biopsychosocial being who responds to environmental stimuli, and health results from nursing actions that lead to predictable changes. These models would be incongruent for contemporary nurses who believe that people are free agents, dynamically interacting with their environment as a whole and capable of making rational decisions, with the nurse's role being to assist clients to explore various options and choose ones that are acceptable with their values and lifestyle.

4. Identify the similarities and differences in client focus, nursing actions, and client outcomes of these models. Nursing models and theories consist of concepts with specific definitions and statements that describe how the concepts are interrelated. Some propose specific nursing actions and expected client outcomes. The major concepts guide which data are collected during the assessment and how those data are organized to identify and interpret bio-behavioral patterns

and determine nursing diagnoses. Nursing models also guide development of the nursing care plans and designate desired outcomes to evaluate. By comparing various models, nurses recognize which ones are congruent with their values and beliefs about nursing and offer the best fit with the client's health concerns.

5. Practice applying the models and theories to clients with different health concerns to determine which ones best fit specific situations and guide nursing actions that will achieve desired client outcomes. The nurse explores specific models in depth and may analyze their usefulness before implementing them. By comparing several models and examining the attributes of the client, the focus of nursing actions, and the proposed outcomes, the nurse will acquire a more in-depth understanding of different models. Each nursing model describes different areas for assessment, unique nursing diagnoses, and specific nursing interventions to assist the client toward health. The nurse must decide which models and theories are most appropriate for each client. Which one offers the best fit for the client's health concerns? Selecting appropriate models and theories for each unique client health situation requires nurses to use their broad knowledge base from various disciplines, critical thinking skills, clinical expertise, and intuition to identify the best fit between the client's health concerns and nursing models (Fawcett et al., 1992).

APPLICATION OF THEORY-BASED NURSING PRACTICE

The choice of theories and models suitable to the client's health concerns occurs during the initial data assessment process. The initial data focus on the client's primary expressed concerns and how they are related to or affect the client's lifestyle and patterns of living. These data assist the nurse to identify and understand the client's common and unique patterns. The client's view of health, along with past and present lived experiences and future lifestyle and health concerns, are also considered. Using this information, the nurse considers various models and theories from nursing and other disciplines that are relevant to the client's unique health concerns and congruent with the nurse's own beliefs. Then, the nurse selects those models and other theories that best fit the client's situation and health concerns and will systematically direct nursing practice.

The major concepts of the chosen models and theories guide each component of the nursing process, as shown in **Table 17-2**. The concepts serve as categories to guide additional data collection. They suggest, either directly or indirectly, which information is relevant and should be collected. The models and theories assist the nurse to organize, categorize, and interpret pertinent data that illustrate the client's bio-behavioral patterns and identify appropriate nursing diagnoses that are linked to relevant etiological factors.

Nursing and other models and theories guide development of a care plan by suggesting appropriate types of nursing interventions and specific nursing actions. Desired client outcomes are derived from the models and theories and define which changes in the client should be evaluated. For example, if Roy's model is chosen, data about the client's physiological needs, self-concept, role mastery, and interdependence, along with related stimuli, would be collected and used to identify adaptive and maladaptive behavioral patterns. The nurse who uses Orem's self-care model would assess and judge clients' ability to meet their universal and developmental self-care requisites and whether they had any health deviations. From analysis of these data, the nurse would diagnose self-care deficits and determine appropriate nursing plans for partial, compensatory, or health education nursing care. Nursing care plans are based on the model and describe the

TABLE 17-2	Theory-Based Nursing Practice	
Component	**Nursing Process Use**	**Nursing Model Use**
Assessment	Describes how to collect data	Guides which data to collect
Diagnosis	Describes how to process data	Guides organizing, categorizing, and interpreting data
	Provides format for nursing diagnosis	
	Describes *how* to plan	Provides concepts for nursing diagnosis
	Facilitates development of care plan unique to client	Guides *what* to plan
		Designates appropriate types of nursing interventions
Implementation	Describes phases of implementation	Directs model-specific nursing actions
Evaluation	Identifies *how* to evaluate	Guides *what* to evaluate
General	Requires accountability through use of systematic approach to nursing practice	Enhances accountability of theory-based practice
	Process enhances continuity of care	Provides a comprehensive, coherent approach to care of client

client's desired outcomes, along with nursing actions to achieve the client's outcomes. Nurses who use Johnson's behavioral systems model would consider ways to nurture, protect, or stimulate the client to facilitate health, whereas the Neuman's healthcare systems model assists the nurse to explore ways to reduce stressors within the three levels of disease prevention.

Some nurses believe that family models complement nursing models and provide a more holistic and comprehensive perspective of clients and their health concerns. Selection of a family model occurs after the nurse gathers preliminary data about the family and identifies unique and common patterns in those data. Then the nurse decides whether the family as context or family as client would be more appropriate and best fit the client's situation. Also, the nurse's perception and definition of family and health guide the selection of a family model. For example, a pediatric nurse who works in an outpatient clinic may choose Orem's self-care model to guide care of a 9-year-old child with an ear infection and the mother's treatment of the child. Friedman's family system model may complement Orem's model and enhance understanding of the family's structure and functions. The nurse may also use Erikson's developmental framework to help the mother recognize and encourage her child's normal developmental behaviors. Pain management theories may also be applied to reduce the child's earache.

This example illustrates how nurses examine and judge the value of various models and theories and select those that are most congruent and useful and best fit the client's health concerns and the nurse's perspective of practice. Gradually, nurse practitioners develop an expertise in selecting theories and models that are appropriate and relevant to their client's health concerns and congruent with their own views of advanced practice.

CONCLUSION

This chapter described the importance and value of applying models and theories from nursing and other disciplines in advanced nursing practice. Issues related to the nursing theory–practice gap were discussed, along with concerns about using only one nursing model in practice and about integrating models and theories from other disciplines with nursing models and theories. The structure of nursing knowledge was explained, as was the need for a perspective transformation to occur prior to implementing theory-based nursing practice. Critical thinking, logical reasoning, and creatively applying nursing models and theories were emphasized. Different types of nursing, family, community, and other models and theories were discussed. Finally, the process of selecting and applying models and theories was thoroughly described.

In the last few decades, the emergence of nursing models and theories has illuminated several nursing paradigms and explicated their underlying assumptions, beliefs, and values that guide nursing practice. The science of nursing and empirical patterns of knowing is represented by these nursing models and their theories. Application of models and theories from nursing and other disciplines depends on nurses having a broad knowledge base and understanding how models and theories are interrelated. Empowerment of nurses through perspective transformation and the use of nursing models and theories is essential. They provide the framework for critical thinking within the context of nursing and guide the reasoning that professional nurses need to survive in an era of cost containment and evidence-based practice. Use of models and theories from nursing and related health disciplines enables nurses to demonstrate accountability for their decisions and actions through scientific explanation and provides a coherent approach to theory-based nursing practice.

DISCUSSION QUESTIONS

1. List the reasons to apply nursing, family, and other theories to advanced practice. What are some underlying concerns about applying theories in nursing practice?

2. Based on the review in this chapter of nursing, family, and other disciplines' theories, choose at least one theory to investigate further. Use the five guidelines for selecting models and theories for nursing practice and evaluate the theory's applicability for your current practice. Was the theory applicable, or do you need to search for a different one?

3. How does the structure of nursing knowledge relate to nursing's metaparadigms?

4. How can applying theory to practice enhance one's critical thinking skills?

5. What is the process and what are the pitfalls of the process for selecting and applying appropriate nursing, family, and other disciplines' models and theories to advanced nursing practice?

REFERENCES

Aggleton, P. J., & Chalmers, H. (1986). *Nursing models and the nursing process.* Basingstoke, UK: Macmillan.

Alligood, M. R. (1997a). Models and theories: Critical thinking structures. In M. R. Alligood & A. Marriner-Tomey (Eds.), *Nursing theory: Utilization and application* (pp. 31–45). St. Louis, MO: C. V. Mosby.

Alligood, M. R. (1997b). Models and theories in nursing practice. In M. R. Alligood & A. Marriner-Tomey (Eds.), *Nursing theory: Utilization and application* (pp. 15–30). St. Louis, MO: C. V. Mosby.

Anderson, E. T., McFarlane, J. M., & Helton, A. (1986). Community as client: A model for practice. *Nursing Outlook, 3*(5), 220.

Beavers, W. R., & Voeller, M. N. (1983). Family models: Comparing and contrasting the Olson circumplex model with the Beavers systems model. *Family Process, 22,* 85–98.

Benner, P., & Wrubel, J. (1989). *The primacy of caring.* Menlo Park, CA: Addison-Wesley.

Chinn, P. L. (1997). Why middle-range theory? *ANS, 19*(3), viii.

Christensen, P. J., & Kenney, J. W. (1996). *Nursing process: Application of conceptual models* (4th ed.). St. Louis, MO: C. V. Mosby.

Cody, W. K. (1996). Drowning in eclecticism. *Nursing Science Quarterly, 9*(3), 86–88.

Cradock, S. (1996). The expert nurse: Clinical specialist or advanced practitioner? In Gary Rolfe (Ed.), *Closing the theory–practice gap: A new paradigm for nursing.* Oxford, UK: Butterworth-Heinemann.

Curran, D. (1985). *Stress and the healthy family.* Minneapolis, MN: Winston Press.

Duvall, E. M. (1977). *Marriage and family development* (5th ed.). Philadelphia: Lippincott.

Fawcett, J. (1995). Implementing conceptual models in nursing practice. In J. Fawcett (Ed.), *Analysis and evaluation of conceptual models of nursing* (3rd ed.). Philadelphia: F. A. Davis.

Fawcett, J. (1997). Conceptual models of nursing, nursing theories, and nursing practice: Focus on the future. In M. R. Alligood & A. Marriner-Tomey (Eds.), *Nursing theory: Utilization and application* (pp. 211–221). St. Louis, MO: C. V. Mosby.

Fawcett, J., Archer, C. L., Becker, D., Brown, K. K., Gann, S., Wong, M. J., et al. (1992). Guidelines for selecting a conceptual model of nursing: Focus on the individual patient. *Dimensions of Critical Care Nursing, 11*(5), 268–277.

Field, P. A. (1987). The impact of nursing theory on the clinical decision making process. *Journal of Advanced Nursing, 12,* 563–571.

Firlet, S. I. (1985). Nursing theory and nursing practice: Separate or linked? In J. McCloskey & H. K. Grace (Eds.), *Current issues in nursing* (pp. 6–19). Boston: Blackwell Scientific Publications.

Friedman, M. M. (1992). *Family nursing: Theory and practice* (3rd ed.). New York: Appleton & Lange.

Goeppinger, J., Lassiter, P. G., & Wilcox, B. (1982). Community health is community competence. *Nursing Outlook, 30*(8), 464.

Kenney, J. W. (1996). Relevance of theory-based nursing practice. In P. J. Christensen & J. W. Kenney (Eds.), *Nursing process: Application of conceptual models* (4th ed., pp. 1–23). St. Louis, MO: C. V. Mosby.

Kim, H. S. (1994). Practice theories in nursing and a science of nursing practice. *Scholarly Inquiry for Nursing Practice: An International Journal, 8*(2), 145–158.

Loveland-Cherry, C. J. (1989). Family health promotion and health protection. In P. Bomar (Ed.), *Nurses and family health promotion: Concepts, assessment, and interventions.* Baltimore, MD: Williams & Wilkins.

Marks-Moran, D., & Rose, P. (Eds.). (1997). *Reconstructing nursing: Beyond art and science.* Philadelphia: Bailliere Tindall.

Mayberry, A. (1991). Merging nursing theories, models, and nursing practice: More than an administrative challenge. *ANS, 15,* 44.

McCubbin, M. A., & McCubbin, H. I. (1993). Families coping with illness: The resiliency model of family stress, adjustment and adaptation. In C. B. Danielson, B. Hamel-Bissell, & P. Winstead-Fry (Eds.), *Families, health and illness: Perspectives on coping and intervention* (pp. 21–65). St. Louis, MO: C. V. Mosby.

McKay, R., & Segall, M. (1983). Methods and models for the aggregate. *Nursing Outlook, 31*(6), 328.

McKenna, H. (1997a). Choosing a theory for practice. In H. McKenna (Ed.), *Nursing theories and models* (pp. 127–157). New York: Rutledge.

McKenna, H. (1997b). Applying theories in practice. In H. McKenna (Ed.), *Nursing theories and models* (pp. 158–189). New York: Rutledge.

Meleis, A. I. (1993). *Nursing research and the Neuman model: Directions for the future.* Panel discussion conducted at the Fourth Biennial International Neuman Systems Model Symposium, Rochester, NY.

Meleis, A. I. (1997). *Theoretical nursing: Development and progress* (3rd ed.). Philadelphia: Lippincott.

Mezirow, J. (1979). Perspective transformation. *Adult Education, 28*(3), 100–110.

Mitchell, G. (1992). Specifying the knowledge base of theory in practice. *Nursing Science Quarterly, 5*(1), 6–7.

Moos, R. H., & Billings, A. G. (1982). Conceptualizing and measuring coping resources and processes. In L. Goldberger & S. Breznitz (Eds.), *Handbook of stress.* New York: Free Press.

Olson, D. H., Russell, C. S., & Sprenkle, D. H. (1983). Circumplex models of marital and family systems: VI. Theoretical update. *Family Processes, 22,* 69–83.

Paul, R. W., & Nosich, G. M. (1991). *Proposal for the national assessment of higher-order thinking* (revised version). Washington, DC: United States Department of Education, Office of Educational Research and Improvement, National Center for Education Statistics.

Pender, N. J. (1987). *Health promotion in nursing practice.* New York: Doubleday.

Rogers, M. E. (1989). Creating a climate for the implementation of a nursing conceptual framework. *Journal of Continuing Education in Nursing, 20*(3), 112–116.

Shamansky, S. L., & Pesznecker, B. (1981). A community is . . . *Nursing Outlook, 29*(3), 182–185.

Smith, M. C. (1994). Beyond the threshold: Nursing practice in the next millennium. *Nursing Science Quarterly, 7*(1), 6–7.

Sorrentino, E. A. (1991). Making theories work for you. *Nursing Administration Quarterly, 15*(3), 54–59.

Spiracino, P. (1991). The reciprocal relationship between practice and theory. *Clinical Nurse Specialist, 5*(3), 138.

Stevenson, J. (1977). *Issues and crises during middlescence.* New York: Appleton-Century-Crofts.

Timpson, J. (1996). Nursing theory: Everything the artist spits is art? *Journal of Advanced Nursing, 23,* 1030–1036.

Wright, L. M., & Leahey, M. (1994). *Nurses and families: A guide to family assessment and intervention* (2nd ed.). Philadelphia: F. A. Davis.

CHAPTER 18

Knowledge Development in Nursing: Our Historical Roots and Future Opportunities

Susan R. Gortner

CHAPTER OBJECTIVES

1. Trace the historical development of American nursing research in the past century.

2. Discuss projections for nursing research in the 21st century and how they will influence advanced practice nursing.

INTRODUCTION

The purpose of this chapter is to provide an historical overview of nursing research in the past century and to offer projections on where our science will be headed in the 21st century. For the overview, a number of reviews were drawn upon (Abdellah, 1970; DeTornyay, 1976; Gortner & Nahm, 1977; Lindeman, 1975a) with reliance on the last citation, which surveyed published nursing literature from 1900 to 1975. In the last two decades, other analyses of published research have been carried out (Brown, Tanner, & Patrick, 1983; Jacobsen & Meininger, 1985; Moody et al., 1988), including an impressive first encyclopedia of nursing research (Fitzpatrick, 1998). Research agendas and priorities have been developed by the American Nurses Association Commission (American Nurses Association Commission, 1976) and Cabinet on Nursing Research (American Nurses Association

Source: Reprinted from *Nursing Outlook, 48*(2), Susan R. Gortner, "Knowledge Development in Nursing: Our Historical Roots and Future Opportunities," 60–67; copyright 2000, with permission from Elsevier.

Cabinet, 1985), by the Academy of Nursing Ad Hoc Group on Knowledge Generation (Oberst, 1986; Stevenson & Woods, 1986b), and by consultant groups to the Division of Nursing's research program (Barnard, 1980; Gortner, 1980a) and to the former National Center for Nursing Research (Bloch, 1988). Research publications of the nursing schools at the University of California–Los Angeles (UCLA; Research, 1998), University of California–San Francisco (UCSF; Science, 1999), and the University of Maryland (*Advancing the Science*) were used to formulate contemporary research questions. As such, they are illustrative rather than representative. Projections for the 21st century have been drawn from the author's reflections on our science (Gortner, 1980a, 1980b, 1984, 1991; Gortner & Schultz, 1988), from Donaldson's seminal paper marking the 25th anniversary of the American Academy of Nursing (1998), and from the latest research agenda of the National Institute of Nursing Research (Grady, 1999). Comments will be made on how our practice has been affected through research and by that applications did not occur, when perhaps they should have. Examples will be from projects personally known to the author.

THE EARLY YEARS

Nursing practice and issues arising from practice have influenced research topics since the time of Nightingale.

While practice issues have varied since then, some early concerns regarding quality of care and qualified caregivers transcended the 19th and 20th centuries and have continued into the 21st century. It is no accident that the development of formal programs of nursing education was seen as the means to improve practice. Historical perspectives on nursing and nursing research may be depicted as follows.

In the early 1900s, concern was for improvement of the public's health; major communicable diseases of childhood and adulthood were prevalent; maternal/child health had yet to benefit from prenatal care and improved obstetrical practices. Most surgery was done in the home. The literature in our professional journals addressed problems associated with tuberculosis, meningitis, scarlet fever, and other infectious diseases. In 1913, the committee on public health nursing of the National League for Nursing Education discussed its concern about infant mortality, prevention of blindness, and the problem of unlicensed midwives. The committee believed that the nursing profession should recognize its role in the prevention of unnecessary deaths among infants and in the prevention of unnecessary blindness, and that intelligent care of the sick must involve "some knowledge of the scientific approach to disease . . . causes and prevention. . . ." (Gortner & Nahm, 1977).

During the 1920s, the first case studies appeared; they were used both as a teaching tool for students and as a record of patient progress. Nursing care plans for specific patient groups and procedures also appeared (e.g., use of turpentine stupes), and continued to be used until recently as a means to standardize and improve practice—medical as well as nursing. The case approach as a major research and teaching model in clinical nursing practice paralleled the use of case studies in medical practice and research. These case studies were used to describe unusual patient situations or symptoms and to report on the effects of nursing and medical therapies with groups of patients.

According to personal interviews with the late Lucile Petry Leone,[1] the need for systematic evaluations of nursing procedures had its origins in the post-Depression years. The Depression forced the graduate nurse out of the home and into the hospital and, at the same time, the first postgraduate nursing programs began to develop (Gortner & Nahm, 1977).

The war years prompted the collection of national data on nursing needs and resources (types, numbers, and uses of nurses). In the immediate postwar years, the federal government, assisted by professional nursing organizations and foundations, provided funds and staff to establish resources for nursing, such as the Division of Nursing Resources of the United States Public Health Service, which was created in 1948. Its staff carried out studies on nurse supply and distribution, job satisfaction and turnover, requirements for public health nursing services, personnel costs, and costs for collegiate nursing education. These studies were widely used throughout the United States, frequently in conjunction with federal staff consultation and training. A 5-year study of nursing functions and activities was begun by the American Nurses Association in 1950, resulting in functions, standards, and qualifications for practice (1959), as well as the publication *Twenty Thousand Nurses Tell Their Story* (Hughes et al., 1958). Also noteworthy during this time was the W. K. Kellogg Foundation Nursing Service Administration Research Project, in which faculty from 12 universities worked with Finer at the University of Chicago to determine needs for administrative science and skills in nursing (Finer, 1952). Thus the period between 1930 and 1960 concentrated on the components of professional nursing practice and how best to secure them.

Focus on the organization and delivery of nursing services was given a boost when the Division of Nursing Resources initiated a small competitive research grant and fellowship program in 1955. Lucile Petry Leone, former director of the cadet nurse corps and then chief nurse officer and assistant surgeon general in the Public Health Service, convinced the U.S. Surgeon General and the director of the National Institutes of Health (NIH) to allocate $500,000 for grants and $125,000 for fellowships from the NIH budget. These programs were the precursors to the National Center for Nursing Research and the current National Institute for Nursing Research (Gortner & Nahm, 1977).

In 1952, the journal *Nursing Research* came into being. Its first few issues contained a section entitled the "Research Reporter," in which areas suitable for research were noted; guest editorials emphasized the need for grassroots support of nursing research by hospitals, agencies, and schools. Lucile Petry Leone's editorial in the Fall 1955 issue summarized the types of studies needed in nursing, based on a staff paper she had prepared earlier. These types included studies of nursing care most essential to patient recovery; the nature of the therapeutic relationship; analysis and optimal use of nursing skills; and efforts to reduce staff turnover rates and student drop-out rates. Her thinking provided a visionary public platform for nursing research (Leone, 1955).

Virginia Henderson's 1956 guest editorial noted that studies of the nurse outnumbered studies of practice by 10 to 1, that more than half of the doctoral theses were carried out in the field of education, and that the "responsibility for designing its methods is often cited as an essential characteristic of a profession" (Henderson, 1956, p. 99). Six years later, the first Nurse Scientist Graduate Training Grants were awarded to universities offering resources in one or more basic science departments for preparation through the doctorate. The first grant awards were to the Boston University School of Nursing for training in biology, psychology, and sociology, and to the University of California School of Nursing for training in sociology. The next fiscal year, three additional grants were awarded—one to the UCLA School of Nursing for study in sociology; one to the University of Washington School of Nursing for graduate study in anthropology, microbiology, physiology, and sociology; and the third to Western Reserve University School of Nursing for study in biology, physiology, psychology, and sociology.[2] Subsequently, grants were made to schools of nursing at the University of Kansas, Teachers College-Columbia University, University of Pittsburgh, University of Arizona,

University of Colorado, University of Illinois, and briefly, New York University (the grant program was terminated in 1975). Required interdepartmental seminars helped to define the boundaries of nursing science for the early grantees. It is not surprising that nurse scientist graduate training settings later developed into PhD programs in nursing (Gortner, 1991).

In the early 1960s, establishment of the American Nurses Foundation's grants program helped to address the demand for more practice-related studies. The foundation published the priorities that would guide its funding decisions: effects of performance of nursing acts on the patient (i.e., nursing procedures and outcomes); effects on nursing of changing patterns of nursing care and changing health needs; and nursing in different process categories (American Nurses Foundation, 1960).

Ellwynne Vreeland, the first chief of the federal research branch, wrote Chief Nurse Officer Lucile Petry Leone in 1959 that studies were needed to further development of nursing theory by identifying the scientific content of nursing, by seeking and experimenting with new concepts of nursing (e.g., motivation— "finding out why nurses can 'bring back' patients who have given up and who fail to respond to careful medical treatment"), and by carefully studying the nursing care given by expert practitioners (e.g., the specifics of expert nursing) (Vreeland, 1959).

Soon the specifics of expert nursing became apparent as several university schools of nursing undertook studies of the nursing process, patient responses to care, and behavioral phenomena. The Yale study of nursing effects on postoperative vomiting became widely cited because of its experimental design and findings suggesting that nurse counseling had a positive effect (Dumas & Leonard, 1963). UCLA nursing investigators studied recovery stages from myocardial infarction (Coston, 1960; interviews with cardiologists revealed no clear demarca-

tion of stages appropriate for nursing detection), breastfeeding (Disbrow, 1963), rooming-in (Ringholz & Morris, 1961), and pain relief (Moss & Myer, 1966). These became among the first practice-related studies to be published in the new journal, *Nursing Research.*

At UCSF, sociologists Strauss and Glaser combined talents with nurse investigator Quint to study hospital personnel's views on death and dying (Glaser & Strauss, 1965). Quint's seminal study (1967) of the experiences of women undergoing radical mastectomies was to launch a scientific career that Donaldson (1998) has termed "pathfinding." Studies at the University of Washington in the early 1960s focused on nursing services for psychiatric, tubercular, alcoholic, and maternity patients; variables included professional attitudes, activities, and accountability for patient care (Gortner & Nahm, 1977). Batey's later expertise in research resource development was an outgrowth of her study with Julian of organizational patterns in psychiatric settings (Batey & Julian, 1964). One of the earliest controlled attempts to document the effects of nursing intervention on the clinical progress of chronically ill adults was carried out by nursing investigators (Little & Carnevali, 1967).

At Presbyterian–University of Pennsylvania Medical Center, a project carried out between 1963 and 1967 in a special facility, the coronary care unit, demonstrated significant reductions in patient morbidity and mortality through continuous monitoring and prompt treatment by expert nurses (Meltzer et al., 1969). This project, which had been supported by the fledgling research grant program of the Division of Nursing Resources, was to become the model of coronary care nursing nationwide. It was also among the first reports of nursing research to be published in *Journal of the American Medical Association.*

Thus the real thrust of nursing research began in the 1960s, as a function of the vision of nursing leaders such as Lulu Wolf Hassenplug,

Helen Nahm, Mary Tschudin, Hildegard Peplau, Virginia Henderson, Lucile Petry Leone, Ellwynne Vreeland, Faye Abdellah, and Jessie Scott, and thanks to the availability of both public and private funds to support the studies and train nurses in research. I joined the division staff in 1966 to aid in the review of the Nurse Training Act of 1964. In 1967, I was appointed executive secretary to the Research in Patient Care Review Committee, the outside group of scientists charged with determining the scientific merit of research proposals submitted from investigators throughout the United States. During my time as staff scientist and later as branch chief for research grants and fellowships, we attempted to nourish the growing enterprise of nursing research nationwide through staff consultation, conferences, research development grants, nurse scientist graduate training grants, and individual research fellowships. We publicized the grant programs (Gortner, 1973), urged scientific accountability for the profession (Gortner, 1974c) as a practice profession (Gortner, 1974b), and early on attempted to show the contributions of research to patient care with a proposed classification, which named nursing research a "science of practice" (Gortner, Bloch, & Phillips, 1976).

To recapitulate, knowledge development in nursing began in earnest only 40 years ago, primarily in university schools of nursing where nurse scientist graduate training was ongoing in alliance with other disciplines, but also in medical centers such as the City of Hope, where Geraldine Padilla was director of research; at Luther Hospital in Eau Claire, Wisconsin, where Carol Lindeman was in charge; and at the Loeb Center for Nursing at Montefiore, under the direction of Gwenrose Alfano. The Loeb Center for Nursing, which demonstrated that cost-effective care could be rendered to elders in a nursing center, was not seen as an innovation until such practice innovations were publicized by the American Academy of Nursing. Why the lag in impact of this research?

Annual research conferences sponsored by the American Nurses Association and later by the regional nursing research societies provided forums for investigators to present their findings and learn the importance of subjecting their results to public scrutiny (Gortner & Nahm, 1977). The art of the critique developed gradually; communality and collegiality joined communication and publication as hallmarks of our research efforts, and greater sophistication among nursing's investigators and clinicians resulted in greater intradisciplinary and interdisciplinary collaboration.

THE TRANSITION YEARS

I have termed the period from 1965 to 1985 "transitional" because it was during this time that professional nursing took on major leadership activities to influence federal policy for nursing education and research. The American Nurses Association established a Commission on Research in 1971; the Council of Nurse Researchers was created in 1972. In a paper presented at the first program meeting of the council in 1973, I described the increasing concern that research financed by the federal government be related to major health priorities, stating that "there is no mistaking the trend toward greater legislative specification of science in the health fields" (Gortner, 1974a). The scientist audience was urged to develop research priorities for nursing research.

In response, Lindeman (1975a) undertook a Delphi survey of priorities in clinical nursing research through the Western Interstate Commission on Higher Education, with Division of Nursing support. Respondents rated items on the quality of care, nursing role, nursing process, and the research process. Patient welfare concerns, particularly items related to nursing interventions to mitigate stress and pain, and to provide patient education and support to frail elders, also were cited (Lindeman, 1975b).

When President Richard Nixon impounded nurse training act, research, and fellowship funds in 1973, all federal support for fellowships and training grants was halted. The president was taken to court by a coalition of nursing organizations and forced to release the funds in 1974. The Division of Nursing held several invitational conferences on nurse scientist graduate training and doctoral personnel needs. Commission members traveled to Washington, D.C., in 1975 to meet with legislators and federal program staff—the first such contacts to be made by what was later to become the nursing research advocacy group. In my capacity as branch chief, I was asked to meet with commissioners to present program needs, vital information for program development and funding that had been embargoed as a result of closure of all public information offices in 1971. Although we could not publish grant and fellowship information, we could respond to requests for information about the programs. To their credit, grantees understood this constraint and found opportunities to request program information. Thus the commission was able to develop priorities for research training and research and set goals for accomplishing them, including funding levels (American Nurses Association Commission, 1976).

Health science research training authorization was restored with the passage of the National Research Service Awards Act in 1974; two years later, primarily through Connie Holleran's efforts, the Division of Nursing research training programs were included (Gortner, 1979). Publication of a review of research grants awarded (Abdellah, 1970) was followed by two historical overviews of nursing research (Lindeman, 1975a; DeTornyay, 1976); two new research journals, *Research in Nursing and Health* and *The Western Journal of Nursing Research* appeared in 1978. The 94th Congress specified $5 million for research projects in nursing and $1 million for research fellowships to be spent during 1977 and 1978, the first

time funds for nursing research had been earmarked in the appropriation. Until then and since 1964, nursing research funds had been allocated along with nurse training act funds, although that act dealt exclusively with training to address the quality and quantity of professional nurses (Gortner, 1979).

This somewhat awkward allocation process and the difficulty health provider legislation was experiencing in the 1970s led to open discussions by nurse scientists and educators regarding the need to locate the nursing research programs within the research environment of the National Institutes of Health. The discussions were frank and heated: Well-respected deans worried that such a relocation would fracture federal nursing; others worried that nursing research could not mature if not nourished within the institute structure. Legislators were sympathetic and passed legislation (Public Law 99-158) authorizing a new center at the National Institutes of Health; it came into being in 1986 after a successful override of a presidential veto, in main attributed to nurse scientist lobbying efforts, including the persuasive efforts of the entire membership of the American Heart Association Council on Cardiovascular Nursing, which was meeting in Washington, D.C., at the time. Council Chairperson Marie Cowan adjourned us to go on the Hill. We did, and the entire California delegation was visited (including the senate office of then Senator Pete Wilson, who voted to override the veto).

Coincidental with the establishment of the national center was the continuing work both of the American Nurses Association Cabinet on Nursing Research and the scientist group in the American Academy of Nursing. The cabinet published *Directions for Nursing Research: Toward the 21st Century* in 1985, setting out goals, priorities, and strategies along with the dollar amounts to achieve them. The next year the American Academy of Nursing held its annual meeting in Kansas City, with the program theme "Nursing in the Year 2000: Setting the Agenda for Knowledge Generation and Utilization." Stevenson and Woods (1986b) provided a synthesis of the focus group priorities both for the new national center and for research in the next two decades. These priorities focused first on fundamental knowledge development about clinical problems, followed by clinical therapeutics to test interventions, along with increasing emphasis on health promotion, health status and functioning, the family, and vulnerable populations and age groups. Scientific knowledge synthesis was aided by the beginning of a series of annual reviews of nursing research under the direction of Werley and Fitzpatrick.

Oberst (1986), at the same Academy conference, provided a thoughtful insight into a possible Year 2000 research agenda:

> The heart of the problem may lie in the almost total absence of basic research into the nature of the phenomena we wish to influence. We know very little about patterns of fatigue and sleep or about the nature of immobility, confusion, or anorexia. We cannot expect to intervene to prevent or control a problem such as incontinence, for instance, without basic knowledge of the natural history of that condition in a variety of contexts.

Oberst also spoke to the extreme biophysical derangement associated with organ transplantation, microsurgery, and aggressive chemotherapy protocols, asking whether health providers fully understood the short-term and long-term physical and psychological effects of these events and their meaning for patients and families. This problem has continued to interest investigators. Mishel and Murdaugh (1987) studied an opportunistic sample of heart transplantation patients and families; this study is one of the finest examples of grounded theory methodology published. Jenkins is among others studying the effects of aggressive protocols on quality of life (*Advancing the Science*).

The transition years also saw the development of research on primary care and evaluation of nurse practitioner programs. Research was directed toward three aspects: (1) understanding the influence of structural variables on nurse practitioner performance (e.g., access to settings); (2) identifying personal and professional characteristics contributing to successful performance as a nurse practitioner; and (3) specifying the nature of clinical judgments used by nurse practitioners and physicians working collaboratively in patient care management to assign patients either to a nurse or to a physician and then reassign responsibilities as changes in health status occur. How do the management plans differ? This last question addresses the elusive nature of the nurse–patient encounter (the initial plan, examination, questioning, priority setting, treatment, and evaluation) (Gortner, 1979). Ford and Silver (1968) evaluated the post-training activities of skilled pediatric nurses and found that these nurses could handle independently three-fourths of clinical visits in a rural station, with high patient satisfaction being reported regarding counseling and health monitoring.

Lewis and Resnik (1967) evaluated the use of adult nurse practitioners at the University of Kansas medical clinic with similar findings. To their disappointment, the program was discontinued after grant funding ceased. The Veterans Administration (VA) South Hill Clinic in Los Angeles became the site of a second attempt to demonstrate the effectiveness of nurse practitioners in managing adult chronic conditions, this time those of veterans. Charles Lewis had just come to UCLA, Theresa Cheyovich was a visionary nursing chief at the Clinic, and I represented the "Feds" in the first interagency agreement signed by the VA with another federal agency. Two UCLA-trained PRIMEX nurses (UCLA was the original PRIMEX training site), one of whom was a former VA clinic nurse, undertook caseloads released by then 33 VA physicians, who had been painstakingly persuaded by Lewis to participate in the project. One nurse, in particular, was able to effect major changes in the health status and outcomes of her veteran caseload. Examining her encounters, we discovered that she "contracted" with patients on a weekly basis, and used social persuasion and professional skills to bolster patient confidence in their own health management (Cheyovich, Lewis, & Gortner, 1976). Ultimately, the experiment was so successful that the VA proceeded thereafter to train and place nurse practitioners in many of its settings. Here is still another example of how nursing research has impacted practice.

NURSING RESEARCH BECOMES NURSING SCIENCE

What also occurred during this transition period was a shift in thinking from research to science—that is, a recognition that what we had thought was nursing science was really research, the tool of science. Nursing science was depicted as a human science that had the additional requirement of intervention or clinical therapy. Nursing research was redefined "as the discrete and aggregated investigations that constitute the professions' modes and foci of inquiry" (Gortner, 1980b). The phenomena of interest to nursing were already being documented through research to become tentative propositions about human health and illness, vulnerable population groups (the aged, the chronically ill, women, children, infants), and illness recovery processes and risk factors. A seminal essay by Donaldson and Crowley (1978), "The Discipline of Nursing," clarified our thinking on what might become our knowledge domains and syntax. Meleis's inaugural Helen Nahm lecture (1980) on nursing scholarship heralded both the scientific and theoretical developments that were to occur in the next two decades. Clinical science was seen as focusing on human problems and treatment modalities; fundamental science was characterized as having no immediate utility but rather

being devoted to understanding basic processes across a wide variety of disciplines (Gortner, 1980b).

The last period of knowledge development in the 20th century witnessed an explosion of fundamental and clinical science activities in nursing. How these phenomena came about is described next.

NURSING SCIENCE COMES OF AGE

Our science came into maturity during the past decade and a half as a result of several factors.

First, emphasis began to shift from discrete studies to aggregates of studies—the precursors of programs of research. This shift initially was encouraged by the Division of Nursing's Nursing Research Emphasis Grant Program, in which areas of concentration, such as vulnerable populations and health across the life span, were suggested as topics to be coupled with graduate education (Holzemer & Gortner, 1988). The program at UCSF concentrated on two of these areas and solicited proposals from faculty that would both extend knowledge and involve and excite graduate students; it was funded and renewed for 5 years.

Second, schools of nursing began to recruit doctorally prepared faculty with excellent research preparation and programmatic interests that fit with concentrations of research within the school. University nursing schools featured "centers of excellence," in which faculty effort and talent were aggregated, acknowledging that selectivity was required to achieve excellence.

Third, educational programs in many universities maintained sufficient stability that faculty time and effort could be redirected toward research. That is, curriculum revisions seemed to reach a plateau. Collaboration and colleagueship began to replace competitiveness and solo investigations.

Fourth, external competition for research support increased as grant success was forthcoming from both public and private agencies;

in the university systems, extramural support is one criterion for advancement up the faculty ranks. At UCSF, the first successful investigators received a bottle of champagne; later beer, and then soda, sufficed.

Fifth, arguments over appropriate methods, whether experimentation, description, and/or interpretation, waxed heatedly and then seemed to wane, as many of us put our energies into substantive activities, whether empirical investigations or philosophic musings, or both, as was the case with me.

Sixth, scientists such as Lindsey, Cowan, Donaldson, Woods, Shaver, Brooten, Norbeck, and Dracup, to name but a few, took the brave step of becoming deans, thereby reinforcing the science enterprise in their settings. With this momentum and influx of prepared scientist nurses, some of whom had been exposed to philosophers in their graduate programs, came debate about the nature of nursing science, what should be the prevailing worldview and research approach. We spent a great of time speaking and writing about empiricism, phenomenology (later hermeneutics), critical theory, and feminism, among other topics. Post-positivists, of which I am one, were maligned for speaking to the components of "good science" such as credibility, reproducibility, and rigor (Gortner, 1991).

The knowledge development group at the American Academy of Nursing program meeting in 1986 attempted to implement a cease-fire between the received and perceived views of science, endorsing pluralism (Stevenson & Woods, 1986a). Meleis (1987) called for a "passion for substance" rather than a passion for method; and I attempted to formulate a philosophy of science for nursing that would embrace values (Gortner, 1990). Notions about nursing research and its substantive activity also have been formulated throughout the years by Ellis (1970), Batey (1971), Barnard (1982), and Shaver (1985). The following represents but one definition of nursing science, drawing on

Barnard (1980; *Research Spanning*, 1998) and Donaldson and Crowley (1998):

> Nursing science, as a form of human science, has as its object of analysis the human organism, with particular reference to human response states in health and illness and health across the life span. Its aim is to generate a body of knowledge that can define patterns of behavior associated with normal and critical life events such as catastrophic illness; depict changes in health status and predict how these are brought about; and along with other scientific fields, determine the principles and laws governing life states and processes. (Gortner, 1984)

In the decades of knowledge development documented in this review, nursing has identified with tasks and technology and has characterized itself as a compassionate human service; it has taken as its subject matter the ecology of human health and human responses to health illness. While these conceptualizations may appear sequential, based on historical literature, in reality they are concurrent.

The researchable components of human health across the life span comprise indicators of health status, biological and behavioral factors contributing to health and illness, culture, environment, and treatment outcomes. These components were visible in the National Center for Nursing Research's (1988) national nursing research agenda, which was developed after an invitational conference on research priorities in nursing science at which 50 nurse scientists were present. To establish the agenda, priorities were selected on the basis of the existing knowledge base, opportunities, areas of low emphasis in other institutes, marketability, and available scientific personnel. These priorities were staged as follows: I—"HIV-Positive Clients, Partners and Families" and "Prevention and Care of Low-Birth-Weight Infants"; II—"Long-Term Care and Symptom Management and Information Systems"; and III—"Health Promotion" (in which the most critical issues for study are the fundamental psychosocial mechanisms underlying maintenance of health promotion behaviors) and "Technology Dependency Across the Lifespan" (Bloch, 1988).

Ten years later, the National Institute of Nursing Research (NINR) distributed a statement on strategic planning for the 21st century with this definition of research (not science!):

> Nursing research addresses the issues that examine the core of patients' and families' personal encounters with illness, treatment, disease prevention. NINR's primary activity is clinical research and most studies involve patients. The basic science is linked to patient problems.
>
> . . . Nursing research is essential in defining and confronting the compelling health and illness challenges of the 21st Century. (Grady, 1999)

These challenges include risk reduction, promotion of healthy lifestyles, enhanced quality of life for persons with chronic conditions, and care for persons at the end of life. These areas are familiar; they have remained persistent for more than 30 years. The National Institute for Nursing Research has identified the following scientific goals for the next 5-year period:

1. Identify research opportunities that will achieve scientific distinction within the scientific and practice communities and within NIH as a result of their significant contributions to health:
   - End-of-life/palliative care research
   - Chronic illness experiences
   - Quality of life and quality of care issues
   - Health promotion and disease prevention
   - Telehealth interventions
   - Implications of generic advances
   - Cultural and ethnic considerations to decrease health disparities

2. Identify future opportunities for high-quality, cost-effective care for patients and contribute to the scientific base of nursing practice through research on:
   - Chronic illness (arthritis, diabetes) and long-term care, including family care
   - Health promotion and risk behaviors
   - Cardiopulmonary health and critical care
   - Neurofunction and sensory conditions
   - Immune response and oncology
   - Reproductive and infant health

3. Communicate research findings

4. Enhance research training opportunities

These initiatives are already incorporated into the research programs of many university schools of nursing. I reviewed the research publications from the schools of nursing at the UCLA (*Research Spanning,* 1998), UCSF (*The Science of Caring,* 1999), and the University of Maryland (*Advancing the Science*) in preparation for the original presentation on which this chapter is based. The scientific topics in these settings include vulnerable populations, cardiovascular and other illnesses, symptom management, chronic pain, health promotion/illness prevention, risk reduction, quality of life, the family in health and illness, women's health, and nursing therapeutics (including intensive cardiac monitoring, coaching for recovery, and "kangaroo care"). As examples:

- Is pain relief universal or are there gender differences? (Miakowski & Levine, UCSF)
- Does an ischemia monitoring protocol result in improved patient outcomes? (Drew et al., UCSF)
- What is the relationship between daytime fatigue and sleep disturbance in women? (Lee, UCSF)
- Does a collaborative intervention (advanced practice nurses and community peer advisors) improve outcomes for cardiac elders? (Rankin, UCSF)

- What is the role of exercise in heart failure patients? (Dracup et al., UCLA)

- Can an intervention with low-income adolescent mothers reduce HIV risk and improve health outcomes? (Koniak-Griffin, UCLA)

- Which chromosomal abnormalities result from environmental toxins and affect reproductive health? (Robbins, UCLA)

- What is the quality of life experience of women with differing stages of lung cancer? (Sarna, UCLA)

- Can kangaroo care be as effective in ventilated infants as in premature infants? (Ludington, University of Maryland)

- What are the effects of estrogen on platelet function after cerebral ischemia? (Kearney, University of Maryland)

- How do aggressive treatment modalities affect health status and quality of life? (Jenkins, University of Maryland)

In the study write-ups, investigators often revealed how their interests originated. Many investigators were and are advanced practice nurses. As such, they have credibility both as clinicians and as scientists. Not surprisingly, then, their research findings have had an impact on practice by encouraging family-sensitive care in several settings;[3] by enhancing patient self-confidence and self-efficacy through coaching, counseling, and performance;[4] by advocating improved critical care heart monitoring procedures;[5] by encouraging early discharge of low-birth-weight infants;[6] and by providing for sensory stimulation of the neonate, including skin-to-skin contact.[7] Whereas nursing investigators have not always received the publicity given medical investigators, this bias is changing slowly as more nurses are appointed and elected to public office, and as more become members of scientific and governmental advisory groups. The media recogni-

tion awards given annually by the American Academy of Nursing also have been instrumental in raising the veil of public ignorance. Schorr and Kennedy's (1999) splendid pictorial of 100 years of American nursing is a cause for celebration!

Whereas the areas of concentration some 20 years ago tended to reflect one dominant knowledge domain (for example, the psychosocial), today the biophysical, particularly biology and genetics, are reflected in the investigations noted earlier and elsewhere. This phenomenon may have been encouraged by the report of the National Center for Nursing Research biological task force, which stated: "the implications for the interface of nursing science with the biological sciences as a basis for research and its subsequent findings for practice are tremendous" (Hinshaw, Sigmon, & Lindsey, 1991). It also may be a natural development of better understanding that nursing problems cannot be solved within one knowledge domain; most involve multiple and complex factors (Gortner, 1984; Gortner & Schultz, 1988).

FUTURE OPPORTUNITIES

In preparing for this last section, I queried several colleagues throughout the United States about where the future might lead us. Invariably, the responses included the following pathways: (1) to reexamine the impact of organizational structures on nursing effectiveness, (2) to continue to examine fundamental processes underlying human responses to health and illness, (3) to take the lead with family health, (4) to continue study of end-of-life and palliative care, and (5) to have an impact on health policy. I would add one more consideration to which I would assign considerable urgency: (6) to identify the biobehavioral factors (in epidemiologic terms, the host factors) that explain much of illness and associated behavior. These factors will frame *why* questions (e.g., why is it that personal recovery beliefs are such a powerful predictor of cardiac surgical outcomes along with the usual pathophysiologic markers?) that will bring our science into increasing respect within the greater medical science community at the National Institutes of Health and elsewhere.

Donaldson's "Breakthroughs in Nursing Research" presentation, given at the 25th Anniversary of the American Academy of Nursing in 1998, identified "pathfinders" who created a new realm of nursing research or reconceptualized an existing realm of nursing research (1998). Many were already working in the previously mentioned areas 30 years ago. Noting that nursing has the "brilliance in family health," she encouraged us to know well the human genotype project, to recognize the environment as the social context for health, and to strengthen the bridge between public health and person/family health. To these mandates, I would add this one: to strengthen collaborations (between nursing and other disciplines and within nursing) and continue to address fundamental problems at the biobehavioral interface.

Two additional opportunities need mentioning. Nursing has a proud heritage of safe and effective midwifery service that has affected health legislation for Medicaid and rural health, but still has not removed barriers to hospital practice (Diers & Burst, 1983). What may be needed here are collaborative teams of obstetrical fellows and midwives in some forward-thinking health science settings who will become "pacesetters" in collaborative practice.

Fagin's (1998) guest editorial in *Nursing Outlook* on the changing burden of care brought on by managed care pleads with us in academia to know what it is like at the bedside. Without documentation of the effects of management on the burden of care, we may not save our workforce. Burden of care has been an issue for us and for housestaff throughout this century. To become clinically refreshed, I undertook a day of practice 20 years ago on a cardiovascular surgery unit. I had forgotten what it was like to leave lunch half-eaten in the staff room. What made this experience bearable was the professional support provided by my mentors, two cardiovascular clinical nurse specialists, with whom I collaborated in clinical research on cardiac surgery recovery.[8]

In conclusion, tribute is paid to readers who are pacesetters in clinics, hospitals, private practice, public health, and academia every day of their professional lives. Those of us now white-haired are grateful that you are where you are and are doing what you do. The future is really ours, as it was years ago!

ACKNOWLEDGMENT

I gratefully acknowledge the contribution of Rebecca Wilson-Loots, academic program analyst, Department of Family Health Care Nursing, University of California–San Francisco, for her assistance with the original paper.

DISCUSSION QUESTIONS

1. How has the history of nursing research influenced the status of nursing research today?

2. Browse the website of the National Center for Nursing Research. What are its current goals and future strategies?

3. Go the website of your specialty organization and determine its research agenda for the future. Does the organization publish research studies?

NOTES

1. Lucile Petry Leone spent many hours with the author and the late Helen Nahm in the writing of the overview of nursing research. She died on Thanksgiving Day, 1999.

2. The first Doctor of Nursing Science program (in psychiatric nursing) was offered by Boston University; the second was offered at the University of California–San Francisco. The first PhD program in nursing was

begun by New York University, to be followed by the program at the University of Pittsburgh.

3. Suzanne Feetham, Kathleen Dracup, and Catherine Gilliss are among the pioneers in family nursing research, along with Lorraine Wright of Canada, Sally Rankin, Maribelle Leavitt, and Kit Chesla. These individuals and others have studied families in acute and chronic illness.

4. Louise Jenkins and Susan Gortner were among the first to employ self-efficacy as a variable in patient recovery; Sally Rankin, Diane Carroll, Mariead Hickey, Virginia Carrieri, and Marylin Dodd are among others who have studied self-efficacy in clinical populations.

5. Barbara Drew has been the pioneering investigator in this aspect of critical care nursing.

6. Eileen Hasselmeyer, Mary Neal, and Kathryn Barnard were the original pioneers in studies of neonate stimulation, followed by Anderson, Whalberg, and Ludington, among others.

7. Dorothy Brooten is credited for demonstrating the cost-effectiveness of care for low-birth-weight infants.

8. The author is indebted to Patricia Sparacino, cardiovascular surgery nurse specialist at the Medical Center, University of California–San Francisco, and Julie Shinn, clinical coordinator in cardiovascular surgical nursing at Stanford University Medical Center. Both are internationally known clinicians/scholars and academy members.

REFERENCES

Abdellah, F. B. (1970). Overview of nursing research 1955-1968. *Nursing Research, 19,* 6–17, 239–252.

Advancing the science of nursing: Vol. 11. (1997–1999). Baltimore, MD: University of Maryland School of Nursing.

American Nurses Association. (1959). *Functions, standards and qualifications for practice.* New York, NY: Author.

American Nurses Association Cabinet on Nursing Research. (1985). *Directions for nursing research: Toward the twenty-first century.* Kansas City, MO: American Nurses Association.

American Nurses Association Commission on Nursing Research. (1976). *Nursing research: Toward a science of health care. Priorities for research in nursing.* Kansas City, MO: American Nurses Association.

American Nurses Foundation. (1960). Research—pathway to future progress in nursing care. *Nursing Research, 9,* 4–7.

Barnard, K. E. (1980). Knowledge for practice: Directions for the future. *Nursing Research, 29,* 208–212.

Barnard, K. (1982). The research cycle: Nursing, the profession, the discipline. In *Communicating nursing research: Vol. 15. Nursing science in perspective.* Boulder, CO: Western Interstate Commission for Higher Education.

Batey, M. (1971). Conceptualizing the research process. *Nursing Research, 20,* 296–301.

Batey, M., & Julian, J. (1964). Staff perceptions of state psychiatric hospital goals. *Nursing Research, 12,* 89–92.

Bloch, D. (1988). *Report of the national nursing research agenda for the participants in the conference on research priorities in nursing science, January 27–29, 1988* [unpublished]. Bethesda, MD: National Center for Nursing Research.

Brown, J. S., Tanner, C. A., & Patrick, K. P. (1983). Nursing's search for scientific knowledge. *Nursing Research, 32,* 29–32.

Cheyovich, T. K., Lewis, C. E., & Gortner, S. R. (1976). *The nurse practitioner in an adult outpatient clinic.* Washington, DC: Health Resources Administration. HEW Publication No. (HRA) 76-29.

Coston, H. M. (1960). Myocardial infarction: Stages of recovery and nursing care. *Nursing Research, 9,* 178–184.

DeTornyay, R. (1976). *Nursing research in the bicentennial year.* Boulder, CO: Western Interstate Commission for Higher Education.

Diers, D., & Burst, H. V. (1983). Effectiveness of policy related research: Nurse-midwifery as case study. *Image Journal of Nursing Scholarship, 15,* 68–74.

Disbrow, M. A. (1963). Any mother who really wants to nurse her baby can do so. *Nursing Forum, 2,* 39–48.

Donaldson, S. (1998). *Breakthrough in nursing research.* Invited presentation. Proceedings of the 25th

Anniversary of the American Academy of Nursing, Acapulco, Mexico.

Donaldson, S., & Crowley, D. (1978). The discipline of nursing. *Nursing Outlook, 26,* 113-120.

Dumas, R. G., & Leonard, R. C. (1963). The effect of nursing on the incidence of postoperative vomiting. *Nursing Research, 12,* 12-15.

Ellis, R. (1970). Values and vicissitudes of the scientist nurse. *Nursing Research, 19,* 440-445.

Fagin, C. (1998). Nursing research and the erosion of care [guest editorial]. *Nursing Outlook, 46,* 259-260.

Finer, H. (1952). *Administration and the nursing services.* New York, NY: Macmillan Company.

Fitzpatrick, J. J. (Ed.). (1998). *Encyclopedia of nursing research.* New York, NY: Springer.

Glaser, B. G., & Strauss, A. L. (1965). *Awareness of dying (Observation series).* Chicago, IL: Aldine Publishing.

Gortner, S. R. (1973). Research in nursing. The federal interest and grant program. *American Journal of Nursing, 73,* 1052-1053.

Gortner, S. R. (1974a). The relations of scientists with professional and sponsoring organizations and with society. In M. Batey (Ed.), *Issues in research: Social, professional, and methodological. Selected papers from the first American Nurses Association Council of Nurse Researchers program meeting.* Kansas City, MO: American Nurses Association.

Gortner, S. R. (1974b). Research for a practice profession. *Nursing Research, 24,* 193-197.

Gortner, S. R. (1974c). Scientific accountability in nursing. *Nursing Outlook, 22,* 764-768.

Gortner, S. R. (1979). Trends and historical perspective. In F. S. Downs & J. W. Fleming (Eds.), *Issues in nursing research.* New York, NY: Appleton-Century-Crofts.

Gortner, S. R. (1980a). Nursing research: Out of the past and into the future. *Nursing Research, 29,* 204-207.

Gortner, S. R. (1980b). Nursing science in transition. *Nursing Research, 29,* 180-183.

Gortner, S. R. (1984). Knowledge development in a practice discipline: Philosophy and pragmatics. In C. Williams (Ed.), *Nursing research and policy formation: The case of prospective payment.* Kansas City, MO: American Academy of Nursing.

Gortner, S. R. (1990). Nursing values and science: Toward a science philosophy. *Image Journal of Nursing Scholarship, 22,* 101-105.

Gortner, S. R. (1991). Historical development of doctoral programs: Shaping our expectations. *Journal of Professional Nursing, 7,* 45-53.

Gortner, S. R., Bloch, D., & Phillips, T. P. (1976). Contributions of nursing research to patient care. *Journal of Nursing Administration, 6,* 22-28.

Gortner, S. R., & Nahm, H. (1977). An overview of nursing research in the United States. *Nursing Research, 26,* 10-32.

Gortner, S. R., & Schultz, P. R. (1988). Approaches to nursing science methods. *Image Journal of Nursing School, 20,* 22-24.

Grady, P. (1999, September 16-18). Strategic planning for the 21st century. *Proceedings of the National Institute for Nursing Research State of the Science Congress.* Washington, DC.

Henderson, V. (1956). Research in nursing practice—When? *Nursing Research, 4,* 99.

Hinshaw, A. S., Sigmon, H. D., & Lindsey, A. M. (1991). Interfacing nursing and biologic science. *Journal of Professional Nursing, 7,* 264.

Holzemer, W. L., & Gortner, S. R. (1988). Evaluation of the nursing research emphasis/grants for doctoral programs in nursing grant program 1979-1984. *Journal of Professional Nursing, 4,* 381-386.

Hughes, E. D., et al. (1958). *Twenty thousand nurses tell their story.* Philadelphia, PA: JB Lippincott.

Jacobsen, B. S., & Meininger, J. C. (1985). The designs and methods of published nursing research: 1956-1983. *Nursing Research, 34,* 306-312.

Leone, L. P. (1955). The ingredients of research. *Nursing Research, 4,* 51.

Lewis, C. E., & Resnik, B. A. (1967). Nurse clinics and progressive ambulatory patient care. *New England Medical Journal, 277,* 1236-1241.

Lindeman, C. A. (1975a). Delphi survey of priorities in nursing research. *Nursing Research, 24,* 434-441.

Lindeman, C. A. (1975b). Priorities in clinical nursing research. *Nursing Outlook, 23,* 693-698.

Little, D. E., & Carnevali, D. (1967). Nurse specialist effect on tuberculosis: Report on a field experiment. *Nursing Research, 16,* 321-326.

Meleis, A. I. (1980). *The age of nursing scholarliness: Now is the time. The inaugural Helen Nahm Research Lecture.* San Francisco, CA: University of California, San Francisco School of Nursing.

Meleis, A. I. (1987). Revisions in knowledge development: A passion for substance. *Scholarly Inquiry Nursing Practice Institute Journal,* 1-19.

Meltzer, L. E., Pinneo, R., Ferrigan, M. M., Kitchell, J. R., Ipsen, J., & Bearman, J. (1969). *Intensive coronary care: An analysis of the system and the acute phase of myocardial infarction.* New York, NY: Charles Press.

Mishel, M., & Murdaugh, C. (1987). Family adjustment to heart transplantation. *Nursing Research, 36,* 332-338.

Moody, L. E., Wilson, M. E., Smythe, K., Schwartz, R., Tittle, M., & VanCort, M. L. (1988). Analysis of a decade of nursing practice research: 1977–1986. *Nursing Research, 37,* 374–379.

Moss, F. T., & Myer, B. (1966). The effects of nursing interaction upon pain relief in patients. *Nursing Research, 15,* 303–306.

Oberst, M. T. (1986). Nursing in the year 2000: Setting the agenda for knowledge generation and utilization. In G. Sorenson (Ed.), *Setting the agenda for the year 2000: Knowledge development in nursing.* Kansas City, MO: American Academy of Nursing.

Quint, J. (1967). *The nurse and the dying patient.* New York, NY: Macmillan.

Research spanning the life cycle: Vol. 15. (1998, Fall). Los Angeles: University of California, Los Angeles School of Nursing.

Ringholz, S., & Morris, M. (1961). A test of some assumptions about rooming-in. *Nursing Research, 10,* 196–199.

Schorr, T., & Kennedy, M. S. (1999). *100 years of American nursing: Celebrating a century of caring.* Philadelphia, PA: Lippincott Williams & Wilkins.

The science of caring: Vol. 11. (1999, Spring). San Francisco, CA: University of California, San Francisco School of Nursing.

Shaver, J. (1985). A biopsychosocial view of human health. *Nursing Outlook, 33,* 187–191.

Silver, H. K., Ford, L. C., & Day, L. R. (1968). The pediatric nurse practitioner program: Expanding the role of the nurse to provide increased health care for children. *Journal of the American Medical Association, 204,* 298–302.

Stevenson, J. S., & Woods, N. (1986a). Nursing science and contemporary science: Emerging paradigms. In G. Sorenson (Ed.), *Setting the agenda for the year 2000: Knowledge development in nursing.* Kansas City, MO: American Academy of Nursing.

Stevenson, J. S., & Woods, N. (1986b). Strategies for the year 2000: Synthesis and projections. In G. Sorenson (Ed.), *Setting the agenda for the year 2000: Knowledge development in nursing.* Kansas City, MO: American Academy of Nursing.

Vreeland, E. (1959, February). Memorandum to Lucile Petry Leone, chief nurse officer. Some frontiers for nursing research.

CHAPTER 19

Research: How Health Care Advances

Harry A. Sultz and Kristina M. Young

CHAPTER OBJECTIVES

1. Define and recognize the focus of different types of research and how each type contributes to the advancement of knowledge about health and the healthcare system.

2. Describe the functions and goals of the Agency for Healthcare Research and Quality and how to access information pertinent to advanced nursing practice.

3. Recognize the interface of health research and policy and of research and quality improvement.

4. Discuss future challenges for healthcare research and the impact they will have on advanced practice nursing.

INTRODUCTION

The last half of the 20th century saw a remarkable growth of scientifically rigorous research in medicine, dentistry, nursing, and the other health professions. The change from depending on the clinical impressions of individual physicians and other healthcare practitioners to relying on the statistical probability of accurate findings from carefully controlled studies is one of the most important advances in scientific medicine. No longer is the literature of the health professions filled with subjective anecdotal reports of the progress of treatment in one or more individual cases. Now readers of peer-reviewed professional journals can monitor the progress of basic science or clinical or technologic discoveries with confidence, knowing that published findings are, with few exceptions, based on research studies that have been rigorously designed and conducted to yield statistically credible results.

In contrast, the ever-growing volumes of reports of medical developments that appear in the popular media are often premature and, depending on the source, may be cause for skepticism. The imprudent publication of inadequately or unproven therapies, the sensationalizing of minor scientific advances, and the promotion of fraudulent devices and treatments create unrealistic expectations that often result in disappointments, mistreatment, and costly deceptions.

From both professional and public perspectives, the continuing research yield of new technologies and clinical advances creates ongoing challenges of evaluation, interpretation, and potential applications.

This chapter explains the focus of different types of research and discusses how each type contributes to the overall advances in health and medicine. Health services research—a newer field that addresses the workings of the healthcare system rather than specific problems of disease or disability—is described. The offices and goals of its major funding source, the federal Agency for Healthcare Research and Quality, are listed. Finally, research into the quality of medical care, the problems being addressed, and the research challenges of the future are discussed.

TYPES OF RESEARCH

Research studies conducted by those in the professional disciplines fall into several categories. Basic science research is the work of biochemists, physiologists, biologists, pharmacologists, and others concerned with sciences that are fundamental to understanding the growth, development, structure, and function of the human body and its responses to external stimuli. Much of basic science research is at the cellular level and takes place in highly sophisticated laboratories. Other basic research may involve animal or human studies. Whatever its nature, however, basic science research is the essential antecedent of advances in clinical medicine.

Clinical research focuses primarily on the various steps in the process of medical care—the early detection, diagnosis, and treatment of disease or injury; the maintenance of optimal physical, mental, and social functioning; the limitation and rehabilitation of disability; and the palliative care of those who are irreversibly ill. Individuals in all the clinical specialties of medicine, nursing, allied health, and related health professions conduct clinical research, often in collaboration with those in the basic sciences. Much of clinical research is experimental, involving carefully controlled clinical trials of diagnostic or therapeutic procedures, new drugs, or technologic developments.

Clinical trials test a new treatment or drug against a prevailing standard of care. If no standard drug exists or if it is too easily identified, a control group receives a placebo or mock drug to minimize subject bias. To reduce bias further, random selection is used to decide which volunteer patients are in the experimental and control groups. In a double-blind study, neither the researchers nor the patients know who is receiving the test drug or treatment until the study is completed and an identifying code revealed.

Research studies have a number of safeguards to protect the safety and rights of volunteer subjects. Studies funded by governmental agencies or foundations are subject to scrutiny by a peer-review committee that judges the scientific merit of the research design and the potential value of the findings. Then a hospital-based or institutional review board checks for ethical considerations and patient protections. Finally, volunteer subjects must receive and sign an informed consent form that spells out in clear detail the potential risks or side effects and the expected benefits of their participation. Volunteers must weigh any potential risks against the likelihood that, by participating in research, they will receive state-of-the-art care and close health monitoring and will contribute to the advancement of science.

EPIDEMIOLOGY

Epidemiology, or population research, is concerned with the distribution and determinants of health, diseases, and injuries in human populations. Much of that research is observational; it is the collection of information about natural phenomena, the characteristics and behaviors of people, aspects of their location or environment, and their exposure to certain circumstances or events.

Observational studies may be descriptive or analytical. Descriptive studies use patient records, interview surveys, various databases, and other information sources to identify those factors and conditions that determine the distribution of health and disease among specific populations. They provide the details or characteristics of diseases or biologic phenomena and the prevalence or magnitude of their occurrence. Descriptive studies are relatively fast and inexpensive and often raise questions or suggest hypotheses to be tested. They usually are followed by analytic studies, which try to explain biologic phenomena by seeking statistical associations between factors that may contribute to a subsequent occurrence and the occurrence itself.

Some analytic studies attempt, under naturally occurring circumstances, to observe the differences between two or more populations with different characteristics or behaviors. For instance, data about smokers and nonsmokers may be collected to determine the relative risk of a related outcome such as lung cancer, or a cohort study may follow a population over time, as in the case of a Framingham, Massachusetts, study. For years, epidemiologists have been studying a cooperating population of Framingham to determine associations between such variables as diet, weight, exercise, and other behaviors and characteristics related to heart disease and other outcomes. These observational studies are valuable in explaining patterns of disease or disease processes and providing information about the association of specific activities or agents with health or disease effects.

Experimental Epidemiology

Observational studies are usually followed by experimental studies. In experimental studies, the investigator actively intervenes by manipulating one variable to see what happens with the other. Although they are the best test of cause and effect, such studies are technically difficult to carry out and often raise ethical issues. Control populations are used to ensure that other nonexperimental variables are not affecting the outcome. Like clinical trials, such studies may raise ethical issues when experiments involve the use of a clinical procedure that may expose the subjects to significant or unknown risk. Ethical questions also are raised when experimental studies require the withholding of some potentially beneficial drug or procedure from individuals in the control group to prove decisively the effectiveness of the drug or procedure.

Other Applications of Epidemiologic Methods

Because the population perspective of epidemiology usually requires the study and analysis of data obtained from or about large-scale population samples, the discipline has developed principles and methods that can be applied to the study of a wide range of problems in several fields. Thus the concepts and quantitative methods of epidemiology have been used not only to add to the understanding of the etiology of health and disease, but also to plan, administer, and evaluate health services; to forecast the health needs of population groups; to assess the adequacy of the supply of health personnel; and, most recently, to determine the outcomes of specific treatment modalities in a variety of clinical settings.

Advances in statistical theory and the epidemiology of medical care make it possible to analyze and interpret performance data obtained from the large Medicare and other insurance databases. Many of the findings of inexplicable geographic variations in the amount and cost of hospital treatments and in the use of a variety of healthcare services resulted from analysis of Medicare claims data and other large health insurance databases.

HEALTH SERVICES RESEARCH

Until the last two decades, most research addressed the need to broaden understanding of health and disease, to find new and more effective means of diagnosis and treatment, and, in effect, to improve the quality and length of life. For the two decades after World War II, supply-side subsidy programs dominated federal healthcare policy. Like other subsidy programs, Medicare and Medicaid were politically crafted solutions rather than research-based strategies. Nevertheless, those major healthcare subsidy programs were the driving forces behind the rise of health services research. The continuous collection of cost and utilization data from these programs revealed serious deficiencies in the capability of the healthcare system to deliver efficiently and effectively the knowledge and skills already at hand. In addition, evidence was growing that the large variations in the kinds and amounts of care delivered for the same conditions represented unacceptable volumes of inappropriate or questionable care and too much indecision or confusion among clinicians about the best courses of treatment. Health services research was born of the need to improve the efficiency and effectiveness of the healthcare system and to determine which of the healthcare treatment options for each condition produces the best outcomes.

AGENCY FOR HEALTHCARE RESEARCH AND QUALITY

Ever since John Wennberg documented large differences in the use of medical and surgical procedures among physicians in small geographic areas in the late 1980s, a number of similar studies have brought the value of increasingly more costly health care into serious question. Wennberg noted that the rate of surgeries correlated with the numbers of surgeons and the number of hospital beds, rather than with differences among patients.

Specifically, Wennberg found that per-capita expenditures for hospitalization in Boston were consistently double those in nearby New Haven, Connecticut.[1-3] Widely varying physician practice patterns provided little direction as to the most appropriate use of even the most common clinical procedures. In addition, adequate outcome measures for specific intervention modalities generally were lacking.

This problem did not escape the attention of the 101st Congress. The development of new knowledge through research has long been held as an appropriate and essential role of the federal government, as evidenced by the establishment and proactive role of the National Institutes of Health. When it became clear that the indecision about the most appropriate and effective ways to diagnose and treat specific medical, dental, and other conditions was contributing to unacceptably large variations in the cost, quality, and outcomes of health care, federal legislation was passed to support the development of clinical guidelines. The Agency for Health Care Policy and Research (AHCPR) was established in 1989 as the successor to the National Center for Health Services Research and Health Care Technology. It was one of eight agencies of the Public Health Service within the Department of Health and Human Services.

AHCPR was responsible for updating and promoting the development and review of clinically relevant guidelines to assist healthcare practitioners in the prevention, diagnosis, treatment, and management of clinical conditions. The authorizing legislation directed that panels of qualified experts be convened by AHCPR or by public and not-for-profit private organizations. These panels were to review the literature that contained the findings of numerous studies of clinical conditions and, after considering the scientific evidence, to recommend clinical guidelines to assist practitioner and patient decisions about appropriate care for specific clinical conditions.[4]

The agency's priority activities included funding two types of research projects: patient outcome research teams and literature synthesis projects or meta-analyses. Both the patient outcome research teams and the smaller literature synthesis projects identified and analyzed patient outcomes associated with alternative practice patterns and recommended changes where appropriate. During its decade-long existence, AHCPR supported studies that resulted in a prodigious array of publications focused on patient care and clinical decision making, technology assessment, the quality and costs of care, and treatment outcomes. Although no longer directly involved in producing clinical practice guidelines, the agency assists private-sector groups by supplying them with the scientific evidence they need to develop their own guidelines.

Several changes occurred in the mandate of AHCPR after its 1989 inception. The agency narrowly escaped the loss of funding and possible elimination in 1996 after incurring the wrath of national organizations of surgeons. In keeping with its original mission, AHCPR issued clinical guidelines. One such guideline discouraged surgery as a treatment for back pain on the grounds that it provided no better outcomes than more conservative treatments. Organizations of angry surgeons led a lobbying effort that convinced key members of Congress that the agency was exceeding its authority and establishing standards of clinical practice without considering the expertise and opinions of the medical specialists involved.[5]

The dispute was resolved when AHCPR agreed to function as a "science partner" with public and private organizations by simply assisting in developing knowledge that could be used to improve clinical practice. The agency pledged to no longer produce clinical guidelines but rather to focus instead on funding research on medical interventions and analyzing

the data that would underlie the development of clinical guidelines. The guidelines themselves would be generated by medical specialty and other organizations.

Subsequently, the Healthcare Research and Quality Act of 1999 was passed, which retitled the AHCPR to the Agency for Healthcare Research and Quality (AHRQ) and changed the title of the administrator to director. The mission of AHRQ is to (1) improve the outcomes and quality of healthcare services, (2) reduce healthcare costs, (3) address patient safety, and (4) broaden effective services through establishment of a broad base of scientific research that promotes improvements in clinical and health systems practices, including prevention of disease.[6]

A top priority of AHRQ is getting its sponsored research results and new health information into the hands of consumers. In addition to a number of consumer-oriented publications, the agency provides information to the public via the Internet. Its website, www.ahrq.gov, offers a great deal of healthcare information.

HEALTH SERVICES RESEARCH AND HEALTH POLICY

Health services research combines the perspectives and methods of epidemiology, sociology, economics, and clinical medicine. Although the basic concepts of epidemiology and biostatistics apply, process and outcome measures that reflect the behavioral and economic variables associated with questions of therapeutic effectiveness and cost–benefit ratios are also used. The ability of health services research to address issues of therapeutic effectiveness and cost–benefit comparisons during this period of fiscal exigency contributed to the field's substantial growth and current value.

The contributions of health services research to health policy within recent years are impressive. Major examples include the Wennberg studies of small-area variation in medical utilization, the prospective payment system based on diagnosis-related groups,[7,8] research on inappropriate medical procedures,[9] resource-based relative value scale research,[10-12] and the background research that supported the concepts of health maintenance organizations and managed care.

The RAND Health Insurance Experiment,[13,14] one of the largest and longest-running health services research projects ever undertaken, began in 1971 and contributed vast amounts of information on the effects of cost sharing on the provision and outcomes of health services. Participating families were assigned to one of four different fee-for-service plans or to a prepaid group practice. As might have been expected, individuals in the various plans differed significantly in their rate of use, with little measurable effect on health outcomes. The Health Insurance Experiment was followed by two large research studies: the Health Services Utilization Study and the Medical Outcomes Study. The findings of both gave impetus to the federal support of outcomes research.[15] Determining the outcomes and effectiveness of different healthcare interventions aids clinical decision making, reduces costs, and benefits patients.

QUALITY IMPROVEMENT

Until the last few years, health care's impressive accomplishments made it difficult for healthcare researchers, policymakers, and organizational leaders to acknowledge publicly that poor-quality health care is a major problem within the dynamic and productive biomedical enterprise in the United States. In 1990, after 2 years of study, hearings, and site visits, the Institute of Medicine issued a report that cited widespread overuse of expensive invasive technology, underuse of inexpensive "caring" services, and implementation of error-prone procedures that harmed patients and wasted money.[16,17]

Although these conclusions from so prestigious a body were devastating in their significance to healthcare reformers, they were hardly news to health services researchers. For decades, practitioners assumed that quality, like beauty, was in the eye of the beholder and, therefore,

was unmeasurable except in cases of obvious violations of generally accepted standards. The medical and other healthcare professions had promoted the image of health care as a blend of almost impenetrable, science-based disciplines, leaving the providers of care as the only ones capable of understanding the processes taking place. Thus only physicians could judge the work of other physicians. Such peer review-based assessment has always been difficult for reviewers and limited in effectiveness. Peer review recognizes that only part of medical care is based on factual knowledge; a substantial component of medical decision making is based on clinical judgment. Clinical judgment entails combining consideration of the potential risks and benefits of each physician's internal list of alternatives in making diagnostic and treatment decisions with his or her medical intuition regarding the likelihood of success based on the condition of each patient. Under these complex and often inexplicable circumstances, physicians are repelled by the notion of either judging or being judged by their colleagues.

That is why, until recently, quality assurance—whether in hospitals or by regulatory agencies—was focused on identifying only exceptionally poor care. This practice, popularly known as the bad apple theory, was based on the presumption that the best way to ensure quality was to identify the bad apples and remove or rehabilitate them. Thus, during the 1970s and 1980s, quality assurance interventions only followed detection of undesirable occurrences. For example, flagrant violations of professional standards had to be in evidence before professional review organizations required physicians to begin quality improvement plans. Of course, physicians were guaranteed due process to dispute the evidence.

Focusing on isolated violations required a great deal of review time to uncover a single case that called for remedial action. In addition, it was an unpleasant duty for reviewers to assign blame to a colleague who might soon be on a committee reviewing their own records. Most importantly, such an inspection of quality represented a method that implicitly defined quality as the absence of mishap. Clinician dislike of quality assurance activities during the 1970s and 1980s was well founded: The processes were offensive and had little constructive impact.

Specifying and striving for excellent care are very recent quality assurance phenomena in the healthcare arena. Just as the automobile and other industries were late giving up supervision as a control mechanism and introducing "quality circles" or teamwork, so hospitals and other healthcare organizations that had long focused on peer-review committees, incident reports, and other negative quality monitoring activities were tardy in embracing this movement.

Health services researchers had known for decades that healthcare quality was measurable and that excellent, as well as poor, care could be identified and quantified. In 1966, Avedis Donabedian[18] characterized the concept of health care as divided into the components of structure, process, and outcomes and the research paradigm of their assumed linkages, all of which have guided quality of care investigators to this day.

Donabedian suggested that the number, kinds, and skills of the providers, as well as the adequacy of their physical resources and the manner in which they perform appropriate procedures, should, in the aggregate, influence the quality of the subsequent outcomes. Although today the construct may seem like a simple statement of the obvious, at the time attention to structural criteria was the major, if not the only, quality assurance activity in favor. It was generally assumed that properly trained professionals, given adequate resources in properly equipped facilities, performed at acceptable standards of quality. For example, for many years the then Joint Commission on Accreditation of Hospitals made judgments about the quality of hospitals on the basis of structural standards, such as physical facilities and equipment, ratios of professional staff to patients, and the qualifications of various personnel. Later, it added process components to its struc-

tural standards. Aspects of process are the diagnostic, treatment, and patient management decisions and their appropriateness in relationship to current knowledge and practice. These quality assessments were directed to process components and did not attempt to determine what happened to the patients as the result of the medical decisions and interventions. Only recently has The Joint Commission included outcomes in its accreditation assessments.

Early landmark quality-of-care studies used implicit and explicit normative or judgmental standards. Implicit standards rely on the internalized judgments of the expert individuals involved in the quality assessment. Explicit standards are those developed and agreed on in advance of the assessment. Explicit standards minimize the variation and bias that invariably result when judgments are internalized. More current studies judge the appropriateness of hospital admissions and various procedures and, in general, associate specific structural characteristics of the healthcare system with practice or process variations.

Another method for assessing the quality of healthcare practices is based on empirical standards. Derived from distributions, averages, ranges, and other measures of data variability, information collected from a number of similar health services providers is compared to identify practices that deviate from the norms. A current popular use of empirical standards is in the patient severity-adjusted hospital performance data collected by health departments and community-based employer and insurer groups to measure and compare both process activities and outcomes. These performance "report cards" are becoming increasingly valuable to the purchasers of care, who need an objective method to guide their choices among managed care organizations, healthcare systems, and group practices. The empirical measures of quality include variables such as the following:

- Timeliness of ambulation
- Compliance with basic nursing care standards

- Average length of stay
- Number of home care referrals
- Number of rehabilitation referrals
- Timeliness of consultation completion
- Timeliness of orders and results
- Patient wait times by department or area
- Infection rates
- Decubitus rates
- Medication errors
- Patient complaints
- Readmissions within 30 days
- Neonatal and maternal mortality
- Perioperative mortality

Normative and empirical standards are both used in studying the quality of health care in the United States. For example, empirical analyses are performed to test or modify normative recommendations. Empirical or actual experience data are collected to confirm performance and outcome improvements after the imposition of clinical guidelines derived from studies using normative standards.

MEDICAL ERRORS

In November 1999, the Institute of Medicine again issued a report on the quality of medical care.[19] Focused on medical errors, the report described mistakes occurring during the course of hospital care as one of the nation's leading causes of death and disability. Citing two major studies estimating that medical errors kill some 44,000 to 98,000 people in U.S. hospitals each year, the Institute of Medicine report was a stunning indictment of the current systems of hospital care. The report contained a series of recommendations for improving patient safety in the admittedly high-risk environments of modern hospitals. Among the recommendations was a proposal for establishing a center for patient safety within the AHRQ. The proposed center would establish national safety goals, track progress in improving safety, and invest in research to learn more about prevent-

ing mistakes.[19] Congress responded by designating part of the increase in the budget for the AHRQ for that purpose.

EVIDENCE-BASED MEDICINE

Evidence-based medicine is defined as "the systematic application of the best available evidence to the evaluation of options and decisions in clinical practice, management and policy-making."[20] Although that statement may appear to be a description of the way physicians and other healthcare providers have practiced since the inception of scientific medicine, it reflects a spreading concern that quite the opposite is true. The wide range of variability in clinical practice, the complexity of diagnostic testing and medical decision making, and the difficulty that physicians have in keeping up with the overwhelming volumes of scientific literature suggest that a significant percentage of clinical management decisions are not supported by reliable evidence of effectiveness.

Although it is generally assumed that physicians are reasonably confident that the treatments they give are beneficial, the reality is that medical practice is fraught with uncertainty. In addition, the ethical basis for clinical decision making allows physicians to exercise their preferences for certain medical theories or practices that may or may not have been evaluated to link treatment to benefits.[21]

Proponents of evidence-based medicine propose that if all health services are intended to improve the health status and quality of life of the recipients, then the acid test is whether services, programs, and policies improve health beyond what could be achieved with the same resources by different means or by doing nothing at all. Evidence is the key to accountability. The decisions made by healthcare providers, administrators, policymakers, patients, and the public need to be based on appropriate, balanced, and high-quality evidence.[21]

The evidence-based approach to assessing the acceptability of research findings considers the evidence from randomized clinical trials involving large numbers of participants to be the most valid. Evidence-based medicine advocates dismiss outcomes research that uses large data files created from claim records, hospital discharges, Medicare, or other sources because the subjects are not randomized. "Outcomes research using claims data is an excellent way of finding out what doctors are doing, but it's a terrible way to find out what doctors should be doing," stated Thomas C. Chalmers, MD, of Harvard School of Public Health, Boston.[22]

In general, most of the investigations reported in the peer-reviewed medical literature have been preliminary tests of innovations and served science rather than providing guidance to practitioners in clinical practice. Only a small portion of those efforts survive testing well enough to justify routine clinical application.[23]

The situation is changing rapidly, however. Articles on evidence-based medicine are appearing with increasing frequency in the medical literature.[23] Cost-control pressures that encourage efforts to ensure that therapies have documented patient benefit, growing interest in the quality of patient care, and increasing sophistication on the part of patients concerning the care that they receive have stimulated acceptance of the concepts of evidence-based medical practice.[23]

OUTCOMES RESEARCH

Given the huge investment in U.S. health care and the inequitable distribution of its services, do the end effects on the health and well-being of patients and populations justify the costs? Insurance companies, state and federal governments, employers, and consumers are looking to outcomes research for information that will help them make better decisions about which kinds of health care should be reimbursed, for whom, and when.

Because outcomes research evaluates results of healthcare processes in the real world of physicians' offices, hospitals, clinics, and homes,

it contrasts with traditional randomized controlled studies that test the effects of treatments in controlled environments. In addition, the research in usual service settings, or "effectiveness research," differs from controlled clinical trials, or "efficacy research," in the nature of the outcomes measured. Traditionally, studies measured health status, or outcomes, with physiologic measurements—laboratory tests, complication rates, recovery, or survival. To capture health status more adequately, outcomes research measures a patient's functional status and well-being. Satisfaction with care also must complement traditional measures.

Functional status includes three components that assess patients' abilities to function in their own environment:

1. Physical functioning
2. Role functioning—the extent to which health interferes with usual daily activities, such as work or school
3. Social functioning—whether health affects normal social activities, such as visiting friends or participating in group activities

Personal well-being measures describe patients' sense of physical and mental well-being—their mental health or general mood, their personal view of their general health, and their general sense about the quality of their lives. Patient satisfaction measures the patients' views about the services received, including access, convenience, communication, financial coverage, and technical quality.

Outcomes research also uses meta-analyses, a technique to summarize comparable findings from multiple studies. More importantly, however, outcomes research goes beyond determining what works in ideal circumstances to assessing which treatments for specific clinical problems work best in different circumstances. Appropriateness studies are conducted to determine circumstances in which a procedure should and should not be performed. Even though a procedure is proved effective, it is not appropriate for every patient in all circumstances. The frequency of inappropriate clinical interventions is one of the major quality-of-care problems in the system. Research is also under way to develop the tools to identify patient preferences when treatment options are available. Although most discussions about appropriateness stress the cost savings that could be achieved by reducing unnecessary care and overuse of services, it is important to remember that outcomes research may be just as likely to uncover underuse of appropriate services.

It is important to recognize that the ultimate value of outcomes research can be measured only by its ability to incorporate the results of its efforts into the healthcare process. To be effective, the findings of outcomes research must first reach and then change the behaviors of providers, patients, healthcare institutions, and payers. The endpoint of outcomes research—that is, the clinical practice guidelines intended to assist practitioners and patients in choosing appropriate health care for specific conditions—must be disseminated in acceptable and motivational ways. With the healthcare industry in a state of rapid and generally unpredictable change, the need to make appropriate investments in outcomes research has become increasingly apparent. The conclusion is now inescapable that the United States cannot continue to spend more than $2 trillion each year on health care without learning much more than is now known about what that investment is buying.[24,25]

PATIENT SATISFACTION

Patient satisfaction has become an important component of the quality of care. Although the subjective ratings of health care received by patients may be based on markedly different criteria from those considered important by care providers, they capture aspects of care and personal preferences that contribute significantly to perceived quality. It has become increasingly important in the competitive market climate of health care that the providers' characteristics, organization, and system attributes important to the consumers be identified and monitored. In addition to caregivers' technical and interpersonal skills, such patient concerns as waiting times for appointments, emergency responses, helpfulness and communication of staff, and the facility's appearance contribute to patient evaluations of health services delivery programs and subsequent satisfaction with the quality of care received.

A number of instruments have been devised to measure patient satisfaction with health care, and most managed care plans, hospitals, and other health services facilities and agencies have adopted one or more to assess patient satisfaction regularly. Some, such as the Patient Satisfaction Questionnaire developed at Southern Illinois University School of Medicine, are short, self-administered survey forms. Others, such as the popular patient satisfaction instruments of the Picker Institute of Boston, Massachusetts, may be used as self-administered questionnaires mailed to patients after a healthcare experience or completed by interviewers during telephone surveys.[26] Whether by mail, direct contact, or telephone interview, questioning patients after a recent healthcare experience is an effective way to both identify outstanding service personnel and uncover fundamental problems in the quality of care as defined by patients. It not only serves the purpose of providing humane and effective care, but it is also good marketing to do everything possible to increase patient satisfaction, maintain patient loyalty, and enhance patient referrals.

RESEARCH ETHICS

In the six decades since World War II, the federal government has invested heavily in biomedical research. The ensuing public–private partnership in health has produced some of the finest medical research in the world. The growth of medical knowledge is unparalleled, and the United States can take well-deserved pride in its research accomplishments.

However, many, if not most, of the sophisticated new technologies address the need to ameliorate the problems of the patients who already have the condition or disease under treatment. Both the priorities and the profits intrinsic to the U.S. healthcare system focus on remedial rather than preventive strategies. Only in the case of frightening epidemics, such as that of polio in the 1940s, AIDS in the 1990s, and H1N1 influenza in 2009, have there been the requisite moral imperatives to fund adequately abundant research efforts that address public health problems. Clearly, much of the recent funding for medical research has failed to fulfill the generally held belief that the products of taxpayer-supported research should benefit not only the practice of medicine, but also the community at large.

CONFLICTS OF INTEREST IN RESEARCH

The increasing amount of research funding emanating from pharmaceutical and medical device companies is of serious concern. Pharmaceutical companies that pay researchers to design and interpret drug trials have been accused of misrepresenting the results or suppressing unfavorable findings. The conflicts that arise in the testing of new drugs and instruments and publishing the results deepen as increasing numbers of studies are shifted from academic institutions to commercial research firms.[27]

For example, in May 2009 the Attorney General of New Jersey issued subpoenas to five major medical device makers for failing to disclose financial conflicts of interest among physicians researching their products. It was learned that physicians who were testing and recommending the use of certain medical devices were being compensated with stock in the companies making those devices.[28]

To compound the problem further, the funding of the U.S. Food and Drug Administration (FDA), which regulates about a fourth of the U.S. economy, has been shifted from the government to the same pharmaceutical companies it is supposed to monitor with damaging effect. Political and pharmaceutical pressures have caused the FDA to stray from its science-based public health mandate. For example, the FDA has been sharply criticized for its alleged failure to monitor adequately the risks of widely advertised and commonly used drugs for the treatment of arthritis.[29] The FDA's handling of clinical trial data collected by pharmaceutical manufacturers to establish the efficacy and safety of their products is a major problem. Although the information collected is necessary for FDA approval of a product, once the product is approved, the FDA does not provide the public with a full report of the drug's safety and efficacy. The withheld information falls into the definition of "trade secrets," and the FDA has taken the position that research data are entitled to protection as proprietary information. That explains the number of recent examples of FDA-approved drugs later discovered to have major safety risks.[30] Clearly, the FDA has to reconsider its position that clinical trial data fall into the classification of "trade secrets."

The most egregious violation of professional ethics is found in the growing body of evidence that physicians at some of the most prestigious of U.S. medical schools have been attaching their names and reputations to scientific publications ghostwritten by employees of pharmaceutical companies. The publications are intended, of course, to boost sales of the pharmaceutical product.[31] The National Institutes of Health, which funds much of the nation's medical research, suggests that the universities involved, rather than the government, should address the problem. Because the universities find it difficult to censure prestigious medical faculty, the problem remains unaddressed.[31]

FUTURE CHALLENGES

Most U.S. healthcare research has been directed toward improving the healthcare system's ability to diagnose and treat injury, disease, and disability among those who seek care. Now, largely because of the influences of managed care, research studies are increasingly focused on identifying and improving the health status of populations. Research priorities are shifting from an individual patient perspective to a population orientation and toward continuous scrutiny of the efficiency and effectiveness of the care delivered.

Basic science research will continue to contribute to the diagnostic and therapeutic efficacy of health care by adding to the knowledge about the human body and its functions. In small but critically important increments, basic science research will unlock many of the secrets of aging, cell growth regulation, mental degradation, and other mysteries of immunology, genetics, microbiology, and neuroendocrinology. The propensity of medicine to use newly obtained knowledge to alter certain physiologic processes, as in the several forms of gene manipulation, will produce new ethical, legal, and clinical issues that then will require further research and adjudication.

Massive databases of gene and protein sequences and structure/function information have made possible a new worldwide research effort called bioinformatics. Bioinformatics research probes those large computer databases to learn more about life's processes in health and disease and to find new or better drugs. It is considered the future of biotechnology.

Of particular interest is research in genomics, the study of genetic material in the chromosomes of specific organisms. The sequencing of the human genome will reshape biology and medicine and lead to significant improvements in the diagnosis of disease and individual responses to drugs.[32]

Similarly, certain advances in clinical medicine and the other health disciplines will result in new and particularly disturbing moral dilemmas. Medical achievements, such as those that permit the maintenance of life in otherwise terminal and unresponsive individuals or the transplantation of organs in short supply that require choosing among recipient candidates when those denied will surely die, generate ex-

tremely complex ethical, economic, religious, personal, and professional issues. Thus much of the basic and clinical research that solves yesterday's problems relating to individual patient care will create new problems to be addressed in the never-ending cycle of discovery, application, and evaluation.

Medical researchers and clinicians are becoming increasingly concerned that health care in the United States is entering a "postantibiotic" era in which bacterial infections will be unaffected by even the most powerful of available antibiotics. Evidence is accumulating that a growing number of microbes, including strains of *Staphylococcus* and *Streptococcus* bacteria, are becoming resistant to common antimicrobials.[33] *Staphylococcus* bacteria are a major cause of hospital infections. According to the Centers for Disease Control and Prevention, these infections are responsible for about 13% of the 2 million infections that occur in U.S. hospitals each year. Overall, infections result in the deaths of as many as 99,000 hospital patients each year.[34]

Although infectious disease epidemiologists and clinical specialists warned for decades that misuse and overuse of antibiotics would result in a host of deadly drug-resistant pathogens, neither physicians nor patients took the warnings seriously, with a widespread belief that the development of new antimicrobial drugs would keep medicine a step ahead of bacterial resistance. Limited development of new antibiotic drugs has failed to keep pace with antibiotic resistance; however, scientists now see promising alternatives in bacterial genetics to address antibiotic resistance.[35]

While researchers address the problems of treating lethal infections, hospitals strive to prevent them. Because bacteria can be transmitted on blankets, clothing, walls, medical equipment, and by hand, hospitals are implementing rigorous infection control and surveillance policies and new education programs for both providers and patients.

Health services research, in contrast, will continue to focus on the performance of the healthcare system as the basis for proposing or evaluating health policy alternatives. It is interdisciplinary, value-laden research concerned with the effectiveness or benefits of care, the efficiency or resource cost of care, and the equity or fairness of the distribution of care. Documenting the influence of financial incentives that affect both patient and provider, understanding the important relationships of socioeconomic status to health and health care, determining the effects of the training and experience of the healthcare team and the ability of the members to work together, and understanding how these many influences interact are basic to improving the quality of care. Reducing the monumental quandaries in medicine and health care about what works well in which situations is the challenge of health services research and the key to a more effective, efficient, and equitable healthcare system.

Public health research is a related research arena that deserves to receive higher priority and significantly increased political support. If health care is ever to develop a true population perspective rather than an individual patient perspective and reap the health and economic benefits of preventive rather than curative medicine, then epidemiology and public health research must be charged with finding ways to better understand and resolve the huge differences in health, health behaviors, health care, and health system effectiveness among communities and the population groups within them. Epidemiology, the core discipline of public health research, can assess the health problems and the provision of health care for the total population rather than just those who are in contact with health services. Surveillance and monitoring of health conditions and assessing the effect of healthcare measures on the entire population are important factors in formulating health policy, organizing health services, and allocating limited resources.[35] The strategy for identifying and dealing with real or suspected biologic attacks on citizens of the United States will depend heavily on the ability of epidemiologists to identify the common source of such outbreaks, the patterns of transmission, and the outcomes of preventive and remedial efforts.

As health care adds to its traditional focus on theories, disease, and individual patient care, the performance of the healthcare system and the health status of populations, public health, and health services research assume increasing relevance and importance. No matter how well the healthcare system performs for some of the people, it cannot be fully satisfactory until it can provide a basic level of care for all.

REFERENCES

1. Wennberg JE, Freeman JL, Culp WJ, et al. Are hospital services rationed in New Haven or over-utilized in Boston? *Lancet.* 1987;1:1185–1189.
2. Wennberg JE. Which rate is right? *N Engl J Med.* 1986;314:310–311.
3. Wennberg JE, Freeman JL, Shelton RM, et al. Hospital use and mortality among Medicare beneficiaries in Boston and New Haven. *N Engl J Med.* 1989;321:1168–1173.
4. Agency for Health Care Policy and Research, U.S. Department of Health and Human Services. *AHCPR Program Note.* Rockville, MD: Public Health Service; 1990.
5. Stephenson J. Revitalized AHCPR pursues research on quality. *JAMA.* 1997;278:1557.
6. U.S. Department of Health and Human Services, Rockville, MD. Agency for Healthcare Research and Quality: Reauthorization Fact Sheet. Available from http://www.ahrq.gov /About/ahrqfact.htm. Accessed April 16, 2010.
7. Mills R, Fetter RB, Riedel DC, et al. AUTOGRP: an interactive computer system for the analysis of health care data. *Med Care.* 1976;14:603–615.
8. Berki SE. DRGs, incentives, hospitals and physicians. *Health Affairs.* 1985;4:70–76.
9. Chassin MR, Kosecoff J, Park RE, et al. Does inappropriate use explain geographic variations in the use of health care services? A study of three procedures. *JAMA.* 1987;258:2533–2537.
10. Hsiao WC, Stason WB. Toward developing a relative value scale for medical and surgical services. *Health Care Finan Rev.* 1979;1:23–28.
11. Hsiao WC, Braun P, Yntema D, et al. Results and policy implications of the resource-based relative value study. *N Engl J Med.* 1988;319:881–888.

12. Hsiao WC, Braun P, Yntema D, et al. *A National Study of Resource-Based Relative Value Scale for Physician Services: Final Report to the Health Care Financing Administration.* Boston, MA: Harvard School of Public Health; 1988.

13. Newhouse JP. A design for a health insurance experiment. *Inquiry.* 1974;11:5–27.

14. Newhouse JP, Keeler EB, Phelps CE, et al. The findings of the RAND health insurance experiment—a response to Welch et al. *Med Care.* 1987; 25:157–179.

15. Newhouse JP. Controlled experimentation as research policy. In: Ginzberg E, Ed. *Health Services Research: Key to Health Policy.* Cambridge, MA: Harvard University Press; 1991:162–194.

16. Lohr KN. *The Institute of Medicine. Medicare: A Strategy for Quality Assurance, Vol. 1.* Washington, DC: National Academy Press; 1990.

17. Surver JD. Striving for quality in health care: an inquiry into policy and practice. *Health Care Management Review.* 1992:17(4);95–96.

18. Donabedian A. Evaluating the quality of medical care. *Milbank Mem Fund Q.* 1966;44:166–206.

19. Kohn LT, Corrigan JM, Donaldson MS, et al. *To Err Is Human: Building a Safer Health System.* Washington, DC: Institute of Medicine; 1999.

20. Watanabe M. A call for action from the National Forum on Health. *Can Med Assoc J.* 1997;156: 999–1000. Available from http://www.cmaj .ca/cgi/reprint/156/7/999. Accessed September 13, 2009.

21. Marwick C. Federal agency focuses on outcomes research. *JAMA.* 1993;270:164–165.

22. Castiel LD. The urge for evidence based knowledge. *J Epidemiol Commun Health.* 2003;57:482.

23. Hooker RC. The rise and rise of evidence-based medicine. *Lancet.* 1997;349:1329–1330.

24. Reinhardt UE, Hussey PS, Anderson GF, et al. U.S. health care spending in an international context. *Health Affairs.* 2004;23:10–25.

25. Kerr D, Scott M. British lessons on health care reform. *N Engl J Med.* Available from www .nejm.org. Accessed September 12, 2009.

26. Gerteis M, Edgman-Levitan S, Daley J. *Through the Patient's Eyes: Understanding and Promoting Patient-Centered Care.* San Francisco: Jossey-Bass; 1993.

27. Walker EP. HHS report slams FDA's conflict of interest oversight. Available from http://www .medpagetoday.com/PublicHealthPolicy/Clinical Trials/12407. Accessed September 13, 2009.

28. New Jersey Office of the Attorney General. Landmark settlement reached with medical device maker Synthes. Available from http://www .nj.gov/oag/newsreleases09/pr20090505a.html. Accessed September 13, 2009.

29. FDA hearing to determine arthritis drugs' safety. Available from http://today.uchc.edu /headlines/2005/feb05/arthritisdrug.html. Accessed September 12, 2009.

30. Bodenheimer T. Uneasy alliance: clinical investigators and the pharmaceutical industry. *N Engl J Med.* 2000;342:1516–1544.

31. Singer N. Ghosts in the journals. *New York Times.* August 18, 2009:B1–B2. Available from http://www.nytimes.com/2009/08/19/health /research/19ethics.html?_r=1&scp=1&sq=Ghosts %20in%20the%20Journals&st=cse. Accessed September 12, 2009.

32. Human Genome Project information: medicine and the new genetics. Available from http://www .ornl.gov/sci/techresources/Human_Genome /medicine/medicine.shtml. Accessed September 13, 2009.

33. Bren L. Battle of the bugs: fighting antibiotic resistance. Available from http://www.rxlist.com /script/main/art.asp?articlekey=85705. Accessed September 13, 2009.

34. Klevens MR, Edwards JR, Richards C, et al. Estimating health-care associated infections and deaths in U.S. hospitals, 2002. Available from http://www.cdc.gov/ncidod/dhqp/pdf /hicpac/infections_deaths.pdf. Accessed September 13, 2009.

35. Ibrahim MA. *Epidemiology and Health Policy.* Gaithersburg, MD: Aspen; 1985.

CHAPTER 20

Evidence-Based Practice in Health Care

Janet Houser

CHAPTER OBJECTIVES

1. Discuss the importance of evidence-based practice for organizations and advanced practice nurses.

2. Define evidence-based practice.

3. Identify barriers to using evidence in clinical practice.

4. Recognize strategies for implementing evidence-based practice.

5. Foster the use of evidence to meet Magnet standards.

INTRODUCTION

It would seem a foregone conclusion that effective clinical practice is based on the best possible, rigorously tested evidence. The public assumes it, patients expect it, and practitioners profess to value it. Yet it is only in the past two decades that an emphasis on evidence as a basis for practice reached the forefront of health care.

While it may be surprising that assurances of the scientific basis for healthcare practice have been this long in coming, there are many reasons why evidence-based practice (EBP) is a relatively recent effort.

The past decade has seen unprecedented advances in information technology, making research and other types of evidence widely available to healthcare practitioners. Whereas a clinician practicing in the 1980s may have read one or two professional journals a month and attended perhaps one clinical conference in a year, contemporary healthcare professionals have access to a virtually unlimited bank of professional journal articles and other sources of research evidence via the Internet. Technology has supported the rapid communication of best practice and afforded consumers open access to healthcare informa-tion as well. As a result, evidence-based practice is quickly becoming the norm for effective clin-ical practice.

WHAT IS EVIDENCE-BASED PRACTICE?

Evidence-based practice is the use of the best scien-tific evidence integrated with clinical experience and incorporating patient values and prefer-ences, in the practice of professional patient care. All three elements are important. An analogy may be made to a three-legged stool, as depicted in **Figure 20-1**. The triad of rigorous evidence, clinical experience, and patient preferences must be balanced to achieve clinical practices that are both scientifically sound and acceptable to the individuals applying and benefiting from them.

While healthcare practitioners have long used research as a basis for practice, a system-atic approach to the translation of research into practice has been introduced relatively re-cently. The first documented use of the term "evidence-based practice" was less than 2 decades ago. A clinical epidemiologist used the term in a text to describe the way students in medical school should be taught to develop an attitude of "enlightened skepticism" toward the routine application of diagnostic technologies and clinical interventions (Sackett, 1991). The authors described how effective practitioners rigorously review published studies to inform clinical decisions. The goal stated in this publi-cation was an *awareness* of the evidence upon which professional practice is based and a criti-cal *appraisal* of the soundness of that evidence.

The term entered the American literature on a broader stage in 1993, when an article in the *Journal of the American Medical Association* de-scribed the need for an established scientific basis for healthcare decisions (Oxman, 1993). The authors of the article noted that the goal of evidence-based practice is to help practitioners translate the results of research into clinical prac-tice. They emphasized that the scientific practice of health care required sifting through and ap-praising evidence to make appropriate decisions.

Even with the relatively recent birth of the term, evidence-based practice has rapidly be-come an international standard for all health-care practitioners. Using the best scientific evidence as a basis for clinical practice makes in-tuitive sense and joins other science-based pro-fessions in using evidence as a foundation for decision making.

WHAT EVIDENCE-BASED PRACTICE IS NOT

A wide range of activities contribute to evidence-based practice. Many of these activities—review-ing research, consulting expert colleagues, con-sidering patient preferences—are common in clinical practice. However, there are many activi-ties that are *not* considered evidence-based prac-tice, but rather other forms of decision making used to solve problems.

| FIGURE 20-1 | Triad of Evidence-Based Practice |

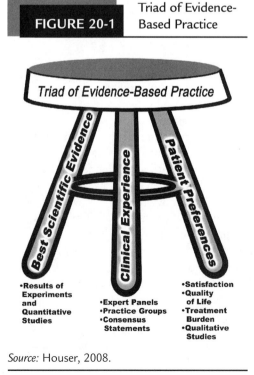

Source: Houser, 2008.

BOX 20-1	Voices from the Field

I was working as the clinical nurse specialist of a busy surgical intensive care unit (ICU) when we received a critically ill patient. He was fresh from cardiac surgery and quite unstable; he needed multiple drugs and an intra-aortic balloon pump just to maintain his perfusion status. He was so sick that we were not able to place him on a special bed for pressure relief. For the first 24 hours, we were so busy trying to keep him alive that we did not even get a chance to turn him.

About 36 hours into his ICU admission, he was stable enough to place on a low-air-loss mattress for pressure ulcer prevention. When we were finally able to turn him, we noted he had a small stage II pressure ulcer on his coccyx. Despite the treatments that we used, the pressure ulcer evolved into a full-thickness wound. He recovered from his cardiac surgical procedure, but unfortunately required surgeries and skin grafts to close the pressure ulcer wound.

The experience I had with this patient prompted me to review the evidence-based practice guidelines we had in place to prevent pressure ulcers in critically ill patients. I wanted to make sure we could prevent this from happening again, but I had a lot of questions. Could we preventively place high-risk patients on low-air-loss mattresses while they were still in the perioperative service? Did we even know the patients who were at risk for pressure ulcers? Which assessment tools did nurses use to assess the patient's risk? When a high-risk patient was identified, which interventions did the nurses use to prevent pressure ulcers? How were the ulcers treated once they appeared?

I was fortunate that my Chief Nursing Officer (CNO) was a strong advocate for evidence-based practice, and she encouraged me to initiate an EBP review of pressure ulcer prevention and treatment. Specifically, I wanted to find out which nursing interventions were supported by research evidence when we were trying to prevent pressure ulcers in the surgical ICU. So I contacted other inpatient units at the hospital to determine what they were doing.

I discovered that the surgical ICU was not different from the other inpatient units. There *was* no standard, evidence-based nursing practice for pressure ulcer prevention. Units were not consistently using the same skin assessment tools, so it was hard to objectively communicate risk from one unit to another. The tools we were using were not necessarily based on research. It was clear that we needed to identify the best available evidence and devise a protocol.

We started by establishing an evidence-based skin care council for the hospital. The team consisted of bedside nurses from all inpatient units and the perioperative service. Initially the council reviewed current nursing skin assessment forms, and we conducted a review of the literature on pressure ulcer prevention and interventions. We discovered the Association for Healthcare Research and Quality (AHRQ) guidelines on pressure ulcer prevention and treatment, a key source of evidence for healthcare practices.

Over the course of the next year, we revised our nursing policy and procedure, incorporating the AHRQ evidence into a treatment guideline. The guideline included a procedure for skin assessment and nursing documentation, and pressure ulcer assessment and treatment decision algorithms. We reviewed skin care products and narrowed down the products to those that were supported by evidence. One

| BOX 20-1 | Voices from the Field *(continued)* |

algorithm helped staff make selections be-tween products that maximized prevention and treatment. Another algorithm guided nurses in the use of therapeutic surfaces (e.g., low-air-loss mattresses) to prevent pressure ul-cers. To monitor our progress, we began quar-terly pressure ulcer prevalence studies. As part of the implementation, we scheduled a skin care seminar featuring a national expert on skin care.

At the beginning of our EBP skin care journey, our pressure ulcer prevalence was 9%.

Since implementing our EBP skin care ini-tiatives, our pressure ulcer prevalence has dropped to 3-5%. The EBP skin care council continues to be active in our hospital. We meet monthly and continue to seek out the best evidence to guide all skin and wound care product decisions, practice guidelines, pro-tocols, and policies. My initial search for a so-lution—based on my experience with one patient—led to improvements in practice that have benefited many patients since then.

—Mary Beth Makic, PhD, RN

Evidence-Based Practice Is Not Clinical Problem Solving

While evidence-based practice is a mechanism for solving clinical problems and making deci-sions about interventions, it is distinct from traditional problem-solving approaches in health care. Conventional decision making about clinical practices relied on expert opin-ion—sometimes achieved by consensus, but rarely through experimentation—combined with "standard practice." Evidence-based prac-tice is a systematic process of reviewing the best available research evidence and then incorpo-rating clinical experience and patient prefer-ences into the mix.

Evidence-Based Practice Is Not Solely Randomized Controlled Trials

Evidence-based practice does not mean choos-ing only those interventions supported by ran-domized controlled trials—although these studies are clearly important in providing guid-ance for effective practices. A somewhat tongue-in-cheek article by Smith and Pell (2006) suggested that we did not need a randomized trial to inform practitioners of the importance

of a parachute as a measure of preventing death when jumping from an airplane (and, in fact, noted the difficulty in recruiting a control group for such a trial!). Evidence-based practice does not rely solely on one type of evidence, but rather is founded on a hierarchy of evidence, with individual studies rated from "strongest" to "weakest" based on the type of design and quality of execution. Evidence can come from many different types of studies in addition to randomized trials.

Evidence-Based Practice Is Not "Cookbook Medicine"

Guidelines based on the best available evidence do not mean that the practitioner has an edict to practice in a single way. In fact, evidence alone is never sufficient to make a specific clinical deci-sion about a specific patient. The clinician needs evidence *plus* good judgment, clinical skill, and knowledge of the patient's unique needs to apply evidence to a specific patient care situa-tion. The definition of evidence-based practice, in fact, holds evidence as only one element of the triad of decision making. Clinical judgment and patient values must be considered when apply-ing the evidence to a single situation.

BOX 20-2	Sacred Cows and Evidence Eagles

Sacred Cow: Cover gowns and shoe covers prevent infections in patients undergoing surgery and other invasive procedures such as bone marrow transplants.

Evidence Eagle: Cover gowns and **shoe covers** worn by caregivers provided no benefit in reducing complications of surgery, including surgical site infections. Outcomes of bone marrow transplants were unaffected by staff wearing cover gowns and shoe covers.

BOX 20-3	Sacred Cows and Evidence Eagles

Sacred Cow: There are more incidents of bleeding, psychiatric illness, and trauma during the full moon.

Evidence Eagle: While the day of the week influences emergency department admission volumes, the phases of the moon have no relationship with the rate of any clinical conditions or traumatic events.

Evidence Is Not the Same as Theory

Theoretical effects must be tested and retested to be determined effective. As late as the early 20th century, physicians still believed that bloodletting was an effective treatment for a host of disorders. This belief was based on the empirical observation that a patient's pulse rate slowed when they were bled and the *theory* that a slower pulse reduced irritation and inflammation. While the empirical observations were accurate—the patient's pulse would slow, indeed, but due to ensuing hypovolemic shock—the theoretical relationship to a therapeutic response was ill founded. Many contemporary healthcare interventions are, unfortunately, based on similar theoretical relationships that have been untested for years. Recent research has refuted many of these theoretical assumptions, including the protective value of hormone replacement therapy, the use of rubbing alcohol to prevent infection in a neonate's umbilical cord, and the use of heat to treat inflammation, among many others.

Evidence-Based Practice Is Not Just Evidence-Based Medicine

The nature and processes of research are likely to be unique for any given profession. Medicine relies on science that is primarily concerned with the cause of disease and effects of treatment. The evidence for medical care, by necessity, focuses on scientific studies that verify and quantify these effects. Medical evidence has been criticized, though, for its sometimes artificial nature. It is a research paradox that the more an experiment is controlled, the less applicability the results will have in the real world. Randomized controlled trials, then, may provide the most rigorous scientific evidence, but that evidence may not apply well to individual patients with a broad range of physical, psychological, and behavioral conditions.

Patient care, in contrast, requires a holistic approach to the care of individuals with physical, psychosocial, and/or spiritual needs. This care is founded on the provider–patient relationship and an appreciation of the patient's unique needs. The evidence for health care, then, will require a broad range of methodologies as a basis for care. This is not to imply that these sources of evidence are not subjected to healthy skepticism and systematic inquiry, but rather that a broad range of evidence is considered as a basis for practice.

THE IMPORTANCE OF EVIDENCE-BASED PRACTICE

Evidence-based practice is important to the healthcare professional for many reasons. At the top of this list is the contribution of evidence to the effective care of patients. Studies have supported the conclusion that patient outcomes are substantially improved when health care is based on evidence from well-designed studies versus tradition or clinical expertise alone. Leufer and Cleary-Holdforth (2009) aggregated outcomes studies related to evidence-based practice changes. A wide range of effects was found in multiple specialties, including orthopedic, cardiovascular, respiratory, and obstetrical outcomes. Evidence-based practices in obstetrics and neonatal care reduced morbidity and mortality, sometimes dramatically. The use of corticosteroids in premature labor, for example, reduced the risk of premature infant death by 20%. A seminal meta-analysis by Heater (1988) demonstrated the impact of evidence-based practices on a range of behavioral, physiological, and psychosocial aspects of patient well-being. The linkage between evidence-based interventions and outcomes is an important one, and determining the scientific support for a practice prior to its implementation makes intuitive sense.

While quantitative studies of cause and effect are limited, there are indications that evidence as a basis for process improvement and leadership practices may benefit the organization as well as its patients (Stetler, 2007). Changes in attitudes, knowledge, and skills related to evidence-based

practices have been demonstrated through testing educational interventions (Varnell, 2008). Evidence-based practice may soon become the norm for both the way care is delivered and the way organizations operate.

Healthcare providers operate in an era of accountability where quality issues, patient safety, and cost concerns are primary drivers of patient care processes. Using evidence to guide practice streamlines patient care (Newhouse, 2007). Practices that are unnecessary are eliminated; ineffective practices are replaced with practices that result in desired outcomes.

Existing practices may even be unintentionally harming patients (as was found in the hormone replacement studies) and so it is ethically unjustified to continue using untested interventions. Evidence can help healthcare professionals avoid making errors in decision making relative to patient care. Using research decreases the need for trial-and-error, which is time-consuming and may be counterproductive. In any case, time is not spent on practices that may be ineffective or unnecessarily time intensive.

Consumers are well informed about their options for personal health care and often resist the traditional, paternalistic approach to health interventions. The public expects that care will be based on scientific evidence, and believes that care processes should routinely lead to high-quality outcomes that are physically and mentally desirable (Aarons, 2009). Healthcare professionals must be able to respond to their patient's questions about the scientific merit of interventions and about the relative benefit of treatment options.

Evidence might come in the form of journal articles, policies, guidelines, professional consensus statements, and standards of practice as well as formalized research. While evidence-based practice implies scientific evidence, the words "relevant" and "rigorous" might be better adjectives to describe the kind of evidence needed by healthcare professionals. Critical skills include the ability to judge both the *type of evidence* that is needed and the *value of that evidence*.

BOX 20-4	Sacred Cows and Evidence Eagles

Sacred Cow: Hydrogen peroxide is an effective antibacterial cleaning agent when applied to wounds. Bubbling of hydrogen peroxide means bacteria are present.

Evidence Eagle: Concentrated **hydrogen peroxide** is caustic and exposure may result in local tissue damage, and can hinder neodermal development, which is necessary for wound healing. The bubbling occurs when hydrogen peroxide is exposed to air, not bacteria.

BOX 20-5	Sacred Cows and Evidence Eagles

Sacred Cow: Neonates and infants should be placed in the prone position during sleep periods to prevent aspiration.

Evidence Eagle: Sleeping in the prone position among blankets and pillows has been discovered to be a primary cause of sudden infant death syndrome through suffocation. Neonates and infants should be placed on their backs with minimal contact with pillows, stuffed animals, or blankets. Warm sleepwear is sufficient to prevent hypothermia.

Healthcare practitioners do not practice in professional isolation, but rather explore what works and does not work using empirical methods. An increased emphasis on evidence-based practice can be viewed as a response to these broader forces in the context of healthcare delivery and a logical progression toward the utilization of research as a basis for patient care decisions.

HOW CAN EVIDENCE BE USED IN HEALTH CARE?

At its best, evidence provides the basis for effective, efficient patient care practices. At a minimum, an evidence-based approach can enhance practice by encouraging reflection on what we know about virtually every aspect of daily patient care. The EBP process need not be onerous and basically includes five elements: (1) formulating an appropriate question, (2) performing an efficient literature search, (3) critically appraising the best available evidence, (4) applying the best evidence to clinical practice, and (5) assessing outcomes of care (Noteboom, 2008). The original question can come from a variety of sources in a healthcare setting and, likewise, there is a wide range of organizational processes for which evidence can improve outcomes.

Evidence can be used as a basis for healthcare processes. Evidence can be incorporated into virtually every phase of the healthcare process. Evidence exists for best practices in the following areas:

- Assessment of patient conditions
- Diagnosis of patient problems
- Planning patient care
- Interventions to improve the patient's function, condition, or to prevent complications
- Evaluation of patient responses to interventions

Evidence can be used as the basis for policies and procedures. While healthcare professionals from different educational programs, backgrounds, and experience may have different ways of delivering patient care, few can argue with the need for best practices. Evidence-based practice provides the foundation for policies and procedures that are tested and found effective (Oman, 2008), as opposed to "the way we've always done it."

Evidence can be used as the basis for patient care management tools. The evidence that is revealed through systematic review of research and other sources of evidence provides an excellent basis for patient care management tools such as care maps, critical paths, protocols, and standard order sets. One of the benefits of patient care management tools is the reduction of variability in practices, and evidence serves as a rational basis for standardized practices.

Evidence can be used as a basis for care of the individual. The complexity of patients who need care in the healthcare system can make the clinician wonder if evidence can ever be applied to an individual patient. It is easy to consider the question, "Is my patient so different from those in the research that results will not help me make a treatment decision?" This question, more than any other, may stand in the way of applying evidence to individual patient care situations. In fact, one study found that the more familiar a patient was to a practitioner, the *less likely* the clinician was to use evidence as a basis for care (Summerskill, 2002).

BOX 20-6	Sacred Cows and Evidence Eagles

Sacred Cow: Oral care is a secondary consideration in patients on ventilators; maintaining a clear airway is the primary preventive method for ventilator-associated pneumonia.

Evidence Eagle: Simple oral care with toothbrush and paste or other means of cleaning the teeth and oral cavity are one of the most effective and primary strategies for reducing the rate of ventilator-associated pneumonia.

As practitioners, we must ask if these assumptions about the uniqueness of patients are in their best interest when it comes to clinical care. Uncertainty is inherent in the healthcare process; evidence helps to quantify that uncertainty. Concern for the uniqueness of the individual patient is not a reason to ignore the evidence, but rather to learn to critically apply it appropriately. Evidence is not intended to be rigid, but rather—as our definition makes explicit—is *integrated* with clinical experience and the patient's unique values to arrive at optimal outcomes.

Evidence in clinical practice is not solely limited to patient care, however. Healthcare professionals might be interested in evidence as it relates to team functioning, the best way to communicate change, organizational models for research utilization, or even the effects of insurance on healthcare usage. Evidence in health care abounds on a variety of topics, and research utilization can improve patient care in a multitude of ways.

Using evidence as a basis for a broad range of clinical practice problems would seem logical. However, there are a variety of reasons that evidence-based practice is yet to be the standard, which is not surprising given the complexity of healthcare delivery.

STRATEGIES FOR IMPLEMENTING EVIDENCE-BASED PRACTICE

Considering the benefits of basing clinical practice on evidence, it would make sense that evidence-based practice be the norm. Unfortunately, this is not the case. There are many reasons why evidence-based practices are the exception rather than the rule. Some of these are limitations created by EBP systems themselves. Some barriers are related to human factors, and still others are related to the organizations within which patient care is delivered. **Table 20-1** lists some of the common barriers to using evidence as a basis for practice.

Organizations do not commonly have systems in place to support clinicians in the development of EBP tools. While there has been a surge in the resources available for practitioners who want to participate in the development of practice guidelines, there has been little in the way of operational models to guide healthcare organizations that want to implement pervasive evidence-based practice (Salbach, 2007).

The complexities of changing practice based on evidence are daunting indeed. Pagogo et al. (2007) studied the barriers and facilitators of evidence-based practice as perceived by healthcare professionals. Seven themes were used to describe both barriers and facilitators:

1. Training and educational support
2. Attitudes toward EBP and research
3. Consumer demand for evidence-based care
4. Logistical and organizational considerations
5. Institutional and leadership support
6. Policies and procedures
7. Access to appropriate evidence

STRATEGIES FOR OVERCOMING BARRIERS

While little can be done to reduce the complexity of contemporary clinical care, some strategies can be applied to improve the rate at which

TABLE 20-1	Barriers to Using Evidence in Clinical Practice
Barrier	**Causes**
Limitations in evidence-based practice systems	Overwhelming amount of information in the literature
	Sometimes contradictory findings in the research
Human factors that create barriers	Lack of knowledge about evidence-based practice
	Lack of skill in finding and/or appraising research studies
	Negative attitudes about research and evidence-based care
	Perception that research is "cookbook medicine"
	Perception that research is only for medicine
	Patient expectations (e.g., demanding antibiotics)
Organizational factors that create barriers	Lack of authority for clinicians to make changes in practice
	Peer emphasis on status quo practice because "we've always done it this way"
	Demanding workloads with no time for research activities
	Conflict in priorities between unit work and research
	Lack of administrative support or incentives

healthcare professionals utilize research as a basis for their practice.

Begin the process by specifically *identifying the facilitators and barriers of EBP practices*. Use of a self-assessment such as that tested by Gale (2009) can help identify organizational strengths and limitations in preparation for an EBP effort.

Education and training can improve knowledge and strengthen practitioners' beliefs about the benefits of EBP (Varnell, 2008). Clinicians may fear that they will appear to lack competence, and knowledge will give them confidence in determining an evidence base for their practice.

One of the most helpful—and difficult—strategies is to *create an environment that encourages an inquisitive approach* about clinical care. The first step in identifying opportunities for best practices is questioning current practice. This can be accomplished by creating a culture in which EBP is valued, supported, and expected.

BOX 20-7	Sacred Cows and Evidence Eagles

Sacred Cow: Women in labor have traditionally been directed to push immediately at 10-cm cervical dilation, which is thought to shorten the second stage of labor, thereby resulting in better outcomes for the neonate.

Evidence Eagle: Passive descent (encouraging mothers to push only when they feel the need) increases the chance that a mother will have a spontaneous vaginal birth, decreases the risk of having instrument-assisted birth procedures, and reduces the amount of time women need to push before the baby is born. By comparison, women who were directed to push at 10 cm had increased rates of fetal oxygen desaturation.

Despite the barriers inherent in implementing evidence-based practice in clinical practice, it is imperative that structures and processes are created that reduce these obstacles. Regardless of the system within which the clinician practices, there is a systematic approach to finding and documenting the best possible evidence for practice. This process involves defining a clinical question, identifying and appraising the best possible evidence, and drawing conclusions about best practice.

EVIDENCE-BASED PRACTICE AND PROFESSIONAL PRACTICE

Assuming all other issues regarding EBP are equal, a final case for practice based on research is that this characteristic typifies a *profession* more than any other. Professions, by definition, require advanced educational preparation, self-regulation, and practice based on a broad body of knowledge. Given that advanced education is being required of every healthcare professional—many now at the practice doctorate level—research-based practice is also imperative to fulfill our obligations as a profession.

This level of professional practice is required for successful achievement of Magnet Recognition, awarded by the American Nurses' Credentialing Center for demonstrating excellence in nursing services. The New Knowledge and Innovation Component makes explicit the expectation that practice is based on high-quality evidence. A summary of the standards related to evidence-based practice appears in **Table 20-2**.

Fundamentally, "to achieve Magnet status, the Chief Nurse Executive needs to create, foster and sustain a practice environment where nursing research and evidence-based practice is integrated into both the delivery of nursing care and the framework for nursing administration decision making" (Turkel, 2005, p. 254). This statement implies that evidence is used in the organization to support a range of professional activities—including direct patient care, staff development, and management. When Magnet candidates are evaluated, reviewers are looking for signs that evidence has been integrated into all areas of professional practice. Some questions asked might be, "When you have a clinical question, how do you resolve it?" and "How has research informed your staff development content and process?"

For nurses to value and recognize the relevance and importance of EBP, they need ongoing, concrete support. Systems for finding, prioritizing, and answering evidence-based practice should be in place with formalized structures and processes. Sufficient resources must be applied to assure success. Magnet standards will lead reviewers to ask, "Are staff members paid for their work on EBP?" and "Do staff members have access to search engines and databases?" Active participation of staff clinicians in identifying areas of concern and finding ways to address them is also critical to meeting Magnet standards. This is the most challenging part of developing integrated EBP systems. A guiding model can help here. One model that demonstrates the integration of evidence-based practice as part of the Magnet recognition process is depicted in **Figure 20-2**. Turkel et al. (2005) laid out the five steps of integrating EBP into daily practice:

Step 1: Establish a foundation for EBP.
Step 2: Identify areas of concern.
Step 3: Create internal expertise.
Step 4: Implement evidence-based practice.
Step 5: Contribute to research evidence.

BOX 20-8   Sacred Cows and Evidence Eagles

Sacred Cow: Inflammatory muscle injuries should be treated in the first 24 hours with ice, and subsequently with heat.

Evidence Eagle: For pure muscle injury, heat increases inflammation. Ice application according to usual protocols reduces inflammation and pain associated with muscle injury throughout the first few days.

Requiring the integration of evidence into practice has increased the amount of research generated in practice settings. Closson (2005) found clear differences in virtually all indices of evidence-based practice in Magnet facilities when compared to non-Magnet facilities. Collaboration with academic researchers, established mechanisms for research study review, use of

TABLE 20-2	Summary of Magnet Standards Relevant to EBP
Standard	Description *Describe and Demonstrate:*
New Knowledge (NK) 1	That nurses at all levels evaluate and use published research findings in their practice.
NK 2	Consistent membership and involvement of a nurse in the institutional review board or other governing body responsible for the protection of human subjects in research; nurse has vote on nursing related protocols.
NK 3	That direct-care nurses support the human rights of participants in research protocols.
NK 4	The structure(s) and process(es) the organization uses to develop, expand, and/or advance nursing research.
NK 4 Empirical Outcomes (EO)	Nursing research studies in the past 2 years, ongoing or completed, generated from the structure(s) and process(es) in NK 4. Provide a table, including: study title; study status; principal investigator name(s) and credentials; role of nurses in study; study scope; study type. Select one completed research study and respond to the four criteria listed in the EO guidelines: 1. Describe the purpose and background. 2. Describe how the work was done. 3. Discuss who was involved and what units participated. 4. Describe the measurement used to evaluate the outcomes and the impact.
NK 5	How the organization disseminates knowledge generated through nursing research to internal and external audiences.
NK 6	The structure(s) and process(es) used to evaluate nursing practice based on evidence.
NK 7	The structure(s) and process(es) used to translate new knowledge into nursing practice.
NK 7 EO	How translation of new knowledge into nursing practice has affected patient outcomes

Source: © 2009 American Nurses Credentialing Center. All rights reserved. Modified and reproduced with the permission of the American Nurses Credentialing Center. Tierney, L. M., McPhee, S. J., & Papadakis, M. A. (2009). *Current medical diagnosis and treatment* (42nd ed., pp. 1647–1649). New York: McGraw-Hill.

| FIGURE 20-2 | Integration of EBP and Magnet Standards |

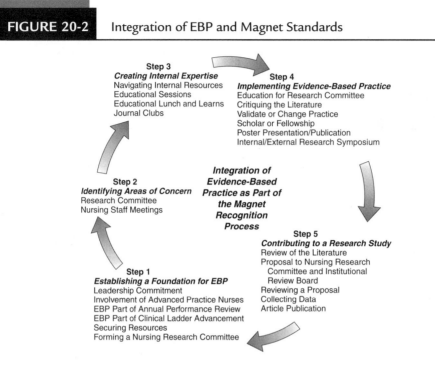

Step 3
Creating Internal Expertise
Navigating Internal Resources
Educational Sessions
Educational Lunch and Learns
Journal Clubs

Step 4
Implementing Evidence-Based Practice
Education for Research Committee
Critiquing the Literature
Validate or Change Practice
Scholar or Fellowship
Poster Presentation/Publication
Internal/External Research Symposium

Step 2
Identifying Areas of Concern
Research Committee
Nursing Staff Meetings

Integration of Evidence-Based Practice as Part of the Magnet Recognition Process

Step 5
Contributing to a Research Study
Review of the Literature
Proposal to Nursing Research
   Committee and Institutional
   Review Board
Reviewing a Proposal
Collecting Data
Article Publication

Step 1
Establishing a Foundation for EBP
Leadership Commitment
Involvement of Advanced Practice Nurses
EBP Part of Annual Performance Review
EBP Part of Clinical Ladder Advancement
Securing Resources
Forming a Nursing Research Committee

Source: Reprinted with permission from Turkel, M., Reidinger, G., Ferket, K., & Reno, K. (2005). An essential component of the Magnet journey: Fostering an environment for evidence-based practice and nursing research. *Nursing Administration Quarterly,* 29(3), 254–262.

| BOX 20-9 | Sacred Cows and Evidence Eagles |

Sacred Cow: Instilling 5 to 10 mL of normal saline before endotracheal suctioning improves oxygenation and removal of secretions by thinning them and stimulating coughing to move secretions out of the lungs.

Evidence Eagle: Oxygen saturation is significantly lower with instillation of saline than with no instillation of saline. When saline was used, returns to baseline oxygenation levels did not occur until 3 to 5 minutes after finishing the suctioning procedure.

findings in practice, resources, and cultural promotion of EBP were all stronger in Magnet than in non-Magnet settings.

This same study also found that no single approach, structure, or system was associated with success. No standard formula can be used to integrate EBP into a professional organization; indeed, there is little agreement on what exactly constitutes an EBP initiative. The processes and systems must mesh with those of the organization, and each will be unique. That said, there are some questions that can be expected of Magnet surveyors, and thoughtful reflection can help an organization's leader determine how they have designed systems to address the issues.

SUMMARY

Evidence-based practice has clear advantages for the contemporary healthcare organization. While there remain many barriers to full implementation of EBP, organizations are finding creative ways to overcome them. The result is a more collaborative, open approach to judging evidence, which values scientific outcomes as well as clinical expertise and patient preferences. Basing evidence on a scientific body of knowledge is critical for the healthcare professions; integrating evidence into daily work is the challenge to be met.

DISCUSSION QUESTIONS

1. After reading the examples of clinical problems In the "Sacred Cows and Evidence Eagles" features, ask a clinical question relevant to your practice and explore the evidence to support an intervention for the problem.

2. What are the barriers that inhibit your use of evidence in the clinical setting? Which strategies might you employ to overcome these barriers?

3. In your clinical practice, which mechanisms are already in place to promote the use of evidence and research?

REFERENCES

Aarons, G., Wells, R., Zagursky, K., Fettes, D., & Palinkas, L. (2009). Implementing evidence-based practice in community mental health agencies: a multiple stakeholder analysis. *American Journal of Public Health, 99*(11), 2087–2095.

Closson, D. (2005). Research activities in Magnet and non-Magnet hospitals. *The 29th Annual MNRS Research Conference,* Session #1211, Scientific Inquiry.

Gale, B., & Schaffer, M. (2009). Organizational readiness for evidence-based practice. *Journal of Nursing Administration, 39*(2), 91–97.

Heater, B. S., Becker, A. M., & Olson, R. K. (1988). Nursing interventions and patient outcomes: A meta-analysis of studies. *Nursing Research, 37*(5), 303–307.

Leufer, T., & Cleary-Holdforth, J. (2009). Evidence-based practice: Improving patient outcomes. *Nursing Standard, 23*(32), 35–39.

Newhouse, R. (2007). Creating infrastructure supportive of evidence-based nursing practice: Leadership strategies. *Worldviews on Evidence-Based Nursing, 4*(1), 21–29.

Noteboom, J., Allison, S., Cleland, J., & Whitman, J. (2008). A primer on selected aspects of evidence-based practice to questions of treatment, Part 2: Interpreting results, application to clinical practice, and self-evaluation. *Journal of Orthopaedic and Sports Physical Therapy, 38*(8), 485–501.

Oman, K. S., Duran, C., & Fink, R. (2008). Evidence-based policy and procedures: An algorithm for success. *Journal of Nursing Administration, 38*(1), 47–51.

Oxman, A., Sackett, D., & Guyatt, G. (1993). Users' guides to the medical literature: I. How to get started. *Journal of the American Medical Association, 270,* 2093–2095.

Pagoto, S., Spring, B., Coups, E., Mulvaney, S., Coutu, M., & Ozakinci, G. (2007). Barriers and facilitators of evidence-based practice perceived by behavioral science health professionals. *Journal of Clinical Psychology, 63*(7), 695–705.

Sackett, D., Haynes, R., Guyatt, G., & Tugwell, P. (1991). *Clinical epidemiology: A basic science for clinical medicine* (2nd ed.). Boston/Toronto/London: Little, Brown.

Salbach, N., Jaglal, S., Korner-Bitensky, N., Rappolt, S., & Davis, D. (2007). Practitioner and organizational barriers to evidence-based practice of physical therapists for people with stroke. *Physical Therapy, 87*(1), 1284–1303.

Smith, G., & Pell, J. (2006). Parachute use to prevent death and major trauma related to gravitational challenge: Systematic review of randomized controlled trials. *International Journal of Prosthodontics, 19*(2), 126–128.

Stetler, C., & Caramanica, L. (2007). Evaluation of an evidence-based practice initiative: Outcomes, strengths and limitations of a retrospective, conceptually-based approach. *Worldviews on Evidence-Based Nursing, 4*(4), 187–199.

Summerskill, W., & Pope, C. (2002). An exploratory qualitative study of the barriers to secondary prevention in the management of coronary heart disease. *Family Practitioner, 19,* 605–610.

Turkel, M., Reidinger, G., Ferket, K., & Reno, K. (2005). An essential component of the Magnet journey: Fostering an environment for evidence-based practice and nursing research. *Nursing Administration Quarterly, 29*(3), 254–262.

Varnell, G., Haas, B., Duke, G., & Hudson, K. (2008). Effect of an educational intervention on attitudes toward and implementation of evidence-based practice. *Worldviews on Evidence-Based Nursing, 5*(4), 172–181.

Youngblut, J., & Brooten, D. (2001). Evidence-based nursing practice: Why is it important? *AACN Clinical Issues, 12*(4), 468–476.

REFERENCES FOR SACRED COWS AND EVIDENCE EAGLES

Shoe and Gown Covers

Duquette-Petersen, L., Francis, M., Dohnalek, L., Skinner, R., & Dudas, P. (1999). The role of protective clothing in infection prevention in patients undergoing autologous bone marrow transplantation. *Oncology Nursing Forum, 26*(8), 1319–1324.

Mayhall, C. (2004). *Hospital epidemiology and infection control* (3rd ed.). Lippincott Williams & Wilkins: Philadelphia, PA.

Effects of the Full Moon

Alves, D. W., Allegra, J. R., Cochrane, D. G., & Cable, G. (2003). Effect of lunar cycle on temporal variation in cardiopulmonary arrest in seven emergency departments during 11 years. *European Journal of Emergency Medicine: Official Journal of the European Society for Emergency Medicine, 10*(3), 225–289.

McLay, R. N., Daylo, A. A., & Hammer, P. S. (2006). No effect of lunar cycle on psychiatric admissions or emergency evaluations. *Military Medicine, 171*(12), 1239–1242.

Román, E. M., Soriano, G., Fuentes, M., Gálvez, M. L., & Fernández, C. (2004). The influence of the full moon on the number of admissions related to gastrointestinal bleeding. *International Journal of Nursing Practice, 10*(6), 292–296.

Zargar, M., Khaji, A., Kaviani, A., Karbakhsh, M., Yunesian, M., & Abdollahi, M. (2004). The full moon and admission to emergency rooms. *Indian Journal of Medical Sciences, 58*(5), 191–195.

Hydrogen Peroxide

Bennett, L., Rosenblum, R., Perlov, C., Davidson, J., Barton, R., & Nanney, B. (2001). An in vivo comparison of topical agents on wound repair. *Plastic and Reconstructive Surgery, 108*(3), 675–687.

Watt, B., Proudfoot, A., & Vale, J. (2004). Hydrogen peroxide poisoning. *Toxicological Reviews, 23*(1), 51–57.

Infants in the Prone Position

American Academy of Pediatrics. (2006). Guidelines for healthy sleep of infants. Retrieved November 2009 from http://www.aap.org/healthtopics/Sleep.cfm.

Oral Care for Ventilator Patients

Coffin, S., et al. (2008). Strategies to prevent ventilator-associated pneumonia in acute care hospitals. *Infection Control and Hospital Epidemiology, 29* (Suppl 1), S31–S40.

Pushing During the Second Stage of Labor

Brancato, R., Church, S., & Stone, P. (2008). A meta-analysis of passive descent versus immediate pushing in nulliparous women with epidural analgesia in the second stage of labor. *JOGNN: The Journal of Obstetrical, Gynecological, and Neonatal Nursing, 37*(1), 4–12.

Simpson, K., & James, D. (2005). Effects of immediate versus delayed pushing during second-stage labor on fetal well-being: A randomized clinical trial. *Nursing Research, 54*(3), 149–157.

Use of Heat for Muscle Injury

Jayaraman, R., et al. (2004). MRI evaluation of topical heat and static stretching as therapeutic modalities for the treatment of eccentric exercise-induced muscle damage. *European Journal of Applied Physiology, 93*(1–2), 30–38.

Instillation of Normal Saline when Suctioning

Rauen, C., Chulay, M., Bridges, E., Vollman, K., & Arbour, R. (2008). Seven evidence-based practice habits: Putting some sacred cows out to pasture. *Critical Care Nurse, 28*(2), 98–102, 104–110, 112–118.

Clinical Scholarship and Evidence-Based Practice

Catherine Tymkow

CHAPTER OBJECTIVES

1. Differentiate between the concepts of clinical scholarship and evidence-based practice.
2. Analyze the hierarchy for evaluating evidence in clinical practice.
3. Identify the different types of research evidence.
4. Explore the steps in the research process.
5. Review methods for critical appraisal of clinical practice guidelines.
6. Discuss approaches for disseminating findings from evidence-based practice.

True scholarship consists in knowing not what things exist,
but what they mean; it is not memory but judgment.
—*James Russell Lowell*

INTRODUCTION

Any discussion of scholarship and evidence-based practice and the doctor of nursing practice (DNP) role must first begin with some essential questions. These include questions as basic as the following: What is scholarship? Are evidence-based practice and clinical scholarship the same thing? How does clinical scholarship differ from the traditional definition of scholarship? Why do we need nursing scholars in practice settings? What is the role of the DNP in clinical scholarship? What are the knowledge resources, tools, and methods necessary to implement and support clinical scholarship and evidence-based practice?

These questions are important ones to consider as healthcare organizations and schools of nursing redefine and expand nurses' roles. If nursing is to maintain a full partnership with medicine in the delivery of health care, the education of nurse leaders and nurses in advanced practice roles must be at a comparable level with other doctorally prepared healthcare practitioners such as MDs, PharmDs, and PsyDs. The merging of nursing leadership skills, evidence-based decision making, and expert clinical care will ensure that nursing has a strong and credible presence in an ever-changing and complex healthcare system.

The DNP degree is a terminal practice degree and is now considered by many healthcare organizations as the preferred degree for nursing leaders involved in the delivery and organization of clinical care and healthcare systems. The DNP's academic preparation, with a strong curricular base in advanced practice principles, experiential learning, intra/interprofessional collaboration, and application of the best clinical research evidence, can best fulfill nursing's goals for leadership in practice and clinical education. In addition, clinical scholarship, including critical inquiry, analysis, synthesis, creativity, and research, must be a distinguishing feature of the DNP's role and expertise.

The purpose of this chapter is to define and explore the meaning of clinical scholarship, to distinguish evidence-based practice from other forms of scholarly activity, to describe the unique role of the DNP in scholarship, and to provide an overview of the language, methodological tools, strategies, and thought processes that are necessary to ensure that nursing's scholarship is useful, significant, and of the highest quality. Entire books are dedicated to research processes, methodologies, and evidence-based practice. This is not the intent of this chapter; rather, it is to explore the concepts, provide resources, and whet the reader's appetite for more in-depth information on the topic.

WHAT IS CLINICAL SCHOLARSHIP?

In Sigma Theta Tau International's (1999) *Clinical Scholarship Resource Paper,* Melanie Dreher, chair of the task force, wrote that "clinical scholarship is about inquiry and implies a willingness to scrutinize our practice" (Dreher, 1999, p. 26). Also, "clinical scholarship is not clinical proficiency, . . . unless we are questioning the reason for its use in the first place . . . ; and neither is it clinical research, although it is informed by and inspires research" (p. 26). Finally, she notes that "clinical scholarship is an intellectual process. . . . It includes challenging traditional nursing interventions, testing our ideas, predicting outcomes, and explaining both patterns and exceptions. In addition to observation, analysis, and synthesis, clinical scholarship includes application and dissemination, all of which result in a new understanding of nursing phenomena and the development of new knowledge" (p. 26).

The American Association of Colleges of Nursing's (AACN) *Position Statement on Defining Scholarship for the Discipline of Nursing* (1999) defines scholarship as "those activities that systematically advance the teaching, research, and practice of nursing through rigorous inquiry that: 1) is significant to the profession, 2) is creative, 3) can be documented, 4) can be replicated or elaborated, and 5) can be peer-reviewed through various methods" (p. 1). Citing the work of Schulman (1993), the National Organization of Nurse Practitioner Faculties (2005) notes further that practice, to be considered scholarship, "must be public, susceptible to critical review and evaluation, and accessible for exchange and use of other members of one's scholarly community" (p. 6).

These definitions are congruent with the evolving definition of scholarship in academia since Boyer's (1990, 1997) groundbreaking work *Scholarship Reconsidered: Priorities of the Professoriate.* Ernest L. Boyer was an American educator, chancellor, and president of the Carnegie Foundation for the Advancement of

Teaching (Carnegie Foundation for the Advancement of Teaching, 1996). Since the publication of *Scholarship Reconsidered* (1990), a new and expanded role for scholarship has emerged in academia that makes the previously mentioned definitions of scholarship more compatible with the goals and processes of practice disciplines. The traditional definition of scholarship in academia did not account for the nuances and rigors of clinical practice knowledge and its application for problem solving and interactive, human engagement (AACN, 2006). Boyer's model (1990, 1997), however, is well suited to scholarship in nursing practice. In Boyer's view, scholarship is not linear; rather, there is a constant, reciprocal, iterative relationship between each of its four aspects. Scholarship embraces the concepts of discovery (building new knowledge through research and careful inquiry to refine existing knowledge), integration (interpreting knowledge through dissemination in various forms), application (using knowledge for problem solving, service, and growth), and teaching (developing and testing instructional materials to advance learning, including the formation and sustaining of an engaging environment for learning between teacher and student) (Boyer, 1990, 1997; Stull & Lanz, 2005).

The AACN's *Essentials of Doctoral Education for Advanced Nursing Practice* (2006) embodies much of Boyer's criteria in the specification of the eight core essentials and specialty focused competencies as the basic underpinnings to be integrated into the DNP curriculum (AACN, 2006). Essential 3 of the core elements is "clinical scholarship and analytic methods for evidence-based practice" (AACN, 2006). In this document the authors state that "scholarship and research are core elements of doctoral education" (AACN, 2006), and, further, that

> [R]esearch doctorates are designed to prepare graduates with the research skills necessary to discover new knowledge in the discipline. However, DNPs engaged in advanced nursing

practice provide leadership for evidence-based practice. This requires competence in knowledge development activities such as the translation of research in practice, the evaluation of practice, activities aimed at improving the reliability of health care practice and outcomes, and participation in collaborative research. (De Palma & McGuire, 2005)

Therefore, DNP programs focus on the translation of new science, its application, and its evaluation. In addition, DNP graduates generate evidence to guide practice.

More recently, the idea that only those with research doctorates (PhD, DNS, and DNSc) should conduct "discovery" research for generating new knowledge has been challenged (Ironside, 2006; Reed & Shear, 2004; Webber, 2008). Webber (2008) asserts that level-appropriate research should be promoted from the baccalaureate through doctoral level because "everyday practice involves daily interaction with an informed public, interpreting the most updated research that is available with the click of a mouse, and identifying phenomena unique to the practice. The only missing piece is the skills necessary to investigate the phenomenon" (p. 468).

As DNP programs have proliferated, the curriculum has evolved to include more focus on research and evidence-based practice. An Internet review of the curricula from several national DNP programs makes it clear that growing numbers of schools are adding courses such as Theory, Research Methods, Discovery and Utilization of Evidence-Based Care, and Translating Evidence into Practice so that graduates have the skills needed to participate in whatever level of research is appropriate to their setting and scholarship goals.

EVIDENCE-BASED PRACTICE AND CLINICAL SCHOLARSHIP: ARE THEY THE SAME?

Scholarship is an evolutionary process that raises the level of the profession through participation in the generation of new knowledge and through scientific and social exchange. "The difference between evidence based nursing practice and scholarship or applied nursing research is that evidence based practice is practice driven" (French, 1999, p. 77). Whereas scholarship was often viewed by many practicing professionals as an add-on, optional activity, evidence-based practice has become a necessity in our current information-based technological age. Computers have given everyone access to both good and bad information. The defining feature of evidence-based practice is the linking of current research findings with patients' conditions, values, and circumstances. In addition, it involves "the conscientious, explicit, and judicious use of current best evidence for making decisions about the care of individuals" (Sackett, Richardson, Rosenberg, & Haynes, 1997, p. 2). Nursing's unique addition to this process must offer a more holistic approach that adds artful practice and ethical standards to the empirics of evidence (Fawcett, Watson, Neuman, Hinton Walker, & Fitzpatrick, 2001).

The work of clinical scholars has increased during the past two decades. A review of published nursing articles from 1986 to 2008 in the Cumulative Index to Nursing and Allied Health Literature (CINAHL) database resulted in 81 published articles with clinical scholarship as the focus. When "evidence-based practice" was added to the search terms, an additional 7 articles were found. When "evidence-based practice" alone was used as the search term, the search returned 3,835 articles published between the years 1993 and 2009. Although not all of the latter were nursing articles, 1,729 articles, or nearly half, were nursing-focused articles.

Holleman, Eliens, van Vliet, and van Acterburg (2006) extensively reviewed six databases, including CINAHL, PubMed, Scirus, Invert, Google, and the Cochrane databases, focusing on the years between 1993 and 2004. In their meta-analysis of the literature on promotion of evidence-based practice (EBP) and professional nursing associations, the authors found

179 articles that addressed EBP activities. Of the 179 articles, 47 dealt with EBP as structural measures (policy, role, quality indicators), 103 with EBP as competence and attitude oriented (e.g., journals, conferences, workshops, research committees), and only 29 with EBP as behavior oriented (care models, guidelines). The increase in EBP articles shows the growing interest and use of evidence to guide practice. Despite this progress, there remain significant gaps in nursing science discovery and application or implementation in practice. The DNP is intended to bridge this gap (McCloskey, 2008).

The principles of EBP were an outgrowth of the work of Dr. Archie Cochrane, a British epidemiologist who criticized the medical profession for not using evidence from randomized clinical trials as a basis for clinical care. He believed that the evidence from these trials should be systematically reviewed and constantly updated to afford patients the best-quality care (Cochrane Collaboration, 2004). Evidence-based practice includes an emphasis on the efficacy of treatments or interventions based on the results of experimental comparison between untreated control groups, treatments, or both. The core principles include (1) formulating the clinical question; (2) identifying the most relevant articles, research, and other best evidence; (3) critically evaluating the evidence; (4) integrating and applying the evidence; and (5) reevaluating the application of evidence and making necessary changes. **Table 21-1** presents the hierarchy of evidence for practice.

That the definition of "evidence-based practice" has been adapted to include provisions for the provider's experience and patient's values in making the ultimate clinical care decisions is in keeping with James Russell Lowell's (1819–1891) definition of scholarship: "True scholarship consists in knowing not what things exist, but what they mean; it is not memory, but judgment." Although Lowell was not a healthcare professional, his definition is applicable to advanced nursing practice. It is through

TABLE 21-1	Hierarchy for Evaluating Evidence for Practice
Level 1 (strongest)	Systematic reviews/meta-analysis of all randomized controlled trials (RCTs); clinical practice guidelines based on RCT data
Level 2	Evidence from one or more RCTs
Level 3	Evidence from a controlled trial; no randomization
Level 4	Case control or cohort studies
Level 5	Systematic reviews of descriptive/qualitative studies
Level 6	Single descriptive or qualitative study
Level 7 (weakest)	Opinions of authorities/experts

Note: All levels assume a well-designed study.

Source: Burns, N., & Grove, S. K. (2009). *The practice of nursing research, appraisal, synthesis, and generation of evidence* (6th ed.). St. Louis, MO: Elsevier Saunders, p. 37. Reprinted with permission.

the incorporation of intuition, observation, theory, research, intelligent analysis, and judgment based on the data that nurses provide care that is truly individualized, reflective, and evidence based. With an increased knowledge of the theory and the tools necessary to critique and translate research into practice, the DNP is in a prime position to affect the delivery of care and to aggregate and translate evidence that can be disseminated to improve overall care and outcomes in a myriad of clinical areas. The translation and dissemination of clinical knowledge form the core of clinical scholarship.

WHAT IS THE ROLE OF THE DOCTOR OF NURSING PRACTICE IN CLINICAL SCHOLARSHIP?

In advanced practice, scholarship should be integrated with practice as a purposeful, systematic, and conscious endeavor. The emphasis is on inquiry, outcomes, and evidence to support practice (Sigma Theta Tau International Clinical Scholarship Task Force, 1999). Because of their education, advanced practice nurses, particularly DNPs, are expected to have mastery

of essential information so that the teaching of staff, patients, and communities becomes a key function of the role. The dynamic nature of health care requires that DNPs be up-to-date on new information, and that they be able to discern nuances in research findings so as to translate those findings in understandable ways that improve care and practice. This requires constant critique and integration and synthesis of new information from various sources into formats that can be disseminated to patients, colleagues, and others.

What distinguishes the role of the DNP from other advanced practice degree holders? The answer is not a simple one; the difference is, in fact, a combination of knowledge, expert skill, and the integration of best research to advance the practice and the profession. This skill comes from additional formal education, experience, and the translation, application, and evaluation of research in practice. Although most practicing nurses are exposed to "research" and "evidence" in practice, the DNP must not only embrace the process but also implement the findings in ways that ultimately change or, at least, improve practice and outcomes. Scholarship is the dissemination of those findings in publications, presentations, and Internet offerings that can be used by others. As envisioned in *The Essentials of Doctoral Education for Advanced Practice Nursing* (AACN, 2006), the DNP program prepares graduates to:

1. Use analytical methods to critically appraise existing literature and other evidence relevant to practice.

2. Lead the evaluation of evidence (existing literature, research findings, and other data) to determine and implement the best evidence for practice.

3. Design and implement processes to evaluate outcomes of practice and systems of care.

4. Design, direct, and evaluate quality improvement initiatives to promote safe, timely, effective, efficient, equitable, and patient-centered care.

5. Evaluate practice patterns against national benchmarks to determine variances in clinical outcomes and population trends.

6. Apply relevant findings to develop practice guidelines and improve practice and the practice environment.

7. Inform and guide the design of databases that generate meaningful evidence for nursing practice.

8. Use information technology and research methods appropriately to:

   - Collect appropriate and accurate data to generate evidence for nursing practice
   - Analyze data from clinical practice
   - Design evidence-based interventions
   - Predict and analyze outcomes
   - Examine patterns of behavior and outcomes
   - Identify gaps in evidence for practice

9. Function as a practice specialist/consultant in collaborative knowledge-generating research.

10. Disseminate findings from evidence-based practice to improve healthcare outcomes.

These objectives encompass the essential skills, tools, and methods necessary to implement and support clinical scholarship and evidence-based practice. They can be distilled into six categories: (1) translating research into practice, (2) quality improvement and patient-centered care, (3) evaluation of practice, (4) research methods and technology, (5) participation in collaborative research, and (6) disseminating findings from evidence-based practice. Each of these areas is discussed in the following sections.

TRANSLATING RESEARCH INTO PRACTICE

The use of evidence to support clinical practice is not a new phenomenon. Medical professionals have relied on data from science, empirical observation, case reviews, and other means for centuries (Monico, Moore, & Calise, 2005). However, as electronic access to sources of data has increased, the amount of evidence available as a basis for clinical practice has often become overwhelming. The key to making best-practice decisions lies in using the best-quality evidence—evidence that is scientifically based and that has been replicated with success in repeated research and application.

Although critical appraisal of research for use in practice is an important aspect of evidence-based practice, it is not the only criterion. Unfortunately, many lack the knowledge and skills on which to base their practice decisions (Pravikoff, Tanner, & Pierce, 2005). Melnyk and Fineout-Overholt (2005) specify three primary knowledge sources for EBP: valid research evidence, clinical expertise, and patient choice. Currently, evidence generated from large-scale randomized controlled trials is considered the gold standard for application in interventions (Fawcett & Garrity, 2009). Depending on the clinical situation and the patient's personal preference, other sources of evidence may be appropriate, including meta-analyses of all relevant randomized controlled trials; EBP guidelines from systematic reviews of randomized controlled trials, case control, or cohort studies; expert opinion; and nursing theory (Fawcett & Garrity, 2009; Melnyk & Fineout-Overholt, 2005).

To understand research evidence that may be used in practice, the following sections on qualitative and quantitative research offer a brief description of the processes and questions to be considered in the evaluation of such research. Exhaustive coverage of every research method is beyond the scope of this chapter. However, the definitions, discussion, and examples are meant to illustrate how different types of research might be applied or used in practice, and how their rigor and adequacy as evidence for practice should be evaluated.

UNDERSTANDING, DISTINGUISHING, AND EVALUATING TYPES OF RESEARCH EVIDENCE

Qualitative Research Evidence

Qualitative research is based on four levels of understanding (Porter, 1996, as cited in Maggs-Rapport, 2001):

1. What is the nature of reality? (Ontology)
2. What constitutes knowledge? (Epistemology)
3. How can we understand reality? (Methodology)
4. How can we collect the evidence? (Methods)

Types of Qualitative Research Studies

There are several kinds of qualitative research studies, including critical social theory, ethnographic studies, grounded theory research, historical research, phenomenological studies, and philosophical inquiry. Each of these methods is discussed briefly so as to provide an overview of the scope and potential uses of qualitative evidence and to provide a basis for evaluating the use of qualitative studies as a basis for changes in practice.

Critical Social Theory

Critical social theory uses multiple research methods as a basis for promoting change in areas where power imbalances exist (Burns & Grove, 2009). Based on the ideas of Horkheimer (1895–1973), Marcuse (1898–1979), Adorno (1903–1969), and Habermas (1929–), critical social theory is based on the belief that individuals should seek freedom from domination (Maggs-Rapport, 2001). Habermas, particularly, believed that people must understand the nature of "constraining circumstances" before they could be liberated from them (Maggs-Rapport, 2001). Another critical social theorist, Giddens (1982, as cited in Maggs-Rapport, 2001), believed that we can understand why people act in certain ways only if we can appreciate the meanings of their actions.

The DNP might use data from critical social theory to identify meaning or patterns of concern where certain societal cultural norms exist in the form of barriers that affect particularly vulnerable populations such as the elderly, the incarcerated, abused women, and the chronically ill. Analysis would necessarily include an examination of the underlying conditions, a critique of the social phenomena, and the discovery and revelation of the social and political injustices embedded in the experience of the population in question that could lead toward removal of barriers (Maggs-Rapport, 2001).

Ethnographic Research

Ethnographic research is used to describe the nature or characteristics of a culture so as to gain insight into the lifeways or behaviors of a group. Distinguishing features are immersion in the participant's way of life (Polit & Hungler, 1997) and the fact that the information gathered speaks for itself, rather than being interpreted or explored for additional meanings (Maggs-Rapport, 2001).

In one ethnographic study, Kovarsky (2008) compared clients' and families' personal experiences of outcomes and interventions with written professional discourse, technical reports, and other conceptualizations of evidence in practice. Unfortunately, the author notes, "the dismissal of subjective, phenomenally oriented information has functioned to marginalize and silence voices . . . of clients when constituting proof of effectiveness," and further, "the current version of EBP needs to be reformulated to include subjective voices from the life-worlds of clients as a form of evidence" (Kovarsky, 2008, p. 47). As one example of an ethnographic approach, Kovarsky proposed the personal experience narrative as a measure of qualitative outcomes and intervention analysis (Kovarsky, 2008, p. 48). Citing a study by Simmons-Mackie and Damico (2001), Kovarsky describes an ethnographic interview with a patient experiencing post-stroke aphasia:

> When asked to comment on life before her stroke, K. [the patient] said: "Before teacher . . . now I don't know . . . .what." and "uh . . . uh . . . always, always . . . uh . . . busy, busy, busy, . . . teachin . . . teachin . . . always, I love it. . . . it's me . . . But now . . . here (points to mouth) talk, not uh . . . teaching." When asked about a typical day, she shrugged and said "nothing . . . here (points to television)" and later added "eat . . . and (points to newspaper) and shows (points to television)." (Simmons-Mackie & Damico, 2001, as cited in Kovarsky, 2008, p. 51)

These statements support an altered level of life activity that cannot totally be accounted for or appreciated in objective technical descriptions of outcomes of disease processes and their sequelae.

The ethnographic narrative is a method of subjective evidence gathering that can enhance the specificity and richness of other research methodologies, including evidence gained from logical positivist approaches such as randomized controlled trials. In particular, DNPs in public health or community health could use this method in conjunction with other, more traditional, forms of evidence to gain a better real-world understanding of the populations they serve.

Grounded Theory Research

Grounded theory research is focused on the influence of interactional processes (identification, description, and explanation) between individuals, families, or groups within a social context (Strauss & Corbin, 1994). It is an observational method that is used to study problems in social settings that are "grounded" in the data obtained from those observations (Burns & Grove, 2009; Glasser & Strauss, 1967). In this regard, grounded theory is an applicable framework for study of a myriad of contexts, situations, and settings.

For example, a study of the implementation of evidence-based nursing in Iran (Adib-Hajbaghery, 2007) sought to distinguish factors influencing the implementation of evidence-based practice in Eastern countries (versus Western countries), particularly Iran. A brief description of this study using the grounded theory approach is presented here. Data collection consisted of purposive sampling of 21 nurses (nine staff and six head nurses in differing clinical settings) with experience in nursing greater than five years. An interview questionnaire consisted of open-ended questions, such as "What is the basis of care you give your patients?" (p. 568), "In your opinion, what is the basis of evidence-based nursing?" (p. 568), and "Can you describe some instances in which you used scientific evidence in nursing?" (p. 568). "Issues were clarified and interviews were audiotaped, transcribed verbatim and analyzed consecutively" (Adib-Hajbaghery, 2007, p. 568). Thirty-six hours of observations and interviews were carried out concurrently and involved observations of those interviewed and others working on the units. According to the procedure identified by Strauss and Corbin (1998), each interview was analyzed before the subsequent interview took place, and the results were coded in three ways: open coding (breaking down, examining, comparing, conceptualizing, and categorizing), axial coding (putting data back together in new ways by linking codes to contexts, consequences, and patterns of interactions), and selective coding (identifying core categories and systematically relating and validating relationships) (Adib-Hajbaghery, 2007). To confirm the credibility of the data, participants were given a full transcript of their responses and a list of codes and themes to determine whether the codes and themes matched their responses. To establish validity, two peer researchers also checked codes and themes using the same procedure as the researcher. The results were that two main categories emerged from the research: (1) the meaning of evidence-based nursing (EBN) and (2) factors in implementation of EBN, including the themes of possessing professional knowledge and experience, having opportunity and time, becoming accustomed, self-confidence, the process of nursing education, and the work environment and its expectations (Adib-Hajbaghery, 2007).

The process and results of grounded theory research and analysis provide rich data for application in practice when paired with evidence from other sources. This is especially true when there is little clinical trial evidence to support the affective dimension of care or practice.

Historical Research

Historical research is a description or analysis of events that have shaped a discipline. Although historical research may not be used directly in practice, it provides the foundation for examination of the discipline and for providing future directions (Burns & Grove; 2009; Fitzpatrick & Munhall, 2001). Often history is handed down in written documents. The Library of Congress's (n.d.) American Memory Collection has original writings, newspaper clippings, photos, and other documents that provide a realistic account of the influence and actions of famous women in history, including nursing leaders. Pictures and other documents showcase the original early work of early nurse leaders such as Lavinia Dock (1858–1956), Margaret Sanger (1879–1966), Clara Barton (1821–1912), and Mary Breckinridge (1881–1965), which provide a basis for advanced nursing practice and can be used by DNPs in education to provide a historical perspective for practice.

Another source of historical research is oral history. Decker and Iphofen (2005) describe a method of oral history research to discover knowledge about, and change within, a profession, particularly as it relates to evidence-based practice. Tropello (2000) used oral history technique in her dissertation, *Origins of the Nurse Practitioner Movement: An Oral History*. The purpose was to gain a better understanding of current advanced nursing practice roles through an exploration of the original movement. Eight participants in the original movement were the primary sources, and the information obtained and transcribed from taped interviews was enhanced by supportive papers, correspondence, and other documents, including secondary sources. One conclusion of the study was that the politics of the 1960s, which emphasized greater freedoms for women and a focus on social programs, helped alleviate healthcare personnel shortages (Tropello, 2000). This movement has paved the way for additional professionalization in nursing, including the evolution of the DNP curriculum. Started as a research project, it became part of the core curriculum under the continuing education division of the School of Nursing at the University of Colorado. The program used a nursing–physician team approach to aid families with limited access to primary providers (Tropello, 2000).

Another oral history intervention project was that of Taft, Stolder, Knutson, Tamke, Platt, and Bowles (2004), who recorded the oral histories of World War II veterans in nursing homes. Themes of patriotism, loss, tense moments, makeshift living, self-sufficiency, and uncertainty were uncovered. The authors' conclusions were that "oral histories, listening[,] and valuing supports, involves, and validates elders" (Taft et al., 2004, p. 38.).

The National League for Nursing (NLN) provides audio and videotapes of nurse theorists whose original work and theory development continue to provide frameworks for advancing nursing practice (Moccia, 1987). For DNPs to prescribe their future, they must have a clear understanding and appreciation for their history so that they can build on and shape evidence-based practice in ways that preserve the essence of nursing.

Phenomenological Research

The aim of a phenomenological (hermeneutic) study is to understand a phenomenon through the recognition of its meaning. Researchers explore an experience as it is lived by the participants in the study. The phenomenon of interest may include any number of experiences, such as death, divorce, pain, or cancer. The researcher collects data and interprets the experiences as they are lived (Burns & Groves, 2009). Phenomenology focuses on the subjective and particular experiences to discern the real truths of any phenomena (Hallett, 1995, as cited in Yegdich, 1999).

One example of a phenomenological study by Marineau (2005) was that of perceptions of telehealth support by an advanced practice nurse for patients discharged from the hospital with acute infections. Because empirical data were insufficient in patients who had previously been enrolled in a quantitative pilot study of telehealth, eidetic phenomenology was used to capture patients' lived experiences after discharge. Theme categories were as follows: initial response, engaging in care, and experiencing the downside. Of the 10 participants in the trial, only one had a negative experience. The study was seen as useful in adding to the understanding of the transitional process of care (Marineau, 2005).

In another phenomenological approach, Maggs-Rapport (2001) used van Manen's (1990) social scientific approach to look at women's immediate response to the phenomenon of egg sharing (donation of one woman's eggs to another woman) after consultation with a clinician and their lived experiences of egg sharing in return for free fertility treatment. The in-depth, open-ended interviews of this technique established a conversational relationship about the meaning of the experience and produced a narrative that "enriches the understanding of the phenomena" (Maggs-Rapport, 2001). Before each description can by transformed into phenomenological language, meaning units must be made of each description (Giorgi, 2000). However, only a small number of descriptions are necessary before the nature of the phenomenon becomes apparent (van Manen, 1990; Giorgi, 2000).

Other studies that utilized the phenomenological approach in advanced practice include studies about the needs of patients and families living with severe brain injury (Bond, Draeger, Mandleco, & Donnelly, 2003); high-risk perinatal experience (Harvey, 1993); the meaning of U.S. childbirth for Mexican immigrant women (Imberg, 2008); the meaning of desire for euthanasia (Mak, 2003); and perimenopausal mental disorders (Rasgon, Shelton, & Halbreich, 2005). Phenomenological techniques with a strong nursing orientation include those of Crotty (1996); Diekelmann, Allen, and Tanner (1989); and Munhall (1994, 2007). Phenomenological studies contribute to the evidence base by enhancing our understanding of the true meaning of patients' experiences and the broader dimensions of a problem, thus aiding in a more holistic perspective in practice.

Philosophical Inquiry

Philosophical inquiry is used to explore the nature of knowledge, values, meaning, and ethical factors related to a question of interest. Although philosophical inquiry is related to theory, it is not the same as theory, which is more specific and concrete (Pesut & Johnson, 2007). Citing Edwards (2001), Pesut and Johnson (2007) describe three "strands" that compose philosophical inquiry: (1) philosophical presupposition, which involves identifying and analyzing presuppositions in nursing (an example might be a concept analysis of nursing practice or advanced practice); (2) philosophical problems, such as what constitutes knowing in a particular situation, or ethical analyses, such as the ethics of caring in situations where nurses' and patients' values conflict; and (3) scholarship, in which nurse theorists' works are examined from a philosophical perspective. In this case, as noted by Burns and Grove (2009), the researcher would "conduct an extensive search of the literature, examine conceptual meaning, pose questions and propose answers including the implications for those answers" (p. 26).

In a practical application of philosophical inquiry, Dorn (2004) described a model, caring-healing inquiry for holistic nursing practice, to guide nursing research and quality improvement in a tertiary hospital. The model, which integrated the values of the hospital, provided the basis for nurses to describe their contributions to care through research and practice improvement. In a partnership between a hospital and university nursing program, a nursing research committee was formed, composed mostly of advanced practice nurses. The group served as an advisory group for program planning and development. The nurse-researcher faculty member facilitated the work of the committee and provided staff development in research and clinical innovation. Knowledge about the process of philosophical inquiry and a focus on value analysis, as demonstrated in these examples, provides DNPs with a basis for facilitating ethical decision making in practice.

Evaluating Qualitative Research Evidence

What are the evaluative questions? Regardless of the type of research design, the general criteria for evaluation of qualitative studies are as follows (Gifford, Davies, Edwards, Griffin, & Lybanon, 2007; Patton, 1990; Russell & Gregory, 2003):

1. Question, purpose, and context: Is the research question clear, the primary purpose and the focus of the study stated, and the context described?
2. Design: Was the design appropriate, were the units of analysis and sampling strategy described, and the sampling criteria clear?
3. Data collection: Which types of data were collected? Were data collection processes systematic and adequately described? How were logistical issues addressed?
4. Data analysis: Was data analysis systematic and rigorous? Which controls were in place?

Which analytical approach or approaches were used? How were validity and confidence in the findings established?

5. Results: Were results surprising, interesting, or suspect? Were conclusions supported by data and explanation (theory)? Were the authors' positions clearly stated?
6. Ethical issues: How were ethical issues and confidentiality addressed?
7. Implications: What is the worth/relevance to knowledge and practice?

Context Matters

In her discussion of evidence-based nursing and qualitative research, Zuzelo (2007) notes that critical appraisal skills are among the most important aspects of the evidence-based movement in health care. Also, the associated terms "relevance" and "best," when applied to practice, are value-laden terms that must be fully explored within the context of nursing practice, so that the unique contribution of nursing is not subsumed into the disease-based medical model of clinical decision making. Additionally, she proposes that "nursing[,] as both a science and an art, needs to assure that qualitative research is as much a part of the considered evidence as quantitative evidence is" (Zuzelo, 2007, p. 484). This is important because qualitative research questions provide an avenue for truly knowing, connecting with patients, and considering individual differences when making clinical decisions. These are the hallmarks of nursing that nurses at every level must retain and that DNPs must foster as role models to ensure that "best practice" does not exclude the best of nursing's perspective.

Quantitative Research Evidence

Steps in the Quantitative Research Process

The important aspect of any quantitative research project is that the project builds on prior results or evidence and that it provides a basis for future research and discovery (Burns &

Grove, 2009). **Figure 21-1** shows the steps in the quantitative research process.

The research problem is often derived from the fact that there is a gap in knowledge that needs to be addressed or described. Research problems or questions often arise from direct observations made in practice. The purpose of the study is to address the problem. To better understand the problem, an extensive literature review must be done to develop an understanding of the nature and scope of the problem and to determine which research has already been done. A framework, map, or theoretical base made up of concepts is developed to provide structure and help the researcher make sense of the findings. The research objectives, questions, or hypotheses set the study limits, in terms of who will be studied, which question(s) will be addressed, and which relationships among variables exist.

The remaining steps are to define the variables in conceptual terms (theoretical meaning) and operational terms (how the variables will be measured or manipulated), explain assumptions (those things we take for granted to be true, whether proven or not), and identify study limitations (any issue within the study that serves to limit a study's generalizability beyond the population or sample studied). Limitations may be weaknesses in the study itself or in the theoretical basis.

Categories and Selection of a Design

Quantitative research may be categorized as experimental, quasi-experimental, or nonexperimental (descriptive or correlational). Quantitative research may be either basic research (as in laboratory studies) or applied (as in clinical research). In an experimental or quasi-experimental study, the researcher actively manipulates the independent variable (treatment or intervention) to see the effect on the dependent variable. In an experimental study, the variables and the setting are highly controlled. In a nonexperimental design, the researcher may simply want to describe or explain a phe-

nomenon or predict a relationship (Burns & Grove, 2009).

Quantitative designs may also be retrospective (the proposed cause and effect have already occurred), prospective (the cause, but not the effect, has occurred), cross sectional (groups in various stages of development are examined), or longitudinal (the same subjects are studied over a period of time). None of the categories are mutually exclusive (Schmidt & Brown, 2009).

The Population and Sample

The population is everyone or everything that meets the criteria for inclusion. The criteria for inclusion may be narrow or broad, depending on the size and scope of the study and the specific research question to be addressed. The sample is a subset of the population and the process for how the subset will be selected. This may be random (all have a better than zero chance of selection), nonrandom (convenience), cross sectional (groups studied over time), or stratified (divided to ensure representation from groups when some variables are known). Often the population and the sample are determined by the method and how accessible the population is to the researcher (Burns & Grove, 2009).

Measurement Instruments

Measurement instruments are tools used by the researcher to answer the operational questions posed in research studies. These tools may be questionnaires, tests, indicators of health status, and a variety of other measurement techniques.

Data Collection, Analysis, and Interpretation

Most data collected in quantitative research studies are coded numerically so that they can be systematically analyzed and interpreted through the use of statistics. A plan for data collection and analysis is an important part of the research process and is crucial to meaningful interpretation of results. Interpretation involves "1) examining the results from data, 2) exploring the significance of findings,

FIGURE 21-1   The Quantitative Research Process

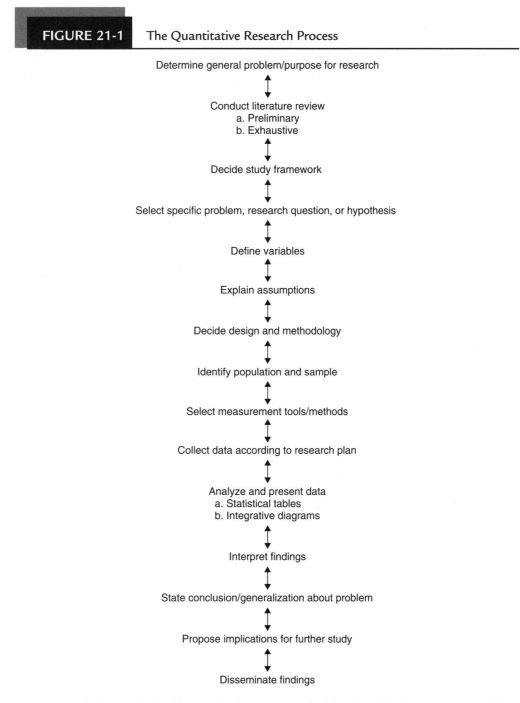

Determine general problem/purpose for research

Conduct literature review
a. Preliminary
b. Exhaustive

Decide study framework

Select specific problem, research question, or hypothesis

Define variables

Explain assumptions

Decide design and methodology

Identify population and sample

Select measurement tools/methods

Collect data according to research plan

Analyze and present data
a. Statistical tables
b. Integrative diagrams

Interpret findings

State conclusion/generalization about problem

Propose implications for further study

Disseminate findings

Source: Burns & Grove (2009). *The practice of nursing research*, 6th ed., p. 37. Elsevier Saunders. Used with permission.

3) forming conclusions, 4) generalizing the data, 5) considering the implications for further study, and 6) suggesting further studies" (Burns & Grove, p. 45). Once interpreted, the researcher synthesizes and reports implications for further study or practice, or both.

This cursory overview of the research process provides the basis for evaluating evidence from research. The reader is referred to a research text for a complete discussion of definitions and the various designs, analyses, and implementation processes.

Evaluating Quantitative Evidence

When a quantitative study is appraised for use in practice, three questions are generally considered: Is the study valid? Is the study reliable? and Is the study applicable in the identified case?

Is the Study Valid?

Specifically, were the methods used scientifically sound? Are the independent (manipulated variable) and dependent variables (observed result) clearly identified? Is the study free from bias or confounding variables?

Bias is a standard point of view or personal prejudice, especially when there is a tendency "to affect unduly or unfairly, or to impose a steady negative potential upon" (*Funk & Wagnalls,* 2003, p. 135). It is an influence or action that distorts or "slants findings away from the expected" (Burns & Grove, 2009, p. 220). In research, bias may occur when participants' characteristics specifically differ from those of the population (Burns & Grove, 2005). This is always possible because volunteers are used for samples. It is less likely to occur, however, if the sampling strategy is well planned and followed and there is random assignment to groups. Bias may also occur if the instruments or measurement tools are faulty, or the data or statistics are inaccurate.

Selection Bias

If a researcher decides to prospectively compare two types of strategies for educating nursing students, such as online instruction and traditional classroom instruction, selection bias may occur if the students are allowed to select which group they enter. Students who select online teaching may be very different from those who choose the traditional classroom experience. Random assignment to the groups minimizes the risk of selection bias.

Gender Bias

Another form of bias is gender bias. Gender bias occurs in research when one gender, more than the other, is used to study research interventions. Timmerman (1999) outlined a procedure for ensuring that research decisions avoid gender bias. The procedure includes critically analyzing the literature, testing gender-specific differences, and identifying researchers' personal biases.

The following example of binge-eating behaviors between men and women illustrates the point. Timmerman (1999), citing Hawkins & Clement (1984) and Spitzer et al. (1992), states "we know that men tend to binge less frequently, consume less during binges and are less distressed by their binge eating behavior than women." And, "in this case, the literature provides justification for either separately studying binge eating behavior in men and women, or, if the sample has both men and women, analyzing the data separately for men and women" (Timmerman, 1999, p. 642).

Table 21-2 lists some gender-based studies. Additional gender-based studies can be found online through the Office on Women's Health of the U.S. Department of Health and Human Services.

Confounding Variables

Confounding occurs when a third variable, either known or unknown, produces the relationship with the outcome instead of the research intervention itself. Or, stated differently, confounding may occur when comparing two groups that may be different in additional ways from the treatment being studied (Leedy &

TABLE 21-2	Gender-Based Studies
Authors and Date of Publication	**Title**
Bernarde, Keogh, & Lima (2007)	Bridging the gap between pain and gender research
Bushnell, Hurn, Colton, Miller, del Zoppo, Elkind, et al. (2007)	Advancing the study of stroke in women Summary and recommendations for future research
Doster, Pardum, Martin, Goven, & Moorefield (2009)	Gender differences, anger expression, and cardiovascular risk
Luttik, Jaarsma, Lesman, Sanderman, & Hagedoorn (2009)	Quality of life in partners of people with congestive heart failure: Gender and involvement in care
Masharani, Goldfine, & Youngren (2009)	Influence of gender on the relationship between insulin sensitivity, adiposity and plasma lipids in lean nondiabetic patients
McCollum, Hansen, Lu, & Sullivan (2005)	Self-care differences in men and women with diabetes
Reeves, Fonarow, Zhao, Smith, & Schwamm (2009)	Quality of care in women with ischemic stroke in the GWTG program

Ormrod, 2010). Randomizing participants to either the intervention or study group helps to eliminate the possibility of confusion because there is an equal chance that extraneous variables will appear equally in both groups, thus minimizing the confounding effect.

One type of confounder is the effect of history. The history effect occurs when an event outside the researcher's control occurs at the same time as, or during, the period of the intervention. For example, in a study of patients with hypertension, a researcher was interested in the impact of a low-salt diet on hypertension levels. A baseline blood pressure was taken; patients were then started on the low-salt diet. However, during the study period, some of these same patients began a rigorous exercise routine, whereas others did not. In this case, the intervening exercise program would make it difficult to attribute the outcome solely to the effect of the intervention. Adding a control group using low-salt diet with exercise, or using statistical tests to control for this confounding variable, would minimize the threat to validity in this study.

In another example of confounding, a researcher was interested in comparing lung cancer and smoking incidence in various regions of the country. In this study, a particular region was seen to have a significantly higher rate of lung cancer death among smokers (15 times higher) than other regions of the country. The confounding factor was the fact that these smokers had also worked in asbestos coal mines for many years. When the researchers controlled for the variable of working with asbestos by removing the confounder, the rate of cancer due to smoking was nearly the same as that in other regions of the country. **Figure 21-2** shows the relationship among the independent variable (smoking) and confounding variable (working in an asbestos coal mine) in relationship to the dependent variable (lung cancer) (International Development Research Center, 2009).

	Interrelationships Among Smoking, Working in an Asbestos Coal
FIGURE 21-2	Mine, and Risk for Lung Cancer in a Cohort/Case Control Study

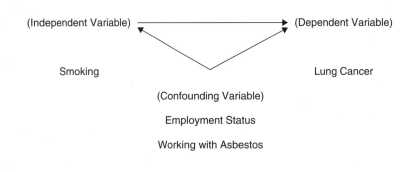

Source: International Development Research Center. (2009). Figure 26.1. http://www.idrc.ca/en /ev-56459-201-1-DO_TOPIC.html. Used with permission of IDRC Canada, www.irdc.ca.

Is the Study Reliable?

The reliability of a study is based on questions such as the following: Does the instrument or test measure what it is supposed to measure? Does it do this consistently? Do the items on the instrument consistently measure the same characteristic? How much consistency is there between raters? (Burns & Grove, 2009; Fain, 2009). Reliability is measured through the use of a reliability coefficient (*r*) and ranges from 00.0 (lowest) to 1.00 (highest). Therefore, the closer a reliability score is to 1.00, the higher the reliability. In most cases a coefficient of 0.80 or higher is considered acceptable if the instrument has already been tested and has been used frequently. If an instrument is new, a reliability coefficient of 0.70 may be acceptable (Griffin-Sobel, 2003, as cited in Schmidt & Brown, 2009). Reliability also focuses on stability (test–retest reliability—whether an instrument yields the same results for the same two people on two different occasions), homogeneity (internal consistency—the extent to which all of the items within a single instrument yield similar results), and equivalence (interrater reliability—the extent to which two or more individuals evaluating the same product or

performance give identical judgments) (Fain, 2009; Leedy & Ormrod, 2010).

A simple example of reliability is seen in the selection of timing devices used in sports events. Timing devices must work consistently each and every time so that competitors are ensured an equal chance of winning. An example of interrater reliability is that of a classroom situation in which two evaluators are trained to use the same tool with a Likert scale to measure student performance on oral presentations.

Are the Results of the Study Applicable in the Identified Case?

Once the science of a study has been appraised and the reliability of results assessed, the next important questions are, Do the results apply to the case of interest? Are the populations in the study and in the proposed population for application similar? If the populations studied are not similar, the significance of results in the study has little value for real-life implementation in a given clinical situation.

Is the effect size sufficient so that application of the study intervention will make a significant difference? The effect size is calculated by determining the mean difference between two groups (intervention and control) and dividing by the standard deviation. It is not the same as the statistical significance, but rather is the size of the difference between two groups. The effect size is often used in meta-analysis for combining and comparing estimates from different studies so as to determine the effectiveness of an intervention. "An effect size is exactly equivalent to the Z-score of a normal standard deviation. For example an effect size of 0.8 means that the score of the average person in the experimental group is 0.8 standard deviations above the average person in the control group, and hence exceeds the scores of 79% of the control group" (Coe, 2002, p. 2). Thus,

Effect Size =

$$\frac{\text{Mean of experimental group} - \text{Mean of control group}}{\text{Standard deviation}}$$

Generally, in evaluating any quantitative study, additional questions include the following: Why was the study done? How was the sample size decided? How were the data analyzed? Were there any surprises or unexpected events that occurred during the study? How do the results of this study compare with others? (Melnyk & Fineout-Overholt, 2005).

The standard of care for practice is increasingly based on scientific evidence. Finding the most current research based on well-conducted clinical trials is an important first step. But how do we evaluate that evidence in practice? Several statistical measures help in the evaluation of study results. **Table 21-3** briefly describes some commonly used statistical tests. An excellent guide to biostatistics is also available from MedPageToday (n.d.).

What happens if the evidence conflicts with patients' values and preferences? What if our

TABLE 21-3 Clinical Statistical Measures

Clinical Statistic	Description
Odds ratio (OR)	The odds of risk for a person in the experimental group having an adverse outcome compared with a person in the control group. An odds ratio of 1 means the event is equally likely in both groups. An odds ratio greater than 1 means the event is more likely in the intervention group than the control group. An odds ratio less than 1 means the event is less likely in the intervention group than the control group. Used most in case control and retrospective studies.
Relative risk ratio (RR)	The risk of an outcome in the intervention/treatment group (Y) compared to the control group (X). RR = Y/X. A relative risk of 1 means there is no difference between the two groups. A relative risk of less than 1 means a smaller potential for the effect to occur in the intervention group than in the control group. Used most in randomized controlled trials and cohort studies.
Relative risk	The percentage of reduction in the treatment group (Y) reduction (RRR) compared with the control group (X). RRR = 1 − Y/X = 100%.
Absolute risk	The difference in risk between the control group (X) reduction (ARR) and the intervention group (Y). ARR = X − Y.
Number needed to treat (NNT)	The number of patients that must be treated over a given period of time to prevent one adverse outcome. NNT = 1/(X − Y).

Source: Long, C. O. (2009). Weighing in on the evidence. In N. A. Schmidt & J. M. Brown (Eds.), *Evidence-based practice for nurses.* Sudbury, MA: Jones and Bartlett, p. 323. Modified with permission.

own experience conflicts with the evidence? The key is that the evidence must be relevant to the problem and tested through application. In addition, some scholars (Fawcett et al., 2001; Kitson, Harvey, & McCormack, 1998; Rycroft-Malone, Seers, Titchen, Harvey, Kitson, & McCormack, 2004) insist that evidence as defined by medicine is too narrowly focused and does not recognize the complexities of nursing practice. They recommend that the definition include the influence of context in the application of evidence (Scott-Findley & Pollack, 2004). This would include findings from qualitative research.

Regardless of the definition, however, once evidence is implemented, the results must be evaluated. Did the evidence support better decision making? Was the patient's care improved? In what way was care or outcomes improved? If they were not improved, why not? (Melnyk & Fineout-Overholt, 2005).

Determining and Implementing the Best Evidence for Practice

A distinguishing feature of evidence-based nursing is that nurses treat and work with patients rather than "work on them" (McSherry, 2002). In addition, nursing's approach is more holistic, so that "effectiveness of treatment" is but one indicator; cost-effectiveness and patient acceptability also matter (McSherry, 2002). According to the Agency for Healthcare Research and Quality (AHRQ, 2002, as cited in Melnyk & Fineout-Overholt, 2005), three benchmark domains must be considered when evaluating evidence: quality, quantity, and consistency. *Quality* refers to the absence of biases due to errors in selection, measurement, and confounding biases (internal validity). *Quantity* refers to the number of relevant, related studies; total sample size across studies; size of the treatment effect; and relative risk or odds ratio strength (causality). *Consistency* refers to the similarity of findings across multiple studies regardless of differences in study design. These considerations make it essential that all types of

evidence be considered when delivering individual care and implementing systems of care. Based on these domains of evidence, a critical appraisal of types of studies can be facilitated and evaluated to determine the best approach for practice.

QUALITY IMPROVEMENT AND PATIENT-CENTERED CARE

In patient care, a process that facilitates continuous improvement is central to an environment that produces changes in practice that are patient centered and focused on care that is both evidence based and of high quality. The process must be based on a commitment by all those involved to change practice, and this commitment must be made in advance so that the research findings are applied early on in the process (French, 1999). As changes are made, they must be continuously evaluated for their impact on care and care systems. The EBP process is consistent with total quality improvement, and often the same resources can be used for both processes.

The steps in the quality management, monitoring, and evaluation processes are based on the work of William Edwards Deming, an American author, professor, statistician, and consultant best known for his work in improving manufacturing production efficiency during World War II. Deming believed that quality is based on continuous improvement of processes and that when work is focused on quality, costs decrease over time (Deming, 1986).

As an advanced practice nurse, the DNP must be constantly attuned and knowledgeable about changes in practice to ensure that current best practice is maintained within the context of empirical evidence and patients' preferences.

Conceptual Frameworks for Evidence and Practice Change

Two conceptual frameworks that help in the promotion and translation of evidence into practice are the PARIHS (promoting action on research implementation in health services) model (Rycroft-Malone et al., 2002) and the AGREE (appraisal of guidelines for research and evaluation) model (AGREE Collaboration, 2001). The PARIHS model, which is based on the work of Kitson, Harvey, and McCormack (1998), suggests that the integration of evidence is based on three factors: the nature of the evidence, the context of the desired change, and the mechanism of facilitating change. This evidence, and its translation for practice, includes practice guidelines and other forms of evidence specific to patient outcomes. The use of randomized controlled trials was central to implementation of this model. The model was revised by Rycroft-Malone et al. (2002) to include research information, clinical experience, and patient choice. In the new conceptualization, which involves continuous improvement of patient care through evidence-based nursing, there was recognition of a need for different types of evidence to answer some clinical questions. Evidence based on one's "professional craft" or experience was part of the evidence contribution (Rycroft-Malone et al., 2004).

Further work by Doran and Sidani (2007) identified gaps in the PARIHS model that led to an intervention framework that specifically addressed indicators for evaluating nursing services, systems, performance measures, and feedback to design and evaluate practice change. The intervention framework incorporates the work of Batalden and Stoltz (1993) and Batalden, Nelson, and Roberts (1994), which identified four categories of information in making care improvements. This information included "clinical (e.g., signs and symptoms), functional (e.g., activities of daily living), satisfaction (e.g., perceived benefit of care) and cost (i.e., both direct and indirect cost to the health care system and the patient)" (Doran & Sidani, 2007, p. 5). **Figure 21-3** depicts Doran and Sidhani's (2007) outcomes-focused knowledge translation intervention framework.

The purpose of the AGREE instrument, as defined by the collaborators, "is to provide a framework for assessing the quality of clinical practice guidelines" (AGREE Collaboration, 2001, p. 2). Further, "by quality . . . we mean the confidence that the potential biases of guideline development have been addressed adequately and that the recommendations are both internally and externally valid, and are feasible for practice. This process involves taking into account the benefits, harms and costs of the recommendations, as well as the practical issues attached to them. Therefore, the assessment includes the judgments about the methods used for developing the guidelines, the content of the final recommendations, and the factors linked to their uptake" (p. 2). The AGREE instrument consists of 23 items organized in six domains: scope and purpose (items 1–3), stakeholder involvement (items 4–7), rigor of development (items 8–14), clarity and presentation (items 15–18), applicability (items 19–21), and editorial independence (items 22–23). The complete instrument and user guide are available for downloading from the Internet.

The nursing faculty at one family nurse practitioner program, the Lienhard School of Nursing at Pace University, used the AGREE instrument to teach family nurse practitioner students how to critically appraise clinical practice guidelines (Singleton & Levin, 2008). In this program, students practice critiquing single studies, systematic reviews, and clinical practice guidelines. **Table 21-4** and **Table 21-5** present an exemplar of a learning activity using the AGREE instrument.

The Johns Hopkins model is another evidence-based model, which was developed as a collaborative effort between Johns Hopkins Hospital and the Johns Hopkins School of Nursing. The model is explained in six sections. Section I introduces the concept—the evolution of EBP—and the role of critical thinking in EBP. Section II describes the components of the model. The model uses the PET process (practice question, evidence, and translation). Section III further explores the PET process in developing EBP projects. Section IV describes

FIGURE 21-3 Outcomes-Focused Knowledge Translation Intervention Framework

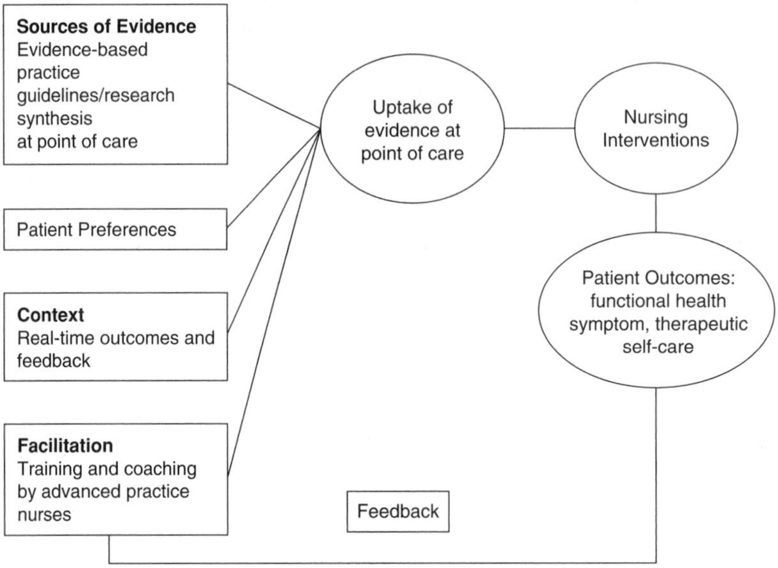

Source: Doran, D. M., & Sidani, S. (2007). Outcomes-focused knowledge translation: A framework for knowledge translation and patient outcomes improvement. *Worldviews on Evidence-Based Nursing*, 4(1), 3–13. Reproduced with permission from Blackwell Publishing, Ltd.

TABLE 21-4 Learning Activity for the Critical Appraisal of Clinical Practice Guidelines

Steps

1. Preparatory reading: Slutsky, J. (2005). Using evidence-based practice guidelines: Tools for improving practice. In B. M. Melnyk & E. Fineout-Overholt (Eds.), *Evidence-based practice in nursing and health-care: A guide to best practice* (pp. 221–227). Philadelphia: Lippincott Williams & Wilkins.

2. Focus for assignment: Academy of Breastfeeding Medicine. (2004). *Breastfeeding the near term infant (35–37 weeks gestation)*. New Rochelle, NY: Author.

3. Work in teams.

4. Obtain the guideline.

5. Use the AGREE instrument to critically appraise the guideline.

6. Report back.

Source: Singleton, J., and Levin, R. (2008). Strategies for learning evidence-based practice: Critically appraising clinical practice guidelines. *Journal of Nursing Education, 47*(8), 380–383. Modified with permission.

TABLE 21-5	Sample Domain and Items from the AGREE Instrument for Critical Appraisal of Clinical Practice Guidelines, with Rating Scale

Scope and Purpose

The overall objective(s) of the guideline is (are) specifically described.

The clinical question(s) covered by the guideline is (are) specifically described.

The patients to whom the guideline(s) is (are) meant to apply are specifically described.

Rating Scale

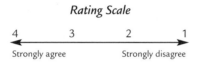

Source: Singleton, J., and Levin, R. (2008). Strategies for learning evidence-based practice: Critically appraising clinical practice guidelines. *Journal of Nursing Education, 47*(8), 380–383. Modified with permission.

the environment necessary for the success of EBP. Section V provides examples of EBP projects. Section VI contains tools used for EBP at Johns Hopkins. A table of contents and sample, including levels of evidence from the model and guidelines, can be downloaded from the Nursing Knowledge International website.

The model and guidelines have "leveled objectives" for baccalaureate-, graduate-, and doctoral-level nursing students. At the doctoral level, the focus is on reviewing, rating, synthesizing, evaluating, and translating evidence at an advanced level (Newhouse, Dearholt, Poe, Pugh, & White, 2008). An example of one evidence-based project, developed by the Neuroscience Nursing Practice Committee, is a question related to the correct procedure for establishing nasogastric tube placement in adult patients. Using the PICO (patient, intervention, comparison, and outcomes) format and levels of evidence, the existing protocol that required insufflations of air was discontinued. A table of the process and levels of evidence is shown in the Johns Hopkins model instructor's guide (Newhouse et al., 2008), available on the Internet.

Designing and Implementing Processes to Evaluate Outcomes of Practice and Systems of Care

As nursing moves practice decisions from those based on tradition to those based on empirical evidence, the advanced practice nurse, particularly the DNP, is in the best position to effect and assess change within the clinical setting. Why? Evidence-based practice and quality management are both practice-driven processes (French, 1999). Each is informed by experience and outcomes that can be directly seen and measured. In most cases, the observations and questions that arise during daily practice provide the basis for the questions, which can be empirically tested and their results implemented and evaluated. The findings of previous research studies can be replicated in a variety of settings with resources that are already in place.

The curriculum of DNP programs includes specialty-focused competencies delineated by specialty nursing organizations, and the core essentials include courses and application experiences in research methods and statistical analysis (AACN, 2006). This education, coupled with advanced clinical knowledge, provides the DNP with the requisites necessary to design and collaborate in studies that can make a practical difference in the delivery of clinical care (French, 1999; Reavy & Tavernier, 2008). **Table 21-6** lists some examples of clinical studies concerning advanced practice nursing interventions and outcomes, as well as studies or interventions designed by DNPs.

The Essentials of Doctoral Education for Advanced Practice Nursing (AACN, 2006) states that "DNP graduates must understand principles of practice management, including conceptual and practice strategies for balancing productivity and quality care" (p. 4). In addition, "they must be able to assess the impact of clinical policies and procedures on meeting the health needs of the patient populations with whom they practice" (p. 4). Also, "they must be proficient in quality improvement strategies and in creating and sustaining changes at the organizational and policy levels" (p. 4).

Quality Improvement Initiatives to Promote Safe, Timely, Effective, Efficient, Equitable, and Patient-Centered Care

The design of quality improvement initiatives must be empirically based and dependent on sources of knowledge that include research evidence, clinical experience, reasoning, authority, quality improvement data, and the patient's situation, values, and experience (Brown, 2005). These are the tools that can help the DNP decide whether the clinical guidelines and scientific evidence are consistent with the context, values, and desires of the patient (Glanville, Schirm, & Wineman, 2000).

For the past century, most outcome measurement has been focused on the outcomes of medical care, particularly negative outcomes. However, in the past several years there has been a greater focus on positive indicators of nursing care delivery (Melnyk & Fineout-Overholt, 2005). The development of nurse-sensitive

patient outcomes (NSPOs) was an outgrowth of public demand for greater accountability by healthcare providers.

Some examples of nurse-sensitive indicators of quality include health-promoting behaviors (Mitchell, Ferketich, & Jennings, 1998), compliance/adherence (Ingersoll, McIntosh, & Williams, 2000), quality of life (Ingersoll et al., 2000), support systems available to assist with caregiver burden (Craft-Rosenburg, Krajicek, & Shin, 2002), trust in care provider (Ingersoll et al., 2000), and length of stay (Hodge, Asch, Olson, Kravitz, & Sauve, 2002). **Table 21-7** presents additional examples of evidence-based outcome indicators.

The success of evidence-based practice depends on asking the right questions at the right time, critically analyzing results of other studies for fit in a given situation, observing for differences in responses, and evaluating. In this regard, quality improvement evaluation is important in advanced practice to ascertain the impact of interventions and their effect on cost-effective care. DNP and advanced practice nurse (APN) interventions are appropriately evaluated on the basis of physiological, psychosocial, functional, behavioral, and knowledge-focused effectiveness (Glanville et al., 2000). The evaluation process involves the selection of appropriate measurement instruments. Glanville et al. (2000) make the point that instruments that measure effectiveness in care processes are not the same as those that measure outcomes. For example, a tool that measures risk for patient infections is not the same tool as one that actually tracks infection rates in a group of postsurgical patients. Similarly, in process management the focus is on which components produce or contribute to practice variations that may ultimately affect, but are not the same as, outcomes (Ingersoll, 2005).

Some basic provisions for an effective outcomes model are to keep the outcomes as short as possible; to use outcomes, not activities or processes; and to use singular, not compound, outcomes (Duignan, 2006). Components of an

TABLE 21-6 Selected Studies of Advanced Practice Nursing Interventions and Outcomes

Advanced Practice Nursing (APN) Interventions and Outcomes

Author and Date of Publication	Design, Sample and Setting	Interventions	Outcome Variables	Findings
Scarbrough & Landis (1997)[a]	Descriptive. 431 patients on three units (FNPs); 821 patients on three units (MDs & RNs). Community hospital; 3-month study.	Evaluated two methods of implementing a hospital-based immunization program. Determined interest, obtained informed consent, administered vaccine, provided education, documented care.	Documentation on patient medication administration record	69 of 431 patients received vaccines in FNP group; 10 of 821 pts. received vaccine in MD/RN group. Conclusion: FNPs administered vaccine at a higher rate.
Naylor et al. (1999)[a]	Randomized controlled trial. Hospitalized adults older than 65 years at discharge. Intervention group (*n* = 177); control group (*n* = 186). Data at 2, 6, 12, and 24 weeks postdischarge at two urban academically affiliated medical centers.	APNs administered standardized discharge protocol for elders at risk for readmission. Included APN visits within 48 hours of admission, every 48 hours during admission, and two home visits within 48 hours of discharge and as needed. On-call availability 24 hours and weekly phone calls.	Readmissions; time to readmission; acute care visits after discharge; functional status; patient satisfaction; cost	Intervention-group patients had fewer hospital days per patient; time to first readmission was prolonged to 24 weeks. Medicare reimbursement was $0.6 million for intervention group versus $1.2 million for control group. No significant differences in acute care visits, functional status, depression, or patient satisfaction. Conclusion: APN-centered discharge plan and home care intervention for at-risk hospitalized older adults promotes positive outcomes and decreases cost.

(continues)

TABLE 21-6 Selected Studies of Advanced Practice Nursing Interventions and Outcomes *(continued)*

Author and Date of Publication	Design, Sample and Setting	Interventions	Outcome Variables	Findings
Burns & Earven (2002)[a]	Descriptive. Patients requiring long-term ventilation in medical intensive care unit (MICU). $N = 669$ patients in 6-year period. Large university medical center.	APNs provided interventions based on pathways from scientific evidence. APNs worked on monitoring patient progress, prevention of complications, and coordinating care.	Length of stay (LOS); duration of ventilation; extubation status; reintubation; complications; discharge placement; cost	Decrease in the mean number of ventilator days; decreased mean LOS; decreased mean MICU LOS; decreased cost. Researchers concluded that APNs were effective in improving a number of outcomes in this population of highly complex patients.
Studies by Doctors of Nursing Practice (DNPs)				
Andrews (2008)	Case study. Rare disease diagnosis: pheochromocytoma genetics, 40-year-old African American man with refractory hypertension presenting to ER.	Holistic evidence-based approach to clinical history taking and evaluation for correct diagnosis.	Lab tests; assessment of diagnostic clues and probability characteristics; genetic pedigree analysis; BP management; surgical intervention; genetic testing	Advanced practice nurses' well-honed evidence-based approach and interview skills allowed them to play a pivotal role in the exploration, diagnosis, and management of this type of complex situation.
Doyle-Lindrud (2008)	Case study. Gestational breast cancer; 33-year-old Asian woman with breast lump and positive pregnancy test. Outpatient cancer center.	Health history and examination; health promotion; anticipatory guidance; collaborative approach to care; chronic disease management.	Lab tests; radiology; long-term follow-up care; psychosocial care; chronic care management	The DNP elements of doctoral competency were illustrated in the evaluation, collaboration, anticipatory planning, and management of care in this complex situation.

TABLE 21-6 Selected Studies of Advanced Practice Nursing Interventions and Outcomes *(continued)*

Author and Date of Publication	Design, Sample and Setting	Interventions	Outcome Variables	Findings
Dohrn (2008)	Case study. HIV treatment for pregnant women in rural Eastern Cape, South Africa, an area with 30–35% HIV prevalence and less than half of facilities providing prevention interventions. Pregnant women enter antenatal care after 24 weeks.	Design of midwifery model of care; interviews; observations; self-assessment of skills and capacity to deliver HIV care.	Voluntary testing and counseling; mother-to-child prevention intervention; antiretroviral treatment; peer counseling; community worker outreach; fast-tracking for antiretroviral therapy; maternity nurse training; anticipatory counseling; early postpartum care/ education; midwife training; nurse mentoring; communication between nurses/MDs; strengthening community worker role.	Study resulted in consensus on model of care for HIV-infected women that included HIV prevention, testing, and management that has the potential to affect qualitatively and quantitatively the health of South Africans by decreasing the number of infants born with HIV, decreasing maternal mortality and the number of AIDS orphans, and improving quality of life.

aFrom Cunningham, R. S. (2004). Advanced practice nursing outcomes: A review of selected empirical literature. *Oncology Nursing Forum, 21*(2), 219–230.

TABLE 21-7	Selected Evidence-Based Outcome Indicators for Advanced Practice Nursing
Outcomes	Examples and Indicators
Patient satisfaction	Ambulatory care: Survey
Risk	Morbidity and mortality: Summary
	Patient falls: Reports
	Medication errors: Medication administration records (MARs); comprehensiveness of exams
Knowledge	Blood pressure medication: Blood pressure control
Condition specific	Postoperative pain: Pain management scale
	Diabetes management: Blood glucose levels
Infection control	Surgical procedures: Hand washing; nosocomial infection rates
Compliance	Fluid restriction: Daily weights
	Prenatal and postpartum visits

effective outcomes management model include the following:

> 1) identification of the problem, 2) scanning the existing evidence and standards of care, 3) identification of benchmark targets, 4) determination and selection of outcomes measuring and monitoring tools, 5) development of specific guidelines to drive care delivery processes, 6) assessment of existing processes, 7) measurement and monitoring of processes and outcomes of care, 8) reporting findings to key stakeholders and decision makers, and 9) refining care delivery processes and data collection techniques based on findings. (Ingersoll, 2005, pp. 314–315)

A significant time commitment is required for designing systems for promoting safe, timely, patient-centered care. However, the benefits are efficiency and effectiveness. Since the Institute of Medicine (IOM) studies, patient safety has been a primary focus of quality improvement initiatives. Safety issues are of concern in every care setting—primary, secondary, and tertiary. A review of the literature from 1995 to 2009 in the Medline and CINAHL databases produced 136

(Medline) and 51 (CINAHL) nursing studies that involved quality improvement projects with safety as a focus. Only 4 studies included the word "evidence" in the title. Topics included studies on drug errors, environment, technology, acute care, pediatrics, critical care, culture, intravenous infusions, long-term care and home health, rural health, legislation and oversight, policy, diabetes, anesthesia, health education, chemotherapy, childhood vaccines, blood and HIV, neuroscience issues, food and drug issues, nurse injury, radiation, emergency services, and behavioral health. In addition to safety issues, a number of studies dealt with issues of timely (24 studies in CINAHL), effective (13,000 studies in CINAHL), and equitable care (467 studies in CINAHL), which are also important dimensions of quality and need to be addressed, especially as they affect safety and quality outcomes. Patient-centered care was addressed in 6,100 CINAHL studies. Direct care providers, including DNPs, must take a lead role in continuing the effort to improve care delivery systems that benefit patients, families, and providers of care.

Using Practice Guidelines to Improve Practice and the Practice Environment

As Goolsby, Meyers, Johnson, Klardie, and McNaughton (2004) have noted, "clinical practice guidelines are protocol-driven, step-wise recommendations for diagnosing, and treating specific conditions, or patient populations" (p. 178). Clinical decision making is grounded in the use of clinical research, expert opinion, and clinical practice guidelines. Further, clinical practice guidelines "minimize differences in practice patterns and the risk of misdiagnosis or treatment failures" (Goolsby, Meyers, et al., 2004, p. 178). Unfortunately, practice guidelines are not always used, for a variety of reasons. Time, communication, involvement, resources, patient expectations, and perceived priority are all facilitators or barriers to the implementation of evidence-based practice guidelines (DiCenso, Cullum, & Ciliska, 1998; Gagan & Hewitt-Taylor, 2004; Lopez-Bushnell, 2002; McCaughan, Thompson, Cullum, Sheldon, & Thompson, 2002; Rutledge & Bookbinder, 2002).

One way to eliminate some of the barriers is through the use of "linkage agents." As described by Cooke et al. (2004), advanced practice nurses (particularly DNPs) are in an excellent position to propose scientifically based recommendations to reduce cost and improve quality, documentation, and outcomes. In developing an institutional change model to promote evidence-based practice with cancer patients, the linking agents from the nursing research department at one hospital functioned as rotating consultants three to four hours per month. The linking agent consultants rotated to clinical units for one hour of monthly case presentation and analysis to assist clinical nurses in translating research into practice. The theoretical framework used was a quality of life model with four domains: psychological, social, physical, and spiritual (Padilla, Ferrell, Grant, & Rhiner, 1990). Each month one or more topics related to the four domains was discussed relevant to a case study. A brief five-minute lecture was presented on EBP principles at the beginning of the session. The program started as a research outreach program and evolved into an EBP program that linked a case study format with critical thinking and practical application. This approach could be modified and used in a variety of clinical practice settings.

EVALUATION OF PRACTICE

> He who every morning plans the transaction of the day and follows out that plan, carries a thread that will guide him through the maze of the most busy life. But where no plan is laid, where the disposal of time is surrendered merely to the chance of incidence, chaos will soon reign.
>
> —*Victor Hugo*

Evaluating practice and changes in practice are essential to the successful implementation of any quality improvement or evidence-based practice initiative. Evaluation is an ongoing process that must start early in a project and be continual. Planning for evaluation is as important as the change itself and must be a systematic process. Classification schemes allow an organized approach to evaluating outcomes. Outcomes may be classified according to population served (e.g., pediatric, adult, geriatric), time (long term, medium term, or short term), or type (care related, patient related, or performance related) (Schmidt & Brown, 2009).

Using Benchmarks to Evaluate Clinical Outcomes and Trends

One method of evaluating practice is to evaluate practice patterns against national benchmarks to determine variances in clinical outcomes and population trends. Benchmarking is "the continual process of measuring services and practices against the toughest competitors in the industry" (Hebda & Czar, 2009). Organizations that regularly collect data on outcomes in health care are state boards of health and the Centers of Medicare and Medicaid Services (CMS). The Joint Commission on

Accreditation of Hospitals (JCAHO; now known simply as The Joint Commission) and the Magnet Recognition Program (American Nurses Credentialing Center, 2005) also have performance measurement standards that are based on quality indicators. In addition to these organizations, many hospitals and healthcare facilities have memberships in organizations that benchmark indicators of quality in specialty services (Schmidt & Brown, 2009).

Nursing services are an important aspect of outcome evaluation and reporting at any healthcare institution because nurses make up such a large part of the healthcare workforce. Effectiveness of nursing care is determined by nurse-sensitive indicators. Nursing administrators are responsible for maintaining evaluation systems and reporting nurse-sensitive outcomes. As leaders in clinical care and outcome evaluation, DNPs must be in the forefront of designing outcome evaluation plans for advanced practice.

DNPs in advanced practice roles are also included in medical outcome working groups within their scope of practice. The American Medical Association–Physician Consortium for Performance Improvement (AMA-PCPI) has performance measures available for 31 topics or conditions (Gallagher, 2009). The general approach to measurement includes six steps: "1) identifying the opportunities for improvement, 2) involving representation from medical specialties and other care disciplines, 3) linking measures to an evidence base, 4) supporting clinical judgment and patient preferences, 5) testing measures, and 6) promoting a single set of measures for widespread use and multiple purpose" (Gallagher, 2009, p. 185). **Table 21-8** contains a brief listing of websites for healthcare outcomes and data.

TABLE 21-8	Websites for Healthcare Outcome Information
Organization	Website
AcademyHealth	http://www.academyhealth.org
Agency for Healthcare	http://www.ahrq.gov/clinic/outcome.htm Research and Quality
Centers for Medicare and Medicaid Services	http://www.cns.hhs.gov/home/rsds.asp
Health Care Excel	http://hce.org
Institute for Healthcare	http://www.ihi.org Improvement
The Joint Commission	http://www.jointcommission.org
National Cancer Institute	http://outcomes.cancer.gov
National Committee for Quality Assurance	http://www.ncqa.org
National Quality Forum	http://www.qualityforum.org
University of Iowa College of Nursing	http://www.nursing.uiowa.edu/excellence/nursing_knowledge /clinical_effectiveness/nocoverview.htm

Source: Rich, K. A. (2009). Evaluating outcomes of innovations. In N. A. Schmidt & J. M. Brown (Eds.), *Evidence-based practice for nurses.* Sudbury, MA: Jones and Bartlett, p. 388. Modified with permission.

Guiding Database Design to Generate Meaningful Evidence for Nursing Practice

A systematic process for collecting patient care and practice data is essential to guide practice. This requires the development of standardized databases to guide outcomes research for practice. Clinical databases from computerized medical records and disease registries exist as the result of documentation of care or research protocols. Outcome data are also available from birth logs, death records, discharge summaries, and clinical pathways. Most important, the outcome must be measurable and the data must relate to the care processes or interventions (Arthur, Marfell, & Ulrich, 2009).

Another useful source of evidence based on outcomes is the National Guideline Clearinghouse (NGC), an initiative of the Agency for Healthcare Research and Quality (AHRQ), the American Medical Association, and America's Health Insurance Plans (AHIP). Users can subscribe to the NGC weekly e-mail update service. The site provides information about new and updated guidelines from the Centers for Disease Control and Prevention (CDC), the National Institute for Clinical Excellence (NICE), the Program for Evidence-Based Care (PEBC), and others. Conference information is also available, as well as food and drug advisory information.

The Cochrane Collaboration Review is another source that provides reprints online of the newest intervention reviews. The Review lists authors and their affiliations; an abstract including background, objectives, search strategies, selection criteria, data collection, and analysis; authors' conclusions; and a plain-language summary. The library contains sections for clinicians, researchers, patients, and policy makers. The Cochrane Library, a collection of medical and healthcare databases, is available online through Wiley InterScience. Podcasts are also available.

These and other evidence-based resources are effective tools to aid in the efficient delivery of evidence-based care. **Table 21-9** provides a brief description of other available databases. The use of these resources is valuable when combined with the best empirical knowledge and judgment. The true measure of their effectiveness is in the evaluation of the outcomes of management and care decisions and delivery processes.

As nursing takes on larger, more autonomous roles in the delivery of health care through advanced practice, the need for accountability will continue to increase. DNPs, with their knowledge of clinical practice, research, and informatics, can best represent advanced practice nursing by participating in and guiding the development of databases that are relevant to the care that DNPs and advanced practice nurses provide. Becoming involved in professional organizations that have quality initiatives is an excellent way for DNPs to become knowledgeable in research that contributes to quality care and the profession. The ANA and specialty organizations such as the Oncology Nursing Society, the Advanced Practice Registered Nurses' Research Network, and the Midwest Nursing Centers Consortium Research Network, a practice-based research network funded by the AHRQ, provide avenues for collaboration and dissemination of information on quality and outcomes (Burns & Grove, 2009).

THE USE OF INFORMATION TECHNOLOGY AND RESEARCH METHODS

Computers have changed the face of clinical care, making them a necessary tool for research and evidence-based practice. They provide efficiency in the inputting of statistical data and the retrieval of the most current information on relevant clinical trial outcomes, supportive research, and accepted practice protocols. It is essential to pay attention to the kind of data that is retrieved and how those data are used to make clinical decisions and evaluate practice.

TABLE 21-9	Evidence Databases
Source	**Content**
ACP Journal Club	Articles reporting original studies and systematic reviews.
Agency for Healthcare Quality and Research	Produces guidelines and technology assessments on selected topics from 12 evidence-based practice (AHRQ) centers.
AIDSLINE	Indexes the published literature on HIV and AIDS. The index includes journal articles, monographs, meeting abstracts and papers, newsletters, and government reports (Fain, 2009).
Bandolier	Reviews literature; offers subjects by medical specialty.
CANCERLIT	Includes cancer literature from journal articles, government reports, technical reports, meeting abstracts and papers, and monographs.
CDC Sexually Transmitted Disease Treatment Guidelines	Includes Web-browsable source with cross-links.
Cochrane Database of Systematic Reviews	"[R]eviews individual clinical trials and summarizes systematic reviews from over 100 medical journals" (Fain, 2009, p. 277).
DynaMed	Point-of-care resource to support clinical decision making.
EPPI	Evidence for Policy and Practice Information and Coordinating Center, Institute of Education, University of London.
Essential Evidence Plus (Formerly InfoPOEMS)	Includes reviews and commentary of recently published articles by the *Journal of Family Practice*.
Evidence-Based Practice at the University of Iowa (http://www .uihealthcare./depts/nursing/rqom /evidencebasedpractice/index.html)	Includes an evidence-based practice toolkit, information about recent evidence-based practice projects, and an evidence-based practice model and resources.
HealthLinks: Evidence-Based Practice (http://healthlinks .washington.edu/ebp)	Includes metasearch engines and links to peer-reviewed journals, a DNP toolkit, and other publications.
HealthSTAR	Indexes materials from books, book chapters, government documents, newspaper articles, and technical reports. The focus is the clinical and nonclinical aspects of healthcare delivery.
HSTAT	Health Services Technology Assessment Text; full-text guidelines.
Joanna Briggs Institute	International institute that provides resources for evidence-based practice for healthcare professionals in nursing, medicine, midwifery, and allied health.
Johns Hopkins Evidence-Based Practice Center Projects	Includes systematic reviews of evidence.

TABLE 21-9	Evidence Databases *(continued)*
Source	**Content**
MD Consult	Includes full-text access to journal articles, textbooks, practice guidelines, patient education handouts, and drug awareness information. MD Consult is a good, quick source for background information on a topic.
Medline	A compilation of information from Index Medicus, Index to Dental Literature, and the International Nursing Index. It includes published research in allied health, biological sciences, information sciences, physical sciences, and the humanities.
MedPage Today	Includes daily research updates, news by specialty, policy news, CMEs, and surveys. Includes an excellent tool, The MedPage Guide to Biostatistics, that can be used as a reference guide when reading research articles.
National Guideline Clearinghouse	Provides nonintegrated evidence-based practice clinical guidelines and recommendations on selected topics from a number of organizations.
Prescriber's Letter	Includes evidence-based information on new drug developments, with links to articles and continuing education offerings.
PubMed	Provides source for queries and evidence-based filters for Medline.
ScHarr	School of Health and Related Research; comprehensive, up-to-date evidence on the Web.
TRIPCeRes	British meta-search engine. Covers 58 different resources for evidence.
University of Minnesota (http://evidence.abc.umn.edu/ebn.htm)	Links and EBP tutorial with case scenarios.

Source: Fain, J. A. (2009). *Understanding evidence-based practice: Reading, understanding and applying nursing research* (3rd ed.). Philadelphia: F. A. Davis, pp. 276–278. Modified with permission.

Collecting Appropriate and Accurate Data

Data and observations from practice can be augmented and strengthened through evidence from clinical trials. There are several electronic databases that provide access to clinical trial data and other peer-reviewed research and outcome data. However, clinical trial data and data from other aggregate sources do not always address the outcomes that can be uniquely attributed to APN/DNP practice. For APN/DNPs to assess and demonstrate their effectiveness, data are needed that reflect what they do. Although the primary goal of outcome data and analysis is to improve care, DNPs in direct practice may be asked to justify their roles in terms of factors such as cost, time, patient outcomes, and revenue generation, among other indicators (Burns, 2009).

Most institutions rely on aggregated data to determine nursing outcomes. Unfortunately, most aggregated data do not show the APN/DNP's specific contribution to the outcomes (Burns, 2009). For this reason it is important that measures be selected that truly reflect the APN/DNP role. This means developing role-sensitive indicators and collecting data that are specific to those indicators in a systematic way. Indicators such as satisfaction with APN/DNP care related to a particular program or procedure that the APN/DNP initiates, controls, or coordinates are better than trying to extrapolate the APN/DNP's role in a multidisciplinary effort. Time savings or clinical outcomes related to a change in practice coordinated by the APN/DNP may also be role sensitive.

A well-designed assessment plan uses a model that considers organizational factors, employee behavior, patient characteristics, patient experience, and outcomes (Minnick & Roberts, 1991, Figure 25.1, as cited in Minnick, 2009). Instruments for measuring outcomes are also a necessary component in the assessment process. A systematic search of the databases mentioned in Table 21-9, such as AHRQ, PubMed, CancerLit, CINAHL, and PsycINFO, may be helpful as a starting place for appropriate measurement tools.

Analyzing Data from Clinical Practice

Data from practice are rich and can be analyzed in a number of ways, depending on the nature of the research question. Computer-based statistical tools such as absolute risk (AR) and absolute risk reduction (ARR) calculations, relative risk (RR) and relative risk reduction (RRR) calculations, number needed to treat (NNT), survival curves, hazard ratios, and sensitivity and specificity are helpful measures for assessing risk of disease in studies of different cohort groups and in aiding clinical decision making. In an excellent article in *Journal of the American Academy of Nurse Practitioners,* Goolsby, Klardie, Johnson, McNaughton, and Meyers (2004) analyzed the implementation of clinical practice guidelines (CPGs) and their outcomes in a hypothetical patient situation. The analysis includes a review of commonly used statistical concepts, including some of those just mentioned, with examples of their application in interpreting and reporting

research. Johnston (2005) also provides a detailed section on statistical measures and their meaning in a chapter entitled "Critically Appraising Quantitative Evidence."

Designing Evidence-Based Interventions

Selecting and defining the problem is one of the most critical steps in the design of any evidence-based intervention. The problem statement provides the direction for the study design and is usually stated at the beginning. Essential to good design is adequate background information that includes a rationale for pursuing an intervention, evidence from research that has already been done on the topic, and the goals to be achieved (Fain, 2009). Depending on the problem to be addressed, evidence-based interventions may be generated from quantitative research, qualitative research, outcome studies, patient concerns and choices, or clinical judgment.

Models serve as good frameworks for design. Several models that were originally designed for research utilization were the historical precursors to evidence-based practice. Four well-known models for research utilization and evidence-based practice include the conduct and utilization of research in nursing (CURN) model (Horsely, Crane, & Bingle, 1978), the Kitson model (Kitson, Harvey, & McCormack, 1998), the Stetler/Marram model (Stetler, 1994; Stetler & Marram, 1976), and the Iowa model of research utilization (Titler et al., 1994). As evidence-based practice has evolved, these models have been adapted, and other models have been developed. Some later models include the ARCC model (Melnyk & Fineout-Overholt, 2002), the Rosswurm and Larrabee model (1999), the Iowa model of evidence-based practice to promote quality care (Titler, 2002), and the Johns Hopkins model (Newhouse et al., 2008). Each of these models has been successful in disseminating research or in facilitating change toward evidence-based practice. **Figure 21-4** shows a schematic of the Iowa model.

FIGURE 21-4 The Iowa Model of Evidence-Based Practice to Promote Quality Care

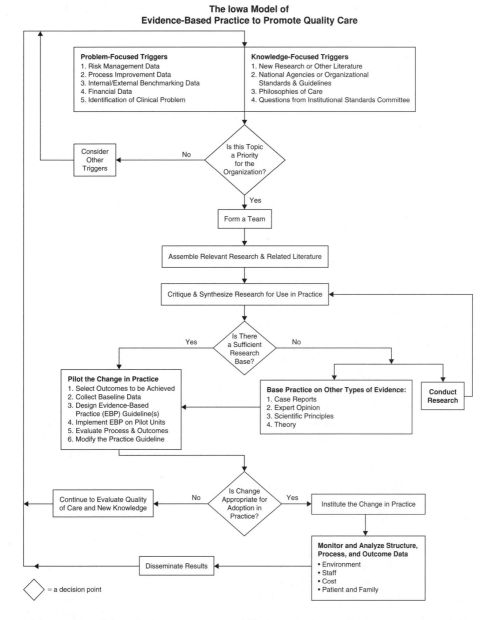

**The Iowa Model of
Evidence-Based Practice to Promote Quality Care**

Source: Titler, M. G., Klieber, C., Steelman, V. J., Rakel, B. A., Budreau, G., Everett, L. Q., et al. (2001). The Iowa model of evidence-based practice to promote quality care. *Critical Care Nursing Clinics of North America, 13*(4), 497–509. Reproduced with permission.

It is beyond the scope of this chapter to detail the specifics of each model. However, although there are nuances and structural differences, all of the models support some form of practice change through the systematic review of research and other evidence, such as clinical practice guidelines, to create a culture of research conduct and research utilization. Certainly, the first step in the design of any practice intervention is to define the clinical practice questions. Once that is accomplished, critical questions include the following: Which patients will be affected? Which treatment or intervention or practice change is involved? Which old practice would need to be discontinued? Which outcomes are expected? (Collins et al., 2008). The next step is to review the evidence, basing the analysis on the hierarchy of evidence (see Table 21-1) and a search of all relevant databases (e.g., Cochrane, CINAHL, National Guideline Clearing House). Once the evidence has been verified, assessing applicability to the population and environment is crucial. Questions to be considered may include the following: Will implementing this practice increase patient safety? Are there ethical or legal considerations? Will other departments or providers be affected? How will the change affect practitioner time? How will patients react to the change? The next step is to develop a plan for the change. Who are the key stakeholders? How will they be apprised and included? Who has final sign-off authority? Is a pilot study indicated before full-scale implementation? Finally, determine the methods of education and communication. How much time, cost, and personnel resources will be needed?

When implementing the plan, the following questions should be considered: Who is responsible for coordinating the effort? Which contingency plans are in place in the event a change must be made? Who is managing issues that may arise? Evaluate the implementation on an ongoing basis. How will feedback be generated? Who will conduct the evaluation? What is the method of analysis? What are the measurement tools? How will results of the evaluation be presented? (Collins et al., 2008). Some specific strategies to promote guideline implementation are outlined by Carey, Buchan, and Sanson-Fisher (2009). **Table 21-10** summarizes their recommendations.

Predicting and Analyzing Outcomes

Often in clinical practice the occurrence of one event in time may be the basis for predicting a future event. In such instances a predictive relationship is established. In this case, the practitioner or researcher is looking for a correlation between the two events that may predict the outcome of a future intervention or occurrence that could be designed to affect or influence the independent variable. Although correlational prediction is not the same as cause and effect, it is stronger than a purely descriptive study (Melnyk & Cole, 2005). This type of study would be appropriate if, for example, the DNP were interested in how a person's initial attitude toward insulin affected compliance with the regimen 3, 6, or 12 months after the therapy began.

Correlation statistics would be used to measure the relationship between the two variables. The results of the correlation could later be used to design interventions, such as educational strategies or follow-up programs, that would help those with negative attitudes toward therapy learn, adapt, and achieve more positive outcomes. Correlational statistics are also used to measure the strength of relationship between two variables. A direct correlation is seen in correlation coefficients between the values of 0 (no correlation) and 1 (large positive correlation) and means that when there is a large change in the value of one predictor, there is a large change in the value of the other predictor; likewise, a small change in one predictor is accompanied by a small change in the other predictor. A relationship that has a correlation coefficient of 0.5 is stronger than 0, but less than 1.0. Conversely, in a negative correlation—between 0 (no correlation) and –1 (large negative correlation)—large changes in the value of

TABLE 21-10	Strategies to Promote Guideline Implementation: Theoretical Constructs and Examples of Application

Strategy	Relevant Constructs	Key Illustrative Examples
Phase 1		
Concrete and specific recommendations	Knowledge, executability, decidability	Concrete and specific recommendations were more likely to be adopted by general practitioners (GPs) than vague, nonspecific recommendations. Observational study. (Grol et al., 1998)
Identify priorities	Goal setting, action planning	Of 228 primary care patients with cardiovascular disease risk factors who made an action plan to identify behavioral change goals, 53% also reported making behavioral change related to their action plan. Descriptive study. (Handley et al., 2006)
Set targets for implementation	Goal setting	
Present a rationale	Beliefs, attitudes, perceived relative advantage	Recommendations compatible with current values were more likely to be adopted by GPs than those perceived as controversial or incompatible with values. Observational study. (Grol et al., 1998)
Highlight clinical norms	Normative beliefs, attitudes, modeling/verbal persuasion	An intervention to improve myocardial infarction care that involved using local medical opinion leaders to influence peers through small-group discussions, informal consultation, and revisions of clinical protocols was compared with performance feedback alone. Hospitals in both groups improved from baseline to follow-up on indicators of quality; however, the improvement was greatest for those allocated to the peer intervention. Randomized controlled trial. (Soumarai et al., 1998)
Orient to the need of the end user	Complexity	Among the guideline characteristics most commonly endorsed to promote use by GPs was "clarity, simplicity and availability of a short format." Descriptive study of 391 GPs. (Watkins et al., 1999)
Phase 2		
Skills training	Skills, knowledge, self-efficacy	Continuing medical education (CME) improves knowledge, skills, attitudes, and patient outcomes. CME that is interactive, uses multimedia, live media, and involves multiple exposures is more effective than other types. Systematic review. (Marinopoulos et al., 2007)

(continues)

TABLE 21-10	Strategies to Promote Guideline Implementation: Theoretical Constructs and Examples of Application *(continued)*	
Strategy	Relevant Constructs	Key Illustrative Examples
Phase 2 (continued)		
Social influences	Normative beliefs, attitudes, modeling, verbal persuasion	The use of local opinion leaders in hospital settings can be effective in promoting evidence-based practice. Systematic review of 12 studies. (Doumitt et al., 2007)
Environmental influences	Cues to action, environmental triggers	Guideline adherence improved due to the implementation of a computerized clinical decision aid that gave clinicians real-time recommendations for venous thromboembolism prophylaxis. Time series study. (Durieux et al., 2000)
Patient-mediated	Knowledge, skills, and attitudes of patients	Patient requests for a new drug and patient acceptability were cited as contributing to decisions to prescribe a new drug in approximately 20% of cases. Descriptive study. (Prosser, Almond, & Walley, 2003)
Feedback	Positive/negative reinforcement; goal setting; skill development	Audit and feedback are effective strategies for improving care, particularly when baseline adherence to the recommended practice is low. Systematic review of 118 studies. (Jamtvedt et al., 2006)
Incentives	Positive/negative reinforcement	Five of six studies examining physician-level incentives, and seven of nine studies examining provider group–level incentives demonstrated partial or positive effects on quality indicators. Systematic review. (Peterson et al., 2006)
Phase 3		
Pilot testing with iterative refinement of implementation strategies	Perceived advantages; beliefs; trialability	Breakthrough collaborative model intervention that involved a series of iterative plan–do–study–act cycles was found to be effective in improving care for chronic heart failure. Quasi-experimental, controlled study. (Asch et al., 2005)

Source: Carey, M., Buchan, H., & Sanson-Fisher, R. (2009). The cycle of change: Implementing the best-evidence clinical practice. *International Journal for Quality in Health Care, 21*(1), 37–43. Reproduced with permission.

one predictor would be accompanied by small changes in the other, or small changes in one would be accompanied by large changes in the other. Therefore, a negative correlation coefficient of -0.6 shows a stronger negative relationship between two variables than a coefficient of 0, but not as strong as a coefficient of -1.0 (Lanthier, 2002).

An example of this kind of analysis is shown in a correlation study on salary and income levels. **Table 21-11** shows salary levels and corresponding years of education. **Figure 21-5** shows an example of a correlation scatter plot, with years of education on the *y* axis and income on the *x* axis. Each point on the plot shows one person's answers to the questions regarding years of education and income. In a positive correlation such as this, the line is always in the upward direction. In another example, **Table 21-12** and **Figure 21-6** show a negative relationship between grade point average (GPA) and number of hours watching television. The scatter plot (Figure 21-6) shows the direction of the line when the correlation is negative. In these cases, the researcher is measuring conditions that already exist and looking for relationships—either positive or negative.

Examining Patterns of Behavior and Outcomes

Although much of the research and evidence for practice is focused on cause and effect, patterns of behavior, dispositions, and attitudes are also outcomes that require examination. Behavioral theories can be classified as intrapersonal (individual), interpersonal (relational), and community based. The stages of change model (Prochaska & DiClemente, 1986), the health belief model (Rosenstock, 1966), and the theory of reasoned action (Fishbein & Ajzen, 1980) are useful in examining behaviors and their relationship to outcomes.

One way of examining data is through the use of aggregated data derived from large data sets. Organizations such as AHRQ, the CDC,

the National Institute for Child Health and Development (NICHD), and the National Institutes of Health (NIH) have large national data sets from various sources, such as quality of life surveys, hospital discharge data, and infection control data. The data sets can be accessed or purchased to allow researchers to develop clinical, behavioral, or interventional outcome questions that can be statistically analyzed. The advantage of this kind of analysis is that the data sets are large enough to provide an adequate sample and effect size from which to generalize intervention effects. AHRQ also maintains a database of comparative effectiveness reviews that synthesizes information from the most current studies on numerous diseases through the Evidence-Based Practice Centers (AHRQ, 2009).

In addition to aggregated evidence, clinical trial data, and comparative effectiveness reviews, some innovative healthcare systems are bringing "'practice-based evidence' to the bedside or work setting in aggregate form so that providers have the most up-to-date information available on outcomes before evidence based interventions are begun" (Lambert & Burlingame, 2009, p. 1). As an example, this kind of decision support has been trialed in the Mental Health Services Centers for the state of Utah. The state partnered with an outcomes measurement vendor (OQ, LLC) to provide aggregated evidence from clinical trials and laboratory research that resulted in a five-minute self-report outcome measurement for patients in any setting—outpatient, inpatient, or residential. Adult patients use a handheld personal digital assistant (PDA), computer kiosk, or paper survey to report information to clinicians based on the domains of symptomatic distress, interpersonal relations, and functional ability. Adolescents and parent/guardians provide information on age-normed questionnaires. The scoring is derived from empirically tested software that alerts the provider that a patient is at risk for a less than optimal outcome from treatment and gives the

TABLE 21-11 Salary and Years of Education

Participant	Income	Years of Education
#1	125,000	19
#2	100,000	20
#3	40,000	16
#4	35,000	16
#5	41,000	18
#6	29,000	12
#7	35,000	14
#8	24,000	12
#9	50,000	16
#10	60,000	17

Source: Lanthier, E. (2002). Correlation. http://www.nvcc.edu/home/elanthier/methods/correlations-samples.htm. Copyright 2002 by Elizabeth Lanthier, PhD. Reproduced with permission.

FIGURE 21-5 Regression Scatter Plot, Salary, and Education in Years

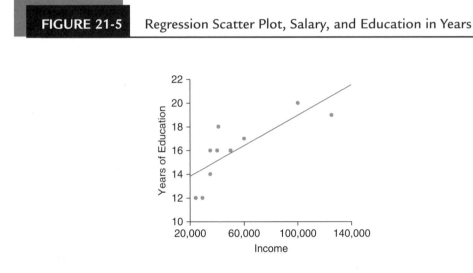

Source: Lanthier, E. (2002). Correlation. http://www.nvcc.edu/home/elanthier/methods/correlations-samples.htm. Copyright 2002 by Elizabeth Lanthier, PhD. Reproduced with permission.

TABLE 21-12	Grade Point Average and TV Use	
Participant	GPA	TV Use (hr/wk)
#1	3.1	14
#2	2.4	10
#3	2.0	20
#4	3.8	7
#5	2.2	25
#6	3.4	9
#7	2.9	15
#8	3.2	13
#9	3.7	4
#10	3.5	21

Source: Lanthier, E. (2002). Correlation. http://www.nvcc.edu/home/elanthier/methods/correlations-samples.htm. Copyright 2002 by Elizabeth Lanthier, PhD. Reproduced with permission.

FIGURE 21-6	Regression Scatter Plot, Hours of Television Use, and Grade Point Average

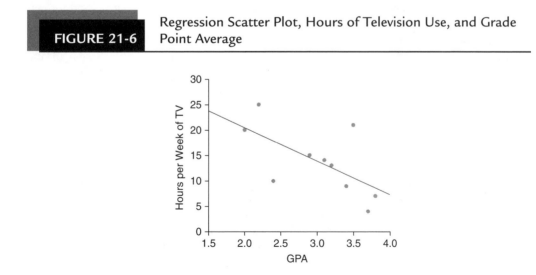

Source: Lanthier, E. (2002). Correlation. http://www.nvcc.edu/home/elanthier/methods/correlations-samples.htm. Copyright 2002 by Elizabeth Lanthier, PhD. Reproduced with permission.

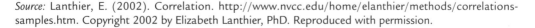

care provider options for consideration using a clinical decision support tree. According to the designers, the advantage of this kind of tracking is that the system provides immediate evidence-based support for direct patient care. Furthermore, it provides a method for storing data for future review, evaluation, and benchmarking (Lambert & Burlingame, 2009). Use and expansion of this kind of system to document and support clinical practice and scholarship would be an easy transition for nurses who are familiar with the use of PDAs "to support the application of current standards, and knowledge for clinical decision making" (Stroud, Erkel, & Smith, 2005).

Identifying Gaps in Evidence for Practice

In a systematic analysis of reviews published by the Joanna Briggs Institute between 1998 and 2002, high-quality evidence to support nursing interventions was not evident (Averis & Pearson, 2003). Further, the report identified considerable gaps in the evidence base available for nurses in relation to 22 discrete areas of practice that were examined in the analysis. However, the impetus to improve patient safety generated by the IOM reports *To Err Is Human* (Kohn, Corrigan, & Donaldson, 2000), *Crossing the Quality Chasm* (IOM, 2001), and *Health Professions Education: A Bridge to Quality* (IOM, 2003) and the availability of support for EBP through educational restructuring and systems support are increasing.

Nevertheless, gaps in the evidence remain. Research by nurses and family physicians suggests that a translational model to fill the gaps is necessary (Armson et al., 2007; Gumei, Tiedje, & Oweis, 2007). One such model, developed in Canada, uses a small, self-formed group-discussion format within local communities. The impetus for this model was the need to stay competent in view of the vast amount of medical information currently available. In these groups a facilitator guides physicians' discussion using sample patient cases and prepared modules on selected clinical topics. The groups have been ongoing for 15 years and have attracted international interest (Armson et al., 2007; Kelly, Cunningham, McCalister, Cassidy, & MacVicar, 2007). Nurses engage in similar forums in hospital grand rounds, within their professional specialty organizations, and at regional and national conferences. However, collaborative engagement needs to be broader and more systematic. DNPs are in an excellent position to initiate this kind of practice-based dialogue in community-based practice settings.

The American Nurses Association, the American Association of Colleges of Nursing, the National Organization of Nurse Practitioner Faculties, and professional nursing organizations in each specialty all have agendas for advancing research and evidence for practice in their respective areas. As examples, the American Academy of Nurse Practitioners, Nurse Practitioner Associates for Continuing Education (NPACE), and the Practicing Clinicians Exchange provide excellent forums for translating current research into practice and for networking with peers about research and clinical outcome information.

The Joint Commission, the National Database of Nursing Quality Indicators, and individual hospital report cards may be used as sources of research or outcome analysis to identify gaps in care delivery or in patient or staff education in particular institutions or practice groups. Examples include adverse events, smoking cessation, rates of adherence to best practice, blood glucose control, patient satisfaction rates, time spent with patients, tests ordered, and number of consultations (care related); knowledge, functional status, and access to care (patient related); and collaboration, technical quality, exam comprehensiveness, and adherence to guidelines (performance related) (Kleinpell, 2009). Within these and other categories, the gaps may be identified through the development of a specific plan based on target areas of APN practice. Planning questions should include the following: What exactly can be measured? How can it be measured? What will be done with the information? When should it be done? (Kleinpell, 2007). **Figure 21-7** shows a sample timeline for outcome assessment.

As advanced practice nursing evolves into the DNP role, it will be imperative that direct care providers, senior-level nurse executives, and doctorally prepared nurse educators take lead roles in quality improvement to positively affect patient safety (O'Grady, 2008). Identifying, testing, and disseminating information about nurse-sensitive quality indicators is essential to close the gap in quality care delivery. All advanced practice nurses prepared at the clinical doctorate level must be involved in this effort.

PARTICIPATION IN COLLABORATIVE RESEARCH

It is a credit to the profession of nursing and its leaders that there are several evidence-based practice centers in the United States: the American Nurses Association National Center for Nursing Quality, Sigma Theta Tau International, the National Institute of Nursing Research (NINR) at the NIH, and centers at many of the major university schools of nursing. However, as O'Grady (2008) notes, turf battles have limited collaboration. On the macro level, "APN organizations along with governmental and private research enterprise must come together to develop a research plan that identifies the most critical research questions" (O'Grady, 2008, p. 12). On the micro and macro levels, APNs individually and as a group must "demonstrate specific clinical performance and patient outcomes" (O'Grady, 2008, p. 12). This means "clearly distinguishing APNs in the context of interdisciplinary practice" (O'Grady, 2008, p. 12). Individual studies can demonstrate gaps in care in smaller samples, but the time has come for a more comprehensive and collaborative agenda for research that focuses on such issues as roles, function, outcomes, access improvements for vulnerable populations, interdisciplinary collaboration impacts, cost effectiveness, safety, and other indicators. To discover gaps in

FIGURE 21-7 Timeline for Outcome Assessment of APN Practice

Identify indicators	Baseline data	Review literature: develop path, protocols, orders, data collection tool	Choose processes: educate and implement	Review initial data monthly: adjust and reevaluate plan	Review data quarterly: adjust and reevaluate plan
← 1 month →	← 2 months →	← 3 months →	← 1 month →	← Monthly Over 3 months →	← As scheduled →

Source: Kleinpell, R. M. (2007, May). APNs invisible champions? *Nursing Management, 38*(5), 18–22. Adapted with permission.

care that are of concern to APNs/DNPs, nurses must have representatives from their ranks on research decision-making bodies. The AHRQ is positioned to take the lead in outcomes research, whereas the NIH focuses on biomedical aspects of disease management (O'Grady, 2008). To have their voices heard and their studies funded and disseminated, DNPs must use the power of their professional organizations to garner positions on national and international research collaboratives.

Participating in collaborative research is an excellent way for advanced practice nurses to resolve clinical dilemmas and highlight their expertise through well-constructed questions that interest scientists and engage professional peers within and outside nursing. The dynamic nature of scientific evidence and the speed with which it is now possible to generate new knowledge through the use of technology demand that all care providers combine their expertise to interpret, plan, and evaluate the outcomes of interventions based on these new discoveries. Collaboration "implies collective action toward a common goal in a spirit of trust and harmony" (D'Amour, Ferrada-Videla, San Martin-Rodriquez, & Beaulieu, 2005). Even within nursing, specialization demands collaboration between peers and patients to resolve complex clinical dilemmas if patients are to be treated holistically instead of as a collection of organ systems. In fact, as Nolan (2005) notes, patients must be included as "shapers of knowledge and action" (p. 329).

Nursing now has a body of knowledge, separate and unique from that of medicine, that provides the basis for unique contributions to science and to the care of individuals. At the same time, "nursing scholarship remains contextual and contingently situated" (Fairman, 2008). Nurses have shown in practice that they are creative and capable of managing changing circumstances and dynamic cultural milieus, thereby ensuring that advanced practice nurses with both research and clinical skills are in a prime position to function as practice consul-

tants in collaborative knowledge-generating research (AACN, 2006). This role is illustrated in the following example.

A DNP was a voluntary member of an advisory board of a suburban primary healthcare network that provided care to uninsured patients. The members of the board were very interested in ascertaining information about the effectiveness of the organization and its efforts to provide cost-effective, timely primary care. A question of particular interest was, Are emergency department visits decreased by the offering of this service? If they are, how much cost is actually saved? The DNP collaborated with the organization's administrator and developed an initial research question and a preliminary plan for presentation to a grant funding agency. The DNP researched the literature and took the preliminary plan to her institution's research group; with the help of a colleague from the college's health administration program, the DNP designed a study that was submitted to a grant funding agency that specialized in grants to medical centers and community health agencies. The agency did not fund the grant that year. However, the following year the original proposal was reframed as a cohort study, "Emergency Room Usage Among Uninsured Patients with Access to a Primary Care Provider" (Tymkow, Shen, and MacMullen, 2006), and resubmitted as a subproject of a much larger NIH grant that was funded. A primary aim of the larger National Center on Minority Health and Health Disparities (NCMHD) grant was to build capacity for research in healthcare disparities through mentoring by senior-level researchers (Samson, 2006). The DNP who was a mentee became the primary investigator, working with two co-investigators on this project. At this writing, the data collection has been completed and the results are being analyzed and will be presented to the agency. Although this was a small pilot study, the researchers hope to use the data gathered from the pilot for a larger study involving additional primary providers of care to uninsured patients. In this case the DNP is functioning as a member of a collaborative multidisciplinary research team.

In another example of collaborative research, Oman, Duran, and Fink (2008) describe a collaborative EBP project to institute evidence-based policy and procedure development at the University of Colorado Hospital using the hospital's evidence-based multidisciplinary practice model. The model established the evidence base through valid and current research and through other forms of evidence or benchmark data, including cost-effectiveness analysis; pathophysiology; retrospective or concurrent chart review; quality improvement and risk data; international, national, and local standards; infection control data; patient preferences; and clinical expertise. The more sources that are added to the research core, the stronger the evidence. However, all sources are contributory to the evidence.

The Evidence-Based Practice Council used the levels of evidence of Stetler (1994) to guide the process of gathering evidence. As described by Oman et al., since there was nothing addressing policy and procedure in the literature, the members identified steps and created an algorithm to describe the process. Once developed, the algorithm was piloted on the units using six nurse champions, mentored by a researcher. The champions and researcher reviewed an orthostatic vital sign policy that was scheduled for update. After obtaining 12 research-based articles, eight clinical articles, one national guideline, and anecdotal recommendations, the group was divided into subgroups, and each person was assigned two reports to review using a standardized critique form. Each nurse was responsible for reading the articles, completing the critique form (with levels of evidence), and presenting the findings at a journal club. The policy being reviewed was checked for references and levels of evidence by the research scientist. A comparison of agreement between the policy author and reviewers was then determined, and the percentage of agreement between reviewer and author tabulated. Only clinically based policies were reviewed. This process is a good example of how collaboration between practice and education could be merged in any number of areas.

Whether collaboration involves clinical research or quality improvement, DNPs in clinical and leadership roles are key stakeholders in the process. As identified in the IOM report *Crossing the Quality Chasm* (IOM, 2001), communication and collaboration are requisites to the achievement of quality systems and patient outcomes. These skills are also a necessary part of a culture of collaboration that begins in educational programs and continues in the professional work setting. Collaborative efforts may include small, unit-based or practice-based efforts or large, systemwide initiatives. These efforts have been driven by consumer demand for excellence, accountability, and transparency in quality care, patient safety, and patient satisfaction (Freshman, Rubino, & Chassiakos, 2010). In any collaborative initiative, three levels of expertise are required: system leadership, including the authority to implement change; clinical technical expertise (guidance and know-how); and day-to-day leadership (details of the system) (Baker, Reising, Johnson, Stewart, & Baker, 1997, cited in Freshman, Rubino, & Chassiakos, 2010).

DISSEMINATING FINDINGS FROM EVIDENCE-BASED PRACTICE

A primary reason for disseminating research is to use the findings to improve practice and improve health outcomes. Communicating the results of research and evidence-based practice trials is the culminating step of the research and research utilization processes. It is one of the most important steps—if not *the* most important step—in research and the application of research in practice, because it is the communication of research findings that provides the basis for meaningful critique, development of new questions, and testing of research evidence in practice (Lyder & Fain, 2009).

The methods used to communicate evidence from practice trials are similar to those used for communicating research findings: journal publications, podium or poster presentations, Internet webinar sessions, media communications, journal clubs, and community presentations. However, the forums for dissemination may be broader because the audience of interest may be more diverse, including those with practice, research, and community development interests. In addition, the choice of method for communicating information depends on a number of important factors. For example, a journal publication may be personally advantageous to the author, but the time from submission to actual publication and dissemination may delay utilization of important evidence-based treatments in practice. Oral reports at national conferences may facilitate timelier dissemination. Webinars may be the fastest way to disseminate information, but may not reach all the desired audiences. Journal clubs are useful forums for discussions of research findings in academic settings. Reports of community-based studies to advisory boards or media venues may also become the basis for further research and political support that help nonprofit and other community organizations. Nevertheless, because theory, research, and practice must be constantly intertwined, the circular and reciprocal relationship among these elements must be apparent regardless of where the research is presented (McEwen & Wills, 2007).

Preparing a Journal Publication

Preparing a journal article for publication is time consuming and at times tedious, but the rewards of feeling that you have made a contribution and seeing your work in print are worth the effort. Once the topic for an article has been established, the next step is that of selecting the journal. Peer-reviewed journals have the most rigorous review criteria. Therefore, publication in one of these journals is considered to be more credible. The actual content will be determined by the editorial guidelines of the journal, which may be found in the "Information for Authors" section of the journal. In most cases, the guidelines may also be obtained from the journal's website. Generally, the submission requirements cover technical details such as page length, margins, font style and size, reference format, use of graphics and figures, and method of submission. It is very important to follow the submission requirements because many journals will not review articles that are not submitted in the correct format.

Once submitted, articles in peer-reviewed journals are blind (anonymously) reviewed by several reviewers. It is not uncommon for the review process to last several weeks or months, and articles may be rejected, accepted with revisions, or accepted. It is common to have articles returned for revision. The key to success is to be persistent, correct those things that can be corrected, give an explanation for those that cannot, and return the submission in the agreed-upon time frame.

Preparing a Research Presentation

Regardless of where or how evidence is reported, the essential element is that it combines the knowledge and values of the study patients or population with practitioner expertise and the best in available and current research evidence. Reporting evidence also requires knowledge of the audience and their needs. Specifically, the presenter must ask: What is the specific content to be addressed? How will the audience use the information? What is the knowledge level of those who are to receive the information? What is the time allowed for the presentation? Which audiovisual resources are available for the presentation? Once these questions have been answered, specific learning objectives should be developed in order to guide and organize the presentation.

Table 21-13 shows an outline for presentation of research study findings. Important points of each aspect of the study can be displayed as a PowerPoint presentation to aid in

TABLE 21-13	Outline for Research Presentation

I. Introduction

II. Purpose of the study

III. Theoretical framework

IV. Hypothesis

V. Design

    A. What kind of study

    B. Intervention

    C. Sample

        1. Population

        2. Inclusion/Exclusion criteria

    D. Instruments

VI. Analysis

    A. Method

    B. Types of statistical tests used

VII. Findings

VIII. Discussion

IX. Implications

    A. Research

    B. Clinical practice

maintaining the presentation within the designated time frame and keep the audience focused on the important elements of the presentation. **Table 21-14** lists some useful websites concerning PowerPoint presentations.

Preparing a Poster Presentation

Disseminating information from scholarship—original research, practice innovations, clinical projects—through poster presentations has become an accepted medium for the exchange of ideas in a more personal and less formal environment than the podium presentation. It is both efficient and effective. Presenters and participants have the freedom to engage in a dialogue that allows for education, clarification, and networking. Posters also allow for the formatting of data in creative ways. As Berg (2005) notes, "imagery can be substituted for words and this is a powerful way to convey information" (p. 245). Like any presentation, posters require preparation. The following steps are essential.

Plan Ahead

A good poster presentation takes considerable time. The planning stage is a most important step. In this stage, considerable thought should be given to the message you are trying to convey. What is the purpose? The format for a research presentation will be different from that of a practice innovation. Is the conference only for nurses, only for advanced practice nurses, or for a multidisciplinary audience? How much background information or detail do you need to include? Is the audience generally familiar with the topic or not? If they are, don't include familiar details, but if they aren't, don't make

TABLE 21-14	Resources and Websites for Developing Multimedia and PowerPoint Presentations

Vanderbilt University
http://www.vanderbilt.edu/cft/resources/teaching_resources/technology/presentation

University of Wisconsin
http://www.cew.wisc.edu/accessibility/tutorials/pptmain.htm

University of South Florida
http://etc.usf.edu/presentations/web

WebAim
http://www.webaim.org/techniques/powerpoint/alternatives.php

the information so specific that those who are not familiar with the topic will be put off. Avoid using abbreviations that only a select audience will understand. These and other considerations specific to the venue should be thought about during the planning stage (Berg, 2005; Hardicre, Devitt, & Coad, 2007).

Decide on Layout and Format

Most people read top to bottom, and left to right. This is the usual sequence for poster layout. Generally, the layout for a research poster presentation is as follows: title, abstract, introduction, methods, results, discussion, and acknowledgments. If the presentation is a practice innovation, the layout will be different. The innovation is usually in the center, with explanatory text at the periphery or below the diagram or explanation of the protocol or change (Hardicre et al., 2007). References are also included, as in the research poster. "The poster should be easy to read from a distance of up to 6 feet. Section heads should be at least 40 pt. and supporting text 32 pt." (Halligan, 2005, p. 49). Titles should be short, with letters two to three inches high (Berg, 2005).

Determine the Content

If the purpose of the poster is to display a research project, it will not be the same as one that is designed to describe a clinical innovation. The content of the research poster should follow the guidelines established by the conference guidelines. If the study is funded by an outside or government agency, some grant-funded studies require specific wording of the acknowledgment; this should be determined during the poster planning. If an abstract is required, it should include the main purpose of the study, be clearly worded, and be succinct. A key component is to keep it simple because posters "show," they do not "tell" (Miracle, 2008).

Clinical project content will vary according to the specific topic and scope. The title for either a research study or clinical innovation should be creative, but, most important, it should accurately reflect the content of the project. The title banner should also include authors and affiliations in order of authorship and/or contribution to the effort. In many instances the organizational logo will be included as well (Hardicre et al., 2007).

Prepare a Brief Presentation

"The poster is a story board of information" (Jackson & Sheldon, 1998, as cited in Hardicre et al., 2007, p. 398). However, it also gives the presenters an opportunity to present themselves. As with any kind of communication, you want to convey confidence and knowledge. Preparing a short presentation script or handouts for participants allows you to organize your thoughts and prepare for possible questions. The handouts are always welcomed by participants, who are inundated with information during a conference. Be sure to include your name and contact number or attach a business card so that participants may contact you with questions. This is a very effective networking tool (Miracle, 2008).

Media Communications

Communicating with large audiences is often facilitated through professional media communications. This kind of communication is essential when there is a major event or change, such as a policy to be initiated. It is usually best to engage the resources of a professional organization to make the preliminary contact and to aid in constructing the message.

Journal Club Presentations

Another way to facilitate the communication of evidence-based research is through journal club presentations. Journal clubs are not new, especially in academic and many professional settings. However, using them to facilitate evidence-based practice is a more recent development, especially as a forum for clinical guideline development (Kirchoff & Beck, 1995, as cited in McQueen, Miller, Nivison, & Husband, 2006). In a small survey study of the use of journal clubs to determine changes in practice, McQueen et al. (2006) found that journal clubs were effective in "1) focusing staff on clinical evidence in discussions, 2) increasing confidence as they became more aware of evidence, and, 3) bridging the evidence-practice gap" (p. 315). Additionally, with the aid of the Internet, evidence-based articles or studies can be posted in advance and facilitated online, increasing the possibility of wider participation. In one pilot study of this format, nurses in New Zealand branded the journal club's website and the articles for discussion. An article is posted for one month and removed on the Friday before the following month's posting (Trim, 2008). **Table 21-15** presents an outline of a journal club.

Whether live or Internet-based, journal clubs provide a mechanism for promoting professional debate, increasing confidence, and, most important, improving practice and quality care (Sheratt, 2005, as cited in McQueen et al., 2006). With their educational background and advanced skills, DNPs are in an excellent position to implement this kind of strategy in a collaborative, interdisciplinary format.

SUMMARY

Scholarship and evidence-based practice are not the same, but each has elements that support the other. Scholarship involves research and application, as does evidence-based practice. Whereas scholarship may be a joint or singular effort, evidence-based practice requires teamwork and collaboration. The outcome of scholarship is a scholarly product, a new way of thinking, or a change in awareness about a subject or phenomenon—an end in itself. Evidence-based practice is based on the scholarship of research and evidence gathering and synthesis. It is a means for improving care for patients or effecting a change in a system that results in better care for patients, providers,

---

TABLE 21-15 Online Journal Club

Outline of the Journal Club

1. A specific clinical question is chosen.

2. All evidence-based literature related to the question is derived from online databases.

3. A reference list of all literature for review is generated.

4. High-level-evidence RTCs and systematic reviews are critiqued and given more weight than quasi-experimental case studies and opinions.

5. Participants critically appraise the relevant literature before attending the journal club.

6. Journal club discussions center on the critical appraisal of evidence found for clinical interventions.

7. Implications for practice and further research are discussed, with key findings recorded in minutes.

8. A resource folder that includes a reference list of resource critiques, guidelines for practice, treatment resources, standardized assessments, disease management strategies, and gaps in evidence is created.

9. A system for ongoing evaluation of outcomes and changes in practice is developed and communicated.

Source: McQueen, J., Miller, C., Nivison, C., & Husband, V. (2006). An investigation into the use of a journal club for evidence-based practice. *International Journal of Therapy and Rehabilitation, 13*(7), p. 313. Modified with permission.

and communities. It is a transformation of knowledge to new levels of understanding and integration. Changing to a model of evidence-based practice does not just happen; it requires the integration of a number of skills, including the use of good research and the synthesis of best information and other "evidences," including patient choice and professional expertise at its core. The DNP, with the advantage of expertise in practice built on a strong base of education and knowledge, is—and will continue to be—in the forefront of this movement to transform care.

DISCUSSION QUESTIONS

1. How will the Iowa model of evidence-based practice help to promote quality care in the clinical practice setting?

2. Which role will the advanced practice nurse play in intradisciplinary and interdisciplinary collaborative research teams?

3. As an advanced practice nurse leading a research team, which strategies would you employ to encourage your team members to critically appraise research articles?

REFERENCES

Adib-Hajbaghery, M. (2007). Factors facilitating and inhibiting evidence-based practice in Iran. *Journal of Advanced Nursing, 58*(6), 566–575.

Agency for Healthcare Research and Quality. (2002). Systems to rate the strength of scientific evidence, summary (Technical Report No. 47). Retrieved from http://www.ahrq.gov/clinic/epcsums/strengthsum.htm

Agency for Healthcare Research and Quality. (2009). Evidence-based practice centers. Retrieved from http://www.AHRQ.gov/clinic/epc

AGREE Collaboration. (2001). AGREE instrument. Retrieved from www.agreecollaboration.org/instrument

American Association of Colleges of Nursing. (1999). Position statement on defining scholarship for the discipline of nursing. Retrieved from http://www.aacn.nche.edu/Publications/positions/scholar.htm

American Association of Colleges of Nursing. (2006). The essentials of doctoral education for advanced nursing practice. Retrieved from http://www.aacn.nche.edu/DNP/pdf/Essentials.pdf

American Nurses Credentialing Center. (2005). Magnet recognition program overview. Retrieved from http://www.medscape.com/partners/ancc/public/ancc

Andrews, T. (2008). Under pressure for a diagnosis: A case study review of pheochromocytoma genetics. *Clinical Scholars Review: The Journal of Doctoral Nursing Practice, 1*(2), 96–100.

Armson, H., Kinzie, S., Hawes, D., Roder, S., Wakefield, J., & Elmslie, T. (2007). Translating learning into practice. *Canadian Family Physician, 53*(9), 1477–1485.

Arthur, R., Marfell, J., & Ulrich, S. (2009). Outcomes measurement in nurse-midwifery practice. In R. M. Kleinpell (Ed.), *Outcome assessment in advanced practice nursing* (2nd ed.). New York: Springer.

Asch, S. M., Baker, D. W., Keesey, J., Broder, M., Schonlau, M., Rosen, M., et al. (2005). Does the collaborative model improve care for chronic heart failure? *Medical Care, 43*(7), 667–675.

Averis, A., & Pearson, A. (2003). Filling the gaps: Identifying nursing research priorities through the analysis of completed systematic reviews. *JBI Reports, 1*(3), 49–126.

Baker, C. M., Reising, D. L., Johnson, D. R., Stewart, R. L., & Baker, S. D. (1997). Organizational effectiveness: Toward an integrated model for schools of nursing. *Journal of Professional Nursing, 13*(4), 246–255.

Batalden, P. B., Nelson, E. C., & Roberts, J. S. (1994). Linking outcome measurements to continual improvement: The serial "V" way of thinking about improving clinical care. *Journal of Quality Improvement, 20*(4), 167–180.

Batalden, P. B., & Stoltz, P. K. (1993). A framework for the continual improvement of healthcare: Building and applying professional and improvement knowledge to test changes in daily work. *Joint Commission Journal of Quality Improvement, 19*(10), 424–447.

Berg, J. A. (2005). Creating a professional poster presentation: Focus on nurse practitioners. *Journal of the American Academy of Nurse Practitioners, 17*(7), 245–248.

Bernarde, S. F., Keogh, E., & Lima, M. L. (2007). Bridging the gap between pain and gender research: A selective literature review. *European Journal of Pain, 12*(4), 427–440. doi: 10.1016.j.ejpain.2007.08.007

Bond, A. E., Draeger, C. R., Mandleco, B., & Donnelly, M. (2003). Needs of family members of patients with severe traumatic brain injury. *Critical Care Nurse, 23*(4), 63–71.

Boyer, E. L. (1990). *Scholarship reconsidered: Priorities of the professoriate.* The Carnegie Foundation for the Advancement of Teaching. San Francisco: Jossey-Bass.

Boyer, E. L. (1997). *Scholarship reconsidered: Priorities of the professoriate* (rev. ed.). The Carnegie Foundation for the Advancement of Teaching. San Francisco: Jossey-Bass.

Brown, S. J. (2005). Direct clinical practice. In A. B. Hamric, J. A. Spross, & C. M. Hanson (Eds.), *Advanced practice nursing: An integrative approach* (3rd ed., pp. 143–185). Philadelphia: W. B. Saunders.

Burns, N., & Grove, S. K. (2005). *The practice of nursing research: Conduct, critique, and utilization* (5th ed.). St. Louis, MO: Elsevier Saunders.

Burns, N., & Grove, S. K. (2009). *The practice of nursing research, appraisal, synthesis, and generation of evidence* (6th ed.). St. Louis, MO: Saunders.

Burns, S. (2009). Selecting advanced practice nurse outcome measures. In R. M. Kleinpell (Ed.), *Outcomes assessment in advanced practice nursing* (2nd ed.). New York: Springer.

Burns, S. M., & Earven, S. (2002). Improving outcomes for mechanically ventilated medical intensive care unit patients using advanced practice nurses: A 6-year experience. *Critical Nursing Clinics of North America, 14*(3), 231–242.

Bushnell, C. D., Hurn, P., Colton, C., Miller, V. M., del Zoppo, G., Elkind, M. S., et al. (2007). Advancing the study of stroke in women: Summary and recommendations for future research from an NINDS-Sponsored Multidisciplinary Working Group. *Stroke, 38*(5), e10.

Carey, M., Buchan, H., & Sanson-Fisher, R. (2009). The cycle of change: Implementing the best-evidence clinical practice. *International Journal for Quality in Health Care, 21*(1), 37–43. Retrieved from http:www//medscape.com/viewarticle/587379

Carnegie Foundation for the Advancement of Teaching. (1996). *Ernest L. Boyer (Ninety-first Annual Report of the Carnegie Foundation for the Advancement of Teaching).* Princeton, NJ: Author.

Cochrane Collaboration. (2004). *Cochrane reviewers' handbook.* London: The Cochrane Group.

Coe, R. (2002, September). *It's the effect size, stupid: What effect size is and why it is so important.* Paper presented at the Annual Conference of the British Educational Research Association, University of Exeter, England. Retrieved from http://www.leeds.ac.uk./educol/documents/0002182.htm

Collins, P. M., Golembeski, S. M., Selgas, M., Sparger, K., Burke, N., & Vaughn, B. B. (2008, January 25). Clinical excellence through evidence-based practice: A model to guide practice changes. *Topics in Advanced Practice E-Journal.* Retrieved from http://www.medscape.com/viewarticle/567682

Cooke, L., Smith-Idell, C., Dean, G., Gemmill, R., Steingass, S., Sun, V., et al. (2004). "Research to practice": A practical program to enhance the use of evidence-based practice at the unit level. *Oncology Nursing Forum, 31*(4), 825–832.

Craft-Rosenburg, M., Krajicek, M. J., & Shin, D. (2002). Report of the American Academy of Nursing Child–Family Expert Panel: Identification of quality and outcome indicators for maternal child nursing. *Nursing Outlook, 50*(2), 57–60.

Crotty, M. (1996). *Phenomenology and nursing research.* Melbourne, Australia: Churchill Livingstone.

D'Amour, D., Ferrada-Videla, M., San Martin-Rodriquez, L., & Beaulieu, M. D. (2005). The conceptual basis for interprofessional collaboration: Core concepts and theoretical frameworks. *Journal of Interprofessional Care, 19*(suppl 1), 116–131.

Decker, S., & Iphofen, R. (2005). Developing the profession of radiography: Making uses of oral history. *Radiography, 11*(4), 262–271.

Deming, E. W. (1986). *Out of crisis.* Cambridge, MA: MIT Press.

De Palma, J. A., & McGuire, D. B. (2005). Research. In A. B. Hamric, J. A. Spross, & C. Mittenson (Eds.), *Advanced nursing practice: An integrative approach* (3rd ed.). Philadelphia: Elsevier Saunders.

DiCenso, A., Cullum, N., & Ciliska, D. (1998). Implementing evidence-based nursing: Some misconceptions. *Evidence-Based Nursing, 1*(2), 38–39.

Diekelmann, N. L., Allen, D., & Tanner, C. A. (1989). *NLN criteria for appraisal of baccalaureate programs: A critical hermeneutic analysis.* New York: National League for Nursing.

Dohrn, J. (2008). Scaling up HIV treatment for pregnant women: Components of a midwifery model of care as identified by midwives in Eastern Cape, South Africa. *Clinical Scholars Review: The Journal of Doctoral Nursing Practice, 1*(1), 50–54.

Doran, D. M., & Sidani, S. (2007). Outcomes-focused knowledge translation: A framework for knowledge translation and patient outcomes improvement. *Worldviews on Evidence-Based Nursing, 4*(1), 3–13.

Dorn, K. (2004). Caring-healing inquiry for holistic nursing practice: Model for research and evidence based practice. *Topics in Advanced Practice Nursing E-Journal, 4*(4). Retrieved from http://www.medscape.com/viewarticle/496363

Doster, J. A., Purdum, M. D., Martin, L. A., Goven, A. J., & Moorefield, R. (2009). Gender differences, anger expression, and cardiovascular risk. *Journal of Nervous and Mental Diseases, 197*(7), 552–554.

Doumitt, G., Gattelliari, M., Grimshaw, J., & O'Brien, M. A. (2007). Local opinion leaders: Effects on professional practice and healthcare outcomes. *Cochrane Database Systematic Review, 4,* Art. No. CD000125. doi: 10.1002/14651858.CD000125.pub3

Doyle-Lindrud, S. (2008). Gestational breast cancer. *Clinical Scholars Review: The Journal of Doctoral Nursing Practice, 1*(1), 23–31.

Dreher, M. (1999). Clinical scholarship: Nursing practice as an intellectual endeavor. In Sigma Theta Tau International Clinical Scholarship Task Force, *Clinical scholarship resource paper* (pp. 26–33). Retrieved from http://www.nursingsociety.org/aboutus/PositionPapers/Documents/clinical_scholarship_paper.pdf

Duignan, P. (2006). Outcomes model standards for systematic outcome analysis. Retrieved from http://www.parkerduignan.com/oiiwa/toolkit/standards1.html

Durieux, P., Nizard, R., Ravaud, P., et al. (2000). A clinical decision support system for prevention of venous thromboembolism: Effect on physician behavior. *Journal of the American Medical Association, 283*(21), 2816–2821.

Edwards, S. D. (2001). *Philosophy of nursing: An introduction.* New York: Palgrave.

Fain, J. A. (2009). *Reading, understanding and applying nursing research* (3rd ed.). Philadelphia: F. A. Davis.

Fairman, J. (2008). Context and contingency in the history of post World War II scholarship in the United States. *Journal of Nursing Scholarship, 40*(1), 4–11.

Fawcett, J., & Garrity, J. (2009). *Evaluating research for evidence-based nursing practice.* Philadelphia: F. A. Davis.

Fawcett, J., Watson, J., Neuman, B., Hinton Walker, P., & Fitzpatrick, J. (2001). On nursing theories and evidence. *Journal of Nursing Scholarship, 33*(2), 115–119.

Fishbein, I., & Ajzen, M. (1980). *Understanding attitudes and predicting social behavior.* Englewood Cliffs, NJ: Prentice Hall.

Fitzpatrick, M. L., & Munhall, P. L. (2001). Historical research: The method. In P. L. Munhall (Ed.), *Nursing research: A qualitative perspective* (3rd ed.). Sudbury, MA: Jones and Bartlett.

French, P. (1999). The development of evidence-based nursing. *Journal of Advanced Nursing, 29*(1), 72–78.

Freshman, B., Rubino, L., & Chassiakos, Y. R. (2010). *Collaboration across the disciplines in health care.* Sudbury, MA: Jones and Bartlett.

Funk & Wagnalls new international dictionary of the English language (comprehensive millennium ed.). (2003). Chicago: Ferguson.

Gagan, M., & Hewitt-Taylor, J. (2004). The issues involved in implementing evidence based practice. *British Journal of Nursing, 13*(20), 1216–1220.

Gallagher, R. M. (2009). Participation of the advanced practice nurse in managed care and quality initiatives. In L. A. Joel (Ed.), *Advanced practice nursing: Essentials of role development* (2nd ed.). Philadelphia: F. A. Davis.

Giddens, A. (1982). *Profiles and critiques in social theory.* London: Macmillan.

Gifford, W., Davies, B., Edwards, N., Griffin, P., & Lybanon, V. (2007). Managerial leadership for nurses' use of research evidence: An integrative review of the literature. *World Views on Evidence Based Practice, 4*(3), 126–145.

Giorgi, A. (2000). Concerning the application of phenomenology to caring research. *Scandinavian Journal of Caring Science, 14*(1), 11–15.

Glanville, I., Schirm, V., & Wineman, N. M. (2000). Using evidence-based practice for managing clinical outcomes in advanced practice nursing. *Journal of Nursing Care Quality, 15*(1), 1–11.

Glasser, B. G., & Strauss, A. (1967). *The discovery of grounded theory.* Chicago: Aldine.

Goolsby, M. J., Klardie, K. A., Johnson, J., McNaughton, M. A., & Meyers, W. (2004). Integrating the principles of evidence-based practice into clinical practice. *Journal of the American Academy of Nurse Practitioners, 16*(3), 98–105.

Goolsby, M. J., Meyers, W. C., Johnson, J. A., Klardie, K., & McNaughton, M. A. (2004). Integrating the principles of evidence-based practice: Prognosis and the metabolic syndrome. *Journal of the American Academy of Nurse Practitioners, 16*(5), 178–186.

Griffin-Sobel, J. P. (2003). Evaluating an instrument for research. *Gastroenterology Nursing, 26*(3), 135–136.

Grol, R., Dalhuijsen, J., Thomas, S., Veld, C., Rutten, G., & Mokkink, H. (1998). Attributes of clinical guidelines that influence use of guidelines in general practice: Observational study. *British Medical Journal, 317*(7162), 858–861.

Gumei, M. K., Tiedje, L. B., & Oweis, A. (2007). Vaginal or cesarean birth: Toward evidence based practice. *American Journal of Maternal Child Nursing, 32*(6), 388.

Hallett, C. (1995). Understanding the phenomenological approach to research. *Nurse Researcher, 3*(2), 55–56.

Halligan, P. (2005). Poster perfect. *World of Irish Nursing and Midwifery, 13*(8), 49.

Handley, M., MacGregor, K., Schillinger, D., Sharifi, C., Wong, S., & Bodenheimer, T. (2006). Using action plans to help primary care patients adopt healthy behaviors: A descriptive study. *Journal of the American Board of Family Medicine, 19*(3), 224–231.

Hardicre, J., Devitt, P., & Coad, J. (2007). Ten steps to successful poster presentation. *British Journal of Nursing, 16*(7), 398–401.

Harvey, S. (1993). The genesis of the phenomenological approach to advanced nursing practice. *Journal of Advanced Nursing, 18*(4), 526–530.

Hawkins, R. C., & Clement, P. F. (1984). Binge eating: Measurement problems and a conceptual model. In R. E. Hawkins, W. J. Fremouw, & P. F. Clement (Eds.), *The binge–purge syndrome: Diagnosis, treatment, and research* (pp. 229–251). New York: Springer.

Hebda, T., & Czar, P. (2009). *Handbook of informatics for nurses and healthcare professionals* (4th ed.). Upper Saddle River, NJ: Pearson/Prentice Hall.

Hodge, M. B., Asch, S. M., Olson, V. A., Kravitz, R. L., & Sauve, M. J. (2002). Developing indicators of nursing quality to evaluate nurse staffing ratios. *Journal of Nursing Administration, 32*(6), 338–345.

Holleman, G., Eliens, A., van Vliet, M., & van Acterburg, T. (2006). Promotion of evidence based practice by professional nursing associations: Literature review. *Journal of Advanced Nursing, 53*(6), 702–709.

Horsely, J. A., Crane, J., & Bingle, J. D. (1978). Research utilization as an organizational process. *Journal of Nursing Administration, 8*(7), 4–6.

Imberg, W. C. (2008). *The meaning of U.S. childbirth for Mexican immigrant women* (Doctoral dissertation). Available from ProQuest Dissertations and Theses database. (UMI No. 3318193)

Ingersoll, G. (2005). Generating evidence through outcomes management. In B. M. Melnyk & E. Fineout-Overholt (Eds.), *Evidence-based practice in nursing and healthcare: A guide to best practice.* Philadelphia: Lippincott Williams & Wilkins.

Ingersoll, G. L., McIntosh, E., & Williams, M. (2000). Nurse sensitive outcomes of advanced practice. *Journal of Advanced Nursing, 32*(5), 1272–1281.

Institute of Medicine. (2001). *Crossing the quality chasm: A new health system for the 21st century.* Washington, DC: National Academies Press.

Institute of Medicine. (2003). *Health professions education: A bridge to quality.* Washington, DC: National Academies Press.

International Development Research Center. (2009). Confounding. Retrieved from http://www.idrc.ca /en/ev-1-201-1-DO_TOPIC.html

Ironside, P. M. (2006). Reforming doctoral curricula in nursing: Creating multiparadigmatic, multipedagalogical researchers. *Journal of Nursing Education, 45*(2), 51–52.

Jackson, K. I., & Sheldon, J. M. (1998). Poster presentation: How to tell a story. *Pediatric Nurse, 10*(9), 36–37.

Jamtvedt, G., Young, J. M., Kristofferson, D. T., O'Brien, M. A., & Oxman, A. D. (2006). Audit and feedback: Effects on professional practice and healthcare outcomes. *Cochrane Database of Systematic Reviews, 2,* CD000259.

Johnston, L. (2005). Critically appraising quantitative evidence. In B. M. Melnyk & E. Fineout-Overholt (Eds.), *Evidence-based practice in nursing and healthcare: A guide to best practice.* Philadelphia: Lippincott Williams & Wilkins.

Kelly, D. R., Cunningham, D. E., McCalister, P., Cassidy, J., & MacVicar, R. (2007). Applying evidence in practice through small group learning: A qualitative exploration of success. *Quality in Primary Care, 15*(2), 93–99.

Kirchoff, K., & Beck, S. (1995). Using the journal club as a component of the research utilization process. *Heart and Lung: The Journal of Acute and Critical Care, 24*(3), 246–250.

Kitson, A., Harvey, G., & McCormack, B. (1998). Enabling the implementation of evidence-based practice: A conceptual framework. *Quality in Healthcare, 7*(3), 149–158.

Kleinpell, R. M. (2007, May). APNs invisible champions? *Nursing Management, 38*(5), 18–22.

Kleinpell, R. M. (2009). Measuring outcomes in advanced nursing practice. In R. M. Kleinpell (Ed.), *Outcome assessment in advanced nursing practice* (2nd ed.). New York: Springer.

Kohn, L. T., Corrigan, J. M., & Donaldson, M. S. (2000). *To err is human: Building a safer health system.*

A report of the Committee on Quality of Health Care in America, Institute of Medicine. Washington, DC: National Academies Press.

Kovarsky, D. (2008). Representing voices from the life-world in evidence-based practice. *International Journal of Language and Communication Disorders, 43*(S1), 47–57.

Lambert, M. J., & Burlingame, G. M. (2009). Measuring outcomes in the state of Utah: Practice based evidence. *Behavioral Healthcare, 27,* 16–20. Retrieved from http://www.behavioral.net

Lanthier, E. (2002). Correlation. Retrieved from http://www.nvcc.edu/home/elanthier/methods/correlations-samples.htm

Leedy, P. D., & Ormrod, J. E. (2010). *Practical research: Planning and design.* Boston: Pearson.

Library of Congress. (n.d.). American memory collection. Retrieved from http://memory.loc.gov/ammem/index.html

Lopez-Bushnell, K. (2002). Get research-ready. *Nursing Management, 33*(11), 41–44.

Lowell, J. R. (1819–1891). Scholarship. Retrieved from http://quotationsbook.com/quote/22196

Luttik, M. L., Jaarsma, T., Lesman, I., Sanderman, R., & Hagedoorn, M. (2009). Quality of life in partners of people with congestive heart failure: Gender and involvement in care. *Journal of Advanced Nursing, 65*(7), 1442–1451. Epub April 30, 2009.

Lyder, C., & Fain, J. A. (2009). Interpreting and reporting research findings. In J. A. Fain (Ed.), *Reading, understanding, and applying research* (3rd ed., pp. 233–250). Philadelphia: F. A. Davis.

Maggs-Rapport, F. (2001). "Best research practice": In pursuit of methodological rigour. *Journal of Advanced Nursing, 35*(3), 373–383.

Mak, Y. (2003). Use of hermeneutic research in understanding the meaning of desire for euthanasia. *Palliative Medicine, 17*(5), 395–402.

Marineau, M. L. (2005). *Exploring the lived experience of individuals with acute infections transitioning in the home with support by an advanced practice nurse using telehealth* (Doctoral dissertation). University of Hawaii at Manoa. (UMI Order No. AA13198369)

Marinopoulos, S. S., Dorman, T., Ratanawongsa, N., Wilson, L. M., Ashar, B. H., Magaziner, J. L., et al. (2007). Effectiveness of continuing medical education. *Evidence Reports in Technology Assessment, 14,* 1–69.

Masharani, V., Goldfine, I. D., & Youngren, J. F. (2009). Influence of gender on the relationship between insulin sensitivity, adiposity, and plasma lipids, in lean nondiabetic patients. *Metabolism.* Advance online publication. Retrieved from http://www.ncbi.nlm.nih.gov/pubmed/19604524

McCaughan, D., Thompson, C., Cullum, N., Sheldon, T. A., & Thompson, D. R. (2002). Acute care nurses' perceptions of barriers to using research information in clinical decision-making. *Journal of Advanced Nursing, 39*(1), 46–60.

McCloskey, D. J. (2008). Nurses' perceptions of research utilization in a corporate health care system. *Journal of Nursing Scholarship, 40*(1), 39–45.

McCollum, M., Hanson, L. S., Lu, L., & Sullivan, P. W. (2005). Gender differences in diabetes mellitus and effects on self-care activity. *Gender Medicine, 2*(4), 246–254.

McEwen, M., & Wills, E. M. (2007). *Theoretical basis for nursing* (2nd ed.). Philadelphia: Lippincott Williams & Wilkins.

McQueen, J., Miller, C., Nivison, C., & Husband, V. (2006). An investigation into the use of a journal club for evidence-based practice. *International Journal of Therapy and Rehabilitation, 13*(7), 311–316.

McSherry, R. (2002). *Evidence informed nursing: A guide for clinical nurses.* London: Routledge.

MedPage Today. (n.d.). Guide to biostatistics. Retrieved from http://www.medpagetoday.com/Medpage-Guide-to-Biostatistics.pdf

Melnyk, B., & Cole, R. (2005). Generating evidence through quantitative research. In B. Melnyk & E. Fineout-Overholt (Eds.), *Evidence-based practice in nursing and healthcare* (pp. 239–281). Philadelphia: Lippincott Williams & Wilkins.

Melnyk, B., & Fineout-Overholt, E. (2002). Putting research into practice. Rochester ARCC. *Reflections on Nursing Leadership, 28*(2), 22–25.

Melnyk, B., & Fineout-Overholt, E. (2005). *Evidence-based practice in nursing and healthcare.* Philadelphia: Lippincott Williams & Wilkins.

Minnick, A. (2009). General design and implementation challenges in outcomes assessment. In R. M. Kleinpell (Ed.), *Outcomes assessment in advanced practice nursing* (2nd ed.). New York: Springer.

Miracle, V. (2008). Effective poster presentations. *Dimensions of Critical Care Nursing, 27*(3), 122–124.

Mitchell, P. H., Ferketich, S., & Jennings, B. M. (1998). Quality health outcomes model. *Image: Journal of Nursing Scholarship, 30*(1), 43–36.

Moccia, P. (1987). *Nursing theory: A circle of knowledge* [Videorecording]. New York: National League for Nursing.

Monico, E. P., Moore, C. L., & Calise, A. (2005). The impact of evidence based medicine and evolving technology on the standard of care in emergency medicine. *Internet Journal of Law, Healthcare and Ethics, 3*(2).

Munhall, P. (1994). *In women's experience.* New York: National League for Nursing.

Munhall, P. (2007) A phenomenological method. In P. L. Munhall (Ed.), *Nursing research: A qualitative perspective* (4th ed.). Sudbury, MA: Jones and Bartlett.

National Organization of Nurse Practitioner Faculties. (2005). Nurse practitioner faculty practice: An expectation of professionalism. Retrieved from www.nonpf.org/FPStatement2005final.pdf

Naylor, M. D., Brooten, D., Campbell, R., Jacobsen, B. S., Mezey, M. D., Pauley, M. V., et al. (1999). Comprehensive discharge planning and home follow-up of hospitalized elders: A randomized clinical trial. *Journal of the American Medical Association, 281*(7), 613–620.

Newhouse, R. P., Dearholt, S. L., Poe, S. S., Pugh, L. C., & White, K. M. (2008). *Johns Hopkins nursing evidence-based practice model and guidelines: Instructor's guide.* Indianapolis, IN: Sigma Theta Tau International.

Nolan, M. (2005). Reconciling tensions between research, evidence-based practice and user participation: Time for nursing to take the lead. *International Journal of Nursing Studies, 42*(5), 503–505.

O'Grady, E. T. (2008). Advanced practice registered nurses: The impact on patient safety and quality. In *Patient safety and quality: An evidence-based handbook for nurses.* Retrieved from http://www.ahrg .gov/qual/nurses/bk/docs/O'Grady.E-Aprn.pdf

Oman, K. S., Duran, C., & Fink, R. (2008). Evidence-based policy and procedures: An algorithm for success. *Journal of Nursing Administration, 38*(1), 47–51.

Padilla, G. V., Ferrell, B., Grant, M. M., & Rhiner, M. (1990). Defining the content domain of quality of life for cancer patients with pain. *Cancer Nursing, 13*(2), 108–115.

Patton, M. Q. (1990). *Qualitative evaluation and research methods* (2nd ed.). Newbury Park, CA: Sage Publications.

Pesut, B., & Johnson, J. (2007). Reinstating the "Queen": Understanding philosophical inquiry in nursing. *Journal of Advanced Nursing, 61*(1), 115–121.

Peterson, L. A., Woodward, L. D., Urech, T., Daw, C., & Sookanan, S. (2006). Does pay-for-performance improve the quality of health care? *Annals of Internal Medicine, 145*(4), 265–272.

Polit, D. F., & Hungler, B. P. (1997). *Essentials of nursing research: Methods, appraisal, and utilization* (4th ed.). Philadelphia: Lippincott-Raven.

Porter, S. (1996). Qualitative research. In D. F. S. Cormack (Ed.), *The research process in nursing* (3rd ed., pp. 113–122). Oxford: Blackwell Science.

Pravikoff, D. S., Tanner, A. B., & Pierce, S. T. (2005). Readiness of U.S. nurses for evidence-based practice. *American Journal of Nursing, 105*(9), 40–51.

Prochaska, J. O., & DiClemente, C. C. (1986). Toward a comprehensive model of change. In W. R. Miller and N. Heather (Eds.), *Treating addictive behaviors: Processes of change.* New York: Plenum Press.

Prosser, H., Almond, S., & Walley, T. (2003). Influences on GP's decision to prescribe new drugs: The importance of who says what. *Family Practice, 20*(1), 61–68.

Rasgon, N., Shelton, S., & Halbreich, U. (2005). Perimenopausal mental disorders: Epidemiology and phenomenology. *CNS Spectrums: The International Journal of Neuropsychiatric Sciences, 10*(6), 471–478.

Reavy, K., & Tavernier, S. (2008). Nurses reclaiming ownership of their practice: Implementation of an evidence-based model and process. *Journal of Continuing Education in Nursing, 39*(4), 166–172.

Reed, P., & Shear, N. C. (2004). *Perspectives on nursing theory* (4th ed.). Philadelphia: Lippincott Williams & Wilkins.

Reeves, M. J., Fonarow, G. G., Zhao, X., Smith, E. E., Schwamm, L. H., & Get with the Guidelines Stroke-Steering Committee and Investigators. (2009). Quality of care in women with ischemic stroke in the GWTG program. *Stroke, 40*(4), 1127–1133. doi: 10:1161./Stroke AHA.108.543/57

Rosenstock, I. M. (1966). Why people use health services. *Milbank Fund Quarterly, 44,* 94–127.

Rosswurm, M. A., & Larrabee, J. (1999). A model for change to evidence based practice. *Image: Journal of Nursing Scholarship, 31*(4), 317–322.

Russell, C., & Gregory, D. (2003). Evaluation of qualitative research studies. *Evidence-Based Nursing, 6*(2), 36–40.

Rutledge, D. N., & Bookbinder, M. (2002). Processes and outcomes of evidence-based practice. *Seminars in Oncology Nursing, 18*(1), 3–10.

Rycroft-Malone, J., Kitson, A., Harvey, G., McCormack, B., Seers, K., Titchen, A., et al., (2002). Ingredients for change: Revisiting a conceptual framework. *Quality and Safety in Health Care, 11*(2), 174–180.

Rycroft-Malone, J., Seers, K., Titchen, A., Harvey, G., Kitson, A., & McCormack, B. (2004). What counts as evidence in evidence-based practice? *Journal of Advanced Nursing, 47*(1), 81–90.

Sackett, D. L., Richardson, W. S., Rosenberg, W. T., & Haynes, R. B. (1997). *Evidence-based medicine: How to practice and teach evidence-based medicine.* New York: Churchill Livingstone.

Samson, L. (2006). *Building capacity for health disparities research.* Grant 1P20MD001816-01 from the National Center on Minority Health and Health Disparities, National Institutes of Health, Bethesda, MD.

Scarbrough, M. L., & Landis, S. E. (1997). A pilot study for the development of a hospital based immunization program. *Clinical Nurse Specialist, 11*(2), 70–75.

Schmidt, N., & Brown, J. M. (2009). *Evidence-based practice for nurses: Appraisal and application of research.* Sudbury, MA: Jones and Bartlett.

Schulman, L. S. (1993). Teaching as community property: Putting an end to pedagogical solitude. *Change, 25*(6), 6–7.

Scott-Findley, S., & Pollack, C. (2004). Evidence, research and knowledge: A call for conceptual clarity. *Worldviews on Evidence Based Nursing, 1*(2), 92–97.

Sheratt, C. (2005). The journal club: A method for occupational therapists to bridge the theory–practice gap. *British Journal of Occupational Therapy, 68*(7), 301–306.

Sigma Theta Tau International Clinical Scholarship Task Force. (1999). Clinical resource paper. Retrieved from www.nursingsociety.org/aboutus /PositionPapers/Documents/clinical_scholarship _paper.pdf

Simmons-Mackie, N. N., & Damico, J. S. (2001). Intervention outcomes: Clinical applications of qualitative methods. *Topics in Language Disorders, 21*(4), 21–36.

Singleton, J., & Levin, R. (2008). Strategies for learning evidence-based practice: Critically appraising clinical practice guidelines. *Journal of Nursing Education, 47*(8), 380–383.

Soumarai, S. B., McLauglin, T. J., Gurwitz, J. H., Guadagnoli, E., Hauptman, P. J., Borbas, C., et al. (1998). Effect of local medicine opinion leaders on quality of care for acute myocardial infarction. *Journal of the American Medical Association, 279*(17), 1358–1363.

Spitzer, R. L., Devlin, M., Walsh, B. T., Hasin, D., Wing, R., Marcus, M., et al. (1992). Binge eating disorder: A multi-site field trial of the diagnostic criteria. *International Journal of Eating Disorders, 11*(3), 191–203.

Stetler, C. B. (1994). Refinement of the Stetler/ Marram model for application of research findings to practice. *Nursing Outlook, 42*(1), 15–25.

Stetler, C. B., & Marram, G. (1976). Evaluating research findings for applicability in practice. *Nursing Outlook, 24*(9), 559–563.

Strauss, A., & Corbin, J. (1994). *Basics of qualitative research: Grounded theory procedures and techniques.* Newbury Park, NJ: Sage Publications.

Strauss, A., & Corbin, J. (1998). *Basics of qualitative research: Techniques and procedures for developing grounded theory.* Thousand Oaks, CA: Sage Publications.

Stroud, S. D., Erkel, E. A., & Smith, C. A. (2005). The use of personal digital assistants by nurse practitioner students and faculty. *Journal of the American Academy of Nurse Practitioners, 17*(2), 67–75.

Stull, A., & Lanz, C. (2005). An innovative model for nursing scholarship. *Journal of Nursing Education, 44*(11), 493–497.

Taft, L. B., Stolder, M. E., Knutson, A. B., Tamke, K., Platt, J., & Bowles, T. (2004). Oral history: Validating contributions of elders. *Geriatric Nursing, 25*(1), 38–43.

Timmerman, G. M. (1999). Using a women's health perspective to guide decisions made in quantitative research. *Journal of Advanced Nursing, 30*(3), 640–645.

Titler, M. G. (2002). Use of research in practice. In G. LoBiondo & J. Haber (Eds.), *Nursing research methods: Critical appraisal and utilization* (5th ed.). St. Louis, MO: Mosby.

Titler, M. G., Klieber, C., Steelman, V., Goode, C., Rakel, B., Barry-Walker, J., et al. (1994). Infusing research into practice to promote quality care. *Nursing Research, 43*(5), 307–313.

Trim, S. (2008). Journal club offers new opportunities. *Kai Tiaki Nursing New Zealand, 14*(11), 23.

Tropello, P. G. D. (2000). *Origins of the nurse practitioner movement: An oral history* (Doctoral dissertation). Rutgers, State University of New Jersey-New Brunswick, and University of Medicine and Dentistry of New Jersey. (UMI Order No. AAI9970979)

Tymkow, C., Shen, J. J., & MacMullen, N. (2006). Project 2: Emergency room usage among uninsured patients with access to a primary care provider. In L. Samson (Ed.), *Building capacity for health disparities research.* Grant 1P20MD001816-01 from the National Center on Minority Health and Health Disparities, National Institutes of Health, Bethesda, MD.

van Manen, M. (1990). *Researching lived experiences: Human science for an action sensitive pedagogy.* Albany, NY: State University of New York Press.

Watkins, C., Harvey, I., Langley, C., Gray, S., & Faulkner, A. (1999). General practitioners' use of guidelines in the consultation and their attitudes to them. *British Journal of General Practice, 49*(438), 11–15.

Webber, P. B. (2008). The Doctor of Nursing Practice degree and research: Are we making an epistemological mistake? *Journal of Nursing Education, 47*(10), 466–472.

Yegdich, T. (1999). In the name of Husserl: Nursing in pursuit of the things-in-themselves. *Nursing Inquiry, 7*(1), 29–40.

Zuzelo, P. R. (2007). Evidence-based nursing and qualitative research: A partnership imperative for real-world practice. In P. L. Munhall (Ed.), *Nursing research: A qualitative perspective* (4th ed.). Sudbury, MA: Jones and Bartlett.

PART 5

The Role of Race, Culture, Ethics and Advocacy in Advanced Nursing Practice

The fifth section of this book covers other core concepts as recommended by the AACN for advanced practice nursing knowledge—namely, diversity and ethics. Diversity in this context incorporates two complementary issues: diversity of the population cared for by nurses and diversity of the nursing workforce itself. As the U.S. population moves a more diverse and pluralistic society, the nursing profession is being challenged to develop greater cultural competence.

In Chapter 22, Washington lays out a background for understanding the migration patterns that have resulted in the multicultural, multiethnic, and multilingual society now found in the United States. The works of two nurse theorists, Leininger and Purnell, have shaped the thinking of the nursing profession related to cultural diversity and cultural competence. Washington reviews their work as a

foundation for the reader to apply their theories to practice.

Chapter 23 considers diversity from the perspective of African American history and its influence on the nursing profession. Further, Hill integrates the social and nursing history into a discussion of racial and ethnic disparities in health care.

In Chapter 24, Shi and Singh provide a comprehensive overview of the major characteristics of select U.S. population groups whose members face challenges and barriers in accessing healthcare services. These groups include racial/ethnic minorities, children and women, persons living in rural areas, the homeless, the mentally ill, and individuals with HIV/AIDS. The health needs of these population groups are summarized, and the services available to them are described. The gaps that currently exist between these population groups and the rest of the population indicate that the nation must make significant efforts to address the unique healthcare disparities of U.S. subpopulations.

In Chapter 25, Pozgar introduces basic ethics concepts and definitions. Scattered throughout this chapter are examples of ethical situations the reader can use to apply ethical principles to nursing practice.

Chapter 26 comprises a discussion by Twomey concerning the ANA Code of Ethics for Nurses. The nursing profession, as guided by this code of ethics, maintains a pursuit of excellence in practice, research, and education. Readers are encouraged to purchase the entire code with the interpretative statements for their professional libraries.

CHAPTER 22

Moving Toward a Culturally Competent Profession

Deborah Washington

CHAPTER OBJECTIVES

1. Discuss how the current multicultural, multiethnic, and multilingual patient population influences nursing practice.
2. Define cultural competence.
3. Apply Leininger's theory of transcultural nursing to the role of the advanced practice nurse.

INTRODUCTION

Historically, nursing has put great effort into establishing itself as a separate and unique discipline. This has meant overcoming challenges to boundaries and functions of practice as well as defining illness and wellness phenomena appropriate to the scope of practice. Over time, the domain of nursing has been clarified through a series of steps, resulting in a recognizable profession with a distinct approach to the delivery of health care.

The 21st century brings a new set of challenges to the ongoing evolution of the nursing profession. In the United States, for example, census data reflect an unprecedented situation in that non-Western cultures are reshaping the national population. The dominant Euro-American culture has shifted to a more pluralistic one. As a consequence, nursing is confronted with a new and provocative undertaking—to explore the professional tenets of nursing as well as to critique whether the United States has a serviceable healthcare system for the current social order. This chapter explores the increasing importance of culture as a direction for growth in clinical practice and discusses how to incorporate theoretical models into patient care. Culture is large in scope and content and has the potential to influence the domain of knowledge unique to nursing as a discipline focused on the phenomenon of care. Although the influence of culture should not change the basic tenets of practice, a determining factor in care is the inclusion of a person-centered approach to the restoration and maintenance of health.

BACKGROUND

The healthcare setting of the 20th century was the result of conventions that do not reflect the reality of the current millennium. The original healthcare model was designed primarily to serve patients who spoke English, were able to read and write that language, typically had the resources to pay for care, believed in the germ theory of disease, valued biomedical preventive health practices, and acquiesced to the authoritarian model of the patient–healthcare provider relationship. The typical user of health services today no longer matches this image. The current patient population includes a wide array of lifestyles and is multicultural, multiethnic, and multilingual. More specifically, patients may not speak English, much less be able to read or write in their native language. They may be employed, but frequently do not have health insurance. Patients may be refugees, recently arrived immigrants, undocumented workers, or residents not yet acculturated to Western life because of indigenous pride or as a consequence of social isolation.

Human migration continues to be an all-embracing phenomenon. Few countries are unaffected by its trends. In the United States, the foreign-born population increased from 7.90% in 1990 to 11.70% in 2003. Information on immigration in 2003 documents that 305,973 people emigrated from the Americas, 251,296 from Asian nations, and 48,738 from African nations (Global Data Center, 2005). Hispanics surpassed African Americans in the 2000 census and are now the largest minority group in the United States. Non-Hispanic Whites are the slowest-growing group, and some predict they will constitute a smaller percentage of the U.S. population in the future (Day, 2005).

THE DIASPORA

The *diaspora* (Greek for "to scatter") of new populations presents challenges to the host culture. Historically, host communities have the unstated expectation that the new arrivals will assimilate into the dominant culture. Adapting to new social norms often requires disengagement from old traditions, customs, and practices and frequently precipitates a loss of heritage-based identity. Culture shock and isolation related to the new environment generate a sense of dislocation, stress, and anxiety. Support services and appropriate resources are necessary to provide for and maintain the mental and physical well-being of groups seeking to establish themselves in new places (Kim, Cho, Klessig, Gerace, & Camilleri, 2002).

Immigrants familiar with health systems and practices in their country of origin face obstacles that can hinder access to care (Leduc & Proulx, 2004). Therefore, informational resources related to health services are of critical importance for new arrivals. The lack of such information influences decision making and compromises timely contact with needed care. Proficiency with English, an understanding of bureaucratic systems, and the ability to acquire health insurance are determining factors with consequences for the clinical encounter. The complexities of providing care to individuals who are unable to cope with these factors can result in culturally insensitive encounters and result in care that is inappropriate and, in some cases, even dangerous.

The inability to communicate and the negative consequences to quality of care have generated both research and awareness among practitioners. Within the paradigm of healthcare disparities, language and communication have been identified as critical additions to a culturally competent healthcare system. In 1999, the U.S. Department of Health and Human Services, Office of Minority Health, proposed national standards for culturally and linguistically appropriate services in order to establish the importance of these criteria as benchmarks for consumers, providers, and health systems. Fourteen recommendations were formulated, five of which explicitly address the need for language support (**Table 22-1**).

These recommendations are unprecedented. Ramifications for the practice of nursing in all healthcare settings are still to be determined. Safe practice and effective approaches to care are the anticipated outcomes. To include the consumer in full clinical decision making, it is incumbent on the clinician to understand the resource needs of patients from different cultural backgrounds.

LIMITATIONS OF MULTICULTURALISM

Becoming fluent in cultural mores is not easy and can be compromised by assumptions that all people from one geographic area are the same. Separating a culture into its component parts as a guide for understanding the whole culture risks reducing complex meanings into formulas. It also is critical to understand people's perceptions of being marginalized as the "other." Canales and Bowers (2001) described the "other" as:

> . . . Someone who is perceived as different from self. Historically, persons labelled as Other, as them, are categorized primarily according to

how their differences from the societal norm are perceived. Their Otherness is signified by their relational differences; when compared to the "ordinary," "usual" and "familiar" attributes of persons, they appear "different," as Other. It is persons categorized as Other who often reside at the margins of society. (p. 103)

Additionally, variables such as class, education, gender, and religion significantly influence individuals. Although these factors can be generalized as themes of personhood, care must be exercised to prevent their use as a basis for stereotypes. The importance of identifying this information strongly affects the course of events that establish quality of care. Access to the best information available as it relates to the patient has significance for length of stay, appropriate discharge planning, and patient satisfaction.

HEALTH DISPARITIES

The constitution of the World Health Organization (WHO) states:

> Health is a state of complete physical, mental and social well-being and not merely the absence of disease or infirmity. The enjoyment of the highest attainable standard of health is one of the fundamental rights of every human being without distinction of race, religion, political belief, economic or social condition. (World Health Organization, 2006)

Decisive evidence of disparities in health care is attracting attention in the literature. The information provided is focused on comparative

TABLE 22-1	Culturally and Linguistically Appropriate Standards (CLAS)

1. Provide all clients with limited English proficiency access to interpreter services.

2. Provide oral and written notices and signage to clients in their primary language, including the right to an interpreter at no cost.

3. Make available patient education and other materials in the language of the predominant group in the relevant service area.

4. Ensure the language proficiency and skills of the interpreter.

5. Ensure that the language preference and self-identified race/ethnicity of the client is included in the organization's information systems.

data that describe a statistical picture of morbidity and mortality, as well as increased awareness of problems of access to care and quality of care. For example, health status and utilization of services by diverse groups have become familiar parts of the discourse on equity in health care. Access and documented health outcomes illustrate a lack of parity between defined populations. However, the lack of national standards in service delivery and the paucity of evaluative research hamper explanations of the causes (Horowitz, Davis, Palermo, & Vladek, 2000). Disparities as an area of concern for healthcare providers is supported by studies that underscore inconsistencies between length of life and quality of life associated with specific cultural groups. The number of excess deaths and the difference between rates of death for minority groups as compared with a reference group reveal a situation in health care that warrants attention (LaVeist, Bowie, & Cooley-Quille, 2000). It is possible to extract issues from current research that indicate the need for close and careful observation of extant conditions. The ability to corroborate the implications of these studies with the daily conventions of clinical practice creates the conditions for strategies to address this dilemma.

Coleman-Miller (2000) emphasized the importance of cultural sensitivity training for healthcare providers to counteract the effects of cultural disregard in the form of poor interpersonal relationships, language with culture-based meanings, and ineffective services. Nontraditional health system designs that serve to improve or advance respectful attention to the needs of a multicultural population must be substantiated with more evaluative research. The significance of this is clear when due consideration is given to the need to delineate the function of factors such as racism and discrimination on health outcomes, despite an inherent discomfort with the concept. A restructuring of the healthcare delivery system driven by budgetary constraints has mobilized entrants into environments where previously they may not have been encountered in great numbers (Williams & Rucker, 2000). This can result in personal and professional challenges for any clinician.

CULTURE AND WESTERN HEALTH CARE

Culture can be a facilitator or a barrier to health care (Searight, 2003), and belief systems can sway an individual's use of information (IOM, 2002). Western biomedicine tends to dismiss non-Western approaches to healing because many of them do not base disease causality in germ theory or practice the scientific method. Many non-Western societies find the Western emphasis on pathophysiology and biomedicine to be problematic. The biomedical definition of absence of disease fails to acknowledge the interrelationship of body, mind, and spirit. In *The Spirit Catches You and You Fall Down*, Fadiman (1997) captures this cultural clash. The lack of understanding between doctors and a Hmong family led to tragedy. Lia, a child diagnosed with severe epilepsy, eventually died from complications; her parents did not understand how important the medication was, and the healthcare team did not understand the complex cultural customs of the Hmong.

Cultural interpretations of the value of abandoning natal beliefs in favor of more dominant customs can be life altering. For instance, in Haitian culture, the power of a spirit that rides or possesses a believer is used to explain changes in personality (Holcomb, Parsons, Giger, & Davidhizar, 1996). In Western culture, the ability to medicalize behavior considered outside the norm endows professional experts with civil power (Reddy, 2002).

These differences in belief practices beg several questions:

- Which culturally relevant treatments maintain health and well-being?
- Is the definition of health and well-being a moving target—does it mean different things to different cultures?

- Is quality care based on the Western biomedical model? What is the role of the traditional healer?
- Which frame of reference does a culturally competent clinician use to answer these questions?

The answers have the potential to place the clinician in an ethical dilemma. The ability to offer a proven best treatment is not simply a function of perspective or worldview. Scientific facts exist and are the basis for evidence-based practice. However, biomedicine does have the capacity to coexist with other belief systems. Therefore, a plan of care that coordinates treatment options, taking into consideration cultural values and customs, can be negotiated.

NURSING LENS OF THE MULTICULTURAL PROFESSIONAL

The impact of culture on nursing must be considered from another perspective if the topic and the profession are to be examined with new vision. The Western model dominates nursing identity and definition (Herdman, 2001). This has evolved into describing the field as science as well as art. In spite of this dual interpretation, however, science and its methods are explicitly positioned as the most desired path to knowledge within the discipline. Observation and experiments are the foundation used to develop tenets of practice, and a knowledge base framed as unique to the profession is the goal of what has become a prolonged endeavor.

Nevertheless, there is also a non-Western perspective on the discipline. From this aspect, nursing can be a formal or an informal concept. This specific differentiation is determined by the infrastructure that validates the role function. When tasks and activities in a particular society are solely the result of an apprenticed experience accepted by the general community, cultural rituals and traditions often dominate. However, when the role is the consequence of an educational regimen controlled by a professional body that confers the status of licensure,

there are accustomed methods and procedures resulting from discipline-specific conventions that must be followed. Historically, the scientific approach has carried the designation of modern, and consequently is more highly valued. This has essentially negated the usefulness and importance of learning accessed through the customs, rituals, and traditions of other cultures and societies. These paths to knowledge should be explored for the value they offer to the complementary part of nursing customarily known as its art. The nursing lens of the multicultural professional has much to offer to this part of nursing, which has been deemphasized in the pursuit of its scientific identity.

Ethnic identity influences all of the domains of nursing: person, health, environment, and nursing. In exploring ethnicity as culture, Phinney (1996) suggested that such factors as values and attitudes were assumed to describe the cultural characteristics of a specific group. This perspective was portrayed in a study conducted by Struthers (2001) that explored nursing from a Native American point of view. Here, caring and holism, among other dimensions, were delineated culturally. Caring involved the elements of humor and partnership; holism included balance and the use of nonverbal interaction. Pang and colleagues (2004) compared Chinese, American, and Japanese nurses' understanding of ethical responsibilities. Interestingly, there were different degrees of value placed on statements related to respect. Chinese nurses gave higher marks to language related to respect for nurses, Japanese nurses gave higher marks to respect for patients, and American nurses gave higher value to statements related to respect for individual rights. Pang and colleagues also examined the experience of nursing practice in Chinese culture. The concept of nursing was rooted in the philosophical principles of the society and the nuances of the associated language. For example, Chinese terms that describe good practice include "truthfulness," "responsibility," and "service," along with "understanding" and "knowledge" in conjunction with the actions of "protect" and "interact." Chen (2000) points out that cultural values influenced by relevant philosophical and religious beliefs are by their nature embedded in attitudes related to health in Chinese culture. To merge these cultural ideologies into a universal understanding of the concepts to nurse or to be a nurse holds great promise for the next steps as the profession continues to develop.

CULTURALLY COMPETENT CARE

An overall definition of culture and a description of its basic elements outline the basis for group identity. Leininger and McFarland (2002) offer a broad-based definition that describes culture as a "way of life belonging to an individual or a group that reflects values and customs taught and learned generationally" (p. 9). In her transcultural nursing model, Leininger (2001) includes religious, kinship, social, political and legal, economic, educational, technologic, and cultural values as components of culture.

The individual with a distinct cultural viewpoint has a dynamic and integral relationship with the nurse who provides culturally congruent care. Cultural competence has many definitions in the literature. However, in essence, it is a compilation of the clinical skills and professional behaviors of a healthcare provider focused on the cultural values, beliefs, and perceptions of the consumer while both are engaged in the therapeutic relationship. Cultural competence is an aspect of nursing that will move the profession to its next developmental phase.

Leininger (2001) defines culture care preservation or maintenance as follows:

> . . . those assistive, supporting, facilitative, or enabling professional actions and decisions that help people of a particular culture to retain and/or preserve relevant care values so that they can maintain their well-being, recover from illness, or face handicaps and/or death. (p. 48)

Nursing has continuously acknowledged the status of the individual. Recognition of the cultural life, values, and beliefs of persons is simply an expansion of that attention. The nursing assessment, problem list, diagnosis, progress note, or discharge plan can be effective only if cultural influences are addressed. This viewpoint is in deference to the concept of cultural autonomy. The dimension of the individual experience is characterized by such concepts as acculturation, the implementation and acceptance of customs different from the primary culture; assimilation, the blending of one culture with another; and cultural autonomy, the ability to retain principal identity in the presence of one or more dominant groups (see **Figure 22-1**).

Cultural autonomy upholds the importance of the valued presence of customs, conventions, and folkways of all cultures within any given society without the pressure to assimilate. The imperative of one culture should not be the cause for dismissal of another.

In contrast, acculturation denotes an ability to adapt to the rules and conventions of a society different from the country of origin. The

FIGURE 22-1 Aspects of Culturally Competent Care

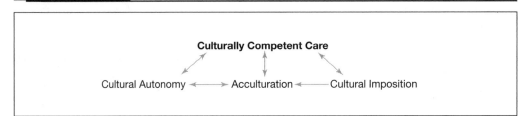

newcomer must manage culture shock and develop survival skills that allow for an effective level of function in new and unfamiliar surroundings. Navigating the healthcare system is one of those skills. The culturally competent provider must organize appropriate resources to enable proficient and uncompromising care. Meeting the needs of the unacculturated challenges system design and tests the justification for and the philosophy in support of care delivery. Explanations for professional practice must be grounded in findings more substantive than mere tradition to avoid the entanglements of ethnocentrism. Providing rationale for current methods prompts analysis and objective application of practice principles.

Cultural imposition imposes the way of life of one culture on that of another. It necessitates a belief in the superiority of the prevailing manner of living and conveys compulsory adherence to accepted norms. However, if any culture and its way of life are to endure, the cultural imposition of one group must be offset by the cultural autonomy of the other. This is the point that underpins the complexities associated with multiculturalism in a pluralistic society. It can be especially problematic in a healthcare situation. In this context, those recently arrived and unaccustomed to the attitudes and values of the culture to which they are not yet accustomed initially present as a problem-solving task in the clinical encounter. Under these circumstances, culturally controlled values and norms can become the focus of intervention as a first step in managing treatment.

THE SUBSTANCE OF NURSING: THEORY AND CULTURE

Nursing theory is the source of discipline-specific concepts. Theory suggests explanations for what nursing does that differentiate it from other branches of knowledge. Theory explains why nurses act as they do and describes how nurses should use those explanations to assist maintenance or restoration of health and well-

being. The influence of culture in this schema deserves exploration.

Transcultural Nursing

Cultural diversity, or multiculturalism, is a social construct of increasing importance to the understanding of healthcare quality. Clarification of the influence of culture on the domains of nursing will be a sign of the next evolutionary stage of the profession. Issues that will move nursing forward include the influence of culture in defining excellence in patient care and the significance of culture as an applied intervention for the improvement of health.

When the concept of transcultural nursing was introduced in the 1950s, it was not viewed as relevant to nursing practice (Leininger, 1978), perhaps because nursing theory was young or because of the hegemonic views of the Euro-American culture of the time. Because the nursing profession is dynamic, it reflects the social needs and conscience of any given era (Henderson, 1966); thus the profession has come to embrace the pioneering efforts of Madeleine Leininger and her conceptualization of transcultural nursing.

Leininger defined transcultural nursing as "a formal area of study and practice focused on comparative human-care differences and similarities of the beliefs, values and patterned lifeways of cultures to provide culturally congruent, meaningful, and beneficial health care to people" (Leininger & McFarland, 2002, p. 6). Culture is the facilitator through which the nurse can understand and support individual needs. The full range of anthropological constructs (for example, language, group history, religion, and politics) are used as reference for a more fully developed understanding of every person and the circumstances of each individual life.

Transcultural nursing provides a holistic approach to understanding each individual within the context of the various influences on that unique life. The sunrise model includes information on the following factors: education, economic, political and legal, kinship and social, religious and philosophical, and technological. This biographical history captures the important details of a patient's life. These details, in turn, provide a comprehensive depiction of the individual that serves to enhance care based in knowledge with both depth and abundant detail. Such detail implements a process for increasing familiarity with those who are dissimilar and decreases anxiety related to contact with the unknown for the healthcare provider and patient alike.

Transcultural nursing also possesses an implicit advantage. Many of the concepts that identify a holistic approach to care enable the building of an authentic relationship between patient and provider. In the practice domain, socially sensitive issues related to bias, prejudice, cultural imposition, cultural blindness, and cultural pain become part of the definition of culturally congruent care. Cultural conflict is an expected development when dissimilar groups who have minimal contact find it necessary to interact. Transcultural nursing supplies a knowledge base by which disharmony can effectively be addressed. For example, Leininger (2001) formulated a concept to describe the psychological and emotional distress experienced by patients when healthcare providers demonstrate a lack of concern for the cultural beliefs and customs of others.

As defined by Leininger and McFarland (2002), "cultural pain refers to suffering, discomfort, or being greatly offended by an individual or group who shows a great lack of sensitivity toward another's cultural experience" (p. 52). Understanding an individual within the context of his or her worldview is the crux of the presence or absence of cultural pain. As an example of emotional distress, cultural pain is associated with hurtful memories, damaging words that evoke those memories, insults, and indignities. It must be acknowledged that what is considered hurtful from one standpoint

may not be understood as such from another. Although inflicting cultural pain is not always intentional or conscious, insensitivity can be enmeshed in a lack of awareness. Concomitant understanding and social blunders often are associated with inadequate knowledge related to cultural triggers that are well known to the insider but less so to the outsider. The resulting distress should not be dismissed by the person hurt simply because the deed was not intended. The prevention of a recurrence is more important and requires an exploration of context and meaning from all relevant perspectives. For example, it is a particular affront to an African American to have his or her smile described as a "big, toothy grin." This can be understood within the context of racist caricatures from the pre–civil rights era. Another example would be the individual who speaks accented English and becomes sensitized to questions about citizenship status.

Understanding the elements of culture in an approach to care that is holistic is a demonstration of cultural competence. As nursing continues to refine the relevance of culturally competent care to its domain of knowledge, an understanding of cultural pain will contribute to an understanding of the impact of diversity on the healthcare system and the clinical encounters that are part of the environment of care.

Elements of culture are a route of communication to generate collaboration between a patient, family, or community and the chosen provider. Separating a culture into its component parts to guide the understanding of a particular people is a more complex process than simple fact finding. Insight that assigns meaning is necessary if the nature and significance of culture are to have value in the care experience.

Purnell's Model for Cultural Competence

The incorporation of cultural skills and knowledge into clinical practice is facilitated by a well-grounded reference, making the gathering of information more manageable. Many culturally based assessment tools for gathering information are very detailed. A busy practitioner would not attempt to collate, at one time, all the information suggested by the instrument. However, the culturally prepared clinician would be mindful of important specifics suggested by these tools that would enhance the quality and usefulness of the information collected.

Larry Purnell developed a conceptual model for the culturally competent provider in 1995 that was originally intended as a nursing assessment tool (Purnell, 2002). His 12 domains of culture (2000) are relevant guideposts for the initial health history (see **Table 22-2**).

A guide of this nature helps to focus the interview process and draws attention to key elements of each unique cultural perspective. When information is clustered in this way, a useful care plan can be formulated from synthesized information. If this framework is used, some foreknowledge of the cultural group is required to support a focused interview process that remains timely and is not haphazard. Not all questions need to be asked. Clinical judgment should guide the clinician. For example, once the issue of communication has been resolved, for the African American patient with a chief complaint of chest pain the initial assessment would most likely include the domains of healthcare practices and practitioners, high-risk behaviors, biocultural ecology (i.e., physical features), and nutrition to determine the most essential information for this complaint. The culturally prepared practitioner would be aware of the following:

- Prominence of cardiovascular disease among African Americans
- Possibility of traditional practices and self-adjusted dosage of medication
- Ability to metabolize medications
- Soul food
- Social history of African Americans as context for clinical encounter

CONCLUSION

Cultural diversity, or multiculturalism, is a social construct of increasing importance in understanding healthcare quality. Clarification of the influence of culture on the domains of nursing will be an indication of the next evolutionary stage of the profession. What is the influence of culture in defining excellence in patient care? What is the significance of culture as an applied intervention for the improvement of health? What is the impact of culture on interpersonal and therapeutic relationships?

Culture can be a paradigm for worldviews. In transcultural nursing, these paradigms utilize anthropological concepts to inform a nursing perspective on health and illness beliefs that originate in the cultural life of a given society. Culture is the facilitator through which nurses can understand and support individual needs. The full range of anthropological constructs (e.g., language, group history) is used as a reference for a more fully developed understanding of every person and the context of each individual life and worldview.

Leininger and McFarland (2002) give an orientational definition of worldview as "the way an individual or group looks out on and understands their world about them as a value, stance, picture, or perspective about life or the world" (p. 83). Blacks, Hispanics, Asians,

TABLE 22-2	Purnell's Model of Cultural Domains
Heritage	Communication
Family roles	Workforce issues
Biocultural ecology	High-risk behaviors
Nutrition	Pregnancy
Death rituals	Spirituality
Healthcare practices	Healthcare practitioners

American Indians, and Caucasians have had vastly divergent social experiences in the United States. These experiences are so disparate that perspectives often are polarized. Empathy and increased cultural knowledge of other ethnic heritages are essential to the promotion of positive and more trusting clinical encounters. However, active questions stimulate discourse on Western definitions of what constitutes good care. For example, the Western philosophies of self-care and out-of-bed activity are representative of differing perspectives on wellness behavior.

As a topic of research, the value of culturally competent care to the patient remains unclear and undefined. For example, some practitioners contend that it is possible to generate a sense of well-being for a patient without undue attention to issues of culture. Also, long-established practices reframed as issues of culture (e.g., referrals to spiritual caregivers or dietary consults) can be viewed as standard procedure as opposed to culture-specific care. However, cultural customs that conflict with policy and procedures (e.g., newborn-naming customs of Cambodians call for a wait of one week and the naming is done by grandparents) are clear illustrations that cultural knowledge does indicate the need for new precedents.

Culture is a form of identity. Identity is a complex concept that involves the explication of factors that, among other things, characterize cultural heritage. The ongoing exploration of the meaning of cultural identity is poised to enhance the functioning of our pluralistic society. History has shown cultural heritage can be a highly charged domain of inquiry when it involves race and ethnicity. However, knowledge-based methods of care underpin the type of practice competence that includes awareness of the human dimensions of diversity. The proficient healthcare provider is sensitive to the distinctions of difference and models a nursing process that promotes the reciprocal relationship between culture and quality care.

DISCUSSION QUESTIONS

1. Discuss each of the following questions:
   a. Which culturally relevant treatments maintain health and well-being?
   b. Is the definition of health and well-being a moving target? Does it mean different things to different cultures?
   c. Is quality care based on the Western biomedical model? What is the role of the traditional healer?
   d. Which frame of reference does a culturally competent clinician use to answer these questions?

2. Describe a client situation in which culture misunderstanding and/or differences were evident. What was the influence of culture in achieving or not achieving the patient care outcome? What was the impact of culture on interpersonal and therapeutic relationships?

3. Apply Leininger's theory of transcultural nursing to advanced nursing practice.

REFERENCES

Canales, M., & Bowers, B. (2001). Expanding conceptualizations of culturally competent care. *Journal of Advanced Nursing, 36*(1), 102–111.

Chen, Y. (2000). Chinese values, health and nursing. *Journal of Advanced Nursing, 36*(2), 270–273.

Coleman-Miller, B. (2000). A physician's perspective on minority health. *Health Care Financing Review, 21*(4), 45–56.

Day, J. C. (2005). National population projections. Retrieved February 2, 2005, from http://www .census. gov/population/www/pop-profile/natproj .html

Fadiman, A. (1997). *The spirit catches you and you fall down.* New York: Farrar, Straus, Giroux.

Global Data Center. (2005). United States: Inflow of foreign-born population by country of birth, 1986 to 2003. Available at http://www.migration information.org/GlobalData/countrydata/data.cfm

Henderson, V. (1966). *The nature of nursing: A definition and its implications for practice, research, and education.* New York: Macmillan.

Herdman, E. (2001). The illusion of progress in nursing. *Nursing Philosophy, 2*(1), 4–13.

Holcomb, L. O., Parsons, L. C., Giger, J. N., & David-hizar, R. (1996). Haitian Americans: Implications for nursing care. *Journal of Community Health Nursing, 13*(4), 249–460.

Horowitz, C. R., Davis, M. H., Palermo, A. G., & Vladek, B. C. (2000). Approaches to eliminating sociocultural disparities in health. *Health Care Financing Review, 21*(4), 57–74.

Institute of Medicine (IOM). (2002). *Speaking of health: Assessing health communication strategies for diverse populations.* Washington, DC: Institute of Medicine.

Kim, M. J., Cho, H., Klessig, Y., Gerace, L., & Camilleri, D. (2002). Primary health care for Korean immigrants: Sustaining a culturally sensitive model. *Public Health Nursing, 19*(3), 191–200.

LaVeist, T. A., Bowie, J. V., & Cooley-Quille, M. (2000). Minority health status in adulthood: The middle years of life. *Health Care Financing Review, 21*(4), 9–21.

Leduc, N., & Proulx, M. (2004). Patterns of health services utilization by recent immigrants. *Journal of Immigrant Health, 6*(1), 15–27.

Leininger, M. (1978). *Transcultural nursing: Concepts, theories, and practices.* New York: Wiley.

Leininger, M. (2001). The theory. In M. Leininger (Ed.), *Culture care diversity and universality* (pp. 5–68). Sudbury, MA: Jones and Bartlett.

Leininger, M., & McFarland, M. (2002). *Transcultural nursing: Concepts, theories, research, practice.* New York: McGraw-Hill.

Pang, S., Wong, T., Wang, C., Sheng, Z., Zhi Jun, C., Helen, Y., et al. (2004). Towards a Chinese definition of nursing. *Journal of Advanced Nursing, 46*(6), 657–670.

Phinney, J. (1996). When we talk about American ethnic groups, what do we mean? *American Psychologist, 31*(9), 918–927.

Purnell, L. (2000). A description of the Purnell model of cultural competence. *Journal of Transcultural Nursing, 11*(1), 40–46.

Purnell, L. (2002). The Purnell model of cultural competence. *Journal of Transcultural Nursing, 13*(13), 193–196.

Reddy, S. (2002). Temporarily insane: Pathologising cultural difference in American criminal courts. *Sociology of Health and Illness, 24*(5), 667–687.

Searight, H. (2003). Bosnian immigrants' perceptions of the United States healthcare system: A qualitative interview study. *Journal of Immigrant Health, 5*(2), 87–93.

Struthers, R. (2001). A conceptual framework of nursing in Native American culture. *Journal of Nursing Scholarship.* Retrieved August 5, 2004, from the HighBeam Research Database.

Williams, D. R., & Rucker, T. D. (2000). Understanding and addressing racial disparities in health care. *Health Care Financing Review, 21*(4), 75–90.

World Health Organization. (2006). Constitution of the World Health Organization. Retrieved November 2, 2007, from http://www.who.int /governance/eb/who_constitution_en.pdf

CHAPTER 23

Race, Race Relations, and the Emergence of Professional Nursing, 1870–2004

Patricia St. Hill

CHAPTER OBJECTIVES

1. Review the social and nursing history of the United States as a backdrop for understanding racial discrimination and healthcare disparity.

2. Suggest future initiatives to increase the numbers of minorities in nursing.

3. Discuss future initiatives for decreasing healthcare disparities.

INTRODUCTION

It is widely known that racial and ethnic minorities experience higher rates of illness and disability and die earlier than Whites. The Institute of Medicine, in its 2003 report titled *Unequal Treatment: Confronting Racial and Ethnic Disparities in Healthcare,* stated the obvious—that minorities receive inferior health care. The current national mandate is to end racial and ethnic discrimination in health care by 2010 and to increase the number of minority healthcare providers.

Barriers to ending racial discrimination can best be understood by examining the social history of the United States. Even though health disparities and minority representation in nursing span many races and ethnic cultures, history best documents this for African Americans (Sullivan Commission, 2004). This chapter examines the influence of race and race relations among Blacks and Whites in American society on the developing nursing profession as it emerged from a task-oriented vocation to a profession in its own right. In doing so, the chapter highlights several critical periods and turning points in American history and traces their reverberations and influences on the emerging nursing profession. In closing, the chapter looks to the future and attempts to predict the challenges and rewards faced by professional nursing.

THE CIVIL WAR ERA

A retrospective view of the nursing profession in the United States mirrors the country's existing sociocultural norms, beliefs, and values. Historical documentation of the social climate prior to and during the 1800s explicates the social inequities, unjust laws, and discriminatory practices that Black nurses were subjected to at the dawning of the profession. The works of Carnegie (1986), Staupers (1961), and Hine (1989) make direct linkages between the difficulties and hardships faced by Black nurses in the early years and the prevailing segregationist views of the nursing leadership, nursing organizations, and large segments of American society.

Elmore (1976), speaking to this issue, noted that there are no special records about Blacks from the earliest days of this country and argued that it was difficult to believe that the slave nursemaid did not become the nurse of the time, in her family or her master's family, at least. Similarly, George, Bradford, and Battle (1995) pointed out that a review of nursing history texts showed that Black nurses were rarely mentioned as contributors to the development of the profession.

With the onset of the Civil War, some minor changes occurred, and the historical record, according to Elmore (1976), becomes clearer. During this period, the names of several early Black nurses surface. Among them are Harriet Tubman and Sojourner Truth, both of whom are well known for activities other than nursing, but who are also credited with having cared for wounded soldiers during the Civil War.

Even more widely recognized is Namahyoke Sockum Curtis, who volunteered her services during the Spanish–American War and was assigned as a contract nurse by the War Department. History also shows that she later served as a Red Cross volunteer during the Galveston flood of 1900 and after the San Francisco earthquake in 1906. The ultimate recognition of her work was a government pension and burial at Arlington Cemetery (Elmore, 1976).

Despite the seeming gains and inroads made by this select group of Black nurses, American society remained very much divided along racial lines. In general, the environment for Blacks throughout the 1800s was hostile. In fact, Massey (1934), recounting the sacrifices, struggles, lack of recognition, and adversities faced by Blacks in America, parallels the history of Black nurses in America.

THE SEGREGATION LAWS AND NURSING

Nineteenth-century America was by all measures a hostile, suppressive, and dangerous place for Blacks. The indelible need to dominate and control a perceived inferior group persisted under the guise of the Jim Crow laws, a series of discriminatory laws in the Southern states that called for the separation of the races. Under Jim Crow, segregation of the races was the order of the day. This social custom prevailed and was supported legally in the 1896 Supreme Court ruling of *Plessy vs. Ferguson*. Furthermore, under these laws, the notion of separate but equal was contrived and promulgated to justify the rigid segregation laws that imposed legal punishment on people for consorting with members of another race and that served to divide all of American society, as well as the emerging nursing profession, along racial lines.

The healthcare system post–Civil War to the late 1960s was composed of two separate and unequal systems—one for Whites and a considerably more inferior one for Blacks. As one woman put it:

> Dr. Bailey on Main Street in Greenville was our family physician. There was a separate waiting room for blacks and you had to wait 'til all the

white patients were seen before he'd see the blacks. As long as white patients kept coming in, you kept being pushed further and further back. (Smith, 1999, as cited in Sullivan Commission, 2004, p. 32)

Black nursing students, for the most part, were excluded from White hospital-based nursing programs and were relegated to Black-operated schools, whose curricula and programs have been described as deplorable (Pitts-Mosley, 1995). A select few Blacks were provided limited access to White schools in accordance with strictly enforced institutional quotas. It should also be pointed out that educational barriers and challenges existed in both the Northern and the Southern states for Black women interested in pursuing a nursing career. Pitts-Mosley (1995) noted that although Black codes limiting access to practice opportunities and to institutions of learning were legislated and enforced by law in the Southern states, they also were observed and enforced unofficially in the North, a phenomenon frequently referred to as de facto segregation. For example, the New England Hospital for Women and Children in Boston, Massachusetts, although renowned for having graduated America's first Black trained nurse, Mary Mahoney, in 1879, nonetheless employed the quota system, limiting the number of Blacks admitted each year to two. This number was later altered to include one Black and one Jewish student (Carnegie, 1986).

Between 1886 and 1977, 77 schools for Negroes had been established in 20 states and the District of Columbia (Carnegie, 1986). For the women attending Black-operated programs, many of which were, in actuality, led by White superintendents, curricula and programs were less than adequate. Documented evidence points to curricula deficiencies, lack of resources, and inadequately trained teachers. Admittedly, the majority of nursing schools (both Black and White) operating during the late 1800s and early 1900s were plagued by inadequacies, including poorly designed or nonexistent curricula. This prompted the estab-

lishment of the American Society of Superintendents of Training Schools of Nurses (the Superintendents' Society) in 1893, which later became the National League for Nursing Education (NLNE), and then the National League for Nursing (NLN).

The purpose of the Superintendents' Society was to improve nursing curricula and develop standards of admissions to schools of nursing (Bullough & Bullough, 1978). These actions contributed to the advancement and professionalization of nursing; however, they were of no benefit to Black nurses. For Black, or Negro, schools, the lack of support and recognition from professional nursing organizations such as the NLNE and the American Nurses Association (ANA) undermined their legitimacy and called into question their professional standing. It was not until 1942 that the NLNE offered individual membership to Black nurses, whose many previous attempts to gain membership had been systematically denied (Champinha-Bacote, 1988). In 1948, six years later, the ANA finally extended its membership to Black nurses.

NURSING PRACTICE UNDER THE SEGREGATION LAWS

Upon graduating from nurse training programs, Black nurses faced the challenges of limited practice opportunities and lower wages than their White counterparts. As a general rule, the practice of Black nurses was limited to caring for Black clients either in the home, as private-duty nurses, or in the hospital. The prevailing sentiment was that Black nurses were best suited to care for Black patients (Carnegie, 1986; Staupers, 1961). It was common practice for Black student nurses to care for Black patients in the home, as private duty nurses, without supervision. This practice, although inarguably dangerous and unsafe for both clients and nursing students, was, nonetheless, routine with Black schools that relied on the monies paid to the students (Pitts-Mosley, 1996).

With the establishment of public health nursing at the Henry Street Settlement in 1893, the few Black nurses hired by Lillian Wald, founder and director of the Henry Street Settlement Visiting Nursing Service, were afforded the opportunity to extend their practice into this arena of nursing (Pitts-Mosley, 1996). Still, the pervasive inequities that haunted the profession persisted and were intimately tied to three issues. The first was the educational structure in place for training Black and White nurses separately, which prevented disadvantaged Black nurses from receiving a high-quality education. The second was the administration of separate licensing examinations for Black and White nurses, which served only to further divide the profession along racial lines. The third issue was the exclusion of Black nurses from membership and representation in professional organizations, such as the ANA and the NLNE, hence denying Black nurses and Black nursing practice legitimacy within a system that already had preconceived notions about the competence of Black nursing programs and their graduates.

RACIAL QUOTAS AND THE WARS (1901–1951)

The 20th century was witness to World War I (1914–1918) and World War II (1939–1945), both of which created additional demands for nurses to care for wounded soldiers. Typically, under conditions of a reasonably normal nursing supply, race is one of several characteristics, along with age, education, sex, and marital status, that are taken into account in the hiring and acceptance of nurses. In the face of necessity, such as war, however, the characteristics least relevant to professional performance are dropped, and individuals who can fulfill minimum standards, such as having a license as a professional nurse, get their chance (Goldstein, 1960). In the case of the U.S. military, however, despite its desperate need for nurses to care for wounded soldiers during World War I, the use of Black nurses was not an option. It took the flu epidemic of 1918 to see the first 18 Black

nurses accepted and assigned to army camps in Ohio and Illinois, with other assignments to follow (Elmore, 1976).

In 1943, the Cadet Nurse Corps was established to address the acute nursing shortage caused by World War II. Students who signed on would receive reimbursement for tuition, books, uniforms, and a monthly stipend if they agreed to complete one year of military nursing or civilian nursing for the remainder of the war. By 1944, the corps was recruiting both Black and White nursing students, and 2,000 Black nursing students were enrolled. However, even though the National Nursing Council for War Service urged that all qualified nurses—regardless of race—be appointed to military service, most Black nurses were still denied service. The army set a small quota for the number of Black nurses it was willing to accept; by the end of the war in 1945, there were only 479 Black nurses out of 50,000 members of the Army Nurse Corps (Bellafaire, 2000). Notably, all of them were confined to segregated areas of the South or sent overseas to care for Black troops (Kalisch & Kalisch, 2004). Because the War Department set a quota of 10% for Black troops, recruiting more nurses was problematic, as illustrated by this statement in a rejection letter sent to an applicant for the army: "colored nurses are authorized for assignment only to those stations where colored troops predominate" (Kalisch & Kalisch, 2004, p. 369). The navy did not accept Black nurses until 1945. Kalisch and Kalisch (2004) note that, had both military branches taken advantage of the numbers of Black nurses in the Cadet Nurse Corps, each would have enlisted at least 1,520 nurses.

ORGANIZING FOR STRENGTH

Barred from professional affiliation or membership, especially in the Southern states, Black nurses as early as 1901 realized that the problems of discrimination and segregation they faced could only be overcome through collective action. In 1901, Black graduates of established schools in New York, Washington,

D.C., and Chicago organized alumnae associations. By 1908, under the leadership of Martha Franklin, Black nurses organized at the national level (Carnegie, 1992). The organization, which came to be known as the National Association of Colored Graduate Nurses (NACGN), lasted from 1908 until 1951. The organization's goals were to (Pitts-Mosley, 1995)

- Achieve higher professional standards for Black nurses
- Break down discriminatory practices in schools of nursing, in jobs, and in nursing organizations
- Develop leadership among Black nurses

By the time the NACGN was dissolved in 1951, because its leaders felt that the organization had accomplished its mission and there was no justification for its continued existence, its members had fought discrimination on all fronts. It had fought especially hard for the integration of Black nurses into the ANA (Carnegie, 1992).

Another recognizable strength of the NACGN, although little recognized by prominent White nursing leaders during its early years, was its ability to form alliances with and gain the support of powerful groups and individuals able to further the cause of the Black nurse. For example, Lillian Wald displayed her faith in Black nurses by hiring three Black nurses in the Visiting Nursing Service in New York (Staupers, 1961). Other support for the NACGN came from the National Medical Association (NMA), the Black physicians' professional organization. The NMA invited the NACGN to hold meetings simultaneously in the same cities and published nurses' articles in its journals (Davis, 1999).

LOWERING THE RACIAL BARRIERS

The 1950s through the early 1970s was one of the most turbulent periods in American history. Hallmarked by the enactment of antidiscrimination and civil rights legislation, beginning with the Eisenhower administration in the 1950s and throughout the Civil Rights Movement in the 1960s, parts of American society were ready and willing to embrace desegregation and observe antidiscriminatory laws. The South, however, remained highly resistant to change. The Civil Rights Act of 1964, passed by the Johnson administration, which prohibited racial discrimination in institutions receiving federal funding, dealt a blow to the segregationists.

Within nursing, the winds of change sweeping the nation also were being felt. The gains that had been achieved by Black nurses up to that point, such as the establishment of the NACGN, collaboration with the NMA, acceptance into the military, and integration into the ANA, were about to be expanded. These gains were consistent with the steady and purposeful strides nursing was making toward establishing itself as a profession. This included the initiation of nursing research and nursing theory development (Schultz, 1990). The profession not only backed away from its previous separatist policies, but took decisive action to lower racial barriers and integrate Black nurses into hospitals. Unprecedented studies on the integration of Black nurses into the workforce were undertaken. Several research articles and editorials addressing civil rights and integration issues were published in some of nursing's most prestigious journals (Goldstein, 1960). In an *American Journal of Nursing* article, for example, Goldstein studied how the services of Black nurses were being utilized on the nursing staffs of several hospitals. The study findings suggested that technological know-how and specialized skills were more of a determinant for employment in hospitals than race. Goldstein went on to note that as educational standards in professional nursing were raised, the Black nurse with special preparation could qualify for a position for which preferred personnel (White nurses) were scarce. As such, the technical competence stressed in all nursing jobs became almost the sole criterion for acceptability in highly skilled specialties.

Goldstein made clear, however, that the Black nurse, as a less-preferred type, would lose out on promotions. She went on to assert that the trend toward specific educational requirements for particular positions, such as head nurse, would work to the ultimate advantage of those Black nurses who took advantage of training. Yet in the hospitals studied, Black nurses still faced a status dilemma that needed to be solved for the hospitals to function smoothly. Goldstein urged a deemphasis on race and a greater focus on professional status and skills.

A July 1964 article appearing in the *American Journal of Nursing* entitled "Problems of Integration" reported on the difficulty encountered by the ANA in getting certain districts, such as the New Orleans district, to comply with the ANA's admission policy and practices. The New Orleans district still barred Black nurses from membership. Issuing an ultimatum, the ANA warned the Louisiana State Nurses Association that the state would be disqualified as an ANA constituent if its practices in the New Orleans district were not corrected by January 1, 1965 (Staupers, 1961). Further, advocating on behalf of the Black nurses, a delegate from Michigan called on the ANA to help districts not only to admit Black nurses, but to help them participate. Staupers also examined the integration of Black nursing in the United States. The April 1965 copy of the *American Journal of Nursing* included an article on how two nurses had integrated a nursing staff that had long been completely segregated.

From the 1950s to the 1970s, there was a significant shift in nursing's race and race relations policies, which had once intentionally erected barriers that excluded Black nurses from membership in professional nursing organizations, from participation in the mainstream of nursing, and from equal access to hospital-based employment.

THE NURSING SHORTAGE AND MINORITY CONSIDERATIONS

The new millennium has brought with it a tremendous shift in the demographics of the nursing workforce. Just as nursing has seemed to be emerging as a true science- and research-based profession, evidenced by the successful integration of nursing theory, research, and practice (Schultz, 1990), it is now experiencing one of the largest and most serious nursing shortages ever.

In 2002, the Health Resources and Services Administration estimated that 30 states had shortages of registered nurses in 2000. It predicted that these shortages will intensify over the next 20 years. In February 2004, the U.S. Bureau of Labor Statistics predicted that more than 1 million new and replacement nurses will be needed by 2012. In a similar vein, reports from the American Association of Colleges of Nursing (AACN) have predicted a 20% shortage of registered nurses by 2020, translating into a shortage of more than 400,000 registered nurses nationwide (AACN, 2004).

Factors contributing to this gloomy outlook include: (1) lower enrollments in schools of nursing (enrollments in 2001 were 17% lower than in 1995); (2) a shortage of faculty in schools of nursing, which is expected to increase dramatically in the next decade; (3) the increasing age of nurses due to the aging baby-boom generation and the lowered numbers of people entering the profession; and (4) burnout and dissatisfaction, as reported in several studies (AACN, 2004).

Evidence shows that staffing shortages contribute to increased mortality. A landmark study by Aiken, Clarke, Cheung, Sloane, and Silber (2003) found that nurses reported greater job dissatisfaction and emotional exhaustion when they were responsible for more patients than they could care for safely. They also found that burnout and job dissatisfaction predicted nurses' intentions to leave their jobs within a year. Similarly, Goodin (2003) conducted an integrative review of the literature and found that, in addition to the reasons for the shortage presented earlier, the lingering poor image of nursing and the wide range of professional occupations now open to women also contribute to the nursing shortage. Substantiation of Goodin's findings came from the National Sample Survey of Registered Nurses (U.S. Department of Health and Human Services, 2001). The National Sample Survey showed that in March 2000, a total of 135,696 registered nurses were not employed in nursing, with a total of 72,568, or 53%, employed in non–health-related occupations. This survey found that the two most important reasons for the prevailing nursing shortage were inconvenient working hours (44.9%) and poor salaries (35.4%).

To fill the nursing gap, the recruitment of minorities into the profession seems a logical step. However, because of the many career options now available to women and the public's unfavorable perception of nursing as a career choice, particularly in minority communities, few minority youngsters are choosing nursing as a career. In fact, statistical data emanating from the U.S. Department of Health and Human Services (U.S. DHHS, 2003) show that members of minority groups, although accounting for about 30% of the U.S. population, make up a mere 12% of the current nursing workforce. These dismal minority statistics, viewed in light of existing nurse shortages and the recognition of minorities as viable additions to the nursing workforce, have prompted legislative action at several governmental levels aimed at narrowing the remaining racial disparities in professional nursing.

GOVERNMENT INTERVENTION

Corrective actions aimed at increasing the number of minorities choosing to pursue nursing as a career came in the form of 16 nursing workforce diversity grant awards from the DHHS in June 2003, totaling nearly $3.5 million to support nursing education opportunities for individuals from disadvantaged backgrounds. The grants were slated to fund scholarships or stipends and preentry preparation and retention activities for disadvantaged students, including students from racial and ethnic minority groups that are underrepresented among registered nurses. Minority enrollment

in the nursing schools that received the grants averaged 38%, about double the national average of 19%. According to U.S. DHHS Secretary Tommy G. Thompson, "these schools and programs have proven their ability to enroll and graduate competent, skilled health care workers, which is important in expanding access to health care for all Americans" (U.S. DHHS, 2003, p. 1). He went on to note that the grants would encourage minority students to enter the field of nursing and help alleviate the critical shortage. In July 2004, DHHS announced an additional $15.5 million to expand and strengthen the nursing workforce, with $5.4 million earmarked for the Nursing Workforce Diversity Program (U.S. DHHS, 2004).

NURSING INTERVENTION

Several prominent nursing organizations are at the forefront of this move toward increasing minority recruitment into professional nursing. The AACN declared that as the United States struggles to find solutions to the current nursing shortage, nursing schools need to strengthen their efforts to attract more men and minority students (AACN Bulletin, 2001). To these ends, the NLN also has been very active by way of its legislative agenda. One element of its legislative package has been asking for increased funding for minority and disadvantaged students.

In an April 26, 2001, testimonial before the National Advisory Council on Nurse Education and Practice (NACNEP), Ruth D. Corcoran, chief executive officer of the NLN, pointed to the NLN's joint and dedicated effort in concert with that of the NACNEP in awakening healthcare stakeholders in academia, the industry, and government to the long-term effects of leaving major portions of our population substantially out of nursing—primarily, ethnic/racial minorities as well as males (Corcoran, 2001).

Further, statistical data emanating from DHHS's Health Resources and Service Administration Bureau of Health Professions shows that even when these underrepresented groups (minorities and men) pursue a nursing education, associate degree programs attract a great percentage of them (U.S. DHHS, HRSA, 2000). Accordingly, Corcoran proposed several recommendations for improving access to nursing education programs for groups traditionally underrepresented in nursing:

1. Creating partnerships among colleges and universities, precollege and college institutions, industry, professional societies, and communities that formulate and maintain effective grassroots career awareness activities for K–12 and reentry students, as well as their teachers, parents, and professional mentors.

2. Commitment in resources and the will to establish the networks and academic enrichment services, which have proved to be labor and time intensive, for successful academic advising, tutoring, and general nurturing of the student.

3. Financial assistance to enable disadvantaged students to pursue nursing studies (Corcoran, 2001).

THE IMPORTATION OF FOREIGN NURSES

One solution to nursing shortages in the United States has historically been the importation of foreign nurses, the majority of whom are people of color coming from underdeveloped and developing countries, such as India, the Philippines, and the Caribbean. Concordant with these recruitment efforts, Congress has passed needed legislation to facilitate the immigration of foreign nurses. For example, the Immigration Nursing Relief Acts of 1986, 1989, and 1990 provided nonimmigrant visas (H-1A) to international nurses hired to fill vacancies in U.S. hospitals (Flynn & Aiken, 2002). Also, the Nursing Relief to Disadvantaged Areas Act of 1999 addressed the nursing shortage in underserved rural and urban areas that are generally difficult to staff. This piece of legislation allowed for the issuance of a maximum of 500

nonimmigrant visas (H-1C) per year to international nurses employed in designated health professional shortage areas, as defined by the U.S. DHHS. Unlike this legislative action, which was viewed as essential and needed, the Immigration Nursing Relief Act, because of political pressure, was allowed to "sunset" (Flynn & Aiken, 2002).

Admittedly, the importation of foreign nurses is a short-term solution to a much larger problem inherent in the U.S. healthcare system (Joel, 1996). Critics, such as the ANA, also question the ethics of importing nurses from other countries during a global nursing shortage. Luring skilled nurses from other countries robs their native countries of talented nurses and increases the global nursing shortage. Additionally, the ANA is concerned about exploiting workers once they begin working in substandard conditions, because many of them are hired to replace American nurses who leave due to deteriorating working conditions (Trossman, 2003).

FACING THE CHALLENGES OF TOMORROW

Gone are the days of Jim Crow and state-mandated segregation laws that curtailed the professional training, practice, and earnings of Black nurses. The major challenge confronting professional nursing today and tomorrow is the disappearance of a qualified replacement nursing workforce to replace the aging baby-boom generation of nurses, the majority of whom are at, or rapidly approaching, retirement age.

Today more than ever before, the doors of opportunity are open to African Americans and other minorities interested in pursuing a nursing career or advanced preparation in nursing. However, the question that remains is whether White nurses and the power structure within nursing are committed and prepared to share the power base in professional nursing with African Americans and other minority nurses. The Cleveland Council of Black Nurses (CCBN) believes that old habits and racial stereotypes are hard to kill. Pointing to the high attrition rates among African American nursing students around the country, the CCBN describes a revolving door syndrome, and notes that the growing body of literature documents the difficulties of African American nursing students. They report feelings of estrangement and isolation on campus; pressure to conform to stereotypes; less equitable treatment by faculty, staff, and teaching assistants; and more faculty racism than other students of color. The CCBN noted a parallel between the occurrences of today and those of yesterday, when White nurse educators and administrators took no responsibility for negative attitudes and discriminatory practices that excluded Blacks from admission into nursing programs and limited their employment opportunities (George, Bradford, & Battle, 1995).

Many predict that the appearance of the future nursing workforce will look quite different. In the final analysis, this may indeed be true. George, Bradford, and Battle (1995) remind us that our tomorrow rests in the minds, hearts, commitments, motivation, and achievements of African American nursing students and nurses, along with the commitment of all nurses, to the values and ideals of the nursing profession.

DISCUSSION QUESTIONS ⎯⎯⎯⎯⎯

1. How have the social and nursing histories in the United States intersected to result in current statistics related to minorities in the profession?

2. Discuss future initiatives to increase the numbers of minorities in nursing in general and advanced practice nursing in particular.

3. Discuss future initiatives for decreasing healthcare disparities for the United States.

REFERENCES ⎯⎯⎯⎯⎯⎯⎯⎯⎯

AACN Bulletin. (2001). Effective strategies for increasing diversity in nursing programs. Retrieved October 7, 2004, from www.aacn.ncheedu /publications/issues/dec01

AACN. (2004). Nursing shortage resource. Retrieved January 12, 2005, from www.aacn.nche.edu /Media/shortageresource.htm#about

Aiken, L. H., Clarke, S. P., Cheung, R. B., Sloane, D. M., & Silber, J. H. (2003). Educational levels of hospital nurses and surgical patient mortality. *Journal of the American Medical Association, 290*(12), 1617-1623.

Bellafaire, J. A. (2000). Black nurses in WWII. Retrieved January 12, 2005, from www.ww2medicine .org/ black.html

Bullough, V. L., & Bullough, B. (1978). *The emergence of modern nursing.* New York: MacMillan.

Carnegie, M. E. (1986). *The path we thread: Blacks in nursing, 1854–1984.* New York: J. B. Lippincott Company.

Carnegie, M. E. (1992). Black nurses in the United States: 1879–1992. *Journal of National Black Nurses' Association, 6*(1), 13–18.

Champinha-Bacote, J. (1988). The Black nurses' struggle toward equality: An historical account of the National Association of Colored Graduate Nurses. *Journal of National Black Nurses' Association, 2*(2), 15–25.

Corcoran, R. D. (2001, April 26). *Testimony of the NLN before the National Advisory Council on Nurse Education and Practice.* Silver Spring, MD.

Davis, A. T. (1999). *Early Black American leaders in nursing: Architects for integration and equality.* Sudbury, MA: Jones and Bartlett.

Elmore, J. A. (1976). Black nurses: Their service and their struggle. *American Journal of Nursing, 76*(3), 435–437.

Flynn, L., & Aiken, L. H. (2002). Does international nurse recruitment influence practice values in U.S. hospitals? *American Journal of Nursing Scholarship, 34*(1), 67–72.

George, V. D., Bradford, D. M., & Battle, A. (1995). Yesterday, today and tomorrow. *Nursing and Health Care Perspectives, 21*(5), 219–227.

Goldstein, R. L. (1960). Black nurses in hospitals. *American Journal of Nursing, 60*(2), 215–218.

Goodin, H. J. (2003). The nursing shortage in the United States of America: An integrative review of the literature. *Journal of Advanced Nursing, 43*(4), 335–343.

Hine, D. C. (1989). *Black women in white: Racial conflict and cooperation in the nursing profession, 1890–1950.* Bloomington: Indiana University Press.

Institute of Medicine. (2003). *Unequal treatment: Confronting racial and ethnic disparities in healthcare.* Washington, DC: Institute of Medicine.

Joel, L. A. (1996). Immigration: Why is it still up for discussion? *American Journal of Nursing, 96*(1), 7–8.

Kalisch, P. A., & Kalisch, B. J. (2004). *American nursing: A history* (4th ed.). Philadelphia: Lippincott Williams & Wilkins.

Massey, E. (1934). The Black nurse student. *American Journal of Nursing, 34*, 608–610.

Pitts-Mosley, M. O. (1995). Despite all odds: A three-part history of the professionalization of Black nurses through two professional nursing organizations, 1908–1995. *Journal of National Black Nurses' Association, 7*(2), 10–19.

Schultz, P. R. (1990, Winter). Milestones in the success of nursing as an emerging discipline. *American Journal of Pharmaceutical Education, 54*, 370–373.

Smith, D. B. (1999). *Health care divided: Race and healing a nation.* Ann Arbor: University of Michigan Press.

Staupers, M. K. (1961). *No time for prejudice: A story of the integration of Negroes in nursing in the United States.* New York: MacMillan.

Sullivan Commission. (2004). *Missing persons: Minorities in the health professions.* Washington, DC: The Sullivan Commission.

Trossman, S. (2003). The global reach of the nursing shortage: The American Nurses' Association questions the ethics of luring foreign-educated nurses to the United States. *Nevada RNformation, 12*(1), 25.

U.S. DHHS. (2001). The registered nurse population: Findings from the 2000 national sample survey. Retrieved January 12, 2005, from http://bhpr.hrsa .gov/healthworkforce/reports/rnsurvey/default.htm

U.S. DHHS. (2003). HHS awards nearly $3.5 million to promote diversity in the nursing workforce. Retrieved October 7, 2004, from http://www.os .hhs.gov/news/press/2003pres/20030602.html

U.S. DHHS. (2004). HHS awards $15.5 million to expand, strengthen nursing workforce. Retrieved October 7, 2004, from http://www.hhs.gov/news /press/2004pres/20040722.html

U.S. DHHS, HRSA. (2000). The registered nurse population: Findings from the national sample survey of registered nurses. Retrieved October 4, 2004, from http://bhpr.hrsa.gov/healthworkforce/reports /rnsurvey/rnss1.htm

CHAPTER 24

Health Services for Special Populations

Leiyu Shi and Douglas A. Singh

CHAPTER OBJECTIVES

1. Identify population groups facing greater challenges and barriers in accessing health care services.

2. Understand the racial and ethnic disparities in health status.

3. Explore the health concerns of America's children and the health services available to them.

4. Discuss the challenges faced in rural health and to learn about measures taken to improve access to care.

5. Analyze the characteristics and health concerns of the homeless population.

6. Develop an understanding of the nation's U.S. mental health system.

7. Comprehend the AIDS epidemic in America, the population groups affected by it, and the services available to HIV/AIDS patients.

INTRODUCTION

Certain population groups in the United States face greater challenges than the general population in accessing timely and needed health care services (Lurie 1997; Shortell et al. 1996). They are at greater risk of poor physical, psychological, social and/or health (Aday 1994). Various terms are used to describe these populations, such as "underserved populations," "medically underserved," "medically disadvantaged," "underprivileged," and "American underclasses." The causes of their vulnerability are largely attributable to unequal social, economic, health, and geographic conditions. These population groups consist of racial and ethnic minorities, uninsured children, women, those living in rural areas, the homeless, the mentally ill, the chronically ill and disabled, and those with human immunodeficiency virus (HIV)/acquired immune deficiency syndrome (AIDS). These population groups are more vulnerable than the general population and experience greater barriers in access to care, financing of care, and racial or cultural acceptance. After presenting a conceptual framework to study vulnerable populations, this chapter defines these population groups, describes their health needs, and summarizes the major challenges they face.

FRAMEWORK TO STUDY VULNERABLE POPULATIONS

The vulnerability framework (see **Exhibit 24–1**) is an integrated approach to studying vulnerability (Shi and Stevens 2010). From a

health perspective, vulnerability refers to the likelihood of experiencing poor health or illness. Poor health can be manifested physically, psychologically, and/or socially. Because poor health along one dimension is likely to be compounded by poor health along others, the health needs are greater for those with problems along multiple dimensions than those with problems along a single dimension.

According to the framework, vulnerability is determined by a convergence of (1) predisposing, (2) enabling, and (3) need characteristics at both individual and ecological (contextual) levels (see **Exhibit 24–2**). Not only do these predisposing, enabling, and need characteristics converge and determine individuals' access to health care, they also ultimately influence individuals' risk of contracting illness or, for those already sick, recovering from illness. Individuals with multiple risks (i.e., a combination of two or more vulnerability traits) typically experience worse access to care, care of lesser quality, and

EXHIBIT 24-1   The Vulnerability Framework

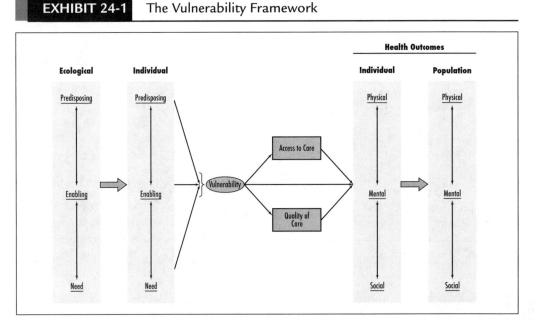

inferior health status than do those with fewer vulnerability traits.

Understanding vulnerability as a combination or convergence of disparate factors is preferred over studying individual factors separately because vulnerability, when defined as a convergence of risks, best captures reality. This approach not only reflects the co-occurrence of risk factors, but underscores the belief that it is difficult to address disparities in one risk factor without addressing others.

The vulnerability model previously presented has a number of distinctive characteristics. First, it is a comprehensive model, including both individual and ecological attributes of risk. Second, this is a general model, focusing on the attributes of vulnerability for the total population rather than focusing on vulnerable traits of subpopulations. Although we recognize individual differences in exposure to risks, we also think there are common, crosscutting traits affecting all vulnerable populations. Third, a major distinction of our model is the emphasis on the convergence of vulnerability. The effects of experiencing multiple vulnerable traits may lead to cumulative vulnerability that is additive or even multiplicative. Examining vulnerability as a multidimensional construct can also demonstrate gradient relationships between vulnerability status and outcomes of interest and, thus,

improve our understanding of the patterns and factors related to the outcomes of interest.

RACIAL/ETHNIC MINORITIES

The 2010 census questionnaire lists 15 racial categories, as well as places to write in specific races not listed on the form (US Census Bureau 2009). These are White, Black, American Indian or Alaska Native, Asian Indian, Chinese, Filipino, Japanese, Korean, Vietnamese, Other Asian, Native Hawaiian, Guamanian or Chamorro, Samoan, Other Pacific Islander, or some other race. The 2010 Census continues the option first introduced in the 2000 Census for respondents to choose more than one race.

The US Census Bureau estimated that, in 2008, over 34% of the US population was made up of minorities: Black or African Americans (12.2%), Hispanics or Latinos (15.4%), Asians (4.4%), Native Hawaiian and Other Pacific Islanders (0.1%), and American Indian and Alaska Natives (0.8%). In addition, 1.5% identified as two or more races (US Census Bureau 2010).

Significant differences exist across the various racial/ethnic groups on health-related lifestyles and health status. For example, in 2006, the percentage of live births weighing less than 2,500 grams (low birth weight) was greatest among Blacks, followed by Asians or Pacific Islanders, American Indians or Native

| EXHIBIT 24-2 | Predisposing, Enabling, and Need Characteristics of Vulnerability |

Predisposing Characteristics	*Enabling Characteristics*	*Need Characteristics*
■ Racial/ethnic characteristics	■ Insurance status (uninsured)	■ Mental health
■ Gender and age (women and children)	■ Homelessness	■ Chronic illness/disability
■ Geographic location (rural health)		■ HIV/AIDS

Americans, Whites, and Hispanics (**Figure 24-1**). Asians and Pacific Islanders were most likely to begin prenatal care during their first trimester, followed by Whites, Hispanics, Blacks, and American Indians or Alaska Natives (**Table 24-1**). Mothers of Asian and Pacific Islander origin are least likely to smoke cigarettes during pregnancy, followed by Hispanics, Blacks, and Whites (**Figure 24-2**). The White adult population is more likely to consume alcohol than other races (**Figure 24-3**). Among women 40 years of age and older, utilization of mammography is the highest among Whites and lowest among Hispanics (**Figure 24-4**).

Black Americans

Black Americans are more likely to be economically disadvantaged than Whites. Likewise, they fall behind in health status, despite progress made during the past few decades. Blacks have shorter life expectancies than Whites (**Figure 24-5**); higher age-adjusted death rates for leading causes of death (**Table 24-2**); higher age-adjusted maternal mortality rates (**Figure 24-6**); and higher infant, neonatal, and postneonatal mortality rates (**Table 24-3**). On self-reported measures of health status, Blacks are more likely to report fair or poor health status than Whites (**Figure 24-7**). In terms of behavioral risks, Black males are slightly more likely to smoke cigarettes than White males (24.6 versus 22.3%), but White females are more likely to smoke than Black females (18.1 versus 15.9%) (**Figure 24-8**), although smoking among Black females has increased. Conversely, Blacks have lower levels of serum cholesterol than Whites (**Table 24-4**).

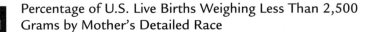

| FIGURE 24-1 | Percentage of U.S. Live Births Weighing Less Than 2,500 Grams by Mother's Detailed Race |

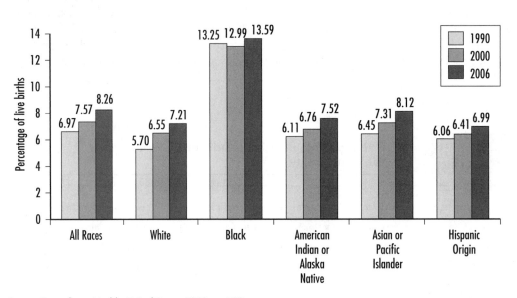

Source: Data from *Health, United States, 2009,* p. 163.

Hispanic Americans

The Hispanic segment of the US population is growing at a significantly higher rate than other population segments. Between 2000 and 2008, the Hispanic segment increased by 33%, compared to the 8% increase in the total population (US Census Bureau 2010). In 2008, the Hispanic population numbered nearly 47 million and is projected to reach 57 million by the year 2015. Hispanic Americans are also one of the youngest groups among Americans. In 2008, the median age among Hispanic Americans was 27.7, compared to 41.1 years for non-Hispanic Whites, and 11.3% are below age 5, compared to 5.6% of non-Hispanic Whites (US Census Bureau 2010). As of 2005, 58.5% of Hispanic Americans 25 years of age and older had completed high school, compared to 87.5% of Whites, and 12% of Hispanic Americans 25 years of age and older had completed college,

| TABLE 24-1 | Characteristics of U.S. Mothers by Race/Ethnicity |

Item	1970	1980	1990	2000	2006
Prenatal Care Begun During First Trimester					
All mothers	68.0	76.3	75.8	83.2	83.2
White	72.3	79.2	79.2	85.0	84.7
Black	44.2	62.4	60.6	74.3	76.0
American Indian or Alaska Native	38.2	55.8	57.9	69.3	69.5
Asian or Pacific Islander	—	73.7	75.1	84.0	84.8
Hispanic origin	—	60.2	60.2	74.4	77.3
Education of Mother 16 Years or Older					
All mothers	8.6	14.0	17.5	24.7	26.6*
White	9.6	15.5	19.3	26.3	27.9*
Black	2.8	6.2	7.2	11.7	13.4*
American Indian or Alaska Native	2.7	3.5	4.4	7.8	8.5*
Asian or Pacific Islander	—	30.8	31.0	42.8	47.1*
Hispanic origin	—	4.2	5.1	7.6	8.7*
Low Birth Weight (Less Than 2,500 Grams)					
All mothers	7.93	6.84	6.97	7.57	8.26
White	6.85	5.72	5.70	6.55	7.21
Black	13.90	12.69	13.25	12.99	13.59
American Indian or Alaska Native	7.97	6.44	6.11	6.76	7.52
Asian or Pacific Islander	—	6.68	6.45	7.31	8.12
Hispanic origin (selected states)	—	6.12	6.06	6.41	6.99

*Data from 2003.

Sources: Data from *Health, United States, 2007,* p. 144; *Health, United States, 2009,* pp. 159, 163.

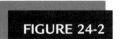

FIGURE 24-2 Percentage of U.S. Mothers Who Smoked Cigarettes During Pregnancy According to Mother's Race

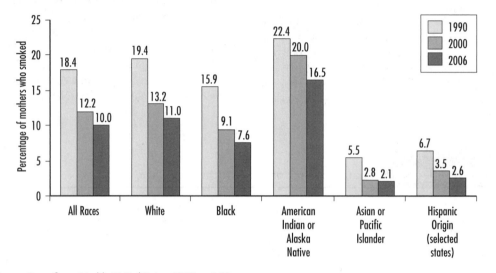

Source: Data from *Health, United States, 2009,* p. 162.

FIGURE 24-3   Alcohol Consumption by Persons 18 Years of Age and Over

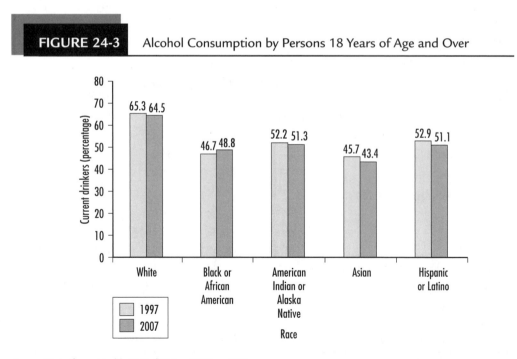

Source: Data from *Health, United States, 2009,* p. 286.

FIGURE 24-4 Use of Mammography by Women 40 Years of Age and Over, 2008

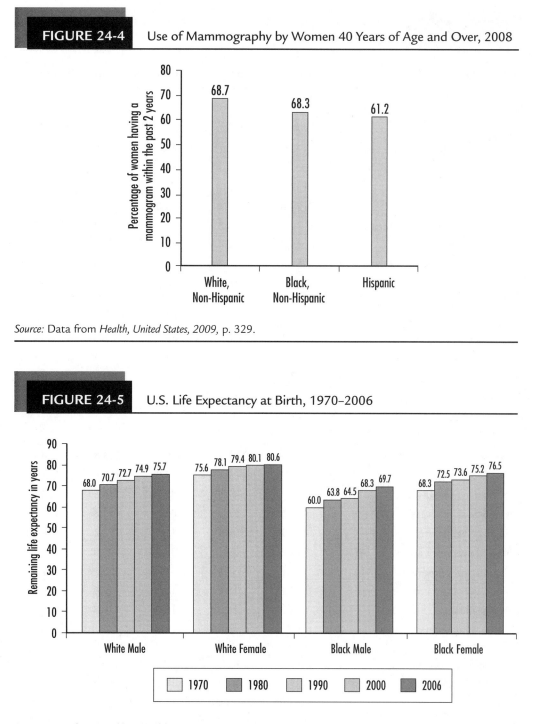

Source: Data from *Health, United States, 2009,* p. 329.

FIGURE 24-5 U.S. Life Expectancy at Birth, 1970–2006

Source: Data from *Health, United States, 2009,* p. 123.

| TABLE 24-2 | Age-Adjusted Death Rates for Selected Causes of Death, 1970–2006 (Deaths per 100,000 Standard Population) |

Race and Cause of Death	1970	1980	1990	2000	2006
All Persons					
All causes	1,222.6	1,039.1	938.7	869.0	776.5
Diseases of the heart	492.7	412.1	321.8	257.6	200.2
Ischemic heart disease	—	345.2	249.6	186.8	134.9
Cerebrovascular diseases	147.7	96.2	65.3	60.9	43.6
Malignant neoplasms	198.6	207.9	216.0	199.6	180.7
Chronic lower respiratory diseases	21.3	28.3	37.2	44.2	40.5
Influenza and pneumonia	41.7	31.4	36.8	23.7	17.8
Chronic liver disease and cirrhosis	17.8	15.1	11.1	9.5	8.8
Diabetes mellitus	24.3	18.1	20.7	25.0	23.3
Human immunodeficiency virus (HIV) disease	—	—	10.2	5.2	4.0
Unintentional injuries	60.1	46.4	36.3	34.9	39.8
Motor vehicle-related injuries	27.6	22.3	18.5	15.4	15.0
Suicide	13.1	12.2	12.5	10.4	10.9
Homicide	8.8	10.4	9.4	5.9	6.2
White					
All causes	1,193.3	1,012.7	909.8	849.8	764.4
Diseases of the heart	492.2	409.4	317.0	253.4	197.0
Ischemic heart disease	—	347.6	249.7	185.6	134.2
Cerebrovascular diseases	143.5	93.2	62.8	58.8	41.7
Malignant neoplasms	196.7	204.2	211.6	197.2	179.9
Chronic lower respiratory diseases	21.8	29.3	38.3	46.0	42.6
Influenza and pneumonia	39.8	30.9	36.4	23.5	17.7
Chronic liver disease and cirrhosis	16.6	13.9	10.5	9.6	9.1
Diabetes mellitus	22.9	16.7	18.8	22.8	21.2
Human immunodeficiency virus (HIV) disease	—	—	8.3	2.8	2.1
Unintentional injuries	57.8	45.3	35.5	35.1	41.0
Motor vehicle-related injuries	27.1	22.6	18.5	15.6	15.4
Suicide	13.8	13.0	13.4	11.3	12.1
Homicide	4.7	6.7	5.5	3.6	3.7

| TABLE 24-2 | Age-Adjusted Death Rates for Selected Causes of Death, 1970–2006 (Deaths per 100,000 Standard Population) *(continued)* | | | | |

Race and Cause of Death	1970	1980	1990	2000	2006
Black					
All causes	1,518.1	1,314.8	1,250.3	1,121.4	982.0
Diseases of the heart	512.0	455.3	391.5	324.8	257.7
Ischemic heart disease	—	334.5	267.0	218.3	161.6
Cerebrovascular diseases	197.1	129.1	91.6	81.9	61.6
Malignant neoplasms	225.3	256.4	279.5	248.5	217.4
Chronic lower respiratory diseases	16.2	19.2	28.1	31.6	28.1
Influenza and pneumonia	57.2	34.4	39.4	25.6	19.6
Chronic liver disease and cirrhosis	28.1	25.0	16.5	9.4	7.0
Diabetes mellitus	38.8	32.7	40.5	49.5	45.1
Human immunodeficiency virus (HIV) disease	—	—	26.7	23.3	18.6
Unintentional injuries	78.3	57.6	43.8	37.7	38.3
Motor vehicle-related injuries	31.1	20.2	18.8	15.7	14.6
Suicide	6.2	6.5	7.1	5.5	5.1
Homicide	44.0	39.0	36.3	20.5	21.6

Source: Data from *Health, United States, 2009,* pp. 190–191, Centers for Disease Control and Prevention, National Center for Health Statistics.

| FIGURE 24-6 | Age-Adjusted Maternal Mortality Rates |

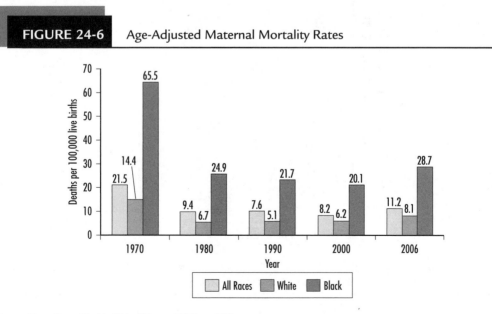

Source: Data from *Health, United States, 2009,* p. 231.

TABLE 24-3	Infant, Neonatal, and Postneonatal Mortality Rates by Mother's Race (per 1,000 live births)											
	Infant Deaths				Neonatal Deaths				Postneonatal Deaths			
Race of Mother	1983	1990	2000	2005	1983	1990	2000	2005	1983	1990	2000	2005
All mothers	10.9	8.9	6.9	6.9	7.1	5.7	4.6	4.5	3.8	3.2	2.3	2.3
White	9.3	7.3	5.7	5.7	6.1	4.6	3.8	3.8	3.2	2.7	1.9	2.0
Black	19.2	16.9	13.5	13.3	12.5	11.1	9.1	8.9	6.7	5.9	4.3	4.3
American Indian or Alaska Native	15.2	13.1	8.3	8.1	7.5	6.1	4.4	4.0	7.7	7.0	3.9	4.0
Asian or Pacific Islander	8.3	6.6	4.9	4.9	5.2	3.9	3.4	3.4	3.1	2.7	1.4	1.5
Hispanic origin (selected states)	9.5	7.5	5.6	5.6	6.2	4.8	3.8	3.9	3.3	2.9	1.8	1.8

FIGURE 24-7	Respondent-Assessed Health Status

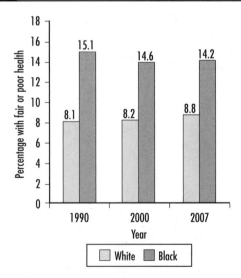

Source: Data from *Health, United States, 1995,* p. 172, Centers for Disease Control and Prevention, National Center for Health Statistics, 1996, and *Health, United States, 2009,* p. 270.

| FIGURE 24-8 | Current Cigarette Smoking by Persons 18 Years of Age and Over, Age Adjusted, 2007 |

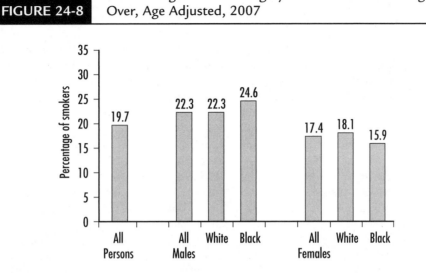

Source: Data from *Health, United States, 2009,* p. 276, Centers for Disease Control and Prevention, National Center for Health Statistics, 2010.

| TABLE 24-4 | Serum Cholesterol Levels Among Persons 20 Years and Older, 2003–2006 |

Sex and Race*	Percentage of Persons 20 Years of Age and Older with Hypertension	Mean Serum Cholesterol Level (mg/dL) of Persons 20 Years of Age and Older	Percentage of Overweight Persons 20 Years of Age and Older
Both sexes	31.3	200	66.7
White			
Male	31.2	198	71.8
Female	28.3	203	57.9
Black			
Male	40.6	193	71.6
Female	44.1	195	79.8

*20–74 years, age adjusted.

Source: Data from *Health, United States, 2009,* pp. 293, 296, 301, Centers for Disease Control and Prevention, National Center for Health Statistics, Division of Health Examination Statistics, 2010.

compared to 28% of Whites (US Census Bureau 2007). In 2007, 20.7% of Hispanic persons lived below the federal poverty level (FPL), compared to 9.0% of non-Hispanic White persons (US Census Bureau 2010).

Many Hispanic Americans experience significant barriers in accessing medical care. Many Hispanic families who immigrated to the United States may not qualify for Medicaid (Rosenbaum and Darnell 1997). This represents a greater problem for those from Central America (79% foreign born) and South America (75% foreign born) than those from Spain (17% foreign born) or Mexico (28% foreign born). Place of birth is also related to Hispanic people's inability to speak English, which is another factor associated with reduced access to medical services (Solis et al. 1990). Low education is related to employment and occupational status. Hispanic Americans have higher unemployment rates than non-Hispanic Whites (12.8 versus 8.8% in 2010; BLS 2010) and are more likely to be employed in semiskilled, nonprofessional occupations (US Census Bureau 2007). Due to the close association between employment status and health insurance, Hispanic Americans are more likely to be uninsured or underinsured than non-Hispanic Whites. In 2007, 31.8% of Hispanic persons were uninsured, compared to 16.3% of non-Hispanic Whites and 17% of non-Hispanic Blacks or African Americans (National Center for Health Statistics 2010). Among Hispanics, 34.7% of Mexican Americans were uninsured, followed by 20.7% of Cubans, 12.8% of Puerto Ricans, and 32.7% of other Hispanics (National Center for Health Statistics 2010).

Homicide was the sixth leading cause of death for Hispanic males in 2006. They have the highest ranking, along with Blacks, for this cause of death (National Center for Health Statistics 2010).

Hispanic Americans are less likely to take advantage of preventive care than non-Hispanic Whites and certain other races.

Hispanic women 40 years of age or older were least likely to use mammography (61.2 versus 68.9% for non-Hispanic Whites and 68.3% for non-Hispanic Blacks; see Figure 24-4). In 2006, fewer Hispanic mothers began their prenatal care during the first trimester than mothers of other ethnic groups (76.7% for Hispanic mothers versus 85.4% for White mothers and 84.8% for Asian and Pacific Islander mothers; see Table 24-1). In 2007, 78% of Hispanic children aged 19–35 months had received the combined series vaccines (4:3:1:3:3:1), compared to 78% of White children, 79% of Asian children, 75% of Black children, and 83% of American Indian and Alaska Native children (National Center for Health Statistics 2010). Among Hispanics 2 years of age and older in 2007, 55.8% had at least one dental visit during a year, compared to 68.7% for non-Hispanic Whites (National Center for Health Statistics 2010).

People of Hispanic origin also experience greater behavioral risks than Whites and certain other racial/ethnic groups. For example, among individuals 18 years of age or older in 2007, a higher proportion of Hispanics were current drinkers than people of other ethnic origins (51.1% for Hispanics versus 48.8% for Blacks and 43.3% for Asians; see Figure 24-3). However, fewer Hispanics smoked, compared to people from other ethnic groups. In 2007, 18.7% of Hispanic males 18 years of age and older identified themselves as "current smokers," compared to 24.1% of non-Hispanic White males and 25.5% of non-Hispanic Black males (National Center for Health Statistics 2010). Among female adults, 9.7% of Hispanics smoked in 2007, compared to 20.7% of non-Hispanic Whites and 17.1% of non-Hispanic Blacks (National Center for Health Statistics 2010).

Asian Americans

Minority health epidemiology has typically focused on Blacks, Hispanics, and American Indians or Alaska Natives because Asian Americans (AAs) have relatively small numbers.

To include the diversity of AAs, the National Center for Health Statistics has expanded the race codes into nine categories: White, Black, Native American, Chinese, Japanese, Hawaiian, Filipino, Other Asian/Pacific Islanders, and other races. But even the category of "Other Asian/Pacific Islander" is extremely heterogeneous, encompassing 21 subgroups with different health profiles. In 2008, Asians accounted for 4.5% of the US population and numbered 13.5 million (US Census Bureau 2010).

AAs constitute one of the fastest-growing population segments in the United States. The percent change in the Asian population was 28% between 2000 and 2008, compared to 5.3% for the population as a whole (US Census Bureau 2010). The US Census Bureau (2010) projects that the AA population will reach 16.5 million by 2015.

In education, income, and health, Asian Americans and Pacific Islanders (AA/PI) are very diverse. In 2008, 88.7% AA/PIs 25 years of age or older had at least 4 years of high school education, compared with 87.1% of non-Hispanic Whites; in addition, the percentage of AA/PIs with a bachelor's degree or higher was 52.6%, compared to 29.8% for non-Hispanic Whites (US Census Bureau 2010). Educational attainment varies greatly among the subgroups. For example, in 1990, 88% of the adults of Japanese descent had graduated from high school, whereas among Vietnamese it was 61% and only 31% among Hmong adults (Kuo and Porter 1998). In 2007, the median income for Asian males (aged 15 years and older) was $37,193, compared to $35,141 for non-Hispanic White males (US Census Bureau 2010). In addition, in 2007, a smaller percentage of Asians (10.2%) lived below the FPL, compared to Whites (10.5%), Blacks (24.5%), and Hispanics (21.5%; US Census Bureau 2010).

The heterogeneity of the AA/PI population is reflected in the various indicators of health status. For instance, a greater percentage of Vietnamese and Korean (17.2 and 12.8%,

respectively) people assess their own health status as fair or poor, compared to people of Chinese, Filipino, and Japanese descent (6.1 to 7.4%) (Kuo and Porter 1998). The incidence of low-birth-weight babies varies greatly, from 4.5% among Chinese to 7% among Filipinos. Cambodian refugees have extremely high rates of posttraumatic stress disorder, dissociation, depression, and anxiety. Although US smoking rates are reported to be lowest among AA/PIs, 92% of Laotians, 71% of Cambodians, and 65% of Vietnamese are smokers (Yoon and Chien 1996). Compared with Whites, Korean-American men have a five-fold incidence of stomach cancer and an eight-fold incidence of liver cancer. Cultural practices and attitudes may prevent AA/PI women from receiving adequate breast cancer screening and prenatal care. A study analyzing National Health Interview Survey data from 1997 to 2000 found that Chinese, Asian Indian, Filipino, and other AA/PI children were more likely to be without contact with a health professional within the past 12 months, compared to non-Hispanic White children. Citizenship/nativity status, maternal education attainment, and poverty status were all significant independent risk factors for health care access and utilization (Yu et al. 2004). Ignorance of this bipolar distribution contributes to the myth of a minority population that is both healthy and economically successful. For example, the 1985 Department of Health and Human Services (DHHS) Task Force Report on Black and Minority Health stated that, as a group, the AA/PI population in the United States is at lower risk of early death than the White population. Such a misunderstanding demonstrates an essential need for more in-depth, ethnic-specific health research.

American Indians and Alaska Natives

In 2008, 3.1 million people identified their race as American Indian or Alaska Native alone, and nearly 4.9 million people identified themselves American Indian or Alaska Native in combination with other races (US Census Bureau 2010). More than one-half live in urban areas (IHS 2010a). According to the Census Bureau, this subpopulation is growing at a rate of 1.7% per year (IHS 2010a). Concomitantly, demand for expanded health care has been on the rise for several decades and is becoming more acute. The incidence and prevalence of certain diseases and conditions, such as diabetes, hypertension, infant mortality and morbidity, chemical dependency, and AIDS- and HIV-related morbidity, are all high enough to be matters of prime concern. Compared to the general US population, Native Americans also have much higher death rates from alcoholism, tuberculosis, diabetes, injuries, suicide, and homicide (IHS 2010b).

It is also no secret that Native Americans continue to occupy the bottom of the socioeconomic strata. American Indians/Alaska Natives are approximately twice as likely to be poor, unemployed, and not to have a college degree, compared to the general populations of the areas in which they live (Castor et al. 2006). A strong positive association exists between socioeconomic status and health status. For example, poverty, not cultural factors, has been found to be associated with the high injury-related mortality rate among Indian children. The effects of Indian poverty are exacerbated by an acute political disempowerment.

The health status of American Indian people appears to be improving, yet it significantly lags behind the health status of the population at large. In the years 1972 to 1974, the mortality rate among Native American expectant mothers was 27.7 per 100,000 live births (Pleasant 2003). By 1996, the occurrence rate was only 6.1%—a 78% drop. Infant mortality also declined from 22.2 per 1,000 births in 1972 to 8.1 per 1,000 births in 2005. Still, Native Americans experience significant health disparities when compared to the general US population. The life expectancy of Native Americans is 4.6 years fewer than the US population as a whole (IHS 2010b). Native Americans die at higher rates

than other Americans from alcohol (519% higher), tuberculosis (500% higher), diabetes (195% higher), unintentional injuries (149% higher), homicide (92% higher), and suicide (72% higher; IHS 2010b).

The provision of health services to American Indians by the federal government was first negotiated in 1832, as partial compensation for land cessions. Subsequent laws have expanded the scope of services and allowed American Indians greater autonomy in planning, developing, and administering their own health care programs. These laws explicitly permit the practice of traditional, as well as Western, medicine.

Indian Health Care Improvement Act

The Indian Health Care Improvement Act was enacted in 1976. This law, and later amendments in 1980, outlined a 7-year effort to help bring American Indian health to a level of parity with the general population. Although appropriations were significantly increased to improve or develop sanitation services, health care programs, and medical facilities, limited fiscal support undermined the Act's goal of achieving health parity for American Indians. Other features of the Act provided for specific funding for programs to improve access to health care for urban Indians and educational scholarships to increase the number of Indian health care professionals. Thus, the Act has at least been successful in minimizing prejudice, building trust, and putting responsibility back into the hands of American Indians.

Indian Health Service

Chapter 6 introduced the federal program administered by the Indian Health Service (IHS). The goal of the IHS is to ensure that Native Americans and Alaska Natives are provided with comprehensive and culturally acceptable health services (Pleasant 2003). The IHS serves the members and descendants of more than 560 federally recognized American Indian and Alaska Native tribes (IHS 2010c). However, the health care needs of a rapidly expanding

American Indian population have grown faster than medical care resources, and most American Indian communities continue to be medically underserved.

IHS is divided into 12 area offices, each responsible for program operations in a particular geographic area. Each area office is composed of branches dealing with various administrative and health-related services. Delivery of health services is the responsibility of 161 tribally managed service units operating at the local level (IHS 2010c). The IHS mandate has been made particularly difficult because the locations of Indian reservation communities are among the least geographically accessible (Burks 1992; Kozoll 1986). Relative isolation and impassable roads continue to present unique challenges.

Over the years, the IHS system has evolved to include not only primary care services but also preventive strategies (Rhodes 1987). Within these environmental, educational, and outreach preventive strategies are special initiatives that focus on areas such as injury control, alcoholism, diabetes, mental health, maternal and child health, Indian youth and children, and elder care (IHS 1999b). Programs have also been established for AIDS, otitis media, and health care database management. Additional proposals include a focus on traditional medicine, domestic violence and child abuse, oral health, sanitation, and new initiatives to improve advocacy for Indian health interests (IHS 1999a). However, despite limitations in the IHS's scope of service, many American Indians do not avail themselves of the system's services.

THE UNINSURED

Chapter 6 discussed the number of uninsured and the reasons why so many Americans have been without health insurance. Although uninsurance among adults has increased, lack of health insurance coverage among children declined from 13.2 to 8.2% in the first 9 months of 2009 (CDC 2009), mainly because of the success of the CHIP program (see Chapter 6).

Nevertheless, 11% of children under the age of 18 remained uninsured (US Census Bureau 2010).

Ethnic minorities are more likely than Whites to lack health insurance. The US Census Bureau (2010) estimated that, in 2007, 32.1% of Hispanic residents were uninsured, compared with 19.5% of Blacks, 16.8% of AAs, and 14.3% of Whites. About 1 in 10 uninsured persons lacks insurance by personal choice (Bennefield 1995). Most of them are young workers in low-paying jobs. Lack of coverage is also more prevalent in the South and the West of the United States, among individuals who lack a high school diploma and the unemployed.

For the most part, the uninsured tend to be poor, less educated, working in part-time jobs, and/or employed by small firms. Many of the poor do not qualify for Medicaid because of stringent means-test criteria. The uninsured also tend to be younger (25–40 years of age) because most of the elderly (65 years of age or older) are covered by Medicare.

Generally, the uninsured are in poorer health than the general population (Donelan et al. 1996). Numerous studies have also shown that the uninsured use fewer health services than the insured (Freeman and Corey 1993). In 2009, 26% of uninsured people reported having no regular source of health care (Kaiser Commission on Medicaid and the Uninsured 2010). Decreased utilization of lower cost preventive services can ultimately result in an increased need for more expensive emergency health care. Even when the uninsured can access health care, they often have serious problems paying medical bills. It used to be a common practice for teaching hospitals, private physicians, and community clinics to provide discounted or even free medical care to the uninsured, but managed care practices have seriously reduced the ability of this social safety net to provide care for the uninsured (Donelan et al. 1996). In 2003, 47% of uninsured people postponed seeking medical care because of cost, compared to 15% of insured people (Kaiser Commission on Medicaid and the Uninsured 2006).

The plight of the uninsured affects those who have insurance. Medical expenditures for uncompensated care to the uninsured was estimated to be $41 million in 2004 (Kaiser Commission on Medicaid and the Uninsured 2006). Much of this cost is absorbed by Medicaid, federal grants to nonprofit hospitals, and charitable organizations.

CHILDREN

In 2007, 29.8% of children under the age of 18 were covered under Medicaid and 59.8% under private insurance (National Center for Health Statistics 2010). Vaccinations of children for selected diseases differ by race, poverty status, and area of residence (**Table 24-5**). White children have greater vaccination rates for diphtheria-tetanus-pertussis (DTP), polio, measles, *Haemophilus influenzae* serotype b (Hib), and combined series than Blacks. Children who come from families with incomes below the federal poverty line or who live in central city areas have lower vaccination rates than those at or above poverty or who live in non-inner city areas.

When children have inadequate access to health care, their ability to learn is compromised. Some children stay home and miss school for long periods when they do not receive needed medical care. Some sick children go to school because of unavailability of child care or inability of working parents to get leave. Once in school, children may also expose other children to contagious illnesses (Wenzel 1996).

In 2007, the United Nations published *The State of the World's Children*, which ties children's health and rights to women's health and rights. This report suggests that greater gender equality will lead to profound and positive impact on children's well-being and development (UN 2007).

Children's health has certain unique aspects in the delivery of health care. Among these are children's developmental vulnerability, dependency, and differential patterns of morbidity

| TABLE 24-5 | Vaccinations of Children 19–35 Months of Age for Selected Diseases According to Race, Poverty Status, and Residence in a Metropolitan Statistical Area, 2007 (%) | | | | | | |

		Race		Poverty Status		Inside MSA	
Vaccination	Total	White	Black	Below Poverty	At or Above Poverty	Central City	Remaining Areas
DTP[1]	85	85	82	81	86	85	85
Polio[2]	93	93	91	92	93	92	93
Measles containing (MMR)[3]	92	92	92	91	93	92	93
HIB[4]	93	93	91	91	93	92	94
Combined series[5]	77	78	75	73	76	75	77

1. Diphtheria–tetanus–pertussis, four doses or more.
2. Three doses or more.
3. Respondents were asked about measles-containing or MMR (measles–mumps–rubella) vaccines.
4. *Haemophilus* B, three doses or more.
5. The combined series consists of four doses of DTP vaccine, three doses of polio vaccine, and one dose of measles-containing vaccine (4 : 3 : 1 : 3 : 3 : 1).

Source: Data from *Health, United States, 2009*, p. 321.

and mortality. Developmental vulnerability refers to the rapid and cumulative physical and emotional changes that characterize childhood and the potential impact that illness, injury, or disruptive family and social circumstances can have on a child's life-course trajectory. Dependency refers to children's special circumstances that require adults—parents, school officials, caregivers, and sometimes neighbors—to recognize and respond to their health needs, seek health care services on their behalf, authorize treatment, and comply with recommended treatment regimens. These dependency relationships can be complex, change over time, and affect utilization of health services by children.

Children increasingly are affected by a broad and complex array of conditions, collectively referred to as "new morbidities." **New morbidities** include drug and alcohol abuse, family and neighborhood violence, emotional disorders, and learning problems from which older generations do not suffer. These dysfunctions originate in complex family or socioeconomic conditions rather than exclusively biological causes. Hence, they cannot be adequately addressed by traditional medical services alone. Instead, these conditions require a continuum of comprehensive services that include multidisciplinary assessment, treatment, and rehabilitation, as well as community-based prevention strategies.

Serious chronic medical conditions, leading to disabling conditions, are less prevalent in children. Estimates of the total number of young people with disabilities range from 5 to 20% of the child population. By the most conservative estimates, at least 3 million children 18 years of age and under are disabled, and 1 million children in the United States have a severe chronic illness. Medical problems in children are usually related to birth or congenital conditions rather than degenerative conditions that affect adults. These differences call for an approach to the delivery of health care that is uniquely designed to address the needs of children.

Children and the US Health Care System

The various programs that serve children have distinct eligibility, administrative, and funding criteria that can present barriers to access. The patchwork of disconnected programs also makes it difficult to obtain health care in an integrated and coordinated fashion. These programs can be categorized into three broad sectors: the personal medical and preventive services sector, the population-based community health services sector, and the health-related support services sector.

Personal medical and preventive health services include primary and specialty medical services, which are delivered in private and public medical offices, health centers, and hospitals. Personal medical services are principally funded by private health plans, Medicaid, and by families' out-of-pocket payments.

The population-based community health services include communitywide health promotion and disease prevention services. Examples are immunization delivery and monitoring programs, lead screening and abatement programs, and child abuse and neglect prevention. Other health services include special child abuse treatment programs and rehabilitative services for children with complex congenital conditions or other chronic and debilitating diseases. Community-based programs also provide assurance and coordination functions, such as case management and referral programs, for children with chronic diseases and early interventions and monitoring for infants at risk for developmental disabilities. Funding for this sector comes from federal programs, such as Medicaid's Early Periodic Screening, Diagnosis, and Treatment (EPSDT) program; Title V (Maternal and Child Health) of the Social Security Act; and other categorical programs.

The health-related support services sector includes such services as nutrition education, early intervention, rehabilitation, and family support programs. An example of a rehabilitation service is education and psychotherapy for children with HIV. Family support services include parent education and skill building in families with infants at risk for developmental delay because of physiological or social conditions, such as low birth weight or very low income. Funding for these services comes from diverse agencies, such as the Department of Agriculture, which funds the Supplemental Food Program for Women, Infants, and Children (WIC), and the Department of Education, which funds the Individuals with Disabilities Education Act (IDEA).

WOMEN

Women are playing an increasingly important role in the delivery of health care. Not only do women remain the leading providers of care in the nursing profession, but they are also well represented in various other health professions, including allopathic and osteopathic medicine, dentistry, podiatry, and optometry (**Figure 24-9**).

Women in the United States can now expect to live almost 8 years longer than men, but they suffer greater morbidity and poorer health outcomes. Morbidity is greater among women than among men, even after childbearing-related conditions are factored out. For instance, nearly 38% of women report having chronic conditions that require ongoing medical treatment, compared to 30% of men (Salganicoff et al. 2005). Women also have a higher prevalence of certain health problems than men do over the course of their lifetimes (Sechzer et al. 1996). Heart disease and stroke account for a higher percentage of deaths among women than men at all stages of life. In contrast to 24% of men, 42% of women who have heart attacks die within a year (Misra 2001). Research has also demonstrated that health problems restrict women's activities by 25% more days each year than they do for men, even when reproductive conditions are statistically controlled. Women are bedridden 35% more days than men are each year because of infectious or parasitic diseases, respiratory

| FIGURE 24-9 | Percentage of Female Students of Total Enrollment in Schools for Selected Health Occupations, 2006–2007 |

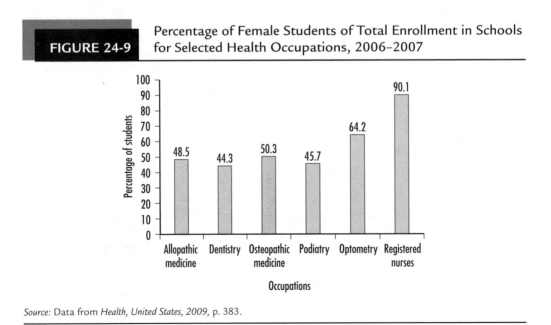

Source: Data from *Health, United States, 2009*, p. 383.

diseases, digestive system conditions, injuries, and other acute conditions (Regier et al. 1988).

According to the 2004 Kaiser Women's Health Survey, 87% of women had at least one visit to a health care provider in the previous year, compared to 74% of men (Salganicoff et al. 2005). Compared to men, women have only a slightly higher mean number of specialty care visits and emergency department visits. However, women have higher annual charges than men do for all types of care, including primary, specialty, emergency, and diagnostic services, indicating that women receive more intensive services (Bertakis et al. 2000).

The differences between men and women are equally pronounced for mental illness. For example, anxiety disorders and major depression affect two to three times as many women as men (Kaiser Family Foundation 2005; Misra 2001). Clinical depression is a major mental health problem for both men and women; however, 6.6% women, compared to 4.4% men, had depression during 2005–2006 (National Center for Health Statistics 2010). An estimated 12% of women in the United States, compared with 7% of men, will suffer from major depression during their lifetime (Misra 2001). Certain other mental disorders also affect more women at different stages of life.

Eating disorders are among the illnesses predominantly affecting women and have been the subject of relatively little rigorous study to date. Up to 3% of women are affected by eating disorders (i.e., anorexia nervosa and bulimia), although between 29 and 38% report dieting at any given time (Misra 2001). At least 90% of all eating disorder cases occur in young women, and eating disorders account for the highest mortality rates among all mental disorders (Misra 2001; Weissman and Klerman 1977).

Some disorders once thought to primarily affect men are now affecting women in increasing numbers. For example, death rates among women who abuse alcohol are 50–100% higher than rates for men who abuse alcohol (Misra

2001). Compared to older men, older women are at substantially greater risk of Alzheimer's disease, a disease responsible for 60–70% of all cases of dementia and one of the leading causes of nursing home placement for older adults (Herzog and Copeland 1985).

Office on Women's Health

The Public Health Service's Office on Women's Health (OWH) is dedicated to the achievement of a series of specific goals that span the spectrum of disease and disability. These goals range across the life cycle and address cultural and ethnic differences among women. The OWH stimulates, coordinates, and implements a comprehensive women's health agenda on research, service delivery, and education across the agencies of the Public Health Service (PHS) that include the National Institutes of Health (NIH), the Centers for Disease Control and Prevention (CDC), the Food and Drug Administration (FDA), and others.

The OWH was responsible for implementing the National Action Plan on Breast Cancer (NAPBC), a major public–private partnership, dedicated to improving the diagnosis, treatment, and prevention of breast cancer through research, service delivery, and education. The OWH also worked to implement measures to prevent physical and sexual abuse against women, as delineated in the Violence Against Women Act of 1994. The OWH is also active in projects promoting breastfeeding, women's health education and research, girl and adolescent health, and heart health.

Within the Substance Abuse and Mental Health Services Administration (SAMHSA), the Office for Women's Services has targeted six areas for special attention: physical and sexual abuse of women; women as caregivers; women with mental and addictive disorders; women with HIV infection or AIDS, sexually transmitted diseases, and/or tuberculosis; older women; and women detained in the criminal justice system. The Women's Health

Initiative, supported by the NIH, took place in more than 50 centers across the country. It was the largest clinical trial conducted in US history, involving over 161,000 women (NIH 2002). It focused on diseases that are the major causes of death and disability among women—heart disease, cancer, and osteoporosis. In 2002, the Women's Health Initiative published a groundbreaking study, finding detrimental effects of postmenopausal hormone therapy on women's development of invasive breast cancer, coronary heart disease, stroke, and pulmonary embolism (NIH 2002). Within the NIH, the National Institute of Mental Health has issued a specific program announcement to broaden the full spectrum of research on issues pertinent to women's health. Both the National Institute on Drug Abuse (NIDA) and the National Institute of Alcohol Abuse and Alcoholism (NIAAA), also within the NIH, support research related to women's health.

Women and the US Health Care System

Women face a distinct disadvantage in employer-based health insurance coverage because they are more likely than men to work part time, receive lower wages, and have interruptions in their work histories. Hence, women are more likely to be covered as dependents under their husbands' plans and are at a higher risk of being uninsured. Women must also place greater reliance on Medicaid for their health care coverage.

Even among women who have health insurance, gaps in benefit coverage discourage them from seeking medical and preventive services. Women are more likely than men to use contraceptives (**Figure 24-10**), but contraceptives are among the most poorly covered reproductive health care service in the United States. As of September 2004, 21 states required private health insurance plans to cover prescription

FIGURE 24-10	Contraceptive Use in the Past Month Among Women 15–44 Years Old, 2002

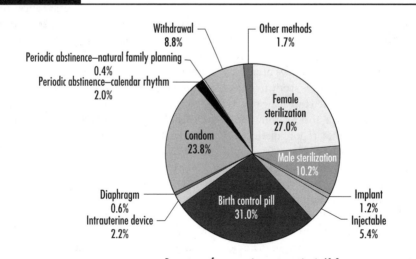

Percentage of women using contraception is 61.9.

Source: Data from *Health, United States, 2009*, pp. 171–172.

contraceptives if they covered other prescription drugs (Kaiser Family Foundation 2004). Many nonsurgical contraceptors, such as diaphragms, Norplant implants, intrauterine devices (IUDs), and oral contraceptives, are either not covered or inadequately covered.

RURAL HEALTH

Poor economic conditions are often reflected in diminished access to health care and poor health of rural citizens (Cohen et al. 1994). Access to health care is affected by poverty, long distances, rural topography, weather conditions, and limited availability of personal transportation.

Geographic maldistribution that creates a shortage of health care professionals in rural settings results in barriers in access to care. Reasons for the maldistribution are discussed in Chapter 4. About 20% of the US population resides in areas where primary care health professionals are in short supply (HRSA Bureau of Health Professions 2002). An estimated 22 million-plus rural Americans live in a federally designated area of primary health care provider shortages (HHS Rural Task Force 2002). The scarcity of health care providers encompasses a broad spectrum of professionals, including pediatricians, obstetricians, internists, dentists, nurses, and allied health professionals (Patton and Puskin 1990). Additionally, rural hospitals tend to be smaller and provide fewer services than urban hospitals. Rural hospitals also face financial hardships because they serve a disproportionately higher number of poor, uninsured, and underinsured patients. Closing of rural hospitals further diminishes access to health care. Rural residents, especially poor residents, seek health care services less frequently throughout their lives than do urban residents (Stratton et al. 1993).

Various measures have been taken to improve access in rural America, including the promotion of the National Health Service Corps (NHSC), the designation of Health Professional Shortage Areas (HPSAs) and Medically Underserved Areas (MUAs), the development of Community and Migrant Health Centers (C/MHCs), and the enactment of the Rural Health Clinics Act. In addition, the Office of Rural Health Policy, within the Health Resources and Services Administration of the US Department of Health and Human Services, was established in 1987 to promote better health care in rural America (HRSA Office of Rural Health Policy 2007).

The National Health Service Corps

The NHSC was created in 1970, under the Emergency Health Personnel Act, to recruit and retain physicians to provide needed services in physician shortage areas. A 1972 amendment created a scholarship program targeting HPSAs. The scholarship and loan repayment program applies to doctors, dentists, nurse practitioners, midwives, and mental health professionals who serve a minimum of 2 years in underserved areas. Since 1972, over 27,000 health professionals have been placed in medically underserved communities in hospitals and clinics (HRSA Bureau of Health Professions 2003). In 2005, the NHSC awarded a record 1,223 loan repayment contracts to health professionals (HRSA Bureau of Health Professions 2007a).

Health Professional Shortage Areas

The Health Professions Educational Assistance Act of 1976 provided the designation criteria for Health Manpower Shortage Areas, later renamed Health Professional Shortage Areas (Fitzwilliams 1977; HRSA Bureau of Health Professions 2007b). The act provided that three different types of HPSAs could be designated: geographic areas, population groups, and medical facilities. A geographic area must meet the following three criteria for designation as a primary care HPSA:

1. The geographic area involved must be rational for the delivery of health services.

2. One of the following conditions must prevail in the area: a) the area has a population

to full-time equivalent primary care physician (PCP) ratio of at least 3,500:1, or b) the area has a population to full-time equivalent PCP ratio of less than 3,500:1 but greater than 3,000:1 and has unusually high needs for primary care services or insufficient capacity of existing primary care providers.

3. Primary care professionals in contiguous areas are overutilized, excessively distant, or inaccessible to the population of the area under consideration (HRSA Bureau of Health Professions 2007c).

A population group can be designated as an HPSA for primary care if it can be demonstrated that access barriers prevent members of the group from using local providers. Medium- and maximum-security federal and state correctional institutions and public or nonprofit private residential facilities can be designated as facility-based HPSAs. HPSAs are classified on a scale from one to four, with one or two signifying areas of greatest need.

Medically Underserved Areas

The primary purpose of the MUA designation, in the HMO Act of 1973, was to target the community health center and rural health clinic programs. The statute required that several factors be considered in designating MUAs, such as available health resources in relation to area size and population, health indices, and care and demographic factors affecting the need for care. To meet this mandate, the Index of Medical Underservice was developed, comprising four variables:

- percentage of population below poverty income levels,
- percentage of population 65 years of age and older,
- infant mortality rate, and
- PCP per 1,000 population. The index yields a single numerical value on a scale from 0 to 100; any area with a value less than 62 (the median of all counties) is designated an MUA. Only one-half of the MUA population lives in a physician shortage area.

Community and Migrant Health Centers

These centers provide services to low-income populations on a sliding-fee scale, thereby addressing both geographic and financial barriers to access. For more than 4 decades, C/MHCs have provided primary care and preventive health services to populations in designated MUAs. These designated areas receive national priority in meeting their health care needs and are targeted for special federal health initiative programs. Traditionally, these areas have had trouble attracting private physicians, particularly in primary care specialties. As a result, C/MHCs heavily rely on nonphysician providers (NPPs) for the delivery of services. The migrant program supports 134 grantees, who run approximately 400 clinics in 40 states and Puerto Rico (HRSA Bureau of Primary Health Care 2007a). They serve approximately 727,000 migrants and seasonal farm workers (HRSA Bureau of Primary Health Care 2007b). Although community health centers must be located in areas designated as MUAs, migrant centers must be located in "high-impact" areas, defined as areas that serve at least 4,000 migrant and/or seasonal farm workers for at least 2 months per year.

The Rural Health Clinics Act

The Rural Health Clinics Act was developed to respond to the concern that isolated rural communities could not generate sufficient revenue to support the services of a physician. In many cases, the only source of primary care or emergency services was NPPs, who were ineligible at that time for Medicare or Medicaid reimbursement. The Act is a reimbursement mechanism that strengthens the financial viability of eligible entities by increasing the opportunities for

Medicare and Medicaid reimbursement. The Act permitted physician assistants (PAs), nurse practitioners (NPs), and certified nurse midwives (CNMs) associated with rural clinics to practice without the direct supervision of a physician; enabled rural health clinics (but not NPPs directly) to be reimbursed by Medicare and Medicaid for their services; and tied the level of Medicaid payment to the level established by Medicare. To be designated as a rural health clinic, a public or private sector physician practice, clinic, or hospital must meet several criteria, including location in an MUA, geographic HPSA, or a population-based HPSA. Over 3,000 rural health clinics provide primary care services to over 7 million people in 47 states (NARHC 2007).

Rural Managed Care

Rural managed care faces demographic, geographic, and infrastructure challenges. The demographic and geographic characteristics of rural communities pose important barriers to managed care. Some rural communities do not have large enough populations to support the array of practitioners and services necessary to provide cost-efficient health care. At the same time, health care needs in rural areas are as great as or greater than those in urban areas because of high rates of chronic disease and other unmet needs. Moreover, rural incomes remain low, making it difficult for managed care plans to generate the revenues that comparable resources might generate in an urban area.

Apart from shortages of physicians and hospitals in rural areas, some rural physicians cannot meet board certification or eligibility requirements imposed by managed care plans. Many physicians practicing in rural areas may find the corporate culture of managed care plans alien. The isolation of rural practice can attract individualistic practitioners who are used to making independent decisions and who are unwilling to be held accountable to a managed care organization (MCO).

THE HOMELESS

Although an exact number is unknown, an estimated 3.5 million people (1.35 million of them children) are likely to experience homelessness in a given year (National Coalition for the Homeless 2006a). Nationally, approximately 26 million people (14% of the US population) are homeless at some point in their lives. Although most homeless persons live in major urban areas, a surprising 19% live in rural areas.

The homeless population includes 43% single men, 17% single women, and 39% children under the age of 18 (National Coalition for the Homeless 2006b). About 33% of the homeless population are families with children (National Coalition for the Homeless 2006b). About 40% of all homeless men are veterans of war (National Coalition for the Homeless 2006b).

Homeless women in particular face major difficulties: economic and housing needs and special gender-related issues that include pregnancy, child care responsibilities, family violence, fragmented family support, job discrimination, and wage discrepancies. Homeless women, regardless of parenting status, should be linked with social services, family support, self-help, and housing resources. Mentally ill women caring for children need additional consideration, with an emphasis on parenting skills and special services for children. Thus, homelessness is a multifaceted problem related to personal, social, and economic factors.

The economic picture of homeless persons is dismal, as would be expected, and suggests that they are severely lacking in the financial and educational resources necessary to access health care. Further, almost one-half of homeless people have not graduated from high school and have been unemployed for 4 years on average. Despite these figures, only 20% receive income maintenance and only 26% have health insurance. These numbers remain low because of federal restrictions that prohibit federal help to those without a physical street address.

The shortage of adequate low-income housing is the major precipitating factor for homelessness. Unemployment, personal or family life crises, rent increases that are out of proportion to inflation, and reduction in public benefits can also directly result in the loss of a home. Illness, on the other hand, tends to result in the loss of a home in a more indirect way. Other indirect causes of homelessness include deinstitutionalization from public mental hospitals, substance abuse programs, and overcrowded prisons and jails.

Community-based residential alternatives for mentally ill individuals vary from independent apartments to group homes staffed by paid caregivers. Independent living may involve either separate apartments or single-room occupancy units (SROs) in large hotels, whereas group homes are staffed during at least a portion of the day and traditionally provide some on-site mental health services (Schutt and Goldfinger 1996).

The homeless, adults and children, have a high prevalence of untreated acute and chronic medical, mental health, and substance abuse problems. The reasons are debatable. Some argue that people may become homeless because of a physical or mental illness. Others argue that homelessness itself may lead to the development of physical and mental disability because homelessness produces risk factors, which include excessive use of alcohol, illegal drugs, and cigarettes; sleeping in an upright position, which results in venous stasis and its consequences; extensive walking in poorly fitting shoes; and grossly inadequate nutrition.

Homeless persons are also at a greater risk of assault and victimization regardless of whether they live in a shelter or outdoors. They are also subject to exposure to extreme heat, cold, and other weather conditions. The homeless are also exposed to illness because of overcrowding in shelters and overexposure to weather.

Barriers to Health Care

The homeless face barriers to ambulatory services but incur high rates of hospitalization.

A high use of inpatient services in this manner amounts to the substitution of inpatient care for outpatient services. Both individual factors (competing needs, substance dependence, and mental illness) and system factors (availability, cost, convenience, and appropriateness of care) account for the barriers to adequate ambulatory services.

Other barriers include accessible transportation to medical care providers and competing needs for basic food, shelter, and income than obtaining health services or following through with a prescribed treatment plan. Homeless individuals who experience psychological distress and disabling mental illness may be in the greatest need of health services and yet may be the least able to obtain them. This inability to obtain health care may be attributable to such individual traits of mental illness as paranoia, disorientation, unconventional health beliefs, lack of social support, lack of organizational skills to gain access to needed services, or fear of authority figures and institutions resulting from previous institutionalization. The social conditions of street life also affect compliance with medical care because of a lack of proper sanitation and a stable place to store medications. They also lack resources to obtain proper food for a medically indicated diet necessary for conditions like diabetes or hypertension.

Federal efforts to provide medical services to the homeless population are primarily through the Health Care for the Homeless (HCH) program. Community health centers supported by the 1985 Robert Wood Johnson Foundation/Pew Memorial Trust HCH program (subsequently covered by the 1987 McKinney Homeless Assistance Act) have addressed many of the access and quality-of-care issues faced by the homeless. In 2004, community health centers served approximately 703,000 homeless patients (HRSA Bureau of Primary Health Care 2007b).

A critical aspect of these programs is outreach, in which teams of health care professionals bring a wide range of services to homeless persons in shelters, hotels, soup lines, beaches and parks, train and bus stations, religious facilities, and other places where homeless people may gather. Such programs help overcome some of the barriers to care. Outreach teams are typically based in health care centers, to which clinicians can refer homeless patients who need additional medical attention. In addition, a walk-in appointment system reduces access barriers at these medical facilities. Medical care, routine laboratory tests, substance abuse counseling, and some medications are provided free of charge to eliminate financial barriers.

The Mental Health Services for the Homeless Block Grant program sets aside funds for states to implement services for homeless persons with mental illness. These services include outreach services; community mental health services; rehabilitation; referrals to inpatient treatment, primary care, and substance abuse services; case management services; and supportive services in residential settings.

Services for homeless veterans are provided through the Department of Veterans Affairs (VA). The Homeless Chronically Mentally Ill Veterans Program provides outreach, case management services, and psychiatric residential treatment for homeless mentally ill veterans in community-based facilities in 45 US cities. The Domiciliary Care for Homeless Veterans Program addresses the health needs of veterans who have psychiatric illnesses or alcohol or drug abuse problems, operating 1,800 beds at 31 sites across the country (US Dept of Veterans Affairs 2006).

The Salvation Army also provides a variety of social, rehabilitation, and support services for homeless persons. Its centers include adult rehabilitation and food programs and permanent and transitional housing.

MENTAL HEALTH

Mental disorders are common psychiatric illnesses affecting adults and present a serious public health problem in the United States (Barker et al. 1989; Klerman and Weissman 1989; Myers et al. 1984; Regier et al. 1988; Romanoski et al. 1992). Mental disorders are the leading cause of disability for people aged 15–44 (NIMH 2007). Mental illness is a risk factor for death from suicide, cardiovascular disease, and cancer. Suicide is currently the 10th leading cause of death in the United States and the 4th leading cause of death among persons aged 18–65. Non-Hispanic White men 85 years of age or older have one of the highest rates of suicide, with 47 suicide deaths per 100,000. American Indian and Alaska Natives are at higher risk for suicides as well, with 14.3 suicide deaths per 100,000 (CDC 2011).

Mental health disorders can be either psychological or biological in nature. Many mental health diseases, including mental retardation (MR), developmental disabilities (DD), and schizophrenia, are now known to be biological in origin. Other behaviors, including those related to personality disorders and neurotic behaviors, are still subject to interpretation and professional judgment. Defining what is and is not normal in a population is difficult and often raises far-reaching moral and ethical issues (Williams 1995).

National studies have concluded that the most common mental disorders include phobias; substance abuse, including alcohol and drug dependence; and affective disorders, including depression. Schizophrenia is considerably less common, affecting an estimated 1.1% of the population (NIMH 2006a).

About one in four adults suffers from a diagnosable mental disorder every year (NIMH 2007). In 2009, 45.1 million adults (18 years of age or older) had a mental illness, including 11 million with severe mental illness (SMI). Among this population, only a small percentage sought care. Prevalence of SMI was higher among women and individuals in the 18–25 age group (NIMH 2008; Substance Abuse and Mental Health Services Administration 2010).

Most mental health services are provided in the general medical sector—a concept first described by Regier and colleagues (1988) as the de facto mental health service system—rather than through formal mental health specialist services. The de facto system combines specialty mental health services with general counseling services, such as those provided in primary care settings, nursing homes, and community health centers by ministers, counselors, self-help groups, families, and friends. Specifically, mental health services are provided through public and private resources in both inpatient and outpatient facilities. These facilities include state and county mental hospitals, private psychiatric hospitals, nonfederal general hospital psychiatric services, VA psychiatric services, residential treatment centers, and freestanding psychiatric outpatient clinics (**Table 24-6**). Total expenditures for mental disorders have increased since 1996, from $35.2 billion to $57.5 billion in 2006 (NIMH 2006a). Per person, the cost was $1,591, including $1,931 per child (NIMH 2006b). Despite the cost of mental health care for individuals with any mental illness, only 37.9% received mental health services and only 60.2% of individuals covered under Medicare Part B received care (Substance Abuse and Mental Health Services Administration 2010). The nation's **mental health system** is composed of two subsystems: one primarily for individuals with insurance coverage or private funds and the other for those without private coverage.

The Uninsured and Mental Health

Patients without insurance coverage or personal financial resources are treated in state and county mental health hospitals and in community mental health clinics. Care is also provided in short-term, acute care hospitals and emergency departments. Local governments are the providers of last resort, with the ultimate responsibility to provide somatic and mental health services for all citizens regardless of ability to pay.

The Insured and Mental Health

For patients who have insurance coverage or personal ability to pay, availability of both inpatient and ambulatory mental health care has expanded tremendously. Inpatient mental health services for patients with insurance are usually provided through private psychiatric hospitals. These hospitals can be operated on either a nonprofit or a for-profit basis. There has been substantial growth in national chains of for-profit mental health hospitals. Patients with insurance coverage are also more likely to receive care through the offices of private psychiatrists, clinical psychologists, and licensed social workers. Mental health services are also provided by the VA and by the military health care system; however, access to these services is limited by eligibility.

TABLE 24-6	Mental Health Organizations (in Thousands), 2004
Service and Organization	Number of Mental Health Organizations
All organizations	2,891
State and county mental hospitals	237
Private psychiatric hospitals	264
Nonfederal general hospital psychiatric services	1,230
Residential treatment centers for emotionally disturbed children	458
All other	702

Source: Data from *Health, United States, 2009,* p. 385.

Managed Care and Mental Health

Managed care has expanded its services into mental health delivery. State and local governments are also contracting with MCOs to manage a full health care benefit package that includes mental health and substance-abuse services for their Medicaid enrollees.

Many health maintenance organizations (HMOs) contract with specialized companies that provide managed behavioral health care, an arrangement called a carve-out. This is mainly because HMOs lack the in-house capacity to provide treatment. Using case managers and reviewers, most of whom are psychiatric nurses, social workers, and psychologists, these specialized companies oversee and authorize the use of mental health and substance abuse services. The case reviewers, using clinical protocols to guide them, assign patients to the least expensive appropriate treatment, emphasizing outpatient alternatives over inpatient care.

Working with computerized databases, a reviewer studies a patient's particular problem and then authorizes an appointment with an appropriate provider in the company's selective network. On average, psychiatrists constitute about 20% of any given provider network, psychologists constitute 40%, and psychiatric social workers constitute another 40%.

Mental Health Professionals

A variety of professionals provide mental health services (**Table 24-7**), including but not limited to psychiatrists, psychologists, social workers, nurses, counselors, and therapists.

Psychiatrists are specialist physicians who specialize in the diagnosis and treatment of mental disorders. Psychiatrists receive postgraduate specialty training in mental health after completing medical school. Psychiatric residencies cover medical, as well as behavioral, diagnosis and treatments. A relatively small proportion of the total mental health workforce consists of psychiatrists, but they exercise disproportionate influence in the system by virtue of their authority to prescribe drugs and admit patients to hospitals.

Psychologists usually hold a doctoral degree, although some hold master's degrees. They are trained in interpreting and changing

| TABLE 24-7 | Full-Time Equivalent Patient Care Staff in Mental Health Organizations, 1998 |

Staff Discipline	Number	Percentage
All patient care staff	531,532	78.1
Professional patient care staff	304,449	44.8
Psychiatrists	28,374	4.2
Other physicians	3,561	0.5
Psychologists	28,729	4.2
Social workers	72,367	10.6
Registered nurses	78,562	11.5
Other mental health professionals	78,854	11.6
Physical health professionals and assistants	14,002	2.1
Other mental health workers	130,551	33.4

Source: Section VI, Chapter 18, Table 7, *Mental Health, United States, 2002.* Ronald W. Manderscheid and Marilyn J. Henderson, eds. Rockville, MD: US Department of Health and Human Services, Substance Abuse and Mental Health Services Administration, Center for Mental Health Services.

the behavior of people. Psychologists cannot prescribe drugs; however, they provide a wide range of services to patients with neurotic and behavioral problems. Psychologists use such techniques as psychotherapy and counseling, which psychiatrists typically do not engage in. Psychoanalysis is a subspecialty in mental health that involves the use of intensive treatment by both psychiatrists and psychologists.

Social workers receive training in various aspects of mental health services, particularly counseling. Social workers are trained at the master's degree level. They also compete with psychologists for patients.

Nurses are involved in mental health through the subspecialty of psychiatric nursing. Specialty training for nurses had its origins in the latter part of the 1800s. Nurses provide a wide range of mental health services.

Many other health care professionals contribute to the array of available services, including marriage and family counselors, recreational therapists, and vocational counselors. Numerous people work in related areas, such as adult day care (ADC), alcohol and drug abuse counseling, and as psychiatric aides in institutional settings.

THE CHRONICALLY ILL AND DISABLED

Chronic diseases are now the leading cause of death in the United States—heart disease, cancer, and stroke account for more than 50% of deaths each year. Seven out of 10 deaths each year are from chronic diseases (CDC 2010a). Heart disease is the number one cause of death in the United States, at 204.3 per 100,000 persons (National Center for Health Statistics 2007). The prevalence of heart disease in 2009 was 12%, which is equal to 26.8 million Americans (National Center for Health Statistics 2009). In 2005, almost 1 in 2 adults had at least one chronic illness, roughly 133 million Americans. This large prevalence of disease results in adverse consequences such as limitations on daily living activities.

The loss in human potential and work days notwithstanding, chronic disease is expensive, incurring more than 75% of the total medical expenditure ($1.4 trillion annually; National Center for Chronic Disease Prevention and Health Promotion 2005). Chronic disease places a huge economic demand on the nation. The estimated annual direct medical expenditures for the most common chronic diseases are $313.8 billion in 2009 for cardiovascular disease and stroke, $89.0 billion for cancer in 2007, and $116 billion for diabetes in 2007 (CDC 2009).

Much of the burden of chronic diseases is the result of four modifiable risk behaviors: physical activity, nutrition, smoking, and alcohol (CDC 2010a). There is a lack of physical activity among the US population, with 23% reporting no leisure-time physical activity at all in the preceding month of the 2008 Physical Activity Guidelines for Americans survey. There has also been a decline in participation of physical education classes among high school students, from 42% in 1991 to 30% in 2007, showing that all age groups do not partake in regular physical activity. The nation also suffers from poor nutrition. Less than 25% of adults and children eat the required five or more servings of fruit and vegetables, although the majority consumes more than the recommended amount of saturated fat (CDC 2009).

Chronic illness can often lead to disability. The chronic conditions most responsible for disabilities are arthritis, heart disease, back problems, asthma, and diabetes (Kraus et al. 1996). The disabled also tend to be covered by public sources (30% by Medicare and 10% by Medicaid), compared to those who have no disabilities, who are more likely to pay for care with private coverage (Kraus et al. 1996).

Disability can be categorized as mental, physical, or social; tests of disability tend to be more sensitive to some categories than others. Physical disability usually addresses a person's mobility and other basic activities performed in daily life, mental disability involves both the cognitive and emotional states, and social disability is considered the most severe disability because management of social roles requires both physical and mental well-being (Ostir et al. 1999). About 19.4% of the noninstitutionalized US population, or 48.9 million Americans, have a disability (Kraus et al. 1996).

The two commonly used measures of disability, activities of daily living (ADLs) and instrumental activities of daily living (IADLs), were covered in Chapter 2. Another tool for assessing disability is the Survey of Income and Program Participation (SIPP), which measures disability by asking participants about functional limitations (difficulty in performing activities such as seeing, hearing, walking, having one's speech understood, etc.), but ADL and IADL scales are more widely used.

Despite the availability of community-based and institutional long-term care services for people with functional limitations, many people are not getting the help they need with the basic tasks of personal care. It is estimated that more than one-third of people with chronic conditions do not receive assistance with ADLs. Consequently, these people do not bathe or shower because of a fear of falling, are unable to follow a dietary regimen, and sustain falls. Ultimately, unmet needs lead to exacerbated health problems, costly treatments, and unnecessary pain and suffering (The Robert Wood Johnson Foundation 1996).

HIV/AIDS

In July 1982, acquired immune deficiency syndrome (AIDS) was officially named a disease. **Figure 24-11** illustrates trends in AIDS reporting. The number of AIDS cases reported increased between 1987 and 1993, decreased between 1994 and 1999, increased between 2000 and 2004, and decreased from 2005 through 2007 (US Census Bureau 2010).

Deaths from AIDS have declined since 1998 and decreased 11.3% between 2003 and 2006,

FIGURE 24-11 U.S. AIDS Cases Reported, 1987–2007

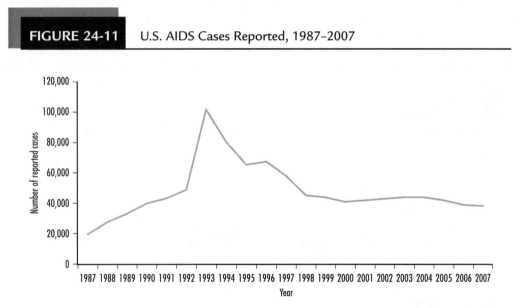

Source: Reprinted from U.S. Centers for Disease Control and Prevention, *Statistical Abstracts of the United States, 2001,* p. 119; and *Statistical Abstracts of the United States, 2007,* p. 120; *Statistical Abstracts of the United States, 2008,* p. 121; *Statistical Abstracts of the United States, 2009,* p. 120; *Statistical Abstracts of the United States, 2010,* p. 122.

from 13,658 to 12,113 (US Census Bureau 2010). Declines in reported AIDS cases between 1994 and 1999 were ascribed to new treatments; decreasing death rates may reflect the fact that benefits from new treatments are being fully realized. Meanwhile, the number of people living with AIDS continues to increase. In 2006, 446,098 people were living with AIDS; in 2001, the figure was 341,332 (CDC 2010b).

AIDS is believed to be caused by the human immunodeficiency virus (HIV). HIV is an unusual type of virus, called a retrovirus, which causes the immune system suppression leading to AIDS. Individuals infected with HIV develop antibodies within a short period but may exhibit no symptoms for many years. Typically, the immune system weakens gradually and the blood level of CD4 cells (a type of white blood cell known as a T-helper/inducer lymphocyte) drops below the normal level of between 1,200 and 1,400/mm. Persons with few CD4 cells are prone to **opportunistic infections**. Symptoms, such as persistent fever, night sweats, and weight loss, begin to occur more often when the CD4 count drops below 500/mm. The development of AIDS is estimated to occur at 11 years on average from the time of HIV infection.

Certain widely recognized risk factors promote the transmission of HIV, including male-to-male sexual contact; male-to-female sexual contact; injection drug use (IDU); blood product exposure; and perinatal transmission from mother to infant during pregnancy, delivery, or possibly during breastfeeding (**Table 24-8**).

Most individuals infected with HIV produce antibodies within 6 to 9 months of exposure, although some people do not form antibodies until 2 to 3 years after exposure to HIV. Consequently, an individual can be exposed to HIV and not develop the antibodies for several years. Further, people may transmit HIV before they know they have been exposed, making transmission unsuspecting. HIV infection was the sixth leading cause of death among persons 25 to 34 years of age in 2006 (US Census Bureau 2010).

For Blacks, Hispanics, and minority women, AIDS/HIV is still a major public health concern. In 2004, males and Blacks continued to have significantly higher rates of HIV/AIDS than females and Whites (**Table 24-9**). Also, only among Black males is HIV infection a leading cause of death (CDC 2010b). In 2007, rates of AIDS cases per 100,000 people were 47.3 in the

TABLE 24-8	Reports of All AIDS Cases: All Years Through 2007		
Sex and Diagnosis	Percentage Distribution	Number of Reported Cases	
All races	100%	1,021,242	
Men who have sex with men	43.6%	445,645	
Injecting drug use	23.1%	235,842	
Men who have sex with men and injecting drug use	6.6%	67,797	
Hemophilia/coagulation disorder	0.5%	5,567	
Heterosexual sex with injecting drug user	3.8%	38,766	
Other heterosexual contact	10.2%	104,086	
Transfusion	0.9%	9,315	
Undetermined	11.2%	114,224	

Source: Data from *Statistical Abstract of the United States, 2010,* p. 122.

Black population, 15.2 in the Hispanic population, 6.9 in the American Indian/Alaska Native population, 5.2 in the White population, 3.6 in the Asian population, and 18.3 in the Native Hawaiian/Other Pacific Islander population (CDC 2007). Blacks accounted for 51% of all HIV/AIDS cases diagnosed in 2007 (CDC 2007). Racial differences in HIV/AIDS infection probably reflect social, economic, behavioral, and other factors associated with HIV transmission risks.

New York and Maryland lead the states in the proportion of individuals afflicted with AIDS, at 24.8 cases per 100,000 population (**Table 24-10**). Vermont has the lowest AIDS rate, at 1.0 per 100,000 population. California has more reported AIDS cases than any other state, followed by New York, Florida, Texas, and Georgia. Vermont has the smallest number of reported AIDS cases, followed by North Dakota and Wyoming (US Census Bureau 2010).

HIV infection has risen to the level of a global pandemic and has become the world's modern-day plague. In 2009, 33.3 million people were estimated to be living with HIV worldwide (UNAIDS 2010). An estimated 2.6 million people acquired HIV in 2009, including 370,000 children younger than 15 years of age (UNAIDS 2010). AIDS caused the deaths of an estimated 1.8 million people, including 260,000 children younger than 15 years of age (UNAIDS 2010). These figures represent a decrease over previous years, but the global HIV/AIDS epidemic is far from under control, particularly in sub-Saharan Africa, where 22.5 million of the world's 33.3 million cases of people living with HIV reside (UNAIDS 2010).

Many public health experts believe that cases of AIDS still remain underreported. The reasons for such underreporting include poor reporting standards in health departments (Selike et al. 1993), physicians desiring to protect the confidentiality of their patients because of the stigma of HIV/AIDS (AIDS Forecasting 1989), lack of physician knowledge about the diagnosis of AIDS (Anonymous 1988), patients' denial

TABLE 24-9 U.S. AIDS Cases Reported Through 2007

Characteristic	All Years		2007	
	Number	Percentage	Number	Percentage
Total	1,018,429	100.0	35,962	100.0
Sex				
Male (13 and older)	810,676	79.6	26,355	73.3
Female (13 and older)	198,544	19.5	9,599	26.6
Children younger than 13 years	9,209	0.9	28	0.1
Race/Ethnic Group				
White	404,465	40.0	10,467	29.3
Black	426,002	42.1	17,507	49.3
Hispanic	169,138	16.7	6,920	19.5
Asian	7,512	0.7	474	.02
Native Hawaiian or other Pacific Islander	720	0.1	76	.04
American Indian/Alaska Native	3,492	0.3	158	.04

Source: Data from *Health, United States, 2009,* p. 252.

			Top and Bottom 10 States for AIDS, According to Cases per
TABLE 24-10			100,000 Population, 2007

Top States	Reported Cases	Cases per 100,000 Population	Bottom States	Reported Cases	Cases per 100,000 Population
California	4,952	13.6	Rhode Island	66	6.3
New York	4,810	24.8	New Hampshire	51	3.9
Florida	3,961	21.8	Maine	46	3.5
Texas	2,964	12.4	Alaska	32	4.7
Georgia	1,877	19.7	Montana	25	2.6
Pennsylvania	1,750	14.1	Idaho	23	1.5
Maryland	1,394	24.8	South Dakota	15	1.9
Illinois	1,348	10.5	Wyoming	13	2.5
New Jersey	1,164	13.5	North Dakota	8	1.3
North Carolina	1,024	11.3	Vermont	6	1.0

Source: Data from *Statistical Abstract of the United States, 2010.*

of the risk behaviors that are likely to transmit HIV, and the absence of or decreased access to health care (Robertson et al. 1974), which prevents the diagnosis of HIV. With the advent of combination antiretroviral therapy, AIDS surveillance data no longer reflect trends in HIV transmission because this therapy has effectively delayed the progression of HIV to AIDS (CDC 1999a).

HIV testing is anonymous or confidential. In anonymous HIV testing, patient-identifying information or other locating information is not linked to the HIV test, whereas, in confidential HIV testing, the test result is linked (CDC 1999c). In September 2006, CDC released new recommendations for HIV testing, which called for routine HIV screening of adults, adolescents, and pregnant women in health care settings in the United States (Branson et al. 2006).

The implementation of rapid HIV testing—versus the previous method, ELISA (enzyme-linked immunosorbent assay)—makes it possible to get early results, permitting the initiation of combined antiretroviral therapy earlier in the disease process. Furthermore, the rapid HIV test may improve the outreach at clinics where testing and counseling are offered together.

Both the rapid HIV test and ELISA require a second testing, using a Western blot or an immunofluorescence assay (IFA) to confirm positive test results. The ELISA test (also known as enzyme immunoassays or EIAs) required special equipment. Blood samples had to be sent to laboratories and test results were not available for 1 or 2 weeks, requiring the clients to make a second visit to the testing site. Many people did not return for their results. The CDC estimated that, in 2000, 31% of patients who tested positive for HIV at public-sector testing points did not return to get their results (Greenwald 2006). With rapid HIV testing, results are available in 5 to 30 minutes, and the test is as accurate as the ELISA. Thus, testing and counseling can be available during the same visit.

Current treatment for HIV/AIDS centers on therapies for slowing the progress of HIV and preventing opportunistic infections (OI), reducing the number of people with HIV who develop and die from AIDS. For example, medications, such as oral antibiotics, are often used to prevent a common pneumonia (pneumocystis carinii or PCP), an OI that often develops in persons with AIDS. Other OIs include tuberculosis, toxoplasmosis, and mycobacterium avium complex (MAC). OIs occur when organisms naturally present in the body get out of control and cause health problems due to a weakened immune system. Protease inhibitors, a combination of new, more effective drugs, are now taken in conjunction with antiretrovirals, the initial drugs used in AIDS/HIV therapy. Combination drug therapy—known as highly active antiretroviral therapy (HAART) or "drug cocktail"—has been more effective because it can reduce the viral load (level of HIV particles circulating in the blood) to extremely low levels; however, the long-term effectiveness of HAART is unknown, and it is extremely expensive. The high cost of HAART makes the treatment unavailable to many patients in the United States and keeps it out of reach in developing countries, where more than 90% of the new HIV infections occur. Also, the complicated drug regimen requires coordination of many pills and doses, which makes it easier to skip medications or doses so that some patients temporarily stop treatment. This lack of regimen adherence not only makes the treatment less effective but also increases the chance of developing a drug-resistant strain of HIV. It is suspected that HIV will eventually develop multidrug resistance. After experiencing improvements in one's condition, complacency may lead to relaxed preventive behavior, which would risk spreading a potential drug-resistant strain of HIV (CDC 1998, 1999b).

HIV Infection in Rural Communities

Spread of HIV into rural communities in the United States has grown. CDC reported 23,615 new cases of AIDS in nonmetropolitan areas of the United States between March 1994 and February 1995 (CDC 1995b). In 1999, 7% of cumulative adult/adolescent AIDS cases were reported from nonmetropolitan areas (CDC 2001).

Rural persons with HIV and AIDS are more likely to be young, non-White, and female and to have acquired their infection through heterosexual contact. Additionally, a growing number of these HIV-infected persons live in the rural South, a region historically characterized by a disproportionate number of poor and minority persons, strong religious beliefs and sanctions, and decreased access to comprehensive health services (CDC 1995a, 1995b; DHHS, Office of Minority Health 2003; Morrison 1993). Trends in new cases of HIV and AIDS in rural areas indicate that poor and non-White residents are disproportionately affected (Aday 1993; Lam and Liu 1994; Rumby et al. 1991).

HIV IN CHILDREN

In the absence of specific therapy to interrupt transmission of HIV, an infected woman has a 25% chance of having a child born with HIV. Therefore, in 1994 and 1995, the US Public Health Service (PHS) began recommending that pregnant women be counseled and voluntarily tested for HIV and that zidovudine (AZT) be given to infected women during pregnancy and delivery, as well as to the infant after delivery. The drop in perinatal transmission rates has been attributed to this strategy, and, in one study, perinatal transmission rates dropped from 21 to 11% after use of AZT, according to PHS guidelines. The number of children with a diagnosis of AIDS who had been perinatally exposed to HIV declined from 122 in 2000 to 47 in 2004 (CDC 2005). The importance of preventing perinatal transmission is underscored by the fact that 91% of all AIDS cases among US children are caused by mother-to-child transmission in pregnancy, labor, delivery, or breastfeeding (CDC 1999d, 1999f). The earliest and most common symptom in HIV-positive children is enlarged lymph nodes, which are often associated with an enlarged spleen (Johnson and Vink 1992). HIV-infected children also have severe and persistent skin infections. Children who are born with AIDS suffer from failure to thrive, the inability to grow and develop as healthy children. Without intervention, this failure to thrive may lead to developmental delays that can have negative lifetime consequences for the child and his or her family.

HIV infection causes morbidity in two different but equally destructive ways. First, viruses like HIV cause illness by direct infection of cells; HIV can infect every organ system in the body and has a particular affinity for cells of the nervous system. Second, as HIV infects and destroys CD4 cells and weakens the immune system, the child becomes increasingly susceptible to various illnesses (O'Hara and D'Orlando 1996).

Family-centered care provides care and support to all immediate family members of children with HIV. It allows health care providers to develop and implement an interdisciplinary treatment plan to manage HIV infection for all children regardless of how they acquired the infection. For example, as the child becomes symptomatic, health care providers may add new therapies to the already prescribed medication regimen. Providers may also perform numerous diagnostic procedures to rule out potential problems or to diagnose a particular disease process to reduce pain and suffering.

HIV in Women

Women are a rapidly growing proportion of the population with HIV/AIDS. In 2004, women made up approximately one-half of HIV/AIDS cases worldwide (WHO 2004). For US women 25 to 44 years of age, HIV/AIDS is a leading cause of death. Between 2001 and 2005, the estimated number of AIDS cases increased 17% for women and 16% for men (CDC 2006a). For women, heterosexual exposure to HIV, followed by IDU, is the greatest cause for exposure. Aside from the inherent risks in IDU, drug use overall contributes to a higher risk of contracting HIV if heterosexual sex with an IDU user occurs or

when sex is traded for drugs or money (CDC 2002). Black and Hispanic minority women are at particular risk. Despite representing less than one-fourth of the total US female population, Black and Hispanic women represent more than three-fourths (79%) of all AIDS cases in women (National Institute of Allergy and Infectious Diseases 2006).

Because of women's position in society, HIV-positive women face many problems not confronted by men with HIV. For instance, the social expectation is that women are the caregivers for those who are ill in the family. As a result, women with HIV often care for their partner or children when they are ill themselves. Domestic violence has been increasingly identified among women living with HIV.

HIV/AIDS-Related Issues

Need for Research

HIV-related research seeks to develop a vaccine to prevent HIV-negative people from acquiring HIV. Researchers are also seeking to develop a therapeutic vaccine to prevent HIV-positive people from developing symptoms of AIDS.

People with HIV/AIDS often belong to groups that differ from each other. For example, women with AIDS may have different concerns than adolescents with AIDS. People with HIV/AIDS represent a broad spectrum of social classes, races, ethnicities, sexual orientations, and genders. Behavioral intervention research, therefore, should focus particularly on populations that are most vulnerable to HIV infection and are in urgent need of preventive interventions. These populations include gay youth and young adults, especially Black and Hispanic; disenfranchised and impoverished women; heterosexual men, again, Black and Hispanic in particular; inner city youth; and out-of-treatment substance abusers and their sexual partners. Research should be aimed not only at the individual but also at the impact of broader interventions (e.g., among drug users or those involved in sexual networks or communitywide groups) that change behavioral norms and, consequently, affect individual behavior (Merson 1996).

Public Health Concerns

AIDS underscores the synergy between poverty and intravenous drug use. The despair commonly caused by poverty is often mitigated only by addictions, such as drug use. Further, control of the HIV epidemic among the poor is hampered by their preoccupation with other problems related to survival, such as homelessness, crime, and lack of access to adequate health care.

Additionally, a relationship exists between the current tuberculosis epidemic and HIV. Indeed, tuberculosis, an opportunistic infection, is the worldwide leading cause of death among HIV-infected people. Tuberculosis in HIV-infected persons is also a particular public health concern because HIV persons are at greater risk of developing multidrug-resistant tuberculosis. Multidrug-resistant tuberculosis is understandably difficult to treat and can be fatal (CDC 1999e, 1999g).

Reducing the spread of AIDS requires the understanding and acceptance of a variety of sexual issues, ranging from the likelihood that even heterosexual men may engage in anonymous homosexual intercourse to the difficulty that adolescents may have controlling their sexual urges. Prejudice against gays and lesbians is manifested as **homophobia**, a fear and/or hatred of these individuals. Homophobia explains the initial slow policy-related response to the HIV epidemic.

A variety of traditional public health measures have been used during the HIV crisis to reduce the spread of HIV, from mass testing for HIV to subjecting the exposed to lifelong quarantine—although quarantine has rarely been used. For several reasons, these traditional measures are much less effective when applied to HIV/AIDS, as opposed to sexually transmitted diseases (STDs), such as gonorrhea or syphilis. The primary purpose for testing for STDs is to limit their spread. This goal is easily accom-plished because the symptoms of STDs appear early and are generally treatable and curable. Testing for the presence of HIV, however, may not limit its spread because many people who learn their HIV status do not change the behaviors that contribute to its spread. Further, HIV has no cure. Current treatments do not affect the transmissibility of HIV, and some treatments are of questionable use for treatment of the symptoms of AIDS. Quarantine has generally not been used to contain the spread of HIV. Because HIV-positive people can transmit HIV throughout their lives, lifetime quarantine is not only legally impossible but also economically unfeasible.

Criminal law has also been used to contain the spread of HIV and to protect public health. For example, several laws nationwide require that those convicted of sex offenses be tested for HIV. Most of these laws, however, are disproportionately enforced against prostitutes. These laws suggest that those who test HIV-positive may receive greater prison sentences; however, it is questionable whether this type of punishment actually reduces the spread of HIV.

Health promotion efforts, including those used to reduce the transmission of HIV, are often hamstrung by many psychosocial and other systematic factors. Some of the psychosocial factors include the fact that humans have a hard time changing their behavior. People have a tendency to justify it. Further, much human behavior is associated with functional needs (e.g., unsafe sex might fulfill a need for intimacy). Because of the strength of these psychosocial factors, knowledge about how HIV is actually transmitted may be too weakly correlated with behavior change. The social learning theory explains that behavior change, first, requires knowledge, followed by a change of attitude or perspective.

Discrimination

HIV-positive people may experience discrimination in access to health care, which could range from refusal of treatment to breach of confidentiality. Even though HIV is difficult to transmit through casual contact, some health care workers often refuse to treat HIV-positive people. Some providers fear losing other patients. A physician who becomes HIV-positive would almost certainly lose patients in his or her practice. Many health care workers simply do not like homosexuals and IV drug users because they do not accept their behavior.

The policies of various government agencies intended to help have also had a discriminatory impact on people with HIV/AIDS. For example, the Social Security Administration has not historically considered many of the HIV-related symptoms of women and IV drug users in adjudicating disability claims. Although the Department of Defense provides adequate medical care to individuals who acquire HIV in the military, recruits who test HIV-positive cannot join the military.

Provider Training

In a study of the HIV-related training needs of health care providers, medical information was identified as the primary training need. Patients with HIV, on the other hand, emphasized that their health care providers needed psychosocial skills, cultural competency, and sensitivity, in addition to medical proficiency. According to HIV patients, the criteria for appropriate care should include providers' attitudes toward patients (e.g., body language denoting respect, treating the consumer as an equal partner in decision making about care) and providers' concern about nonmedical aspects of consumer quality of life (e.g., child care, transportation, and emotional well-being).

Increased knowledge about HIV and personal contact with people who have HIV have improved the attitudes of health care providers toward individuals with HIV and contributed to their willingness to care for people with HIV. Training should encompass not only medical and treatment-related information but also a range of competencies related to interpersonal interaction.

In the area of psychosocial skills, the following characteristics are essential for an effectively trained provider: good communication skills (ability to establish rapport, ask questions, and listen), positive attitudes (respect, empowerment, trust), and an approach that incorporates principles of holistic care. In the area of cultural competence, essential elements include understanding of and respect for the person's specific culture; understanding that racial and ethnic minorities have important and multiple subdivisions or functional units; acknowledging the issues of gender and sexual orientation within the context of cultural competence; and respecting the customs, including modes of communication, of the person's culture. In the area of substance abuse, the following key elements are essential for primary care providers: understanding the complex medical picture presented by a person who suffers both from HIV and addiction; understanding the complicated psychosocial, ethical, and legal issues related to care of addicted persons; and being aware of the personal attitudes about addiction that may impair the providers' ability to give care objectively and nonjudgmentally (e.g., in the administration of pain medication; Gross and Larkin 1996).

The risk of transmission of HIV from an infected health care worker to a patient lies somewhere between 1 in 4,000 and 1 in 40,000 (Pell et al. 1996). Guidelines adopted in the United Kingdom on the management of HIV-infected health care workers encompass three main principles: a duty to protect patients, a duty of confidentiality toward infected health care workers, and the concept that the risk of HIV transmission is restricted to certain exposure-prone procedures from which infected staff should refrain (Pell et al. 1996):

- Infected health care workers should stop performing exposure-prone procedures immediately after diagnosis.

- Patients who have undergone an exposure-prone procedure, when the infected health care worker was the sole or main operator, should be notified of this situation, offered reassurance and counseling, and administered an HIV test if requested.

- If possible, letters to patients should be sent so that they arrive before or on the day of the planned press statement.
- A dedicated local telephone helpline should be established as soon as possible.
- Health care workers have a right to confidentiality, which can be breached only in exceptional circumstances when required in the public interest.

Cost of HIV/AIDS

Medical care for an HIV/AIDS patient is extremely expensive. Pharmaceutical companies claim that the high prices they charge for AIDS drugs are related to their extensive investment in research and development of drugs. At least for HIV/AIDS-related drugs, the government must pay these prices without question. Medicaid covers an estimated 200,000 to 240,000 people with HIV (Kaiser

Family Foundation 2008). In fiscal year (FY) 2008, combined federal and state Medicaid spending on HIV totaled $7.5 billion, making it the largest source of public financing for HIV/AIDS care in the United States. Of this, the federal share was $4.1 billion in FY 2008, or 35% of federal HIV care spending (Kaiser Family Foundation 2008). Lack of insurance and underinsurance represent formidable financial barriers to HIV/AIDS care.

The US government also invests substantial amounts of money in research and development through research supported at NIH and CDC. Government programs spend money in several areas for HIV (**Figure 24-12**).

Much of the cost of medical care for a person infected with HIV is concentrated in the relatively brief period after a diagnosis of full-blown AIDS. From the time of entering HIV care, per person projected life expectancy is 24.2 years, discounted lifetime cost is $385,200, and undiscounted cost is $618,900 for adults who initiate HAART when the CD4 cell count is 350/L. Seventy-three percent of the cost is antiretroviral medications, 13% inpatient care, 9% outpatient

FIGURE 24-12 U.S. Federal Spending for HIV/AIDS by Category, FY 2011 Budget Request

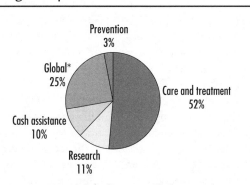

*Categories may include funding across multiple agencies/programs; global category includes international HIV research at NIH.

Source: Adapted from Kaiser Family Foundation. US Federal Funding for HIV/AIDS: The President's FY 2011 Budget Request. HIV/AIDS Policy Fact Sheet, February 2010.

care, and 5% other HIV-related medications and laboratory costs. For patients who initiate HAART when the CD4 cell count is 200/L, projected life expectancy is 22.5 years, discounted lifetime cost is $354,100 and undiscounted cost is $567,000. Results are sensitive to drug manufacturers' discounts, HAART efficacy, and use of enfuvirtide for salvage. If costs are discounted to the time of infection, the discounted lifetime cost is $303,100. Indirect costs include lost productivity, largely because of worker morbidity and mortality. However, other factors affect cost projections associated with the HIV epidemic, including the level of employment of HIV-positive people; regional differences in the cost of care, which is often associated with the lack of subacute care in many parts of the country; and the rate at which HIV spreads.

Containment of escalating medical costs, including the coordination of medical care, is the objective of two HIV-specific efforts: the **Medicaid waiver program** and the Ryan White Comprehensive AIDS Resources Emergency (CARE) Act. Through the Medicaid waiver program, states may design packages of services to specific populations, such as the elderly, the disabled, and those who test HIV positive. At this time, it is unknown whether the program is cost effective.

The passage of the Ryan White CARE Act in 1990 by Congress provided much-needed federal money to develop treatment and care options for persons with HIV and AIDS (Summer 1991). This legislation's main purpose was to provide emergency assistance to cities significantly affected by HIV/AIDS, allowing them to provide an array of testing, counseling, and other services, including case management, to people with HIV/AIDS. Title II of this legislation is administered by states and has been used to establish HIV clinics and related services in areas lacking the resources needed to offer this specialty care. Some public health systems have used Ryan White money to provide HIV and AIDS services in rural communities in which poor or medically underserved persons lack access to adequate care. Through the allocation of Ryan White funds, persons with HIV infection have been provided medical care, medicines, and care coordination within the public health system. The Act focuses on the development of cost-effective service schemes by funding innovative and existing services. Federal spending for Ryan White was estimated to total $2.1 billion in 2007 (Kaiser Family Foundation 2007).

AIDS and the US Health Care System

The course of AIDS is characterized by a gradual decline in a patient's physical, cognitive, and emotional function and well-being. Such a comprehensive decline requires a continuum of care, including emergency care, primary care, housing and supervised living, mental health and social support, nonmedical services, and hospice care. The continuum can encompass elements like outreach and case finding, preventive services, outpatient and inpatient care, and coordination of private and public insurance benefits.

As HIV disease progresses, many persons become disabled or lose their jobs and rely on public entitlement or private disability programs for income and health care benefits. These programs include Social Security Disability Income and Supplemental Security Income, administered by the Social Security Administration. Medicare and Medicaid become primary payers for health care because of the onset of disability and depletion of personal funds.

SUMMARY

This chapter examines the major characteristics of certain US population groups that face challenges and barriers in accessing health care services. These population groups are racial/ethnic minorities, children and women, those living in rural areas, the homeless, the mentally ill, and those with HIV/AIDS. The health needs of these population groups are summarized, and services available to them are described. The gaps that currently exist between these population groups and the rest of the population indicate that the nation must make significant efforts to address the unique health concerns of US subpopulations.

DISCUSSION QUESTIONS ─────────

1. How can the framework of vulnerability be used to study vulnerable populations in the United States?
2. What are the racial/ethnic minority categories in the United States?
3. Compared with White Americans, what health challenges do minorities face?
4. Who are the AA/PIs?
5. What is the Indian Health Service?
6. What are the health concerns of children?
7. Which childhood characteristics have important implications for health system design?
8. Which health services are currently available for children?
9. What are the health concerns of women?
10. What are the roles of the Office on Women's Health?
11. What are the challenges faced in rural health?
12. What measures are taken to improve access to care in rural areas?
13. What are the characteristics and health concerns of the homeless population?
14. How is mental health provided in the United States?
15. Who are the major mental health professionals?
16. How does AIDS affect different population groups in the United States?
17. Which services and policies currently combat AIDS in America?

REFERENCES ─────────

Aday, L.A. 1993. *At risk in America: The health and health care needs of vulnerable populations in the United States.* San Francisco, CA: Jossey-Bass Publishers.

Aday, L.A. 1994. Health status of vulnerable populations. *Annual Review Public Health* 15: 487–509.

Barker, P.R. et al. 1989. *Serious mental illness and disability in the adult household population: United States, 1989.* Hyattsville, MD: National Center for Health Statistics.

Bennefield, R. 1995. Current population reports: Health insurance coverage 1995. Bureau of the Census. [Online]. Available at: http://www.census.gov/prod/99pubs/p60-208.pdf. Accessed October 1999.

Bertakis, K.D. et al. 2000. Gender differences in the utilization of health services. *Journal of Family Practice* 49: 147–152.

Branson, B.M. et al. 2006. Revised recommendations for HIV testing of adults, adolescents, and pregnant women in health care settings. *MMWR* 55, no. RR14: 1–17.

Bureau of Labor Statistics (BLS). 2010. Bureau of Labor Statistics news release dated 11-5-10. Available at: http://www.bls.gov/news.release/empsit.nr0.htm. Accessed November 2010.

Burks, L.J. 1992. Community health representatives: The vital link in Native American health care. *The IHS Primary Care Provider* 16, no. 12: 186–190.

Castor, M.L. et al. 2006. A nationwide population-based study identifying health disparities between American Indians/Alaska Natives and the general populations living in select urban counties. *American Journal of Public Health* 96, no. 8: 1478–1484.

Centers for Disease Control and Prevention (CDC). 1995a. *Facts about women and HIV/AIDS.* Atlanta, GA: CDC.

Centers for Disease Control and Prevention (CDC). 1995b. *HIV/AIDS surveillance report, February.* Atlanta, GA: CDC.

Centers for Disease Control and Prevention (CDC). 1998. Update: HIV counseling and testing using rapid tests—United States, 1995. *Morbidity and Mortality Weekly Report* 47, no. 11: 211–215.

Centers for Disease Control and Prevention (CDC). 1999a. Guidelines for national human immunodeficiency virus case surveillance, including monitoring for human immunodeficiency virus infection and acquired immunodeficiency syndrome. *Morbidity and Mortality Weekly Report* 48, no. RR-13: 2–7.

Centers for Disease Control and Prevention (CDC). 1999b. *Rapid HIV tests: Questions/answers.* Available at: http://www.cdc.gov/nchstp/hiv_aids/pubs/rt/rapidqas.htm. Accessed December 2010.

Centers for Disease Control and Prevention (CDC). 1999c. Anonymous or confidential HIV counseling and voluntary testing in federally funded testing sites—United States, 1995–1997. *Morbidity and Mortality Weekly Report* 48, no. 24: 509–513.

Centers for Disease Control and Prevention (CDC). 1999d. *CDC fact sheet: HIV/AIDS among US women: Minority and young women at continuing risk.* Available at: http://www.cdc.gov/nchstp/hiv_aids/pubs/facts.htm. Accessed December 2010.

Centers for Disease Control and Prevention (CDC). 1999e. *CDC fact sheet: Recent HIV/AIDS treatment advances and the implications for prevention.* Available at: http://www.cdc.gov/nchstp/hiv_aids/pubs/facts.htm. Accessed December 2010.

Centers for Disease Control and Prevention (CDC). 1999f. *CDC fact sheet: Status of perinatal HIV prevention: US declines continue.* Available at: http://www.cdc.gov/nchstp/hiv_aids/pubs/facts.htm. Accessed December 2010.

Centers for Disease Control and Prevention (CDC). 1999g. *CDC fact sheet: The deadly intersection between TB and HIV.* Available at: http://www.cdc.gov/nchstp/hiv_aids/pubs/facts.htm. Accessed December 2010.

Centers for Disease Control and Prevention (CDC). 2001. *National Center for HIV, STD, and TB Prevention. Commentary.* Available at: http://www.cdc.gov/hiv/stats/hasrsupp62/commentary.htm. Accessed December 2010.

Centers for Disease Control and Prevention (CDC). 2002. *CDC fact sheet: HIV/AIDS among African-Americans, key facts.* Available at: http://www.cdc.gov/hiv/pubs/facts/afam.pdf. Accessed April 2003.

Centers for Disease Control and Prevention (CDC). 2005. *HIV/AIDS surveillance report, 2004.* Vol. 16. Atlanta: US Department of Health and Human Services.

Centers for Disease Control and Prevention (CDC). 2006. *HIV/AIDS surveillance report, 2005.* Vol. 17. Atlanta: US Department of Health and Human Services.

Centers for Disease Control and Prevention (CDC). 2007. *HIV/AIDS surveillance report.* Available at: http://www.cdc.gov/hiv/surveillance/resources/reports/2007report/table6b.htm. Accessed December 2010.

Centers for Disease Control and Prevention (CDC). 2009. The power of prevention. Available at: http://www.cdc.gov/chronicdisease/overview/index.htm. Accessed January 2011.

Centers for Disease Control and Prevention (CDC). 2010a. Chronic disease and health promotion.

Available at: http://www.cdc.gov/chronicdisease/pdf/2009-Power-of-Prevention.pdf. Accessed January 2011.

Centers for Disease Control and Prevention (CDC). 2010b. Deaths among persons with AIDS through December 2006. *HIV/AIDS surveillance report*, volume 14, no. 3. Available at: http://www.cdc.gof/hiv/surveillance/resources/reports/2009supp_vol14no3/pdf/table1.pdf. Accessed December 2010.

Centers for Disease Control and Prevention (CDC), National Center for Injury Prevention and Control. 2011. Web-based injury statistics query and reporting system (WISQARS). Available at: www.cdc.gov/ncipc/wisqars. Accessed January 2011.

Cohen, S.E. et al. 1994. The geography of AIDS: Patterns of urban and rural migration. *Southern Medical Journal* 85, no. 6: 599.

Department of Health and Human Services (DHHS), Office of Minority Health. 2003. *HIV impact, AIDS in rural America.* Washington, DC: Government Printing Office. pp. 10–11.

Donelan, K. et al. 1996. Whatever happened to the health insurance crisis in the United States? *Journal of the American Medical Association* 276, no. 16: 1346–1350.

Fitzwilliams, J. 1977. Critical health manpower shortage areas: Their impact on rural health planning. *Agricultural Economic Report* No. 361. Washington, DC: Economic Research Service, Department of Agriculture.

Freeman, H.E., and C.R. Corey. 1993. Insurance status and access to health services among poor persons. *Health Services Research* 28: 531–541.

Greenwald, J.L. et al. 2006. A rapid review of rapid HIV antibody tests. *Current Infectious Disease Reports* 8: 125–131.

Gross, E.J., and M.H. Larkin. 1996. The child with HIV in day care and school. *Nursing Clinics of North America* 31, no. 1: 231–241.

Health Resources and Services Administration (HRSA), Bureau of Health Professions. 2003. National Health Service Corps. Available at: http://nhsc.bhpr.hrsa.gov/about/. Accessed December 2008.

Health Resources and Services Administration (HRSA), Bureau of Health Professions. 2007a. About NHSC. Available at: http://nhsc.bhpr.hrsa.gov/about/history.asp. Accessed December 2008.

Health Resources and Services Administration (HRSA), Bureau of Health Professions. 2007b.

Shortage designation. Available at: http://bhpr .hrsa.gov/shortage/. Accessed December 2008.

Health Resources and Services Administration (HRSA), Bureau of Health Professions. 2007c. Health professional shortage area primary medical care designation criteria. Available at: http ://bhpr.hrsa.gov/shortage/hpsacritpcm.htm. Accessed December 2008.

Health Resources and Services Administration (HRSA), Bureau of Primary Health Care. 2007a. Migrant health centers. Available at: http://bphc .hrsa.gov/migrant/. Accessed December 2008.

Health Resources and Services Administration (HRSA), Bureau of Primary Health Care. 2007b. America's health centers. Available at: http://bphc .hrsa.gov/chc/charts/healthcenters.htm. Accessed December 2008.

Health Resources and Services Administration (HRSA), Office of Rural Health Policy. 2007. Strategic plan 2005-2010. Available at: http://rural health.hrsa.gov/policy/StrategicPlan.asp. Accessed December 2008.

Herzog, D.B., and P.N. Copeland. 1985. Medical progress: Eating disorders. *New England Journal of Medicine* 313, no. 5: 295-303.

HHS Rural Task Force. 2002. Report to the Secretary: One department serving rural America. Available at: http://ruralhealth.hrsa.gov/PublicReport.htm #2001. Accessed December 2008.

Indian Health Service (IHS). 1999a. *A quick look*. Washington, DC: Public Health Service, September: 1.

Indian Health Service (IHS). 1999b. *Fact sheet: Comprehensive health care program for American Indians and Alaskan Natives*. Washington, DC: Public Health Service, October: 1.

Indian Health Service (IHS). 2010a. *Indian population. IHS fact sheet*. Washington, DC: Public Health Service. January 2010.

Indian Health Service (IHS). 2010b. *Indian health disparities. IHS fact sheet*. Washington, DC: Public Health Service. January 2010.

Indian Health Service (IHS). 2010c. *IHS year 2010 profile. IHS fact sheet*. Washington, DC: Public Health Service. January 2010.

Johnson, J.P., and P.E. Vink. 1992. Diagnosis and classification of HIV infection in children. In: *Management of HIV infection in infants and children*. R. Yogev and E. Connor, eds. St. Louis, MO: Mosby-Year Book. pp. 117-128.

Kaiser Commission on Medicaid and the Uninsured. 2006. *The uninsured: A primer*. Available at:

http://www.kff.org/uninsured/upload/7451-021 .pdf. Accessed December 2008.

Kaiser Commission on Medicaid and the Uninsured. 2010. *The uninsured and the difference health insurance makes*. Washington, DC: Kaiser Commission on Medicaid and the Uninsured. September 2010.

Kaiser Family Foundation. 2004. *Health care and the 2004 elections: Women's health policy*. Available at: http://www.kff.org/womenshealth/7184.cfm# repro. Accessed December 2008.

Kaiser Family Foundation. 2005. *Women and health care: A national profile*. Available at: http://www .kff.org/womenshealth/7336.cfm. Accessed December 2008.

Kaiser Family Foundation. 2007. *Fact sheet: The Ryan White Program*. Available at: http://www.kff.org /hivaids/upload/7582_03.pdf. Accessed December 2008.

Kaiser Family Foundation. 2008. *Medicaid and HIV/AIDS. HIV/AIDS policy fact sheet*. Washington, DC: Kaiser Family Foundation. February 2009.

Klerman, G.L., and M.M. Weissman. 1989. Increasing rate of depression. *Journal of the American Medical Association* 261, no. 24: 2229-2235.

Kozoll, R. 1986. Indian health care. In: *New dimensions in rural policy: Building upon our heritage*. Washington, DC: Government Printing Office. pp. 447-480.

Kraus, L.E. et al. 1996. *Chartbook on disability in the United States, 1996. An InfoUse Report*. Washington, DC: US National Institute on Disability and Rehabilitation Research.

Kuo, J., and K. Porter. 1998. *Health status of Asian Americans: United States, 1992-1994*. Advance data from vital and health statistics. Hyattsville, MD: National Center for Health Statistics. no. 298: 1-3.

Lam, N., and K. Liu. 1994. Spread of AIDS in rural America, 1982-1990. *Journal of Acquired Immune Deficiency Syndrome* 7, no. 5: 485-490.

Lurie, N. 1997. Studying access to care in managed care environment. *Health Services Research* 32: 691-701.

Merson, M.H. 1996. Returning home: Reflections on the USA's response to the HIV/AIDS epidemic. *Lancet* 347, no. 9016: 1673-1676.

Misra, D. ed. 2001. *Women's health data book: A profile of women's health in the United States*, 3rd ed. Washington, DC: Jacobs Institute of Women's Health and the Henry J. Kaiser Family Foundation.

Morrison, C. 1993. Delivery systems for the care of persons with HIV infection and AIDS. *Nursing Clinics of North America* 28, no. 2: 317-333.

Myers, J.K. et al. 1984. Six-month prevalence of psychiatric disorders in three communities. *Archives of General Psychiatry* 41, no. 10: 959–967.

National Association of Rural Health Clinics (NARHC). 2007. Available at: http://www.narhc.org/about_us/about_us.php. Accessed December 2008.

National Center for Chronic Disease Prevention and Health Promotion. 2005. *Chronic disease: Overview.* Available at: http://www.cdc.gov/nccdphp/overview.htm. Accessed December 2008.

National Center for Health Statistics. 2007. Deaths: Final data for 2007, table B, national vital statistics report. Hyattsville, MD: Department of Health and Human Services.

National Center for Health Statistics. 2009. Summary health statistics for U.S. adults: National health interview survey, 2009, tables 1, 2. Hyattsville, MD: Department of Health and Human Services.

National Center for Health Statistics. 2010. *Health, United States, 2009.* Hyattsville, MD: Department of Health and Human Services.

National Coalition for the Homeless. 2006a. *NCH fact sheet #2: How many people experience homelessness?* Available at: http://www.nationalhomeless.org/publications/facts/How_Many.pdf. Accessed December 2008.

National Coalition for the Homeless. 2006b. *NCH fact sheet #3: Who is homeless?* Available at: http://www.nationalhomeless.org/publications/facts/Whois.pdf. Accessed December 2008.

National Institute of Allergy and Infectious Diseases. 2006. *Fact sheet: HIV infection in women.* Available at: http://www.niaid.nih.gov/factsheets/womenhiv.htm. Accessed December 2008.

National Institute of Health (NIH). July 9, 2002. *News release: NHLBI stops trial of estrogen plus progestin due to increased breast cancer risk, lack of overall benefit.* Available at: http://www.nhlbi.nih.gov/new/press/02-07-09.htm. Accessed December 2006.

National Institute of Mental Health (NIMH). 2006a. *The numbers count.* Available at: http://www.nimh.nih.gov/publicat/numbers.cfm#Schizophrenia. Accessed December 2008.

National Institute of Mental Health (NIMH). 2006b. Total expenditures for the five most costly health conditions (1996, 2006). Available at: http://www.nimh.nih.gov/statistics/4TOT_MC9606.shtml. Accessed January 2011.

National Institute of Mental Health (NIMH). 2007. *Statistics.* Available at: http://www.nimh.nih.gov/healthinformation/statisticsmenu.cfm. Accessed December 2008.

National Institute of Mental Health (NIMH). 2008. Prevalence of serious mental illness among U.S. adults by sex, age, race in 2008. Available at: http://www.nimh.nih.gov/statistics/SMI_AASR.shtml. Accessed January 2011.

O'Hara, M.J., and D. D'Orlando. 1996. Ambulatory care of the HIV-infected child. *Nursing Clinics of America* 31, no. 1: 179–205.

Ostir, G.V. et al. 1999. Disability in older adults 1: Prevalence, causes, and consequences. *Behavioral Medicine* 24: 147–154.

Patton, L., and D. Puskin. 1990. *Ensuring access to health care services in rural areas: A half century of federal policy.* Essential Health Care Services Conference Center at Georgetown University Conference Center. Washington, DC.

Pell, J. et al. 1996. Management of HIV infected health care workers: Lessons from three cases. *British Medical Journal* 312, no. 7039: 1150–1152, discussion 1152–1153.

Pleasant, R. 2003. Minority health. In: *The Department of Health and Human Services: 50 years of service.* DHHS. pp. 92–95.

Regier, D.A. et al. 1988. One month prevalence of mental disorders in the United States: Based on five epidemiologic catchment area sites. *Archives of General Psychiatry* 45, no. 11: 977–986.

Rhodes, E.R. 1987. The organization of health services for Indian people. *Public Health Reports* 102, no. 4: 361–365.

Robertson, L.S. et al. 1974. *Changing the medical care system: A controlled experiment in comprehensive care.* New York: Praeger Publishers.

Romanoski, A.J. et al. 1992. The epidemiology of psychiatrist-ascertained depression and DSM-III depressive disorders: Results from the Eastern Baltimore Mental Health Survey Clinical Reappraisal. *Psychological Medicine* 22, no. 3: 629–655.

Rosenbaum, S., and J. Darnell. 1997. *An analysis of the Medicaid and health-related provisions of the Personal Responsibility and Work Opportunity Reconciliation Act of 1996 (P.L. 104–193).* Washington, DC: The Kaiser Commission on the Future of Medicaid.

Rumby, R.L. et al. 1991. AIDS in rural Eastern North Carolina. Patient migration: A rural AIDS burden. *AIDS* 5, no. 11: 1373–1378.

Salganicoff, A. et al. 2005. *Women and health care: A national profile.* Menlo Park, CA: The Henry J. Kaiser Family Foundation.

Schutt, R.K., and S.M. Goldfinger. 1996. Housing preferences and perceptions of health and functioning among homeless mentally ill persons. *Psychiatric Services* 47, no. 4: 381–386.

Sechzer, J.A. et al. 1996. Women and mental health. New York: *Academy of Sciences.*

Selike, R.M. et al. 1993. HIV infection as leading cause of death among young adults in US cities and states. *Journal of the American Medical Association* 269, no. 23: 2991-2994.

Shi, L., and G. Stevens. 2010. *Vulnerable Populations in the United States.* 2nd ed. San Francisco, CA: Jossey-Bass Publishers, Inc.

Shortell, S.M. et al. 1996. *Remaking health care in America.* San Francisco, CA: Jossey-Bass Publishers.

Solis, J.M. et al. 1990. Acculturation, access to care, and use of preventive services by Hispanics: Findings from HHANES 1982-84. *American Journal of Public Health* 80 (Suppl): 11-19.

Stratton, T. et al. 1993. *A demographic analysis of nurse shortage counties: Implications for rural nursing policy.* Grand Forks, ND: University of North Dakota Rural Health Research Center.

Substance Abuse and Mental Health Services Administration. 2010. Results from the 2009 National Survey on Drug Use and Health: Mental Health Findings. Rockville, MD: Office of Applied Studies, NSDUH Series H-39, HHS Publication No. SMA 10-4609.

Summer, L. 1991. *Limited access: Health care for the rural poor.* Washington, DC: Center on Budget and Policy Priorities.

The Robert Wood Johnson Foundation. 1996. *Chronic care in America: A 21st century challenge.* Available at: http://www.rwjf.org/files/publications/other/ChronicCareinAmerica.pdf?gsa=1.[O1] Accessed December 2000.

United Nations (UN). 2007. *The state of the world's children 2007.* Available at: http://www.unicef.org/sowc07/docs/sowc07.pdf[O2]. Accessed December 2008.

UNAIDS. 2010. UNAIDS report on the global AIDS epidemic 2010. Available at: http://www.unaids.org/globalreport/Global_report.htm. Accessed December 2010).

US Census Bureau. 2007. *Statistical abstract of the United States, 2007: The National Data Book.* Washington, DC: Government Printing Office.

US Census Bureau. 2009. *The 2010 census questionnaire: Informational copy.* Available at: http://2010.census.gov/2010census/pdf/2010_Questionnaire_Info_Copy.pdf. Accessed April 2009.

US Census Bureau. 2010. *Statistical abstract of the United States, 2010.* Washington, DC: Government Printing Office.

US Department of Veteran Affairs. 2006. *Fact sheet: VA programs for homeless veterans.* Available at: http://www1.va.gov/opa/fact/hmlssfs.asp. Accessed December 2008.

Weissman, M.M., and G.L. Klerman. 1977. Sex differences and the epidemiology of depression. *Archives of General Psychiatry* 34, no. 1: 98-111.

Wenzel, M. 1996. A school-based clinic for elementary school in Phoenix, Arizona. *Journal of School Health* 66, no. 4: 125-127.

Williams, S.J. 1995. *Essentials of health services.* Albany, NY: Delmar Publishers.

World Health Organization (WHO). 2004. *Women and AIDS: Have you heard us today?* Available at: http://www.who.int/features/2004/aids/en/. Accessed December 2008.

Yoon, E., and F. Chien. 1996. Asian American and Pacific Islander health: A paradigm for minority health. *Journal of the American Medical Association* 275, no. 9: 736-737.

Yu, S.M. et al. 2004. Health status and health services utilization among US Chinese, Asian Indian, Filipino, and other Asian/Pacific Islander children. *Pediatrics* 113, no. 1 part 1: 101-107.

CHAPTER 25

Introduction to Ethics

George D. Pozgar

CHAPTER OBJECTIVES

1. Apply basic ethical concepts to advanced nursing practice.

2. Discuss important historical events that have influenced biomedical ethics.

3. Develop an understanding of relevant ethical theories and principles, person values and beliefs, and the concepts of morality that provide a framework for advanced nursing practice.

4. Apply the concept of situational ethics to the practice of advanced nursing.

5. Trace the historical developments of the code of ethics for nursing.

6. Apply ethical theories specific to health care to the role of the advanced practice nurse.

INTRODUCTION

This chapter provides the reader with an overview of ethics and moral principles. *Ethics* and *morals* are derivatives from the Greek and Latin terms (roots) for custom. The intent here is not to burden the reader with the philosophy and arguments surrounding ethical theories, morality, principles, virtues, and values. However, as with the study of any new subject, words are the tools of thought. Therefore, some new vocabulary will be presented to the reader to apply the abstract theories and principles of ethics. One needs to understand the words and the concepts to make practical use of them.

Ethical dilemmas arise when values, rights, duties, and loyalties conflict, and consequently not everyone is satisfied with a particular decision. An understanding of the concepts presented here will help to reduce conflict when addressing ethical dilemmas and making difficult decisions.

ETHICS

> How we perceive right and wrong is influenced by what we feed on.
>
> —*Author Unknown*

Ethics, also referred to as moral philosophy, is the discipline concerned with what is morally good and bad, right and wrong. This term is also applied to any theoretical system of moral values or principles. Ethics is less concerned with factual knowledge than with virtues and values—namely, human conduct as it ought to be, rather than as it actually is.

Ethics is the branch of philosophy that seeks to understand the nature, purposes, justification, and founding principles of moral rules and the systems they comprise. Ethics deals with values relating to human conduct. It focuses on the rightness and wrongness of actions as well as the goodness and badness of motives and ends. Ethics encompasses the decision-making process of determining ultimate actions. It involves how individuals decide to live within accepted and desirable principles and how they live in harmony with the environment and one another.

Microethics involves an individual's view of what is right and wrong based on personal life experiences. Macroethics involves a more global view of right and wrong. Although no person lives in a vacuum, solving ethical dilemmas involves consideration of ethical issues from both a micro and macro ethical perspective.

The term "ethics" is used in three different but related ways, signifying (1) a general pattern or way of life, such as religious ethics (e.g., Judeo-Christian ethics); (2) a set of rules of conduct or moral code, which involves professional ethics and ethical behavior; and (3) philosophi-

cal ethics, which involves inquiry about ways of life and rules of conduct.

The scope of healthcare ethics encompasses numerous issues, including the right to choose or refuse treatment and the right to limit the suffering one will endure. Incredible advances in technology and the resulting capability to extend life beyond what would be considered a reasonable quality of life have complicated the process of healthcare decision making. The scope of healthcare ethics is not limited to philosophical issues but embraces economic, medical, political, social, and legal dilemmas as well.

Bioethics addresses such difficult issues as the nature of life, the nature of death, what sort of life is worth living, what constitutes murder, how we should treat people who are in especially vulnerable and painful circumstances, and the responsibilities we have to other human beings. The following events are some of many that have had a significant impact on healthcare ethics.

1932–1972: Tuskegee Study of Syphilis

The purpose of the Tuskegee study, involving African American men, was to analyze the natural progression of untreated syphilis. The study was conducted from 1932 through the early 1970s. The participants were not warned during the study that there was a cure for syphilis (i.e., penicillin). They believed that they were receiving adequate care and unknowingly suffered unnecessarily. The Tuskegee syphilis study used disadvantaged, rural black men to investigate the untreated course of a disease, one that is by no means confined to that population. We know now that the selection of research subjects must be closely monitored to ensure that specific classes of individuals (e.g., terminally ill patients, welfare patients, racial and ethnic minorities, or persons confined to institutions) are not selected for research studies because of their easy availability, compromised position, or manipulability. Rather, they must be selected for reasons directly related to the research being conducted.

1946: Military Tribunal for War Crimes

In 1946, a military tribunal began criminal proceedings against 23 German physicians and administrators for war crimes and crimes against humanity. As a direct result of these proceedings, the Nuremberg code was established, which made it clear that the voluntary and informed consent of human subjects is essential to research, and that benefits of research must outweigh risks to human subjects involved (Eastern Michigan University, n.d.).

1949: Nuremberg Trials: International Code of Medical Ethics

This code was adopted following numerous experiments conducted by the Nazis on prisoners in concentration camps. Prisoners were exposed to cholera, diphtheria, malaria, mustard gas, yellow fever, typhus, and other horrendous experiments, ultimately claiming thousands of lives. This exploitation of unwilling prisoners as research subjects in Nazi concentration camps was condemned as a particularly flagrant injustice.

1954: First Kidney Transplant

The National Institutes of Health published guidelines on human experimentation. The transplantation of human organs has generated numerous ethical issues (e.g., the harvesting and selling of organs, who should have first access to freely donated human organs, and how death is defined) (A science odyssey, 1998).

1960s: Cardiopulmonary Resuscitation

Prolonging life beyond what reasonably would be expected has generated numerous ongoing ethical dilemmas. Should limited resources, for example, be spent on those who have been determined to be in a comatose vegetative state with no hope of recovery? Or should limited resources be spent on preventive medicine that would improve the quality of life for all?

1964: World Medical Association

In 1964, the World Medical Association established guidelines for medical doctors doing biomedical research involving human subjects. The Declaration of Helsinki is the basis for good clinical practices today (Eastern Michigan University, n.d.).

1968: Harvard Medical School Report on Brain Death Criteria

How does one determine when brain death occurs? In 1968, the Harvard Ad Hoc Committee on Brain Death published a report describing the following characteristics of a permanently nonfunctioning brain, a condition it referred to as "irreversible coma," now known as brain death:

1. Patient shows total unawareness to external stimuli and unresponsiveness to painful stimuli.

2. No movements or breathing: All spontaneous muscular movement, spontaneous respiration, and response to stimuli are absent.

3. No reflexes; fixed, dilated pupils; no eye movement even when hit or turned, or when ice water is placed in the ear; no response to noxious stimuli; no tendon reflexes.

In addition to these criteria, a flat electroencephalogram was recommended as a marker of brain death (Harvard Ad Hoc Committee, 1968).

1970: Paternalism Questioned

As physicians are faced with many options for saving lives, transplanting organs, and furthering research, they also must wrestle with new and troubling choices—for example, who should receive scarce and vital treatment, how to determine when life ends, and what limits should be placed on care for the dying.

1971: Kennedy Institute of Ethics at Georgetown University

In 1971, the Joseph P. and Rose F. Kennedy Institute of Ethics was founded at Georgetown University and became the first academic bioethics center in the world. The Institute provides a comprehensive resource for academicians, ethicists, policy makers, and the general public through its library, programs, and publications. The library can be accessed through its website at http://bioethics.georgetown.edu/databases/.

In addition, it is the home to ethical scholars who lecture at conferences, seminars, symposia, and special programs worldwide. They also serve as consultants on government commissions or committees and testify at government hearings on a wide range of ethical issues. Emerging areas of research and study include racial and gender equality, international justice and peace, and other issues affecting vulnerable populations (Kennedy Institute of Ethics, 2007).

1972: Informed Consent

The case of *Canterbury v. Spence* (1972), set the "reasonable man" standard requiring informed consent for treatment. Patients must be informed of the risks, benefits, and alternatives associated with recommended treatments.

1974: National Research Act

Due to publicity from the Tuskegee Syphilis Study, the National Research Act of 1974 was passed. This act created the National Commission for the Protection of Human Subjects of Biomedical and Behavioral Research. One of the commission's charges was to identify the basic ethical principles that should underlie the conduct of biomedical and behavioral research involving human subjects and to develop guidelines to ensure that such research is conducted in accordance with those principles (*Belmont Report,* 2004).

The commission was directed to consider:

■ The boundaries between biomedical and behavioral research and the accepted and routine practice of medicine

■ The role of assessment of risk–benefit criteria in determining the appropriateness of research involving human subjects

■ Appropriate guidelines for the selection of human subjects for participation in such research

■ The nature and definition of informed consent in various research settings (National Institutes of Health, 1979)

The Food and Drug Administration and the National Institutes of Health internal policy guidelines became federal regulation. As a result of the National Research Act, the National Commission for the Protection of Human Subjects in Biomedical and Behavioral Research was established.

1976: Substituted Judgment

In *In the Matter of Karen Ann Quinlan* (1976), the Supreme Court rendered a unanimous decision providing for the appointment of Joseph Quinlan as personal guardian of his daughter Karen, with full power to make decisions regarding the identity of her treating physicians. Upon the concurrence of the guardian and family, if Karen's physicians concluded that there was no reasonable possibility of her emerging from her comatose condition to a cognitive, sapient state and that her life support apparatus should be withdrawn, they were to consult with the ethics committee of the institution where Karen was then hospitalized. If that consultative body concurred in the prognosis, the life support system could be withdrawn without any civil or criminal liability on the part of any participant, whether it be the guardian, physician, hospital, or others. In addressing itself to the question of possible homicide, the court concluded that there is a valid distinction between withdrawing life support systems in cases such as Karen's and the infliction of deadly harm either on oneself or another person. It saw a difference between Karen's situation and the unlawful killing that is condemned in statutory law. The court denied that the death following withdrawal of treatment would be homicidal. Rather, it would be the result of previously existing natural causes, not from the withdrawal of treatment; and, even if it were considered homicide, it could not be unlawful if done pursuant to the exercise of an explicitly recognized constitutional right.

1978: Establishment of the President's Commission for Study of Ethical Problems in Medicine

The duties of the commission include conducting studies of the ethical and legal implications of the requirements for informed consent to participate in research projects and to otherwise undergo medical procedures; the matter of defining death, including the advisability of developing a uniform definition of death; voluntary testing, counseling, and information and education programs with respect to genetic diseases and conditions, taking into account the essential equality of all human beings, born and unborn; the differences in the availability of health services as determined by the income or residence of the persons receiving the services; current procedures and mechanisms designed to safeguard the privacy of human subjects of behavioral and biomedical research, to ensure the confidentiality of individually identifiable patient records, and to ensure appropriate access of patients to information; and such other matters relating to medicine or biomedical or behavioral research as the president may designate for study by the commission (42 U.S. Code 6A [XVI]).

1990: Physician-Assisted Suicide

Jack Kevorkian, a physician, assisted terminally ill patients in suicide outside the boundaries of the law.

1990: Patient Self-Determination Act

The Patient Self-Determination Act of 1990 was enacted to ensure that patients are informed of their rights to execute advance directives and accept or refuse medical care.

1994: Oregon's Death with Dignity Act

Physician-assisted suicide became a legal medical option for terminally ill Oregonians. The Oregon Death with Dignity Act allows terminally ill Oregon residents to obtain from their physicians and use prescriptions for self-administered, lethal medications.

1996: Health Insurance Portability and Accountability Act

The Health Insurance Portability and Accountability Act of 1996 (Public Law 104-191) was designed to protect the privacy, confidentiality, and security of patient information.

2001: President's Council on Bioethics

The President's Council on Bioethics was created by President George W. Bush in 2001. The council was charged with advising the president on bioethical issues that may emerge as a consequence of advances in biomedical science and technology (President's Council on Bioethics, n.d.).

2003: Human Genome System Became Fully Sequenced

The Human Genome Project, sponsored by the National Institutes of Health, completed the sequencing of the full human genome sequence in April 2003. The next phase in the project is research aimed at improving human health and fighting disease (National Human Genome Research Institute, 2007). The expectation is that genetic and medical research will accelerate at an unprecedented rate with ethical implications and dilemmas arising such as cloning, stem cell transplants, and others.

ETHICAL THEORIES

> Ethics, too, are nothing but reverence for life. This is what gives me the fundamental principle of morality, namely, that good consists in maintaining, promoting, and enhancing life, and that destroying, injuring, and limiting life are evil.
>
> —*Albert Schweitzer (Schweitzer, 1949)*

Ethics seeks to understand and to determine how human actions can be judged as right or wrong. Ethical judgments can be made based upon our own experiences or based upon the nature of or principles of reason. Those who study ethics believe that ethical decision making is based upon theory. Ethical theories attempt to introduce order into the way people think about life and action. The following paragraphs provide a review of the more commonly discussed ethical theories.

Normative Ethics

Normative ethics is the attempt to determine which moral standards should be followed so that human behavior and conduct may be morally right. Normative ethics is primarily concerned with establishing standards or norms for conduct and is commonly associated with general theories about how one ought to live. One of the central questions of modern normative ethics is whether human actions are to be judged right or wrong solely according to their consequences.

General normative ethics is the critical study of major moral precepts of such matters as which things are right, which things are good, and which things are genuine. General normative ethics is the determination of correct moral principles for all autonomous rational beings.

Applied ethics is the application of normative theories to practical moral problems. It attempts to explain and justify specific moral problems such as abortion, euthanasia, and assisted suicide.

Consequential or Teleological Ethics

The consequential or teleological ethics theory emphasizes that the morally right action is whichever action leads to the maximum balance of good over evil. From a contemporary standpoint, theories that judge actions by their consequences have been referred to as consequentialism. Consequential ethics theories revolve around the premise that the rightness or wrongness of an action depends upon the consequences or effects of an action. The theory of consequentialism is based on the view that the

value of an action derives solely from the value of its consequences. The goal of a consequentialist is to achieve the greatest good for the greatest number. It involves asking:

- What will be the effects of each course of action?
- Will they be positive or negative?
- For whom?
- What will do the least harm?

Nonconsequential Ethics

The nonconsequential ethics theory denies that the consequences of an action or rule are the only criteria for determining the morality of an action or rule. In this theory, the rightness or wrongness of an action is based on properties intrinsic to the action, not on its consequences.

Deontological Ethics

Deontological theory focuses on one's duties to others. It includes telling the truth and keeping one's promises. Deontology involves ethical analysis according to a moral code or rules, religious or secular, as presented next.

Religious Ethics

The Great Physician

Dear Lord, You are the Great Physician, I turn to you in my sickness asking for your help.

I place myself under your loving care, praying that I may know your healing grace and wholeness.

Help me to find love in this strange world and to feel your presence by my bed both day and night.

Give my doctors and nurses wisdom that they may understand my illness.

Steady and guide them with your strong hand.

Reach out your hand to me and touch my life with your peace. Amen.

—*University of Pennsylvania Health System*

Religious ethics, as it relates to character and morality, varies from person to person based on one's religious beliefs. Religious beliefs are heavily influenced by the family within which one is born. The more dogmatic the belief, the more likely one will adopt the family's religious beliefs and values.

Often one's religious beliefs can change as circumstances change. What is troublesome to one individual may not be to another person. One's need to survive can change his or her moral character. The extent to which one will adapt to survive can take on the extremes of who we really are and how far we will go to survive.

Religious codes of ethics are based on a particular religion. Biblical ethics, for example, is God centered. Judaism is based on Old Testament scriptures. Christianity is based on both Old and New Testament scriptures. The notion of right and wrong is not so much an object of philosophical inquiry as an acceptance of divine revelation. Moses, for example, received a list of 10 laws directly from God. These laws are known as the Ten Commandments. Some of the commandments are related to the basic principles of justice that have been adhered to by society since they were first proclaimed and published. For some societies, the Ten Commandments were a turning point where essential commands such as "Thou shalt not kill" or "Thou shalt not commit adultery" were accepted as law.

The Ten Commandments

1. I am the Lord thy God, which have brought thee out of the land of Egypt, out of the house of bondage. Thou shalt have no other gods before me.
2. Thou shalt not make unto thee any graven image, or any likeness of anything that is in heaven above, or that is in the earth beneath, or that is in the water under the earth. Thou shalt not bow down thyself to them, nor serve them.
3. Thou shalt not take the name of the Lord thy God in vain.
4. Remember the Sabbath day, to keep it holy.
5. Honor thy father and thy mother: that thy days may be long.
6. Thou shalt not kill.
7. Thou shalt not commit adultery.
8. Thou shalt not steal.
9. Thou shalt not bear false witness against thy neighbor.
10. Thou shalt not covet thy neighbor's house, thou shalt not covet thy neighbor's wife, nor his manservant, nor his maidservant, nor his ox, nor his ass, nor anything that is thy neighbor's.

Spirituality in the religious sense implies that there is purpose and meaning to life; spirituality generally refers to faith in a higher being. For a patient, injury and sickness are frightening experiences. This fear is often heightened when the patient is admitted to a healthcare facility. Healthcare organizations can help reduce patient fears by making available to them appropriate emotional and spiritual support and coping resources. It is a well-proven fact that patients who are able to draw upon their spirituality and religious beliefs tend to have a more comfortable and often improved healing experience. To assist both patients and caregivers in addressing spiritual needs, patients should be provided with information as to how their spiritual needs can be addressed.

Difficult questions regarding a patient's spiritual needs and how to meet those needs are best addressed upon admission by first collecting information about the patient's religious or spiritual preferences. Caregivers often find it difficult to discuss spiritual issues for fear of offending a patient who may have beliefs different from their own. If caregivers know from admission records a patient's religious beliefs, the caregiver can share with the patient those religious and spiritual resources available in the hospital and community.

Secular Ethics

Unlike religious ethics, secular ethics are based on codes developed by societies that have relied on customs to formulate their codes. The Code of Hammurabi, for example, carved on a black

Babylonian column, 8 feet high, now located in the Louvre in Paris, depicts a mythical sun god presenting a code of laws to Hammurabi, a great military leader and ruler of Babylon (1795–1750 BC). Hammurabi's code of laws is an early example of a ruler proclaiming to his people an entire body of laws. The following excerpts are from the Code of Hammurabi.

Code of Hammurabi

5

If a judge try a case, reach a decision, and present his judgment in writing; if later error shall appear in his decision, and it be through his own fault, then he shall pay twelve times the fine set by him in the case, and he shall be publicly removed from the judge's bench, and never again shall he sit there to render judgment.

194

If a man give his child to a nurse and the child die in her hands, but the nurse unbeknown to the father and mother nurse another child, then they shall convict her of having nursed another child without the knowledge of the father and mother and her breasts shall be cut off.

215

If a physician make a large incision with an operating knife and cure it, or if he open a tumor (over the eye) with an operating knife, and saves the eye, he shall receive ten shekels in money.

217

If he be the slave of some one, his owner shall give the physician two shekels.

218

If a physician make a large incision with the operating knife, and kill him, or open a tumor with the operating knife, and cut out the eye, his hands shall be cut off.

219

If a physician make a large incision in the slave of a freed man, and kill him, he shall replace the slave with another slave.

221

If a physician heal the broken bone or diseased soft part of a man, the patient shall pay the physician five shekels in money.

PRINCIPLES OF HEALTHCARE ETHICS

> You cannot by tying an opinion to a man's tongue, make him the representative of that opinion; and at the close of any battle for principles, his name will be found neither among the dead, nor the wounded, but the missing.
> —*E. P. Whipple (1819–1886),*
> *American Essayist*

Ethical principles are universal rules of conduct that identify which kinds of actions, intentions, and motives are valued. Ethical principles core to the ethical practice of medicine are discussed next. These principles assist caregivers in making choices based on moral principles that have been identified as standards considered worthwhile in addressing healthcare-related ethical dilemmas. Ethical principles provide a generalized framework within which particular ethical dilemmas can be analyzed. Caregivers, in the study of ethics, will find that difficult decisions often involve choices between conflicting ethical principles.

Autonomy

> . . . no right is held more sacred, or is more carefully guarded, by the common law, than the right of every individual to the possession and control of his own person.
> —*Union Pacific Ry. Co. v. Botsford (1891)*

The principle of *autonomy* involves recognizing the right of a person to make one's own decisions. *Auto* comes from a Greek word meaning "self" or "the individual." In this context, it means recognizing an individual's right to make his or her own decisions about what is best for himself or herself. Autonomy is not an absolute principle. The autonomous actions of one person must not infringe upon the rights of another.

Respect for autonomy has been recognized in the 14th Amendment to the Constitution of the United States. The law upholds an individual's right to make his or her own decisions about health care. A patient has the right to refuse to receive health care even if such care would be beneficial in saving his or her life. Patients can refuse treatment, refuse to take medications, refuse blood or blood by-products, and refuse invasive procedures regardless of the benefits that may be derived from them. They have a right to have their decisions followed by family members who may disagree simply because they are unable to let go.

What has been mandated by law has been reflected in bioethical thinking. Although patients have a right to make their own decisions, they also have a concomitant right to know the risks, benefits, and alternatives to recommended procedures.

When analyzing an ethical dilemma, caregivers must consider how autonomy and the respect for a patient's wishes affect the caregivers' decision-making processes. Is, for example, the patient's right to self-determination being compromised because of a third party's wishes for the patient?

The caregiver respects the mentally competent decision-making capabilities of autonomous persons and that right of an individual to make his or her own decisions. The eminent Justice Cardozo, in *Schloendorff v. Society of New York Hospital* (1914), stated:

> Every human being of adult years and sound mind has a right to determine what shall be done with his own body and a surgeon who performs an operation without his patient's consent commits an assault, for which he is liable in damages, except in cases of emergency where the patient is unconscious and where it is necessary to operate before consent can be obtained.

What happens when the right to autonomy conflicts with other moral principles, such as beneficence and justice? Conflict can arise, for example, when a patient refuses a blood transfusion considered necessary to save his or her life while the caregiver's principal obligation is to do no harm.

Autonomous decision making can be affected by one's disabilities, mental status, maturity, or incapacity to make decisions. Although the principle of autonomy may be inapplicable in certain cases, a person's autonomous wishes may be carried out through an advance directive and/or an appointed healthcare agent in the event of one's inability to make decisions.

Beneficence

Beneficence describes the principle of doing good, demonstrating kindness, showing compassion, and helping others. In the healthcare setting, caregivers demonstrate beneficence by providing benefits and balancing benefits against risks. Beneficence requires one to do good. Doing good requires knowledge of the beliefs, culture, values, and preferences of the patient—what one person may believe to be good for a patient may, in reality, be harmful. For example, a caregiver may decide that a patient should be told frankly, "There is nothing else that I can do for you." This could be injurious to the patient if the patient really wants encouragement and information about care options from the caregiver. Compassion here requires the caregiver to tell the patient, "I am not aware of new treatments for your illness; however, I have some ideas about how I can help treat your symptoms and make you more comfortable. In addition, I will keep you informed as to any significant research that may be helpful in treating your disease processes."

Paternalism is a form of beneficence. People, often believing that they know what is best for another, often make decisions that they believe are in another person's best interest. Such decisions may involve, for example, withholding information from someone, believing that the person would be better off that way. Paternalism can occur due to one's age, cognitive ability, and level of dependency.

Medical paternalism involves making choices for (or forcing choices on) patients who are capable of choosing for themselves. This directly violates patient autonomy. Physicians are often in situations where they can influence a patient's healthcare decision simply by selectively telling the patient what he or she prefers based on personal beliefs. The problem of paternalism involves a conflict between principles of autonomy and beneficence, each of which is conceived by different parties as the overriding principle in cases of conflict. Conflict between the demands of beneficence and autonomy underlies a broad range of controversies.

Nonmaleficence

Nonmaleficence is an ethical principle that requires caregivers to avoid causing patients harm. Nonmaleficence is not concerned with improving others' well-being but rather with avoiding the infliction of harm. Medical ethics requires healthcare providers to "first, do no harm." In *In re Conroy*, 464 A.2d 303, 314 (N.J.. Super. Ct. App. Div. 1983), the court stated that "the physician's primary obligation is . . . First do no harm." Telling the truth, for example, can sometimes cause harm. If there is no cure for a patient's disease, a healthcare provider may have a dilemma. Should he or she tell the patient and possibly cause serious psychological harm, or should the physician give the patient what he or she considers false hope? Is there a middle ground? If so, what is it? To avoid causing harm, alternatives may need to be considered in solving the ethical dilemma.

The caregiver, realizing that he or she cannot help a particular patient, attempts to avoid harming the patient. This is done as a caution against taking a serious risk with the patient, or doing something that has no immediate or long-term benefits.

The principle of nonmaleficence is broken when a physician is placed in the position of ending life by removing respirators, giving lethal injections, or writing prescriptions for lethal doses of medication. Helping patients die violates the physician's duty to save lives. In the final analysis, there needs to be a distinction between killing patients and letting them die.

Justice

Justice is the obligation to be fair in the distribution of benefits and risks. Justice demands that persons in similar circumstances be treated similarly. A person is treated justly when he or she receives what is due, is deserved, or can legitimately be claimed. Justice involves how people are treated when their interests compete with one another.

Distributive justice is a principle requiring that all persons be treated equally and fairly. No one person, for example, should get a disproportional share of society's resources or benefits. There are many ethical issues involved in the rationing of health care. This is often due to limited or scarce resources, limited access due to geographic remoteness, or a patient's inability to pay for services combined with many physicians who are unwilling to accept patients who are perceived as "no pays" with high risks for legal suits.

Justice and Government Spending

Scarce resources are challenging to the principles of justice. Justice involves equality. Yet equal access to health care, for example, across the United States does not exist. How do you think the government should spend $1 trillion? With 45 million Americans without healthcare insurance, describe the value of the one-time $300–$600 per household giveback from the United States Treasury delivered under the George W. Bush administration. Consider the following questions:

- Should the money have been distributed equally among families?
- Should the money have been distributed equally among all citizens?
- Should the money have been invested and saved for a rainy day?
- Should the money have been used to improve educational programs, build libraries, build state-of-the-art hospitals, or fund after-school programs for disadvantaged youths?
- Should the money have included both savings for that rainy day and funding for the programs described above?
- What would have been the greater good for all?

Injustice for the Insured

> Even if you're insured, getting ill could bankrupt you. Hospitals are garnishing wages, putting liens on homes and having patients who can't pay arrested. It's enough to make you sick.
>
> —*Sara Austin*

Hospitals are receiving between $4 million and $60 million annually in charity funds in New York alone, according to Elizabeth Benjamin, director of the health law unit of the Legal Aid Society of New York City. However, even the insured face injustice. In 2003, almost 1 million Americans declared bankruptcy because of medical issues, accounting for nearly half of all of the bankruptcies in the country. When an insured patient gets ill and exhausts his or her insurance benefits, should the hospital be able to:

- Garnish the patient's wages?
- Place liens on homes?
- Arrest patients who cannot pay?
- Block patients from applying for the hundreds of millions of dollars in government funds designated to help pay for care for those who need it?

Age and Justice

- Should an 89-year-old patient get a heart transplant because he or she is higher on the waiting list to receive a heart transplant than a 10-year-old girl?
- Should a 39-year-old single patient get a heart transplant because he or she is higher on the waiting list to receive a heart transplant than a 10-year-old boy?
- Should a 29-year-old mother of three get a heart transplant because she is higher on the waiting list to receive a heart transplant than a 10-year-old girl?
- Should a 29-year-old pregnant mother with two children get a heart transplant because she is higher on the waiting list to receive a heart transplant than a 10-year-old boy?

Emergency Care

When two patients arrive in the emergency department in critical condition, consider who should get treated first. Should the caregiver base his or her decision on the

- First patient who arrives?
- Age of the patients?
- Likelihood of survival?
- Ability of the patient to pay for services rendered?
- Condition of the patient?

Patients are to be treated justly, fairly, and equally. But what happens when resources are scarce and only one patient can be treated at a time? What happens if caregivers decide that age should be the determining factor as to who is treated first? One patient is saved and another dies. What happens if the patient saved is terminal and has an advance directive in his wallet requesting that no heroic measures be taken to save his life? What are the legal issues intertwined with the ethical issues in this case?

Justice describes how people are treated when their interests compete. Distributive justice implies that all are treated fairly; no one person is to get a disproportional share of society's resources or benefits. This principle raises numerous issues, including how limited resources should be allocated.

When there is a reduction in staff, managers are generally asked to eliminate nonessential personnel. In the healthcare industry, this translates to those individuals who are not directly involved in patient care (e.g., environmental services employees). Is this fair? Is this justice? Is this the right thing to do?

MORALITY

> Aim above morality. Be not simply good; be good for something.
>
> —*Henry David Thoreau*

Morality implies the quality of being in accord with standards of right and good conduct. Morals are deeply ingrained into a culture or religion and are often part of its identity. Morals are ideas about what is right and what is wrong; as examples, killing is wrong, helping the poor is right, easing pain is right, and causing pain is wrong. Morals should not be confused with cultural habits or customs, such as wearing a certain style of clothing. Morality is a code of conduct. It is a guide to behavior that all rational persons would put forward for governing their behavior.

It is important to examine not only what one considers the right thing to do in a given situation, but also why it is the right thing to do. Being morally responsible requires that a person look inward and question his or her own values.

Morality describes a class of rules held by society to govern the conduct of its individual members. A moral dilemma occurs when moral ideas of right and wrong conflict.

Moral judgments are those judgments concerned with what an individual or group believes to be the right or proper behavior in a given situation. It involves assessing another person's moral character based on how he or she conforms to the moral convictions established by the individual and/or group. Lack of conformity typically results in moral censure, condemnation, and possibly derision of the violator's character. What is considered right varies from nation to nation, from culture to culture, from religion to religion, and from person to person. There is no universal morality.

When it is important that disagreements be settled, morality is often legislated. Law is distinguished from morality by having explicit rules and penalties and officials who interpret the laws and apply the penalties. There is often considerable overlap in the conduct governed by morality and that governed by law. Laws are created to set boundaries for societal behavior. They are enforced to ensure that the expected behavior happens (Morality, 2005).

VIRTUES AND MORAL VALUES

The term *virtue* is normally defined as some sort of moral excellence or beneficial quality. In tra-

ditional ethics, virtues are those characteristics that differentiate good people from bad people. Virtues, such as honesty and justice, are abstract moral principles. Properly understood, virtues serve as indispensable guides to our actions. However, they are not ends in themselves. Virtues are merely abstract means to concrete ends. The ends are values—the things in life that we aim to gain or keep. Most individuals have a tendency to focus on values and not virtues. Simply stated, most individuals find it difficult to make the connection between abstract principles (virtues) and that which has value. The relationship between means and ends, principles (virtues) and practice (values) is often difficult to grasp.

A moral value is the relative worth placed on some virtuous behavior. What has value to one person may not have value to another. A value is a standard of conduct. Values are used for judging the goodness or badness of some action. Ethical values imply standards of worth. They are the standards by which we measure the goodness in our lives. Intrinsic value is something that has value in and of itself. Instrumental value is something that helps to give value to something else (e.g., money is valuable for what it can buy).

Values may change as needs change. If one's basic needs for food, water, clothing, and housing have not been met, one's values may change such that a friendship, for example, might be sacrificed if one's basic needs can be better met as a result of the sacrifice. If a mother's estate is being squandered at the end of her life, a financially well-off family member may want to take more aggressive measures to keep the mother alive despite the financial drain on her estate. Another family member who is struggling financially may more readily see the futility of expensive medical care and find it easier to let go. Values give purpose to each life. They make up one's moral character.

All people make value judgments and make choices among alternatives. The values one so dearly proclaims may change as needs change.

Values are the motivating power of a person's actions and are necessary to survival, both psychologically and physically.

We begin our discussion here with an overview of those virtues commonly accepted as having value when addressing difficult healthcare dilemmas. The reader should not get overly caught up in the philosophical morass of how virtues and values differ, but should be aware that virtues and values have been used by many interchangeably. Whether we call compassion a virtue or a value, or both, the importance for our purposes in this text is to understand what compassion is and how it is applied in the healthcare setting.

Commitment

> I know the price of success: dedication, hard work, and an unremitting devotion to the things you want to see happen.
> —*Frank Lloyd Wright*

Commitment is the act of binding oneself (intellectually or emotionally) to a course of action. It is an agreement or pledge to do something. It can be ongoing or a pledge to do something in the future.

Compassion

> Compassion is the basis of morality.
> —*Arnold Schopenhauer*

Compassion in the healthcare setting means a deep awareness of and sympathy for another's suffering. The ability to show compassion is a true mark of moral character. There are those who argue that compassion will blur one's judgment. Detachment, or lack of concern for the patient's needs, however, is what often translates into mistakes that often result in patient injuries. Caregivers need to show the same compassion for others as they would expect for themselves or their loved ones. Those who have excessive emotional involvement in a patient's care may be best suited to work in those settings where patients are most likely to recover and have good outcomes (e.g., maternity units). As with all things in life, there needs to be a comfortable balance between compassion and detachment.

> Never apologize for showing feeling. When you do so, you apologize for the truth.
> —*Benjamin Disraeli*

Conscientiousness

A conscientious person is one who has moral integrity and a strict regard for doing what is considered the right thing to do. An individual acts conscientiously if he or she is motivated to do what is right, believing it is the right thing to do. Conscience is a form of self-reflection on and judgment about whether one's actions are right or wrong, good or bad. It is an internal sanction that comes into play through critical reflection. This sanction often appears as a bad conscience in the form of painful feelings of remorse, guilt, shame, disunity, or harmony as the individual recognizes that his or her acts were wrong. Although a person may conscientiously object and/or refuse to participate in some action (e.g., abortion), that person must not obstruct others from performing the same act if the others have no moral objection to it.

Cooperativeness

Cooperativeness is the willingness and ability to work with others. In the healthcare setting, it is important that caregivers work cooperatively as a team.

Courage

> Courage is the greatest of all virtues, because if you haven't courage, you may not have an opportunity to use any of the others.
> —*Samuel Johnson*

Courage is the mental or moral strength to persevere and withstand danger. "Courage is the ladder on which all the other virtues mount" (Luce, 1979).

Discernment

> Get to know two things about a man—how he earns his money and how he spends it—and you have the clue to his character, for you

have a searchlight that shows up the innermost recesses of his soul. You know all you need to know about his standards, his motives, his driving desires, and his real religion.

—*Robert J. McCracken*

The virtue of discernment is the ability to make a good decision without personal biases, fears, and undue influences from others. A person who has discernment has the wisdom to decide the best course of action when there are many possible actions to choose from.

Fairness

Do all the good you can, By all the means you can, In all the ways you can, In all the places you can, At all the times you can, To all the people you can, As long as you ever can.

—*John Wesley (1703–1791),*
Evangelist and Founder of Methodism²

In ethics, fairness means being objective, unbiased, dispassionate, impartial, and consistent with the principles of ethics. Fairness is the ability to make judgments free from discrimination, dishonesty, or one's own bias.

Fidelity

Nothing is more noble, nothing more venerable, than fidelity. Faithfulness and truth are the most sacred excellences and endowments of the human mind.

—*Cicero*

Fidelity is the virtue of faithfulness, being true to our commitments and obligations to others. A component of fidelity—veracity—implies that we will be truthful and honest in all our endeavors. It involves being faithful and loyal to obligations, duties, or observances. The opposite of fidelity is infidelity, meaning unfaithfulness.

Freedom

Freedom is the quality of being free to make choices for oneself within the boundaries of law. Freedoms enjoyed by citizens of the United States include the freedom of speech, freedom of religion, freedom from want, and freedom from physical aggression.

Honesty/Trustworthiness/Truth-Telling

Lies or the appearance of lies are not what the writers of our Constitution intended for our country—it's not the America we salute every Fourth of July, it's not the America we learned about in school, and it is not the America represented in the flag that rises above our land.

—*Message from the Internet*

The virtue of honesty is possessed by those who do not lie, resulting in their being good. Trust involves confidence that a person will act with the right motives. It is the assured reliance on the character, ability, strength, or truth of someone or something. To tell the truth, to have integrity, and to be honest are most honorable virtues. Veracity is devotion to and conformity with what is truthful. It involves an obligation to be truthful.

Truth-telling involves providing enough information so that a patient can make an informed decision about his or her health care. Intentionally misleading a patient to believe something that the caregiver knows to be untrue may give the patient false hope. There is always apprehension when one must share bad news; the temptation is to gloss over the truth for fear of being the bearer of bad news. To lessen the pain and the hurt is only human. But in the end, truth must win over fear.

At the end of our days, the most basic principles of life, trust and survival, are on trial.

—*Author Unknown*

Healthcare Morass

The declining trust in the United States' ability to deliver quality health care is evidenced by a system caught up in the morass of managed care companies, which have in some instances inappropriately devised ways to deny healthcare benefits to their constituency. In addition, the continuing reporting of numerous medical errors serves only to escalate distrust in the nation's political leadership and the providers of health care.

Physicians find themselves vulnerable to lawsuits, often because of misdiagnosis. As a result, patients are passed from specialist to specialist in an effort to leave no stone unturned. Fearful to step outside the boundaries of their own specialties, physicians escalate the problem by ineffectively communicating with the primary care physician responsible for managing the patient's overall healthcare needs. This can also be problematic if no one physician has taken overall responsibility to coordinate and manage a patient's care.

Politics and Discerning Truth

Truthfulness is just one measure of one's moral character. Unfortunately, politicians do not always set good examples for the people they serve. The following are but a few examples of how political decisions have caused, or have given the appearance of causing, division to the detriment of unity. Discuss the following political decisions and how they have helped to divide the nation by political party.

1964: Gulf of Tonkin

Did President Johnson order U.S. bombers to retaliate for a North Vietnamese torpedo attack that never happened (Cohen & Solomon, 1994)?

2003: Persian Gulf War

Did President George W. Bush have legitimate reasons to believe that Saddam Hussein had weapons of mass destruction? If so, was there a real threat that he would use them against the United States?

2004: Prescription Drugs

Senior citizens who did not have prescription drug coverage through Medicare, found that needed medications were unaffordable. Has this issue been honestly and effectively addressed by our government, or must many of the nation's aging population substitute drugs for food?

Hopefulness

> Hope is the last thing that dies in man; and though it be exceedingly deceitful, yet it is of this good use to us, that while we are traveling through life, it conducts us in an easier and more pleasant way to our journey's end.
> —*François de la Rochefoucauld*

Hopefulness in the patient care setting involves looking forward to something with the confidence of success. Caregivers have a responsibility to balance truthfulness while promoting hope. The caregiver must be sensitive to each patient's needs and provide hope.

Integrity

Integrity involves a steadfast adherence to a strict moral or ethical code and a commitment to not compromise this code. A person with integrity has a staunch belief in and faithfulness to, for example, his or her religious beliefs, values, and moral character. Patients and professionals alike often make healthcare decisions based on their integrity and their strict moral beliefs. For example, a Jehovah's Witness will refuse a blood transfusion because it is against his or her religious beliefs, even if such refusal may result in death. A provider of health care may refuse to participate in an abortion because it is against his or her moral beliefs. A person without personal integrity lacks sincerity and moral conviction, and may fail to act on professed moral beliefs.

Preservation of Life

Medical ethics do not require that a patient's life be preserved at all costs and in all circumstances. The ethical integrity of the profession is not threatened by allowing competent patients to decide for themselves whether a particular medical treatment is in their best interests. If the doctrines of informed consent and right of privacy have as their foundations the right to bodily integrity and control of one's own fate, then those rights are superior to the institutional considerations of hospitals and their medical staffs. A state's interest in maintaining the ethical integrity of a profession does not outweigh, for example, a patient's right to refuse blood transfusions.

Kindness

> When you carry out acts of kindness, you get a wonderful feeling inside. It is as though something inside your body responds and says, yes, this is how I ought to feel.
>
> —*Harold Kushner*

Kindness involves the quality of being considerate and sympathetic to another's needs.

Respect

> Respect for ourselves guides our morals; respect for others guides our manners.
>
> —*Laurence Sterne*

To give and show respect is to show special regard to someone or something. Caregivers who demonstrate respect for their patients will be more effective in helping them cope with the anxiety of their illness. Respect helps to develop trust between the patient and caregiver, and improve healing processes. If caregivers respect the family of a patient, cooperation and understanding will be the positive result, encouraging a team effort to improve patient care.

SITUATIONAL ETHICS

A person's moral values and moral character can be compromised when faced with difficult choices. Why do good people behave differently in different situations? Why do good people sometimes do bad things? The answer is fairly simple: One's moral character can sometimes change as circumstances change; thus the term *situational ethics.*

> Situational ethics refers to a particular view of ethics, in which absolute standards are considered less important than the requirements of a particular situation. The standards used may, therefore, vary from one situation to another, and may even contradict one another (Situational ethics, n.d.).

For example, a decision not to use extraordinary means to sustain the life of an unknown 84-year-old may result in a different decision than it would if the 84-year-old is one's mother. To better understand this concept, consider the desire to live, and the extreme measures one will take to do so. Remember that ethical decision making is the process of determining the right thing to do in the event of a moral dilemma. For example, those who survived the crash of a Fairchild FH-227 twin turboprop airplane on Friday, October 13, 1972, were faced with some difficult survival decisions. The plane, which was crossing the Andes Mountains carrying 40 passengers and 5 crew, disappeared from the modern world, and everyone on board was thought to be dead. However, 72 days later, 16 emerged alive and told their story ("Alive," 2001). They chose to live by feeding off of those who did not live. This is a gruesome picture indeed, but it illustrates to what lengths one may go in certain situations (situational ethics) in order to survive.

THE FINAL ANALYSIS

> People are often unreasonable, illogical and self-centered;
>
> Forgive them anyway.
>
> If you are kind, people may accuse you of selfish, ulterior motives.
>
> Be kind anyway.
>
> If you are successful, you will win some false friends and some true enemies;
>
> Succeed anyway.
>
> What you spend years building, someone may destroy overnight;
>
> Build anyway.
>
> The good you do today, people will often forget tomorrow;
>
> Do good anyway.
>
> Give the world the best you have, and it may never be enough;
>
> Give the world the best you have anyway.
>
> You see, in the final analysis, it is between you and God;
>
> It was never between you and them anyway.
>
> —*Author Unknown*

| CASE STUDY 1 | Can the Physician Change His Mind? |

Walls had a condition that caused his left eye to be out of alignment with his right eye. Walls discussed with Shreck, his physician, the possibility of surgery on his left eye to bring both eyes into alignment. Walls and Shreck agreed that the best approach to treating Walls was to attempt surgery on the left eye. Prior to surgery, Walls signed an authorization and consent form that included the following language:

a. I hereby authorize Dr. Shreck . . . to perform the following procedure and/or alternative procedure necessary to treat my condition . . . of the left eye.

b. I understand the reason for the procedure is to straighten my left eye to keep it from going to the left.

c. It has been explained to me that conditions may arise during this procedure whereby a different procedure or an additional procedure may need to be performed, and I authorize my physician and his assistants to do what they feel is needed and necessary.

During surgery, Shreck encountered excessive scar tissue on the muscles of Walls's left eye and elected to adjust the muscles of the right eye instead. When Walls awoke from the anesthesia, he expressed anger at the fact that both of his eyes were bandaged. The next day, Walls went to Shreck's office for a follow-up visit and adjustment of his sutures. Walls asked Shreck why he had operated on the right eye, and Shreck responded that he reserved the right to change his mind during surgery.

Walls filed a lawsuit. The trial court concluded that Walls had failed to establish that Shreck had violated any standard of care. It sustained Shreck's motion for directed verdict, and Walls appealed. The court stated that the consent form that had been signed indicated that there can be extenuating circumstances when the surgeon exceeds the scope of what was discussed presurgery. Walls claims that it was his impression that Shreck was talking about surgeries in general.

Roussel, an ophthalmologist, had testified on behalf of Walls. Roussel stated that it was customary to discuss with patients the potential risks of a surgery, benefits, and the alternatives to surgery. Roussel testified that medical ethics requires informed consent.

Shreck claimed that he had obtained the patient's informed consent not from the form, but rather based on what he discussed with the patient in his office. The court found that the form itself does not give or deny permission for anything. Rather, it is evidence of the discussions that occurred and during which informed consent was obtained. Shreck, therefore, asserted that he obtained informed consent to operate on both eyes based on his office discussions with Walls.

Ordinarily, in a medical malpractice case, the plaintiff must prove the physician's negligence by presenting expert testimony. One of the exceptions to the requirement for expert testimony is the situation whereby the evidence and the circumstances are such that the recognition of the alleged negligence may be presumed to be within the comprehension of laymen. This exception is referred to as the "common knowledge exception."

The evidence showed that Shreck did not discuss with Walls the possibility that surgery might be required on both eyes during the

CASE STUDY 1　Can the Physician Change His Mind? *(continued)*

same operation. There is evidence that Walls specifically told Shreck he did not want surgery performed on the right eye.

Expert testimony was not required to establish that Walls did not give express or implied consent for Shreck to operate on his right eye. Absent an emergency, it is common knowledge that a reasonably prudent healthcare provider would not operate on part of a patient's body if the patient told the healthcare provider not to do so.

On appeal, the trial court was found to have erred in directing a verdict in favor of Shreck. The evidence presented established that the standard of care in similar communities requires healthcare providers to obtain informed consent before performing surgery. In this case, the applicable standard of care required Shreck to obtain Walls's express or implied consent to perform surgery on his right eye (*Walls v. Shreck*, 2003).

1. Discuss the conflicting ethical principles in this case.
2. Did the physician's actions in this case involve medical paternalism? Explain your answer.

CASE STUDY 2　Virtues and Moral Values: Who Makes the Rules?

Mr. Jones was trying to get home from a long trip to see his ailing wife, who had been ill for several years, suffering a great deal of pain. His flight was to leave at 7:00 P.M. Upon arrival at the airport in New York at 4:30 P.M., he inquired at the ticket counter, "Is there an earlier flight that I can take to Washington, D.C.?" The counter agent responded, "There is plenty of room on the 5:00 P.M. flight but you will have to pay a $200 change fee." The passenger inquired, "Could you please waive the change fee? I need to get home to my ailing wife." The ticket agent responded, "Sorry, your ticket does not allow me to make the change."

The passenger made a second attempt at the gate to get on an earlier flight but the manager at the gate was unwilling to authorize the change, saying, "I don't make the rules."

Mr. Jones decided to give it one more try. He called the airline's customer service center. The customer service agent responded to Mr. Jones's plea: "We cannot overrule the agent at the gate. Sorry, you just got the wrong supervisor. He is going by the book."

1. Should rules be broken for a higher good?
2. Who decides?

CASE STUDY 3   Honesty

Annie, a 23-year-old woman with two children, began experiencing severe pain in her abdomen while visiting her family in May 2002. After complaining of pain to Mark, her husband, in June 2002, he scheduled an appointment with Dr. Roberts, a gastroenterologist, who ordered a series of tests. While conducting a barium scan, a radiologist at Community Hospital noted a small bowel obstruction. Dr. Roberts recommended surgery, and Annie agreed.

Following surgery on July 7, Dr. Brown, the operating surgeon, paged Mark over the hospital intercom as he walked down a corridor on the ground floor. Mark, hearing the page, picked up a house phone and dialed zero for an operator. The operator inquired, "May I help you?"

"Yes," Mark replied. "I was just paged."

"Oh, yes. Dr. Brown would like to talk to you. I will connect you with him. Hang on. Don't hang up," the operator instructed.

Mark's heart began to pound.

"Mark?" Dr. Brown asked.

"Yes."

"Well, surgery is over," Dr. Brown informed him. "Your wife is recovering nicely in the recovery room."

Mark was relieved, but for a moment. "That's good," he said.

Dr. Brown continued, "I am sorry to say that she has carcinoma of the colon."

Mark replied, "Did you get it all?"

"I am sorry, but the cancer has spread to her lymph nodes and surrounding organs," the doctor said.

Mark asked, "Can I see her?"

Dr. Brown replied, "She is in the recovery room but I am sure it will be okay to see her."

Before hanging up, Mark told Dr. Brown, "Please do not tell Annie that she has cancer. I want her to always have hope."

Dr. Brown agreed, "Don't worry, I won't tell her. You can tell her that she had a narrowing of the colon."

Mark hung up the phone and proceeded to the recovery room. Upon entering the recovery room, he spotted his wife. His heart sank into his stomach. Tubes seemed to be running out of every part of her body. He walked to her bedside. His immediate concern was to see her wake up and have the tubes pulled out so that he could take her home.

Later, in a hospital room, Annie asked Mark, "What did the doctor find?"

Mark replied, "He found a narrowing of the colon."

Annie asked, "Am I going to be okay?"

"Yes, but it will take a while to recover," Mark replied.

"Oh, that's good. I was so worried," said Annie. "You go home and get some rest."

"I'll see you in the morning," he said as he left.

Mark left the hospital and went to see his friends, Jerry and Helen, who had invited him for dinner. As Mark pulled up to Jerry and Helen's home, he got out of his car and just stood there looking up a long stairway leading to Jerry and Helen's home. They were standing there looking down at Mark. It was early evening, the sun was setting, a warm breeze was blowing, and Helen's eyes were watering.

(continues)

CASE STUDY 3   Honesty *(continued)*

But for a few moments, it seemed like a lifetime. Mark discovered a new emotion as he stood there speechless. He knew then that he was losing a part of himself. Things would never be the same.

Annie had one more surgery 2 months later in a futile attempt to extend her life.

By November 2002, Annie was admitted to the hospital for the last time. Annie was so ill that even during her last moments she was unaware that she was dying. Dr. Brown entered the room and asked Mark, "Can I see you for a few moments?"

"Yes," Mark replied. He followed Dr. Brown into the hallway.

"Mark, I can keep Annie alive for a few more days or we can let her go."

Mark, not responding, went back into the room. He was now alone with Annie. Shortly thereafter a nurse walked into the room and gave Annie an injection. Mark asked, "What did you give her?"

The nurse replied, "Something to make her more comfortable."

Annie had been asleep; she awoke, looked at Mark, and said, "Could you please cancel my appointment at the university? I will have to reschedule my appointment. I don't think I will be well enough to go tomorrow."

Mark replied, "Okay, try to get some rest."

Annie closed her eyes, never to open them again.

1. Do you agree with Mark's decision not to tell Annie about the seriousness of her illness? Explain your answer.

2. Should the physician have spoken to Annie as to the seriousness of her illness? Explain your answer.

3. Describe the ethical dilemmas in this case (e.g., how Annie's rights were violated). Place yourself in Annie's shoes, the physician's shoes, and Mark's shoes, and then discuss how the lives of each may have been different if the physician had informed Annie as to the seriousness of her illness.

4. In the final analysis, is it possible to say who is right?

DISCUSSION QUESTIONS

1. Discuss the questions posed throughout this chapter.

2. Which common ethical dilemmas do you foresee facing in your new role as an advanced practice nurse?

3. Which ethical theories and principles reviewed in this chapter apply to recent or current ethical issues you have faced in your practice?

4. Apply the ethical decision-making process to these issues.

5. How can the principle of justice raise ethical dilemmas?

6. How can the meaning of virtues and personal values and beliefs influence advanced practice?

7. Identify a situation in which a personal conflict of interest may arise and propose a resolution or actions to resolve the conflict.

8. Describe how what you believe to be the right thing to do might change as circumstances change.

9. Describe how your consultative advice might change based on a patient's needs, beliefs, and family influences.

10. Investigate the ethics committee in your organization and review its purpose, membership, and recent issues discussed in the committee. Attend a meeting and report to your classmates.

11. Discuss the ethical dilemmas involved in the allocation of scarce resources. How would the ethical principles, virtues, and values discussed in this chapter affect how you would allocate scarce resources? How might resolving this issue cause conflict between your personal values and beliefs and organization perspective?

REFERENCES

Alive: The Andes survivors. (2001). Retrieved November 2, 2007, from http://members.aol.com/porkinsr6/alive.html

Belmont report. (2004, October). Presentation for IRB members. Retrieved November 9, 2007, from www.rgs.uci.edu/ora/rp/hrpp/BelmontReport.ppt

Canterbury v. Spence, 464 F.2d 772 (D.C. Cir. 1972).

Cohen, J., & Solomon, N. (1994). 30-year anniversary: Tonkin Gulf lie launched Vietnam War. Retrieved November 2, 2007, from http://www.fair.org/media-beat/940727.html

Eastern Michigan University. (n.d.). Protection and use of human subjects in research. Retrieved November 2, 2007, from http://www.rcr.emich.edu/module1/a_7part1.html

Harvard Ad Hoc Committee on Brain Death. (1968). Brain death. Retrieved November 2, 2007, from http://www.ascensionhealth.org/ethics/public/issues/harvard.asp

In re Conroy, 464 A.2d 303, 314 (N.J. Super. Ct. App. Div., 1983).

In the Matter of Karen Ann Quinlan, 70 N.J. 10 (1976).

Intute: Health and Life Sciences. Retrieved from http://bioresearch.ac.uk/browse/mesh/C0020125L0020125.html

Kennedy Institute of Ethics at Georgetown University. (2007, August). The Kennedy Institute of Ethics. Retrieved November 2, 2007, from http://kennedyinstitute.georgetown.edu/index.htm

Luce, C. B. (1979). *Reader's Digest.*

Morality. (2005). In *Stanford encyclopedia of philosophy.* Retrieved November 2, 2007, from http://plato.stanford.edu/entries/morality-definition/

National Human Genome Research Institute. (2007). The large-scale genome sequencing program: History. Retrieved December 10, 2007, from http://www.genome.gov/25521731

National Institutes of Health. (1979, April). The Belmont Report: Ethical principles and guidelines for the protection of human subjects of research. Retrieved November 9, 2007, from http://ohsr.od.nih.gov/guidelines/belmont.html

Patient Self-Determination Act of 1990, 42 U.S.C. 1395cc(a)(1).

President's Council on Bioethics. (n.d.). Retrieved November 2, 2007, from http://www.bioethics.gov/reports/past_commissions/index.html

Schloendorff v. Society of New York Hospital, 105 N.E. 92, 93 (N.Y. 1914).

Schweitzer, A. (1949). *Civilization and ethics.* New York: Macmillan.

A science odyssey—People and discoveries: First kidney transplant performed. (1998). Retrieved November 2, 2007, from http://www.pbs.org/wgbh/aso/databank/entries/dm54ki.html

Situational ethics. (n.d.). *Wikipedia.* Retrieved November 2, 2007, from http://en.wikipedia.org/wiki/Situational_ethics

Union Pacific Ry. Co. v. Botsford, 141 U.S. 250, 251 (1891).

United States Code, Title 42—The Public Health and Welfare, Chapter 6A—Public Health Service, Subchapter XVI—President's Commission for the Study of Ethical Problems in Medicine and Biomedical and Behavior Research, Section 300v-1. Retrieved November 2, 2007, from http://caselaw.lp.findlaw.com/casecode/uscodes/42/chapters/6a/subchapters/xvi/sections/section_300v-1.html

Walls v. Shreck, 658 N.W.2d 686 (2003).

CHAPTER 26

The Role of Codes of Ethics in Nursing's Disciplinary Knowledge

John G. Twomey

CHAPTER OBJECTIVES

1. Trace the historical developments of the code of ethics for nursing.

2. Apply ethical theories specific to health care to the role of the advanced practice nurse.

INTRODUCTION

Since the inception of modern nursing in the 19th century, considerable thought has been paid to the moral nature of the discipline. A cursory review of the writings of early leaders such as Nightingale highlights efforts to increase the numbers of qualified applicants into nursing. Although the call for "sober, honest, truthful, trustworthy applicants" (Dossey, 2000, p. 222) was based on an emotional desire to keep the ranks of the developing discipline free from scandal, it is now more accurate to describe the ethical core of nursing as being part of its intellectual heritage.

To fully appreciate the role of moral and ethical knowledge in nursing, it is necessary to examine the evolving development of ethics within the greater domain of disciplinary nursing knowledge. This examination requires a familiarity with how a distinct nursing ethic has emerged within the greater umbrella of bioethics. This historical occurrence cannot be fully comprehended without an appreciation of how the intellectual leaders of the discipline centered this development on an informal code of ethics for the profession that eventually became formalized into the current Code of Ethics for Nurses (American Nurses Association, 2001). Additionally, an ongoing issue within this profession of multiple subspecialty practices is whether a single code of ethics can serve a group of professionals with multiple interests and obligations that can pose intriguing individual moral challenges.

VIEWS OF ETHICS FOR NURSING

Founders' Views

Florence Nightingale, the intellectual matriarch of modern nursing, set strict standards of behavior for the women she recruited to her radical model of care. Her then-modern concept of nursing went beyond the traditional view of nursing that was inured with the notion that personal care was limited to the intimate. Generally, such care was delivered by the family or by those in society, usually women, who were forced to provide such intimate care for pay. These circumstances often were shameful for both caregiver and patient, for it meant that either had to leave the familiar bosom of the family and seek or provide services, through pecuniary means, that should have been given, not paid for (Rothman, 1990). Not surprisingly, premodern nursing, for pay, was considered in many societies to be on par with prostitution.

Nightingale's efforts often have been portrayed as persuading society, as well as the group of women recruited to her cause, to accept a notion of women who shared a devotion of intimate caring that divorced the emotion of caring from the physical. Nightingale's best-known works emphasize her drive to merge her strong belief in the emergent 19th-century principles of public health and the scientific basis that such health was founded on with an interesting insistence on behavior that married military discipline with a fervor such as one could find in contemporary religious orders (Church, 1990).

It is not surprising that most accounts of Nightingale's views on moral behavior centered on her beliefs that nurses' personal behaviors were the most important part of the ethical role. Therefore, dress, decorum, and devotion were considered within the auspices of virtue

and came to be how the public perceived how a professional nurse should be judged. But recent examination of Nightingale's correspondence suggests that she struggled to reconcile her public and private personas. Nightingale's much-touted public persona as a woman who sought to consolidate nursing's position through connections with powerful men has come into question. Widerquist (1990) has challenged F. B. Smith's widely accepted characterization of Nightingale's relationships as only being based on a need for power, stating, "they [her relationships] resulted not in a need for power, but from her idealized need for perfection and mutuality, i.e., sympathy, a quality of fellow feeling, with others before she was able to sustain a relationship" (p. 303). This interpretation may provide some evidence that although Nightingale seemed to prefer attention to rule in her nurses, she also viewed the perfect world as one based on virtues that included a spirituality that was embedded in an ethic of nursing care.

Nightingale's views almost completely dominated the vision of professional nursing that immigrated to the United States and elsewhere. Not until well into the 20th century did nursing practice based on her methods go much beyond education and practical nursing interventions. Subsequent American nursing leaders worked with little success to move nursing into modern professional reforms, such as control of entry into practice and nursing knowledge development, during the early genesis of nursing. However, they did confront the need to go beyond the concepts of duty and service as the core values of nursing. Early prominent American nurses such as Lavinia Dock and Annie Goodrich wrote persuasively of the need for nurses to go beyond etiquette in their practice. They called for nurses to recognize that the intimate nature of their practice was a basic ethical concept and, therefore, a core value that necessitated more than superficial physical care (Hamilton, 1994). Hamilton argues that these beliefs ultimately were transformed into the concepts of compassion and caring. However, before they could become the core values of modern nursing, they needed to be separated from their original interpretations of being religious values. The development of ethical knowledge in nursing continually focused on virtues as well as principles. As will be discussed, the evolution of the current Code of Ethics for Nurses is a reflection of this intellectual tradition.

Views on Codes of Ethics

Early nursing leaders did not believe that ethical codes were necessary for the emerging profession. As has been noted, this was not from lack of interest in nurses' behaviors. In fact, leaders' attention focused heavily on nurses' behaviors, but their dictums to both their students and nurses under their direction focused on proper behavior when providing care, not of care directed by ethics. During much of the 20th century, the result was that nursing practice was rule bound in both scientific principles and professional behaviors. This devotion to policy was less the result of proven data, but rather emerged from the inability of nursing to successfully ingrain itself in the developing healthcare system with its members as leaders rather than servants (Ashley, 1976).

Codes of ethics were not a primary part of the emergent health professions in the 19th century. The Hippocratic oath offered a list of behaviors for healers. Historically, its use was limited to those who had knowledge of foreign languages and access to books. The Nightingale pledge (n.d.) offered a similar listing of virtuous behaviors. Some of these behaviors appeared in future nursing codes. Nightingale had no hand in writing the Nightingale pledge, and she herself was famously opposed to external vehicles for guiding nursing behavior, such as licensure by government agencies. Finally, the lack of ethical codes for health professions during the 19th century reflected the absence of formal collective organizations. As professional organizations gained in size and power, their role in the development of ethical codes also increased.

Early American nursing leaders did address the issue of ethical codes, but found the argument for them to be unconvincing. Lavinia Dock and Annie Goodrich argued that ethical behavior was an essence of nursing and could be found within its practice of compassion and human interaction, not slavish devotion to rules. It is not surprising that Dock, with her experience at the Henry Street Settlement House, viewed nursing as a vibrant force that was attributable to the individual care that each nurse gave to her patients (Hamilton, 1994). Goodrich also rejected a code of ethics on the grounds that it took nurses away from compassion as a means and instead directed their efforts toward etiquette (Goodrich, 1932). Presumably, Goodrich did not agree with the code of ethics espoused by Isabel Hampton Robb (1900), as it was clearly a creed of etiquette.

A CODE OF ETHICS FOR NURSING

Ethical codes reflect a range of ethical theories and guidelines. Given the versions that have been presented to nurses, it is useful to consider how those who would use them should interpret the contents of such codes. Ethical guidelines are derived from bioethics. Bioethics draws on the knowledge and processes of ethics to examine health care; as such, it applies to the moral behavior of any person performing actions because he or she has chosen to be a healthcare professional. It may or may not involve patients directly. Nursing ethics and medical ethics are subsets of bioethics that apply to those in the specific professions. All bioethical codes share many similar concepts.

Metaethics: Where Theories Live

The term *metaethics* refers to ethical theories that are applicable to bioethics. Two familiar broad ethical theories that most nurses recognize include deontology and utilitarianism

(Beauchamp & Childress, 2001). Deontology grounds the ethical value of one's actions on the value of the act itself. If an act, like truth-telling, is good as a goal itself, then not adhering to that good is unethical. Therefore, telling a lie is unethical, even if it might ultimately provide a result that most reasonable people would define as good. Utilitarianism states that an act should be judged on how much good it produces. Contrast this view using the prior example.

A number of theories derive some of their base concepts from deontology and utilitarianism. These theories also fit under the metaethical framework. The most commonly recognized theory of bioethics is principled theory. Common concepts or principles such as patient autonomy, risk of harm, or provision of benefits have their base in principled theory. For example, the principle of autonomy has its theoretical underpinning in deontological thought. This thinking holds that a primary good is the respect for personhood; therefore all patients are given respect by allowing them to make fully informed decisions about their care. Principled theory is employed when those people making bioethical decisions weigh the varied principles to assess which principle is most applicable in a particular situation. This theory, though not perfect in its ability to answer all bioethical questions, became the most applied bioethical theory in Western medical culture in the latter half of the 20th century and continues to be an important part of contemporary bioethical discourse (Evans, 2000).

Recently, other theories have ascended in their contributions to ethical discussions, particularly in nursing ethics. Communitarianism is a framework of ethical thought that changes the locus of moral deliberation from the individual (as in the previously discussed theories) to the group within which the decision will be made. Therefore, the patient is recast from being an autonomous individual who is an isolated decision maker to one whose existence is made meaningful by being a member of a group. According to this theory, input from group members in decision making is just as important as that from the individual patient, because group members will be affected by the decision (Beauchamp & Childress, 2001).

Caring, or contextual, ethics provides a framework of ethical thought that grants insights into moral decision making that is appealing to many nurses. According to the theory of caring ethics, bioethical decisions are viewed through the prism of the relationship between the caregiver and the care recipient. Decisions are looked on as a means of maintaining the interdependent bond that a provider has with the patient (Noddings, 2003). Whereas principled theories tend to emphasize patient rights, caring and communitarian theories see the individual as existing more within a nurturing role. This caring relationship places the provider on equal footing with the patient in the decision-making process.

The metaethical level of theories provides the basic reference point for any ethical consideration. It is important to recognize that this level is often unspoken when people put forward their beliefs in a moral discussion. When someone states, "I feel that we should do this because . . ." he or she is saying, "I believe this is an underlying core consideration." The core often lies within a broad theory. Such beliefs can also derive from other theoretical beliefs, such as religious theories on behavior, that often share the same values, such as the importance of providing justice to people.

For metaethical theories to be relevant to practice, their concepts need to be narrowed so that they can be applied to specific situations. The process of bringing theory to practice begins at the next level of analysis: descriptive ethics.

Descriptive Ethics: Where Codes Live

The descriptive level of ethical analysis is best understood as being juxtaposed between the metaethical (theory) level and the level below it, which is referred to as normative ethics, which can be likened to specific rules. Descriptive ethics provides broad descriptions of moral behaviors that are recognizable as coming from the theoretical frameworks already discussed. However, the guidelines that come from this level often have wide latitude and can be interpreted differently by the varied decision makers who use them, particularly when those decision makers approach the frameworks from different perspectives. For instance, both the nursing and medical codes of ethics have proscriptions from abandoning patients that are interpreted differently. Physicians, who have a legacy of operating their practices as businesses, are expected to continue to care for patients under many circumstances, but are allowed to refuse to care for patients who cannot pay them. By contrast, nurses, who come from a legacy of accepting patients who are assigned to them by their employers, have an ethic that allows them to leave the care of a patient only when another nurse will substitute and provide the needed care.

Descriptive ethics interprets the broad theories within understandable language so that the professions can adapt them to their professional needs. Therefore, the principle of justice, which states that people should be given what they deserve, is represented in the first provision of the Code of Ethics for Nurses (ANA, 2001), which states that nursing care is delivered without regard to economic status. Obviously, this statement is open to many interpretations, and how any individual nurse will abide by it depends on the specific professional situation. Indeed, this phrase within the first provision is not elaborated on further by the accompanying interpretive statement, whereas other pieces of the provision are interpreted in detail.

Descriptive ethical statements are heard widely when one is in professional training through formal and informal means of acculturation. New nurses are socialized through the use of such phrases as "to preserve confidentiality," "not to harm patients," "to make sure patients make informed decisions," and other slogans. When examined, such broad sayings provide little direction for the professional, for they are generally presented without context. In the reality of everyday practice, nurses and other healthcare professionals do share information without patients' permission, sometimes do inflict some harm when doing painful procedures, and may purposely allow patients to make decisions that are not fully informed because they agree with the patients' decisions.

However, descriptive ethics is important for several reasons. It provides the professions with valuable weapons in their efforts to win the public's trust and to legitimate the professions as forces in a society's health. The use of descriptive ethics helps the professions to maintain a dynamic legacy of continuous ethical thought by leaving open the predominant theories to interpretation in ways that the professions want their members to present themselves. For example, the 2001 ANA code contains phrases that can be traced back to the original code ratified by the membership more than a half-century ago. The current code uses ethical referents that are well recognized by society and its members to draw attention to the newer, more modern and relevant interpretations that the profession needs in the 21st century (Daly, 1999).

Ethical codes also straddle the third level of ethical analysis—normative ethics. It is important to understand how such movement across the levels of analysis works to provide flexibility for professions as they address issues in their practice.

Normative Ethics: Where Codes Are Interpreted

Normative rules dominate our private and professional lives. They are seen in many forms—ranging from civil regulations, such as traffic laws, to rules and regulations within our work settings. Normative rules can take the form of policies that govern professional practice, such as those specifying which professionals can prepare drug preparations and which ones can administer them. Professional standards of care also can be stated in normative fashion—for example, as evidenced by clinical pathways that dictate specific action given a patient scenario.

It is not difficult to recognize the form that normative ethics takes within the healthcare setting. Specific rules that limit accessibility to patient records, policies that define how much free care will be given to indigent clients, and other written guidelines exemplify normative ethics and display how broader forms of ethics are grounded in practice. Generally, clinicians are comfortable with normative ethical rules because they are easy to understand and can be amended when it appears that contemporary patient care dictates such changes. Consider informed consent policies in today's hospitals that dictate many more points within a stay where patients are asked to give permission for different procedures. The underlying concept of autonomy has a much stricter interpretation today than a generation ago when patients rarely were approached to give consent after signing a general consent form at the admitting office.

Ethical codes are not generally written at the normative level, but because members of professions seek specific guidelines, many professions provide interpretations of the descriptive ethics that codes reflect. As illustrated later in the chapter, the ANA code provides a clear example of how a profession uses its professional code and adjunct policy statements to meet the needs of its members.

THE ROLE OF ETHICAL CODES

The existence of ethical codes for healthcare professionals is a relatively unquestioned phenomenon in current society. A listing on the Illinois Institute of Technology website (http://ethics.iit .edu/codes/health.html) contains dozens of links, some of them going to the base moral code of a given profession or professional subgroup, and others providing interpretations of the individual code. However, one simply cannot accept the premise that such codes exist because each health profession has such distinct ethical positions that they need to articulate them. Instead, codes must be seen as a vehicle for the legitimacy of a health profession itself.

Any group that claims to be a profession will exhibit a number of characteristics. The most common ones are claims to (1) a distinct body of knowledge, (2) control over the entry of members into the profession, and (3) a legitimacy and accountability of the professional group as it serves the needs of the society within which it exists. The latter is represented by the profession having leaders whose main responsibility is to help create an environment in which the profession can (1) educate its members, (2) create knowledge through research that the profession can claim and pass on to its practicing members, and (3) participate in the policy process that society uses to negotiate relationships with the professions.

The means by which a profession accomplishes these tasks is through a leadership group. The collective action and influence of professional organizations are essential to the survival and advancement of a profession. Membership in a professional organization may be voluntary or mandatory. Whether or not a majority of the members have an active bond with the leadership organization, most professional organizations share the following features:

- Support through membership dues
- Some form of acceptance by government authorities as being a legitimate voice for the organization's members
- A relationship with the institutions that prepare and employ the organization's members
- A governance model that allows participation by the organization's members in its decision process
- A permanent staff who conduct the daily business of the profession

The professional group has many challenges when trying to maintain the profession's recognized legitimacy, and an ethical code is often one of the tools it employs. Whereas one might assume that a code is simply the list of directions for a given professional, examination of any professional code provides evidence that part of being a professional in that given field is to accept the values that the group espouses. For example, the third provision of the current ANA code states, "The nurse promotes, advocates for, and strives to protect the health, safety, and rights of the patient." The main goal of this statement is to focus the reader on the object of the sentence, the patient. When this statement was written, the goal of the authors, which was accepted by the professional group, was to underscore that the nursing profession was primarily responsible to its patients, not employers nor third-party payers. In a time of complex professional relationships, the one person a patient can rely on is the (registered) nurse. This is a value that the profession wants the public to see that it strongly embraces.

Thus it is essential to recognize that the code of nursing ethics is commissioned, accepted, and owned by the professional group. It reflects not just moral values, but also the ethical face that the professional wants to present to current society.

THE ANA CODE OF ETHICS

The current code of ethics for nursing was published in 2001. The development of this version of the code began at least 6 years earlier (Daly, 1999). The code's roots are embedded in a half-century of efforts at promulgating an ethical code. Early leaders of American nursing debated the need for a code of ethics for nurses, and early versions of nursing codes of ethics were proposed but not accepted (Fowler, 1999). In 1950, a formal code for nurses was accepted by the ANA (Fowler, 1992). During the next quarter-century, this code was modified several times. For example, the ideas of etiquette and loyalty evolved over time into more professional concepts of professional autonomy and accountability (Scanlon & Glover, 1995). The code was revised again in 1969, and minor revisions occurred in 1976 and 1985 (Daly, 1999).

In 1995, the ANA called together a group of prominent nurse ethicists and asked them whether the 1985 version of the code needed further revision. When they replied affirmatively, the association appointed a task force of practicing and academic nurses to do a total revision of the code (Daly, 1999). The group convened in 1997, and by the time the task force's work was complete and the current code was accepted by the house of delegates of the ANA in 2001, the code had a new title and the 11 provisions of the 1985 code had been reduced to 9. The preface and the interpretive statements had all been rewritten, and an afterword was added. The task force not only debated and rewrote multiple iterations of the new code, but at every stage input was sought from interested parties, such as the state associations that make up the federal structure of the ANA, prominent nurse leaders in nursing education and practice, and subspecialty nursing organizations outside the ANA.

At one point, the adoption of the new code was held up by debate and politics within the organization's house of delegates. A temporary roadblock was generated by a deep schism between the state groups that formed this governance group over issues that the new code addressed, particularly the role of the nurse in collective actions within employment settings. This dispute caused the code to be sent back to the task force for further revision. As evidenced by this example, codes of ethics reflect more than the moral beliefs of the profession; they also are seen as powerful vehicles for professing the values of the profession—which are not always agreed to unanimously by the members of a given group.

READING THE ANA CODE OF ETHICS

When anyone, nurse or layperson, reads the ANA code, it is necessary to remember that it is a descriptive ethical document. This code is not unlike many other professional codes in that it attempts to voice the ethics and values of the profession. All professions have to go beyond the descriptive nature of their codes. These groups get to the normative level whereby their audiences can more easily understand the practicality of their code's messages in several different ways.

The ANA has long chosen to portray its ethical assertions through a three-level mechanism. The first level is the code, with its nine provisions (see **Figure 26-1**). If one retrieves the code online or acquires a copy of the ANA code booklet, then one immediately has access to the accompanying interpretive statements, which offer more specific information to help to

---

FIGURE 26-1 | ANA Code of Ethics

The ANA house of delegates approved these nine provisions of the new Code of Ethics for Nurses at its June 30, 2001, meeting in Washington, D.C. In July 2001, the Congress of Nursing Practice and Economics voted to accept the new language of the interpretive statements resulting in a fully approved revised Code of Ethics for Nurses with Interpretive Statements.

1. The nurse, in all professional relationships, practices with compassion and respect for the inherent dignity, worth and uniqueness of every individual, uniqueness of every individual, unrestricted by considerations of social or economic status, personal attributes, or the nature of health problems.
2. The nurse's primary commitment is to the patient, whether an individual, family, group, or community.
3. The nurse promotes, advocates for, and strives to protect the health, safety, and rights of the patient.
4. The nurse is responsible and accountable for individual nursing practice and determines the appropriate delegation of tasks consistent with the nurse's obligation to provide optimum patient care.
5. The nurse owes the same duties to self as to others, including the responsibility to preserve integrity and safety, to maintain competence, and to continue personal and professional growth.
6. The nurse participates in establishing, maintaining, and improving healthcare environments and conditions of employment conducive to the provision of quality health care and consistent with the values of the profession through individual and collective action.
7. The nurse participates in the advancement of the profession through contributions to practice, education, administration, and knowledge development.
8. The nurse collaborates with other health professionals and the public in promoting community, national, and international efforts to meet health needs.
9. The profession of nursing, as represented by associations and their members, is responsible for articulating nursing values, for maintaining the integrity of the profession and its practice, and for shaping social policy.

Source: Reprinted with permission from American Nurses Association. *Code of Ethics for Nurses with Interpretive Statements.* © 2001 nursebooks.org, American Nurses Association, Silver Spring, MD.

bridge the gap to the normative level. Provision 3, mentioned earlier, has six interpretive statements that begin to detail that the services that nurses provide to their patients include protection of sensitive information (3.1, 3.2) and extend to safeguarding the patient from impaired colleagues (3.6). If one reads any of those interpretive statements, it is clear that they are more specific than the parent provision, but that there is still a lot of latitude and room for interpretation within them.

The ANA also has a third category of statements, which are very normative, called position statements. These statements are policy statements that the organization promotes in several clinical and policy areas, including the areas of ethics and human rights. For example, the position statement on assisted suicide (http://www.nursingworld.org/readroom /position/ethics/etsuic.htm) begins with a strong declaration that nurses should not participate in acts aimed at helping patients end their lives prematurely through any means. However, another position statement on pain relief (http://www.nursingworld.org/readroom /position/ethics/etpain.htm) provides support for nurses to titrate narcotic pain relief to levels that might be lethal if the express goal of the act is to relieve pain, not cause death. The message is that individual nurses will never be able to ask their professional organization to completely answer all ethical questions. What will be found within the code, the interpretive statements, and the position statements are mixes of ethical theory, professional values, and discussions of the competing issues within a given topic so that nurses can apply this guidance to their specific context.

As previously stated, the 2001 code consists of nine provisions. The first three provisions describe the central nursing ethic as being that of the individual nurse providing care to patients. The first provision centers on social justice; the nurse is linked with providing care in an indiscriminate fashion, no matter the economic, racial, social, or value system of the patient he or she encounters. The second provision defines fidelity as a significant value of nursing, but it makes clear in no uncertain terms that the relationship most important to nurses is that with patients. The third provision focuses on the ethical duties of the nurse and specifies that protection of the patient is a major part of nursing. To fully understand these provisions, one must go to the individual interpretive statements. But if one stops momentarily to look closely at these introductory provisions, evident in these three statements of just 75 words, the professional organization puts forth a clear and cogent statement of philosophy: Nurses act without reflecting on the nature of their patient, they protect the patient, and, most importantly, they center their actions on a relational ethic that harkens back to the original nursing value of caring, which does not reduce the patient to just a body with an illness, but views the patient as a holistic being with complex needs that nurses can address (Bishop & Scudder, 1990).

The first three provisions also perform another task for the nursing profession. The 2001 code is another step in the development of nursing's value system, particularly its beliefs about its own moral self. Earlier codes, formal and informal, moved from etiquette to duty. The emphases of such duties often were nurses' supposed colleagues, particularly physicians, who were actually superiors, if not employers. As social values changed, nursing's attention turned to values such as racial justice, and it shifted its loyalties in directions that allowed nurses to focus on the objects of their care, the patient. The value of duty evolved into the concept of advocacy for the patient. But as bioethical views of the nurse–patient relationship moved away from the paternalism of the past, advocacy had to be modified. Thus the interpretive statements accompanying the first three provisions now include language that emphasizes the equal relationship between nurses and their patients. For example, interpretive statements 1.1 through 1.5 focus on issues of human dignity and describe the topic as accommodating issues as specific as pain relief and end-of-life care and as general as self-determination. Interpretive statement 1.5 also notes that such respect extends to relations between all professionals, thereby placing nurses alongside all of their healthcare colleagues in mutually supporting roles. This theme continues in interpretive statements 2.1 through 2.4. These statements play off the provision's broad dictum that the nurse primarily serves the patient by recognizing that a practicing clinician has many claims to his or her time. The statements discuss how to identify and work with possible conflicts of interest and very pointedly note that any party to an ethical problem involving the nurse must have an equitable voice in a proposed solution.

Provision 3 reflects the historical threads that have made up the fabric of the ANA's ethical codes over the years. Over the years, many strong statements about confidentiality have been made at the provision level. The task force working on the 2001 code decided that many patient rights deserved the same level of protection as patient information, and provision 3 addresses the need for nurses to help to protect the autonomy of subjects in research as well as to actively shield patients from impaired professionals or improper practice. Interpretive statement 3.5 is the longest of the interpretive statements; it lays out a clear duty for the nurse to be a whistle-blower, despite the acknowledged risks that acting in such a role places the nurse. This interpretive statement is written in such normative language that it could stand alone as a position statement on this topic.

In provisions 4, 5, and 6, the code shifts a bit as it addresses the nurse as a moral agent who has responsibilities of duty that provide good care in ways that go beyond direct patient care but that are truly within the venue of the profession. Provision 4 is very simple: Nursing care is delivered by nurses, and only nurses are responsible for nursing care that is delivered, even

if that care comes from someone else. Anyone with the faintest familiarity with the history of professionalism in nursing knows that the profession has struggled to control a crucial piece of its discipline, that of entry into practice. The result is that not only are there multiple pathways of entry to the status of a registered nurse, but much nursing care is and has been given by nonregistered nurses. All four of the interpretive statements in provision 4 directly state that the ANA claims responsibility for maintaining the professional and ethical standards that define good nursing practice. In response to calls by other allied medical groups to be involved in providing semiprofessional nursing care, interpretive statement 4.4 directly notes that nursing responsibilities can never be delegated, only specific nursing tasks, and states that only nurses can do that delegating. The ultimate responsibility for any nursing care is always owned by the nurses involved in that care, including those nurse administrators who oversee the setting where care is given.

Provision 5 is a new and unique addition. For the first time in an ANA code of ethics, a statement that the individual nurse has moral worth is proclaimed in a provision. This represents the progression of nursing values through the years and shows that the profession feels comfortable in its development as a scientific discipline. As such, the profession can now more forthrightly assert its humanistic values, not just vis-à-vis the patient, but also as a part of the individual nurse's devotion to the profession, harkening back to the values of nursing's early leaders.

Provision 6 continues this theme of the nurse's responsibility for establishing the proper ethical milieu for the delivery of care, but what happens in this provision is evidence of the moral maturation of modern nursing, as the profession claims once and for all that nurses are not beholden to any other group to prepare the environment where they provide care, nor will they take an ethical backseat to any profession in the overall moral milieu of the healthcare setting. A subtle shift occurs within provision 6. Whereas the focus earlier in the code is on the individual nurse, this provision begins to assign the broader responsibilities that the professional group wishes to claim. Although all of the first eight provisions begin with the statement "The nurse . . . ," the later part of the code focuses more on the profession of nursing and the relationship of the individual nurse to the discipline.

The interpretive statements within provision 6 begin to discuss the duties of the nurse that are not directly patient centered. Interpretive statements 6.1 and 6.2 reiterate that the central virtues of the nursing profession cannot be imparted by the individual nurse without support. Therefore, the code now addresses how the nursing profession must provide assistance to the nurse in ways that allow the nurse to practice in an ethically appropriate manner. The code also makes it clear that the verb "to nurse" applies to the relationship of any nurse in any working relationship. Thus nurse educators have duties to their students, just as nurse administrators have responsibilities to the staff nurses under their authority. Consequently, staff nurses on a chronically understaffed unit have a moral responsibility to provide care that meets acceptable professional and ethical standards. If the usual pattern of care on the unit does not meet these standards, then the nurse administrator has at least equal responsibility to change the situation so that patients are treated safely and with respect.

Interpretive statement 6.3 represents probably the most contentious issue that the profession currently faces. The topic of collective action rights and the role of the ANA in assisting nurses who choose to exercise those rights has rent the fabric of the professional organization within the past decade. Professional nurses have claimed the right to collective bargaining for more than a half-century, with the ANA supporting this right by allowing each state unit to decide individually as to the level of involvement it will have in the matter. However, there is a sharp divide between those state nurses associations that reject this position as a part of professional nursing and those that see it as an absolute good. This disagreement has escalated in recent years as a minority of registered nurses have come to believe that not only do nurses have a right to collective bargaining, but that professional nursing organizations should also make representation of nurses in collective bargaining a primary service. Despite the fact that the ANA has a stated goal and a defined subunit that addresses this issue, the disagreement over this issue has caused some state nurses associations to break away from the parent professional group and create their own group that does not accept the ANA's positions nor its code of ethics.

Therefore, interpretive statement 6.3 should be read as a policy statement from the ANA. It clearly supports the right to collective action and grounds that right within the duties of the registered nurse to ensure good patient care through the creation of a safe and nurturing environment as well within the right of the nurse to practice in a way so that the nurse is not continually morally degraded by having to work in substandard conditions. Reading between the lines, one sees the belief that nurses deserve appropriate compensation and humane workloads. But because the definition of such terms is never clear-cut, and because the professional organization also must represent nurse executives and administrators, provision 6.3 has language that matches the general descriptive tone of the overall code and that leaves the topic of collective action somewhat understated.

The last three provisions of the code should be read as disciplinary statements that continue to claim the place of nursing as a leader in healthcare policy and delivery. The profession, through the ANA, made very determined efforts to place itself in the forefront of such efforts in the last quarter of the 20th century.

Through documents such as the Bill of Rights for Registered Nurses, Nursing's Social Policy Statement, and the Code of Ethics for Nurses, the profession provides evidence of its leadership in providing ethical approaches to patient care (Know Your Rights, 2003).

Provisions 7 through 9 contain much material from past codes. Provision 7 synthesizes material from two of the provisions of the 1976 code regarding nursing's duties to make ongoing contributions to the profession's body of knowledge. The interpretive statements of this provision try to balance the nursing profession's need for sophisticated knowledge through research and expert clinical experience without either shutting the staff nurse out of this dynamic role or by putting the onus on that same person to be "super-nurse." Provision 7 reflects the notion that the profession is moving forward and expects its members to make significant efforts toward disciplinary growth, even if by devoting themselves to personal professional growth at the bedside or just paying dues to the professional organization and attending local organizational meetings.

Provision 8 is a restatement of nursing's historical involvement in worldwide health. The 2001 code goes further, however, by noting that this commitment is made as a full partner with other health professions.

Provision 9, the final statement in the code, is a self-reflective assertion that the ANA is the legitimate voice for registered nurses in the United States and that its current vehicles for portraying the face of nursing are well grounded. The three interpretive statements strongly declare that the association has done its job of providing a forum of debate that continues to give voice to the disparate viewpoints of the nation's largest group of healthcare providers. It also finishes laying out the case for the areas of interest in which nurses should have input. Interpretive statement 9.4 stakes the claim that the professional organization rightfully speaks from valid nursing disciplinary interests when it engages in activities such as lobbying for changes in laws that affect patient health, such as domestic violence laws.

In summary, the Code of Ethics for Nurses is best read as a descriptive document that provides basic guidelines for ethical conduct of nurses engaged in patient care and professional growth. Its equal purpose, like that of other professional ethical codes, is to lay the groundwork for a claim to legitimacy for the profession as a respected group with equal moral standing within the nation's healthcare workforce.

ALTERNATIVE CODES OF ETHICS

A continuing question nurses must consider is the need for alternative codes of ethics within the profession. It is certainly understandable when foreign nursing groups (e.g., the Canadian Nurses Association and the International Council of Nurses) wish to state their own views on nursing ethical standards and develop their own codes that have limited applicability to U.S. registered nurses. In addition, however, many subspecialty nursing organizations in the United States have considered the issue of whether a code of ethics for their group would advance their agenda as well as the welfare of the patients they serve (Peterson & Potter, 2004).

It is debatable whether specialized registered nurses experience ethical issues differently than their colleagues in other areas. In a series of surveys across several nursing specializations, reports from nurses in different clinical specialties did not reflect striking differences between the ethical issues they experienced or how they were resolved. Instead, any differences could be predicted by the type of practice setting (Redman & Fry 1996, 1998a, 1998b). For example, pediatric nurses were concerned about child abuse (Butz, Redman, Fry, & Kolodner, 1998), whereas dialysis nurses reported the topic of ending treatment as a common ethical issue (Redman, Hill, & Fry, 1997).

Where specialty codes may have some contribution to an increased moral climate is when the descriptive level of the proposed code is minimized and the normative guidance to the specialty group and its outside audience is pronounced (Scanlon & Glover, 1995; Scanlon, 2000). An example of such a pathway is the program of the International Society of Nurses in Genetics (ISONG, 2007), which periodically prepares and releases position statements on discrete ethical issues that arise because of advances in genomic knowledge and subsequent impacts on genetic nursing practice, such as in the area of access to genetics services (ISONG, 2003).

CONCLUSION

Codes of ethics for health professionals provide guidance for conduct in patient encounters and justify the discipline's role as professional purveyors of care. The current ANA Code of Ethics for Nurses represents a much needed upgrade of the profession's moral guidelines that strongly states the group's just place as the spokesman for its members. The code stakes the claim to the emergence of nursing as a scientific but humanistic health group that constantly strives to update its knowledge base and has rightfully taken its place within the nation's accepted healthcare leaders. The nursing profession, guided by the Code of Ethics for Nurses, maintains a pursuit of excellence in practice, research, and education. This is evidenced by the accomplishments of the National Institute of Nursing Research at the National Institutes of Health, as well as the many respected colleges of nursing and magnet hospital nursing organizations.

DISCUSSION QUESTIONS ───────

1. What are the historical roots that have led to the development of the current Code of Ethics for Nurses?

2. Read each of the nine provisions and provide examples of how each affects ethical decision making for the advanced nursing practitioner.

3. What are the advantages and disadvantages of nursing subspecialty groups having separate codes of ethics?

REFERENCES ───────────────

American Nurses Association (ANA). (2001). *Code of ethics for nurses with interpretive statements.* Washington, DC: American Nurses Association.

Ashley, J. (1976). *Hospitals, paternalism, and the role of the nurse.* New York: Teachers College Press.

Beauchamp, T. L., & Childress, J. F. (2001). *Principles of biomedical ethics* (5th ed.). New York: Oxford University Press.

Bishop, A., & Scudder, J. (1990). *The practical, moral, and personal sense of nursing.* New York: SUNY Press.

Butz, A. M., Redman, B. K., Fry, S. T., & Kolodner, K. K. (1998). Ethical conflicts experienced by certified pediatric nurse practitioners in ambulatory settings. *Journal of Pediatric Health Care, 12*(4), 183–190.

Church, O. (1990). Nightingalism: Its use and abuse in lunacy reform and the development of nursing in psychiatric care at the turn of the century. In V. Bullough, B. Bullough, & M. Stanton (Eds.), *Florence Nightingale and her era: A collection of new scholarship* (pp. 229–244). New York: Garland.

Daly, B. J. (1999). Ethics: why a new code? Code for nurses. *American Journal of Nursing, 99*(6), 64, 66.

Dossey, B. (2000). *Florence Nightingale: Mystic, visionary and reformer.* Philadelphia: Lippincott Williams & Wilkins.

Evans, J. H. (2000). A sociological account of the growth of principlism. *Hastings Center Report, 30*(5), 31–38.

Fowler, M. D. (1992). A chronicle of the evolution of the code for nurses. In G. B. White (Ed.), *Ethical dilemmas in contemporary nursing practice* (pp. 149–154). Washington, DC: American Nurses Association.

Fowler, M. D. (1999). Relic or resource? The code for nurses. *American Journal of Nursing, 99*(3), 56–57.

Goodrich, A. (1932). *The social and ethical significance of nursing: A series of lectures.* New York: Macmillan.

Hamilton, D. (1994). Constructing the mind of nursing. *Nursing History Review II,* 3–28.

International Council of Nurses. (2005). The ICN code of ethics for nurses. Retrieved November 2, 2007, from http://www.icn.ch/icncode.pdf

International Society of Nurses in Genetics (ISONG). (2007). Position statements. Retrieved November

2, 2007, from http://www.ISONG.org/about/position.cfm

International Society of Nurses in Genetics (ISONG). (2003). Position statement: Access to genomic healthcare: The role of the nurse. Retrieved November 2, 2007, from http://www.ISONG.org/about/ps_genomic.cfm

Know your rights. (2003). Available at http://nursingworld.org/tan/novdec02/rights.htm

Nightingale pledge. (n.d.). Available at http://www.accd.edu/sac/nursing/honors.html

Noddings, N. (2003). *Caring: A feminine approach to ethics and moral education.* Berkeley: University of California Press.

Peterson, M., & Potter, R. L. (2004). A proposal for a code of ethics for nurse practitioners. *Journal of the American Academy of Nurse Practitioners, 16*(3), 116–124.

Redman, B. K., & Fry, S. T. (1996). Ethical conflicts reported by registered nurse/certified diabetes educators. *Diabetes Educator, 22*(3), 219–224.

Redman, B. K., & Fry, S. T. (1998a). Ethical conflicts reported by rehabilitation nurses. *Rehabilitation Nursing, 26*(4), 179–184.

Redman, B. K., & Fry, S. T. (1998b). Ethical conflicts reported by registered certified diabetes educators: A replication. *Journal of Advanced Nursing, 28*(6), 1320–1325.

Redman, B. K., Hill, M. A., & Fry, S. T. (1997). Ethical conflicts reported by certified nephrology nurses (CNNs) practicing in dialysis settings. *American Nephrology Nurses Association Journal, 24*(1), 23–33.

Robb, I. H. (1900). *Nursing ethics for hospitals and private use.* Cleveland, OH: E. D. Kloeckert Publishing.

Rothman, D. J. (1990). The *discovery of the asylum: Social order and disorder in the new republic* (rev. ed.). Boston: Little, Brown.

Scanlon, C. (2000). A professional code of ethics provides guidance for genetic nursing practice. *Nursing Ethics, 7*(3), 262–286.

Scanlon, C., & Glover, J. (1995). A professional code of ethics: Providing a moral compass for turbulent times. *Oncology Nursing Forum, 22*(10), 1515–1521.

Widerquist, J. G. (1990). Dearest Rev'd Mother. In V. Bullough, B. Bullough, & M. Stanton (Eds.). *Florence Nightingale and her era: A collection of new scholarship* (pp. 288–308). New York: Garland.

PART 6

Leadership and Role Transition for the Advanced Practice Nurse

The last four chapters of this book take a different perspective on the role of the advanced practice nurse, looking at personal development of the reader for assuming a new role and leadership in the profession.

In Chapter 27, Barker identifies the importance of having a mentor and suggests how to select a mentor and how the relationship may develop over time. The checklist for selecting a mentor presented in this chapter is a helpful tool for the reader, as are the tools used to identify professional development needs and develop a written plan to achieve them.

Conventional wisdom for all leaders states that to be successful, the individual needs to lead a balanced life. To achieve this goal, both time and stress management are central. Chapter 28 suggests relevant strategies related to these aspects of self-care and offers tools to assist readers in

assessing their own skills and developing strategies to capitalize on their strengths and note opportunities for improvement.

In Chapter 29, Beauvais discusses role transitions for advanced practice registered nurses who assume a direct care provider role. She outlines the pathway from novice to expert nurse practitioner and reviews important strategies for career development, including interviewing skills, portfolio and curriculum vitae development, and involvement in professional organizations. The author's expertise in executive administration lends itself well to her discussion of organizational fit, continued professional development, and credentialing and obtaining hospital privileges.

Lastly, in Chapter 30, Ash and Miller provide an in-depth look at interdisciplinary and interprofessional collaborative teams as means to effect positive health outcomes. Both barriers to successful collaborative teams and factors for successful team development are discussed. Advanced practice nurse leaders educated at both the master's and doctoral levels are uniquely positioned to overcome the workforce and regulatory issues that might otherwise diminish the success of collaborative teams-in particular, those involving participants from the nursing and medicine disciplines.

CHAPTER 27

Leadership Development Through Mentorship and Professional Development Planning

Anne M. Barker

CHAPTER OBJECTIVES

1. Discuss the benefits of having a mentor.
2. List the issues to consider when selecting a mentor.
3. List the phases of the mentor–mentee relationship.
4. Distinguish between mentoring and networking.
5. Identify professional development needs and make a plan to achieve them.

INTRODUCTION

The mentor–mentee relationship is a very special one between two individuals. The benefits of having a mentor, or more than one, are well documented, and one should consider them as one decides to find a mentor or enhance the role a mentor plays in one's career. This chapter can help readers evaluate the mentoring relationship and provide a structure for working with a mentor.

Research regarding mentorship shows that individuals who have a mentor, as compared to those not having a mentor, have

- Increased job satisfaction.
- Higher salaries.
- Enhanced self-esteem and confidence.
- Greater opportunities for promotion and advancement.
- Enhanced role socialization.
- A definitive career plan (Grindell, 2003).

MENTORSHIP MODEL

From the many definitions of a mentor, for this chapter the classic definition proposed by Vance (1982) is used. She defines a mentor as an experienced person who guides and nurtures a less experienced person (the mentee). The mentor is someone who inspires, instructs, nurtures, and encourages the mentee. Vance states that the mentoring relationship is a helping relationship that is special, emotional, intense, and enduring as opposed to shorter term and less intense relationships such as preceptor, sponsor, role model, or peer.

Figure 27-1 illustrates the Barker-Sullivan model of mentorship, which was devised through a review of the literature and through personal experiences of having a mentor and being a mentor. The relationship between the mentor and mentee can best be described as a partnership. In this partnership there is a congruency between the expertise and organizational connections of the mentor and the learning needs of the mentee. As a result of the relationship and interactions between the two, the mentee is energized for self-reflection, learning, and action, leading to professional role development and growth.

At the heart of this relationship there must be mutual trust and respect and open communications (Klein, 2002). The mentee will be

FIGURE 27-1 The Barker-Sullivan Model of Mentor Partnerships

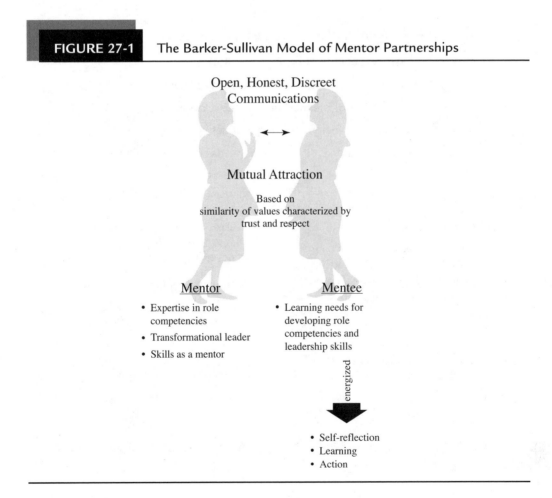

Open, Honest, Discreet
Communications

← →

Mutual Attraction

Based on
similarity of values characterized by
trust and respect

Mentor
- Expertise in role competencies
- Transformational leader
- Skills as a mentor

Mentee
- Learning needs for developing role competencies and leadership skills

energized

- Self-reflection
- Learning
- Action

disclosing sensitive information, exposing weaknesses, and discussing lack of skills and competence in job-related areas. Thus the mentee must feel that he or she can be open and honest and, in return, expect confidential, nonjudgmental, and sensitive feedback from the mentor.

STAGES OF THE MENTOR–MENTEE RELATIONSHIP

The mentor–mentee relationship ideally exists over a long period of time and, therefore, goes through several stages (Anderson et al., 2002). Each stage is discussed next. Readers can use this information to understand what to expect from a mentor–mentee relationship, or, for those who already have a mentor, use the information to assess their relationship.

Stage 1: Selecting a Mentor and Determining Expectations

Mentee-mentor relationships are formed in healthcare organizations in one of two ways, formally or informally. Some organizations have formal, structured mentorship programs established to assist new employees in developing their role. The benefit of a formal mentorship program is that it provides structure and well-defined expectations for both parties, as well as deploying organizational resources, particularly time, for the ongoing development of the relationship (Anderson et al., 2002).

Having a formal mentorship program does not preclude the mentee from initiating other informal mentor relationship(s). In fact, informal mentor relationships are often the best ones because at the heart of the mentor–mentee relationship is an attraction of both people whose personality and values fit. Informal mentor–mentee relationships happen because both the mentor and the mentee wish to work together and share mutual respect and admiration. This may or may not happen when one is assigned a mentor in a formal program.

There are many considerations as one decides who to ask to be a mentor. We offer several guidelines to assist in identifying appropriate individuals. First, one may find that there are several people to consider as mentors. Each of these individuals can bring something different to one's professional growth and development; therefore, no one should rule out having more than one mentor.

Second, we do not recommend choosing a direct supervisor or a potential supervisor. There are several reasons for this, the most important being that since the supervisor serves as an evaluator, the mentee may be reluctant to be vulnerable and share what he or she sees as weaknesses for fear that they will turn up on an official evaluation. However, to be an effective advanced practice nurse, the nurse does need to establish an effective and appropriate relationship with his or her supervisor. Having a mentor can help with this relationship and contribute to professional growth and learning.

A third consideration is whether to ask someone within or outside the organization to serve as a mentor. The pros of having an internal mentor are that the person knows the organization, can help make connections, can observe behaviors and outcomes, and may get indirect feedback about the mentee's performance from others. A mentor external to an organization, however, can offer new insights and different ways of doing things and can help make connections outside the organization.

A final consideration is whether to use a peer mentor or someone in an advanced position other than the supervisor position. The advantages of having a mentor from among peers are that the person is experiencing the issues and needs of the role in a similar way. Their network of connections may be more appropriate. A mentor at a higher level in the organization, however, can provide a broader view of the organization and a different level of connections with others.

In summary, it is worth considering having more than one mentor representing other disciplines, both genders, cultural and generational diversity, and professionals who work in other organizations. **Table 27-1** is a checklist for you to use in selecting someone as a mentor. The

TABLE 27-1 Mentor Selection Checklist

Name of Potential Mentor: _____

Brief explanation of why you are considering this person:_____

Desired Characteristic	Yes	No	Don't Know
1. Does the person have the expert knowledge and skills in the competencies that you need to develop?	❑	❑	❑
2. Is the person a leader by action and by example?	❑	❑	❑
3. Does this person have the ability to guide, coach, and teach you?	❑	❑	❑
4. Is the person respected in the organization?	❑	❑	❑
5. Does the person have access to important organizational information and can he or she help you to direct attention on important issues?	❑	❑	❑
6. Does the person have a network of influential people and is he or she willing to assist you to be visible, credible, and accepted by others in the organization?	❑	❑	❑
7. Is the person willing to work collaboratively with you?	❑	❑	❑
8. Is the person willing to spend the time and energy required for the development of this relationship?	❑	❑	❑
9. Are you comfortable with this person and do you trust him or her to hold confidentiality?	❑	❑	❑
10. Is the person able to provide you with negative as well as positive feedback?	❑	❑	❑
11. Can the person help you identify what you need to learn and provide the structure for learning activities?	❑	❑	❑

Summary statement:

_____

_____

first six questions focus on the person's leadership skills and role expertise. If the answer to any of these questions is "no," then we recommend reconsidering the person as a mentor. However, that person might have several important skills the mentee wishes to learn and the assessment might make it clear of what the potential mentor can and cannot offer. The last five questions relate to the person's ability to be an effective mentor.

After selecting a mentor(s), the next step is to establish ground rules. Borges and Smith (2004) provide a set of strategies to set up expectations for the relationship in this very early stage. First, they suggest setting up the details of when, where, and how long meetings will take place and which other forms of communication, such as email, should be used. Second, the mentee should write down long-term career goals/visions and use this information as a starting point for discussion and planning. The last strategy is to develop specific professional learning goals and personal goals. In the next section we discuss tools for assessing developmental needs and a form for documenting plans for meeting these needs and progress toward goals. In this process the mentee should also consider life goals such as salary, health, family, spiritual needs, and so forth. We believe that an advanced practice nurse must lead a balanced and happy life to be effective. A mentor can help set and pay attention to personal goals and help balance them with professional goals.

Stage 2: Development of Role Competencies

In stage 2, the mentee works on developmental goals by engaging in specific learning activities, with the guidance and support of the mentor. The mentor serves as teacher, advisor, facilitator, coach, and sounding board (Anderson et al., 2002). During this time the mentor connects the mentee to appropriate people both inside and outside the organization and helps the mentee develop the skills, knowledge, and attitudes to be effective.

Stage 3: Growing Independence

As time progresses, the mentee grows in confidence, gains the necessary knowledge and skills to be an effective advanced practice nurse, and demonstrates the attainment of the role competencies. At this point the mentee begins to seek independence, and the mentor role changes to consultant, giving advice only when asked (Anderson et al., 2002).

Stage 4: The Dissolution of the Relationship

In the last stage, the mentee is ready to move on from the relationship and no longer needs the mentor's advice and support. However, often an enduring friendship and colleagueship evolves and is maintained over the course of many years (Anderson et al., 2002).

MENTORSHIP VERSUS NETWORKING

Networking is interacting with individuals within and outside the organization to share ideas, information, and experiences, and to give and get advice. In contrast to mentoring, networking has less sustained interactions with others and is less structured. Having a network of people is as important for professional development as it is to have a mentor.

For networking to be effective, one needs to reflect on networking needs and set up processes to ensure that one interacts with people who can contribute to professional growth and development. First of all, one should think about people in the organization who can provide good insights about the organization, whose personality and values are similar to one's own, whose communication style is compatible, and who might be willing to share. In turn, the advanced practice nurse should think about people in the organization with whom he or she could share experiences and ideas. He or she should think about this broadly and include other disciplines and peers. Next, he or she simply needs to make contact with these people by asking them for coffee or lunch, or to stay after a meeting for a few minutes just to talk or to ask for their advice about a specific issue. As nurses establish a relationship with others, phone calls and email will assist them in maintaining contact even when they are busy. The key here is to be attentive about developing the networks, rather than just letting the relationships emerge. Further, the nurse and the person he or she networks with should establish guidelines for confidentiality, being clear what information can and cannot be shared.

Besides having a network within the organization, everyone should also establish a network of contacts outside the organization. Most often this occurs through professional organizations and meetings. The same thought process put into establishing an internal network should be used for establishing a network of people outside the organization. Contact with others should be made, and the contact should be maintained over time.

A MODEL OF CAREER DEVELOPMENT

In the next section of this chapter, we will discuss a process for assessing career development needs and planning for continual growth. These activities should provide a structure for a mentor and mentee to begin their initial work together. Our goal in this activity is for people to develop certain capabilities, including the following:

- Engaging in self-reflection and self-awareness
- Enhancing self-confidence
- Learning to take a broad systematic view of health care and one's organization
- Learning to work effectively within an organization and with others
- Developing the ability to think critically and creatively
- Engaging in experimental learning

Klein (2002) presents a model of career development that provides a useful framework for reflecting on career development needs. Most professional development programs place an emphasis on the development of individual skills and competencies and learning how the organization works while ignoring the vision and values of the individual and the organization. This model presents a more holistic view; the tools presented here were developed using this framework.

Table 27-2 has four quadrants to consider in looking at career development. Individual and collective aspects are placed along the vertical axis, while internal and external aspects are placed along the horizontal axis. Individual aspects are things to consider about oneself, whereas collective aspects deal with the organization and the larger world.

Quadrants 1 and 2 list individual aspects of career—internal and external, respectively. Quadrant 1 is the internal or self aspects. In this area nurses reflect on their individual values,

TABLE 27-2	Model of Career Development	
	Internal	External
Individual	*Quadrant 1* *Self* ■ Values ■ Purposes ■ Personal meaning	*Quadrant 2* *Your Behaviors* ■ Competencies ■ Skills ■ Knowledge ■ Leadership traits
Collective	*Quadrant 3* *Organizational Culture* ■ Vision ■ Shared values ■ Shared purpose ■ Relationships	*Quadrant 4* *The Environment* ■ Organizational structures and systems ■ Technology ■ The healthcare delivery system

Source: Klein, E. (2002, First Quarter). Missing something in your career? *Reflections on Nursing Leadership*, 41–42. Used with permission.

purposes, and the personal meaning that leadership and their profession have for them. In quadrant 2, the external individual aspects of career development (behaviors) reside and include the competencies and skills needed to perform a job or to obtain advanced positions.

Quadrants 3 and 4 attend to the collective aspects of one's career, both internal and external. In quadrant 3, the internal collective aspects of organizational culture include consideration of the shared values, shared purposes, and relationships that affect how one relates to others in the organization. Quadrant 4, the environment, includes the organizational structures and systems, policies and procedures, and technology in the organization.

It is useful to study Table 27-2 to gain a full understanding of career development needs. No one quadrant stands on its own. For instance, values and beliefs as an individual must be consistent with the values and purposes of the organization. Likewise, the external competencies and skills one develops must be pertinent to and useful for the work environment. These activities can maximize the chances of a good fit between the nurse and the organization, increasing role satisfaction.

PROCESS FOR CAREER DEVELOPMENT PLANNING

Using the career development model, we suggest a four-step career development planning process (Donner & Wheeler, 2001). **Table 27-3** and **Table 27-4** give two tools to integrate these steps with the model:

- Scan the environment (Table 27-3)
- Complete a self-assessment (Table 27-3)
- Create a career vision (Table 27-3)
- Develop a career plan (Table 27-4)

TABLE 27-3	Self-Assessment of Advanced Practice Nursing Development Needs

Section 1: Scan the Environment

1. What are the current realities about advanced practice nursing in your organization, your state, and in the nation? What are the future trends?

2. How do you see your strengths and weaknesses related to the needs of the healthcare environment and the organization and your role as an advanced practitioner?

3. What are the organization's vision and shared values, and how do you contribute to moving them forward?

Section 2: Self-Assessment

1. What are your personal values about your profession and about health care? How do you find meaning and purpose in your career and in your personal life?

2. Which strengths, experiences, and knowledge do you have to build on?

3. Which new experiences or knowledge do you need for the future?

4. What are your limitations?

Section 3: Career Vision

1. Where do you see yourself going?

2. What is stopping you? What are you doing about it?

| TABLE 27-4 | Professional Development Plan |

Goals	Plans	Timelines	Resources

The first section of Table 27-3 asks individuals to scan the environment and look at the organizational culture and the environmental considerations (quadrants 3 and 4 of Table 27-2) discussed in the model. This will help nurses to understand their developmental needs in a broad context of the overall environment of health care and professional nursing.

The second section of Table 27-3 is a self-assessment (quadrants 1 and 2 of Table 27-3) in which users are asked to assess their values and beliefs, skills, and knowledge needed for advanced practice.

In the third section of Table 27-3, users are asked to write down their overall career goal and vision. This will serve as a starting point in initiating conversations with a mentor about goals and learning needs.

PROFESSIONAL DEVELOPMENT PLAN

Based on the self-assessment, Table 27-4 can be used to develop an individualized professional development plan. Space is provided for goals, plans, timelines, and the resources to be used.

It is easy to pass over these activities and exercises, because one already has them in mind, but one of the keys to success is having written goals and plans and reviewing and revising them periodically. Completing these activities and exercises will help one to select a mentor who can assist with learning needs. Further, this self-assessment and plan should be reviewed and revised with a mentor at planned intervals and/or when the mentee has completed a significant accomplishment.

Goal setting has multiple benefits:

- The individual will feel that his or her future is positive and that he or she has control over where he or she is headed.
- The individual knows what he or she wants and how to get there.
- The individual has clear targets to focus on and to guide each day's actions and commitments.
- Daily actions will build into personal successes over time.

DISCUSSION QUESTIONS

1. Who are some individuals you currently know who may be a good mentor for you? Using Table 27-1, assess whether you should approach these persons about mentoring you.

2. Complete Tables 27-3 and 27-4 and discuss the similarities and differences of your plan with your peers.

REFERENCES

Anderson, M., Kroll, B., Luoma, J., Nelson, J., Sheman, K., & Surdo, J. (2002). Mentoring relationships. *Minnesota Nursing Accent, 74*(4).

Borges, J. R., & Smith, B. C. (2004, June). Strategies for mentoring a diverse nursing workforce. *Nurse Leader,* 45–48.

Donner, G. J., & Wheeler, M. M. (2001). Career planning and development for nurses: The time has come. *International Nursing Review, 48*(2), 79–86.

Grindell, C. G. (2003). Mentor managers. *Nephrology Nursing Journal, 30*(5), 517–522.

Klein, E. (2002). Missing something in your career? *Reflections on Nursing Leadership, 30*(1), 41–42.

Vance, C. (1982). The mentor connection. *Journal of Nursing Administration, 12*(4), 7–13.

CHAPTER 28

Managing Personal Resources: Time and Stress Management

Anne M. Barker

CHAPTER OBJECTIVES

1. Discuss the benefits of managing time and stress.
2. List strategies to management time and stress that can enhance work life.

INTRODUCTION

One of the recurring themes in the literature about nursing and the nursing shortage is the need for nurses to lead a balanced life. As one advances his or her career and expertise, this skill becomes even more vital especially when pursuing new goals and developing new expertise. By completing the exercises and assessments in this chapter, the reader should gain a better understanding of his or her strengths and weaknesses regarding time and stress management.

TIME MANAGEMENT

Time is one of the most precious resources that we have and one we can control. To be effective and efficient in one's role as an advanced practice nurse, one needs to manage time so as to spend it in professional activities that are meaningful and effective while at the same time gaining satisfaction and enjoyment in the role.

Benefits of Managing Time

The traditional view of time management is that time is a precious resource that must be managed. However, there is more to time management than only thinking of it as a resource. The most important benefits of time management are as follows (Barker, 1992):

- *Having clarity of mind.* When a nurse manages time well, he or she can have a clear, calm mind when confronted with the multiple demands of his or her role. In the confusion and disorder of daily activities and crises, nurses still must pay attention to the most important aspects of the job. If they are struggling to accomplish daily tasks and to keep on top of their workload, they will not have the peace of mind to reflect on their own practice, be there for others, and act proactively.

■ *Conserving personal energy.* Nurses have a limited amount of energy to use for the achievement of professional and personal goals, no matter how vigorous and energetic they are. Another goal of managing time is to minimize the number of demands on themselves at any one time to assure that they have adequate energy at all times.

■ *Nonverbal messaging about significance.* How nurses spend their time sends a message to others about what they think is important and what they do not think is important. It is in essence "walking the talk" or spending time on important activities.

■ *Contributing to feelings of well-being and happiness.* When an individual manages his or her time, he or she will feel more in control of his or her life, less stressed, and be less likely to experience burnout. In fact, personal success can be measured by how a person spends his or her time and if he or she is spending it on activities that bring meaning, satisfaction, and joy to his or her life.

Consequences of Poor Time Management

The consequences of not managing time well include the following problems:

■ *Being unable to manage oneself.*
■ *Negatively impacting others.* Others in the workplace can be negatively affected if someone does not complete his or her work and projects on time. People often rely on others' input and work to complete their work. It is simply unfair to others not to be timely in submission of one's own work (Barker, 1992).

Time Management: Self-Assessment

This section presents two approaches for assessing time management skills. Those persons who are experiencing any one of the following conditions should pay particular attention to this section:

■ Regularly exceeding the number of required hours spent on the job
■ Regularly taking work home and working in the evenings and on weekends
■ Feeling resentful about the amount of time that one must devote to his or her position
■ Not having clarity of mind
■ Constantly feeling rushed and out of control
■ Not having time for personal reflection and growth

The good news is that people can gain control over their time. Time management experts believe that people waste on average 2–3 hours per day as a result of ineffective use of time (Davenport, 1982). When an individual assesses how he or she uses time and adopts the suggested techniques, that person should be able to capture some of this wasted time for more meaningful and important activities.

We suggest engaging in two activities to assess time management strengths and weaknesses. The first is to do a brief self-assessment (see **Table 28-1**). After completing the assessment, those who score a 3 or less in any area should pay particular attention in their reading about those areas.

The second way for someone to assess how he or she is spending time is to keep a time log for at least 1 week. This is a more detailed assessment but is well worth the effort. It is best to keep a time management log for both organizational time and personal time, since the goal is to have a balance between both aspects of life.

Table 28-2 is a time log format that can be used for completing this activity. Column 1 identifies the beginning and ending time for an

TABLE 28-1 Assessment Tool for Time Management

Use the following scoring system for each answer below.

1 = Never

2 = Rarely

3 = Occasionally

4 = Usually

5 = Always

Place an X in the appropriate column.

	1	2	3	4	5
1. I feel calm and in control of my time.	❏	❏	❏	❏	❏
2. I am aware of fluctuations in my energy level and perform my most challenging tasks when my energy level is at its highest.	❏	❏	❏	❏	❏
3. I spend the majority of my time in meaningful work that contributes to the positive work on my clinical unit.	❏	❏	❏	❏	❏
4. I spend the majority of my time in activities that I find satisfying.	❏	❏	❏	❏	❏
5. I complete my paperwork and projects on time.	❏	❏	❏	❏	❏
6. I follow through on promises I make to my staff, boss, and others.	❏	❏	❏	❏	❏
7. I have written daily goals.	❏	❏	❏	❏	❏
8. I delegate tasks to others in my clinical unit.	❏	❏	❏	❏	❏
9. I assess tasks for their importance and their urgency.	❏	❏	❏	❏	❏
10. I keep a "to do" list and schedule time to complete the tasks on the list.	❏	❏	❏	❏	❏
11. I set aside time each week to complete paperwork and other tasks.	❏	❏	❏	❏	❏
12. I am able to control interruptions.	❏	❏	❏	❏	❏
13. I embrace the philosophy "do today instead of putting off until tomorrow."	❏	❏	❏	❏	❏
14. I set aside time each day for planning.	❏	❏	❏	❏	❏
15. I have written long-term goals.	❏	❏	❏	❏	❏

activity. There should be an entry for every activity switch. In column 2, the individual completing the log states what the activity is and who is involved in this activity with him or her. In column 3, he or she states the purpose of the activity. (This is to help determine if the person is spending time in activities that he or she deems important for the leadership of the unit versus mundane and even unmeaningful tasks.) The user indicates his or her energy level in column 4: L for low, M for medium, and H for high. (The purpose of reflecting on energy level is to analyze whether the individual is doing his or her most important work when his or her energy level is highest.) In column 5, the individual notes whether he or she was interrupted while completing the activity and indicates who interrupted and the reason for the interruption. Each interruption can be rated as very important (VI), important (I), or of little importance (LI).

In the last column, the person includes notes about the effectiveness of how the individual spent his or her time as soon as possible after the event or at the end of the day. One might ask oneself the following questions when completing this column:

- Was this activity directly related to my role in the organization and/or assuring positive patient outcomes?
- Could the task have been done in a better way or delegated?

- Did I spend too much or not enough time on the activity? Was I able to complete the task?
- Was the task performed at the right time in relationship to my energy level?

At the end of the week, the nurse should perform an analysis of the entire week. in addition to the preceding questions, the nurse should ask these questions:

- What percentage of my time is spent in work, family, home, social, spiritual, and physical activities? Do I have the balance of these that I want?
- What percentage of my time is spent in activities that are important or urgent?
- With whom am I spending time, and are they the most appropriate people to help me reach my goals?
- What are my main interruptions? Assess the percentage of time they fall into each of the categories: very important, important, not important. How can I decrease the number of unimportant interruptions?
- What are my biggest time wasters?
- Are there any activities I can reduce or eliminate?
- Is there anything I can delegate to others or simplify?
- Can I save time by grouping related tasks?
- Were there any tasks that I had put off and then felt pressure to complete?

TABLE 28-2   Time Management Log

Time	Activity/ People	Purpose	Energy Level	Interruptions	Effectiveness of the Time Spent

This activity can be completed annually or more often if a time management tune-up is needed. It will help identify areas of improvement and suggest what else can be done in the future. Time management is not easy, and everyone will experience setbacks and days when they will not feel they have managed their time well. It takes constant care and attention to be a good manager of time.

Strategies for Managing Time

Based on the self-assessment and the findings from the time management log, several of the strategies discussed in this section will provide leverage in managing time. The conventional wisdom is that it is using these strategies collectively, not in isolation of one another, that will give the best results (Seaward, 2004).

Goal Setting and Planning

Most time management experts agree that goal setting and planning are the premier time management strategies. In this section, ways to plan for goal achievement are suggested.

First, individuals should write down their goals. Once they have written goals, they should carry them in a day planner, personal digital assistant (PDA), or a handheld computer. They should do two complementary things with these written goals. First, they should look at their goals daily to keep them fresh in their mind. By doing so, they will be more sensitive to opportunities that will help them reach their goals.

At the beginning of each day, individuals should have a list of activities to accomplish that day to move toward their written goals. It is not easy to set realistic daily goals; at first it is common to plan more than one can accomplish, but as time progresses most people will get better at this task. Most important, people should not get frustrated if they do not accomplish every task every day. In fact, one time management principle suggests that a task will consume the time that has been allotted for it. Therefore, planning an aggressive schedule is a

good strategy as long as the person does not get frustrated about not accomplishing everything he or she set out to do.

Barker (1992) suggests a number of guidelines to follow when setting goals:

- Goals should include all aspects of life, including work, family, social, financial, spiritual, physical, and psychological areas.
- Goals should be measurable and achievable, yet challenging.
- In determining realistic goals, organizational constraints, resources, and personal strengths and skills should be considered.
- Time frames for goal completion should be realistic but should not allow for procrastination. Timelines can be reassessed and new deadlines set, and new goals can be added or old ones dropped when appropriate.
- Individuals should reward themselves upon completion of goals.
- People should pursue goals with enthusiasm, even when they are not feeling enthusiastic.

Scheduling

Nurses should have a calendar/day planner/PDA in which to schedule meetings, make plans for time to accomplish tasks, keep goals, and have an ongoing "to do" list. Each day when they review their goals, they should also review their schedule and block in time to accomplish daily tasks and work on long-term goals.

Nurses not only need to see what the schedule for each day is, but also need a broader view of the week and month. They can put deadlines into the planner and block out times to work on projects or paperwork to accomplish them in a timely manner. There are two benefits to doing this: This approach assures that nurses have a plan to get their work completed on time, and they do not have to worry needlessly about when and how they are going to accomplish it.

Prioritizing Tasks: Urgent Versus Important

A useful way of prioritizing a daily list of goals and tasks is to consider whether the task is important or not important and whether it is urgent or not urgent. **Figure 28-1** provides a template to assess the importance and urgency of tasks to help prioritize daily activities accordingly. On the vertical axis is a rating of urgency from low to high; on the horizontal axis is a rating of importance from low to high. The grid prioritizes tasks by importance first and urgency second. The user should place each activity in one of the four quadrants. He or she should first complete the tasks in quadrant I—those that rate a high urgency and high importance score. Next, he or she should complete the activities in quadrant II, which are high in importance but low in urgency. Next, he or she should complete the activities in quadrant III, which are low in importance and high in urgency. Finally, he or she should complete those tasks low in urgency and importance.

Another complementary way to prioritize daily activities is to understand the Pareto principle, also known as the 80/20 rule. This principle suggests that 80% of positive, satisfying outcomes are a result of just 20% of the time spent. In other words, paying attention to important tasks will give 80% of the results. This principle is useful for assigning importance to each task in the grid. It also suggests that even minor changes to time management skills can produce dramatic results.

Delegation

Delegation is an important skill for being able to accomplish one's work and goals. Before a nurse can successfully delegate to others, however, he or she needs to think about his or her attitude and values about delegating. Here are some useful ways to think positively about delegation:

- Delegation is a trust-building activity.
- Delegation builds the confidence and self-esteem of others.
- Delegation unburdens one from routine, mundane tasks to provide the time for important activities and relationship building.
- Delegation helps others to grow, learn, and become leaders as they see more of the big picture.
- Delegation is an important tool in succession planning.
- Delegation can match the right person with the right expertise to the right job.

The process of delegation involves looking at the task(s) a nurse plans to delegate and the people to whom she or he will delegate. Some

---

FIGURE 28-1 Assessing Tasks for Importance and Urgency

	Quadrant III Low Importance High Urgency	Quadrant I High Importance High Urgency
URGENCY	Quadrant IV Low Importance Low Urgency	Quadrant II High Importance Low Urgency

High ↑ URGENCY ↓ Low

Low ← Importance → High

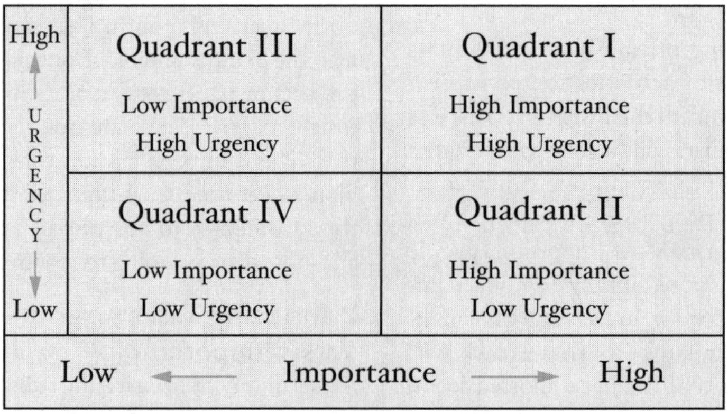

tasks should not be delegated. These items include organizational functions and meetings that the nurse attends or leads, or personnel matters including rewarding people, conflict management, and so forth if they fall within the purview of his or her job. Eliminating these tasks from the delegation possibilities leaves the nurse with a substantial number of routine tasks that he or she might possibly delegate.

The next step is to consider the individuals to whom he or she might delegate. The nurse should judge the expertise, strengths, knowledge, interests, skills, and attitudes of the staff. These should match the job to be done. When delegating, one also needs to be sensitive to the workload of the person to whom one is delegating. Giving the person the ability to negotiate what he or she will do and when it will be done and the appropriate time to complete the delegated task is essential for success.

The process used to delegate is important. First, the person who is being assigned a task needs to understand its importance, why it is being delegated, and what the requirements and guidelines are. He or she will need appropriate information and resources such as time, space, and money to complete the task. He or she should be aware of dates for task completion and periodic evaluation if the task extends over a long time period. As difficult as this may be to delegate, the results of the assignment are more important than the means by which the person completes them, as long as he or she completes the task consistent with organizational policies and works with others in a positive manner.

Throughout the process of task completion, the person who assigned the task must be available to give advice, support, and guidance. Once the task is completed an appropriate reward needs to be given.

Allowing Oneself Private Time

An oft-spoken value for which nurses take great pride is having an open-door policy. There is a difference between having an open-door policy and having the door open all the time. One of the most effective time management strategies is to schedule and set aside time every week to close your door and to get required paperwork and tasks completed. Everyone should review their calendar and find a time when they do not have meetings and book in private time for 2–4 hours per week in one to two blocks of time for the next 6 months.

Controlling Interruptions

On average, we experience one interruption every 8 minutes or approximately seven per hour. In an 8-hour day, that totals around 50–60 interruptions in the day. The average interruption takes approximately 5 minutes. If someone has 50 interruptions in the day and each takes 5 minutes, that totals 250 minutes, or 50% of the workday. Moreover, most people will discover that only about 20% of their interruptions are important or very important. Thus, if an individual experiences 250 minutes of interruptions in a day and 80% have little value, then 3 hours per day is being consumed by interruptions that are not worthy of his or her time (Wetmore, 1999).

This math shows how one can capture time. People should go back over their time logs and try to identify patterns in their interruptions, the time they spend dealing with them, and if there are people who tend to take more of their time than others. After this analysis, they can then set some strategies to decrease their interruptions. For example, if one person interrupts more than others, it might be necessary to schedule time with this person periodically and ask that individual to have a list of items to discuss rather than ask for time on the fly.

Procrastination and Perfectionism

Procrastination—delaying what needs to be done until the last minute—is often referred to as "putting off until tomorrow what I should have done today." Procrastination can take several forms, including knowingly doing something other than what needs to be done;

starting to work on a project, but then stopping work on it, only to have to complete it at the last minute; or doing less difficult tasks rather than the required one (Seaward, 2004). Being aware of a tendency toward procrastination is important in understanding time management skills and strategies. Scheduling, maintaining to-do lists, and adhering to them can help break this habit.

A different, but parallel problem is being a perfectionist. Perfectionists generally get caught up in the details and never see the whole picture; thus they waste time (Seaward, 2004). Further, believing that one should and can be perfect is detrimental to one's self-esteem. No one can be perfect. When an individual holds himself or herself up to a standard of perfection and does not meet this standard, he or she then feels as if he or she failed. Recognizing a tendency to want to be perfect and moderating it is important not only to time management but also to self-esteem.

One way to reduce a need to be perfect is to consider what is good enough. To do this, one must make a judgment about the level of perfection/accuracy required for the specific task.

Managing Communications

Reading and responding to email can consume a large portion of time. Here are several hints for making the task more meaningful and less time consuming:

- One should read email one to two times per day depending on one's schedule and the volume received. One should not have email constantly on and interrupting.

- Individuals should set up folders for emails from important people, about meetings, or tasks to be done.

- Email users should keep the inbox uncluttered by reading and responding to messages, then moving those emails to an appropriate folder if they need to keep them for the future. Otherwise, they should immediately delete emails that do not need to be saved.

- Everyone should respond immediately to emails that need short responses (2 minutes or less) and then move the emails or delete them.

- One should read emails that are marked as urgent first.

- Nurses should sort email by sender and read emails from their boss and other important contacts in the organization next.

- If an email cannot be responded to quickly and one does not have time to answer it, schedule time for a response at a later time. One should print the email as a reminder to follow up.

Managing phone calls is another important time management technique. Phone conversations can be much more pertinent and personal than emails, but everyone should learn to keep their calls to less than 5 minutes. The downside of phone calls is that we often find ourselves playing phone tag, which can be a time waster. When someone leaves a person voicemail, he or she should specify a good time for the person to return the call so as to increase the possibility of being available when the person calls.

A nurse who has a support person who answers the phone should give instructions for how to handle phone calls. Whoever is taking calls should be able to screen calls and refer the caller to the appropriate person. The support person can find out when a convenient time is to return the call or can even schedule a phone appointment if the person keeps the nurse's calendar. The nurse can also instruct on how to communicate availability. For example, saying that "she is not on the unit" is a different message than saying "she is at x meeting and I expect her back in an hour."

STRESS MANAGEMENT

As healthcare professionals, nurses should already be familiar with the physiology of stress and stress-related diseases. Stress management is a life skill. Although it is important to success as an advanced nurse practitioner, much stress management occurs outside the workplace. No doubt nurses already use many different techniques to reduce their stress. In this section we look briefly at occupational stressors and provide some stress management techniques.

Occupational Stress

The National Safety Council (Seaward, 1994) lists many causes of job stress. How someone experiences and reacts to these stressors varies from person to person. **Table 28-3** can be used to assess job-related stress based on the reasons identified by the National Safety Council. After

---

TABLE 28-3 Assessment Tool for Occupational Stress

Use the following scoring system for each answer below.

1 = Never

2 = Rarely

3 = Occasionally

4 = Usually

5 = Always

Place an X in the appropriate column.

	1	2	3	4	5
1. I have too much responsibility with little or no authority.	❑	❑	❑	❑	❑
2. The organization sets unrealistic expectations and deadlines that I am unable to meet.	❑	❑	❑	❑	❑
3. I do not feel adequately trained for my position.	❑	❑	❑	❑	❑
4. I do not feel appreciated.	❑	❑	❑	❑	❑
5. I am not able to voice concerns.	❑	❑	❑	❑	❑
6. I have too much to do with too few resources.	❑	❑	❑	❑	❑
7. I lack a clear understanding of what is expected of me.	❑	❑	❑	❑	❑
8. I have a difficult time keeping pace with technology.	❑	❑	❑	❑	❑
9. The physical environment in which I work has poor lighting, a lot of noise, and poor ventilation.	❑	❑	❑	❑	❑
10. There is the possibility of workplace violence.	❑	❑	❑	❑	❑
11. People in the organization have experienced sexual harassment and racial discrimination.	❑	❑	❑	❑	❑
12. The organization has recently downsized or restructured.	❑	❑	❑	❑	❑
13. Creativity and autonomy are not valued.	❑	❑	❑	❑	❑

an individual completes the assessment, he or she should look closely at items that he or she rated 3 or more before reading the next section.

A Stress Management Model

People have many ways of dealing with stress. Those who read this section should note the techniques that appeal to them. Using a mix of techniques can help readers be more effective in dealing with stress. These techniques fall into three categories: altering behaviors to deal more effectively with stress, avoiding stress, or accepting stress (Tubesing & Tubesing, 1983). We recommend selecting at least one strategy from each category as a beginning point. Some of the techniques require behavioral approaches to managing stress while others require a change of thinking.

The purpose of stress management is to adopt coping skills. Coping is defined as the process of managing demands that are perceived by the person as demanding or exceeding the individual's resources. The purpose of coping skills can be to reduce the harmful effects of the stressor, to be able to better tolerate or adjust to negative events, to maintain a positive self-image, and to keep emotional equilibrium while maintaining satisfying relationships with others (Lazarus, 1999).

Altering Techniques

Many stressors cannot be eliminated, but techniques can be used to alter how one deals with stress:

- Problem solving
- Communication
- Having the right information
- Time management, priority setting, and planning
- Conflict management (Tubesing & Tubesing, 1983; Seaward, 2004)

Avoidance Techniques

A second set of strategies to deal with stress suggests avoiding stress, rather than altering one's reactions to it as just discussed:

- Using an assertive communications style
- Saying "no" and walking away
- Letting go
- Delegating tasks
- Being aware of personal limitations and energy (Tubesing & Tubesing, 1983)

Acceptance Techniques

Acceptance techniques fall into two different categories. The first comprises techniques to build up resistance to stress, and the second includes cognitive approaches to change one's perception of the stress.

Building Resistance to Stress

These techniques are probably most familiar as stress management techniques. They include such things as diaphragmatic breathing, meditation, yoga, music, massage, progressive muscular relaxation, nutrition, physical exercise, engaging in creative activities or hobbies, humor, and prayer.

Changing Perceptions of Stress

A second set of techniques are cognitive ones that help one deal more effectively with stress by changing one's perceptions of both oneself and one's reactions to stress. This set of techniques includes the following measures:

- Being optimistic and positive, rather than negative
- Using visualization and affirmation, including positive self-talk
- Journal writing for self-expression and self-awareness
- Practicing forgiveness (Tubesing & Tubesing, 1983; Seaward, 2004)

DISCUSSION QUESTIONS ——————

1. What are the pros and cons of the time and stress management strategies discussed in this chapter? Do you have others to add that have been successful for you?

2. If you completed a time management log, what were your findings and what strategies will you adapt to improve your time management skills?

3. Review the information regarding stress management. Realistically, how much stress are you experiencing? Which strategies will you try to help you cope with stress?

REFERENCES

Barker, A. M. (1992). *Transformational nursing leadership: A vision for the future.* New York: National League for Nursing.

Davenport, R. (1982). *Making time, making money: A step by step process for setting your goals and achieving success.* New York: St. Martin's Press.

Lazarus, R. (1999). *Stress and emotion: A new synthesis.* New York: Springer.

Seaward, B. L. (1994). *National Safety Council's stress management.* Sudbury, MA: Jones and Bartlett Publishers.

Seaward, B. L. (2004). *Managing stress: Principles and strategies for health and well-being* (4th ed.). Sudbury, MA: Jones and Bartlett Publishers.

Tubesing, N., & Tubesing, D. (1983). *Structured exercises in stress management.* Duluth, MN: Whole Person Press.

Wetmore, D. E. (1999). The big hole in your day. Retrieved February 15, 2005, from http://www.balancetime.com/articles/hole_in_your_day.htm

CHAPTER 29

Role Transition: Strategies for Success in the Marketplace

Audrey Beauvais

CHAPTER OBJECTIVES

1. Discuss strategies to facilitate role transition and acquisition.

2. Conduct a personal, marketplace, and organizational analysis when transitioning to the job market.

3. Identify components of a professional portfolio.

4. Develop a curriculum vitae.

5. Review interviewing skills and techniques.

6. Recognize opportunities to foster professional development following graduation.

INTRODUCTION

Advanced practice nurses first began working in the United States more than four decades ago (Lindblad, Hallman, Gillsjo, Lindblad, & Foerstrom, 2010; U.S. Department of Health and Human Services Health Resources and Services Administration, 2010). Currently, nurse practitioners are an established professional group in approximately 30 countries and on every continent (Lindblad et al.). Sources estimate that there are between 140,000 and 158,000 nurse practitioners in the United States, which is more than a 12% increase over the numbers reported 4 years earlier (American Academy of Nurse Practitioners, 2010a; U.S. Department of Health and Human Services Health Resources and Services Administration).

Nurse practitioners are in great demand as they provide cost-effective, high-quality, patient-centered health care in a wide variety of settings to a diverse range of consumers (American Academy of Nurse Practitioners,

2007; Bryant-Lukosius & DiCenso, 2004). Nurse practitioners are well equipped and prepared to provide the patient-centered care that is vital to achieving the current and upcoming primary care needs of the United States (American Academy of Nurse Practitioners, 2007). Nurse practitioners are a viable answer to the developing movement toward health and wellness that has been promoted by the consumer need and demand (American Academy of Nurse Practitioners, 2010b). Of interest, the American Academy of Nurse Practitioners has reported that nurse practitioners are the fastest-growing professional group within the primary care labor force. Furthermore, this professional organization predicts that demand for nurse practitioners will continue to increase because they offer a practical solution to the problem of fewer doctors going into the area of family practice (American Academy of Nurse Practitioners, 2010c).

To meet the demand for nurse practitioners, it is essential that they be given the tools necessary to promote a successful transition into advanced nursing practice. The transition from the student nurse practitioner role to the employed nurse practitioner is a critical time. During nurse practitioner programs, students proceed through a step-like progression of clinical knowledge and clinical skills as well as encounter significant life transitions in their social and professional status (Barton, 2007). Identifying and distinguishing the transitional experiences will help nurse practitioners know what to expect (Barton). As such, this chapter discusses the specific transitional phases the nurse practitioner can expect to encounter as well as practical strategies that can facilitate the graduate's professional adjustment to the role of advanced practice nursing (Cleary, Matheson, & Happell, 2009).

If nurse practitioners are to meet the market demand, then they will need to have knowledge and skills that will enable them to obtain a suitable employment. This chapter is intended to help nurse practitioners who are entering the job market by addressing how to find employment opportunities, how to complete several different assessments to prepare the nurse practitioner for the job market, how to develop a professional portfolio, and how to apply for a job. Considering that some nurse practitioner specialties have noted difficulty with retention (Pye, 2011), the nurse practitioner-organization fit assessment discussed in this chapter will be of particular interest.

Once they are employed, it is essential that nurse practitioners put structures and strategies in place to promote their growth and development. To this end, the chapter identifies ways to foster the nurse practitioner's professional development. After all, continuing professional development should be part of all nurse practitioners' lifelong learning plan.

TRANSITIONING ROLES

The role transition from registered nurse to advanced practice nurse can be a challenging journey (Cleary et al., 2009; Spoelstra & Robbins, 2010). Having realistic expectations about the new roles and responsibilities will help alleviate the nurse practitioner's angst associated with this evolution (Cleary et al.). Experiencing a positive transition between roles will help facilitate the advanced practice nurse's ability to achieve independency, self-sufficiency, and influence over his or her professional practice (Cleary et al.). In addition, it will help foster a sense of worth and identity within the profession of nursing (Cleary et al.).

The role transition from registered nurse to advanced practice nurse begins during the educational preparation and goes right through the first few years of practice (Barton, 2007). Some scholars have proposed that this transition happens in a three-stage composite model of social, cultural, and professional components that involve identity loss, transitional role evolution, and incorporation into clinical practice (Barton, 2007). The following subsections briefly describe the three components.

Identity Loss Phase

Identity loss happens early in nurse practitioners' educational program (Barton, 2007). Nurse practitioner students become cognizant that they are both novice student nurse practitioners and experienced, practicing, professional nurses (Barton; Spoelstra & Robbins, 2010). For the student nurse practitioners to progress in their transition, it is necessary for the students to re-examine and separate from their prior career status (Barton). However, nurse practitioner students often attend school part-time (Baron; Lindblad et al., 2010). Hence, it is difficult for them to completely disengage from their previous professional role, as they are functioning in that role as part of their ongoing nursing employment (Barton; Lindblad et al.). This duality can enhance the feeling of identity loss (Barton; Lindblad et al.; Spoelstra & Robbins, 2010). The perception of identity loss is advanced through these learning transitions, which enable the students to acquire new knowledge and skills that affect their clinical practice within their current nursing role (Barton; Lindblad et al.; Spoelstra & Robbins). Interestingly, during this phase nurse practitioner students tend to have intensified consciousness of the anxieties among their colleagues, which can help foster cohesion and a unique group identity (Barton).

Transitional Role Evolution

The uncertainty of nurse practitioner professional identity can increase as student nurse practitioners cope with the increasing duality of roles (Barton). During the transition role evolution phase, student nurse practitioners experience a sense of role limbo and at times feel invisible and/or inept (Barton). Fortunately, during this stage, student nurses have developed a strong sense of community and group identity (Barton). This mutual support is critical, as they often experience opposition and aggression from professionals in the healthcare field (Barton). The camaraderie and support from fellow peers allows them to become competent in their new skill sets (Barton). The transition

phase and sense of community often emerge at the midpoint of the academic preparation (Barton). After this time, the sense of unity gradually decreases as the students anticipate graduation from the program (Barton). This trend helps foster resocialization into the new professional role as the students grow individually and develop their new identities (Barton). The end of the transition phase is denoted by the students' independence and self-reliance as well as decreased group cohesion (Barton).

Incorporation Phase

During the incorporation phase, which begins during the latter part of nurse practitioners' studies, students begin to resolve their issues regarding their new role in their clinical practice (Barton). By the time their studies are completed, APNs have increased confidence and security in their new clinical role (Lindblad et al., 2010). Throughout this phase, students start to look at practical problems and begin to select role models (Barton). These role models may be from both the medicine and nursing disciplines, allowing the nurse practitioner to take various traits and develop them into the new role construct (Barton). During this stage, their relationships with their medical peers change (Barton). For example, nurse practitioners may begin to describe a reciprocal trust and confidence between themselves and the general medical practitioners who serve as their role models and supervisors (Lindblad et al.). The medical staff become aware of the skills the nurse practitioner has acquired and note those areas in which the nurse practitioner requires additional guidance (Lindblad et al.). This changing clinical relationship tends to support mutual admiration and increasing collegiality (Barton).

Students' licensure exam is perceived as the final initiation and source of legitimacy of their new clinical role (Barton). Although they are still novices who are developing their professional identity in clinical practice, after passing their licensing examination they are qualified nurse practitioners.

STRATEGIES FOR A SUCCESSFUL TRANSITION

A successful transition begins with competent, knowledgeable nurse practitioners who demonstrate critical thinking, self-awareness, and effective interpersonal and leadership skills. To promote successful role transition, nurse practitioners should utilize a framework that emphasizes evidence-based practice, research, collaboration, and consultation as a way to inform nursing practice (Spoelstra & Robbins, 2010). Additionally, nurse practitioners must provide patient care that is grounded in evidence and theory while viewing the patient holistically and deserving of comprehensive treatment (Spoelstra & Robbins). Finally, nurse practitioners need to demonstrate comprehension and exemplification of professional responsibilities (Spoelstra & Robbins). To be successful, nurse practitioners will need to demonstrate leadership skills grounded in ethical values. Not only will they need to be knowledgeable in their area of clinical practice, but they will also have to communicate effectively with others, identify goals, determine effective strategies to accomplish those goals, role-model professional behavior, and collaborate with others to improve patient and financial outcomes (Spoelstra & Robbins).

Ideally, nurse practitioners' academic programs will implement strategies to help foster the development of the previously mentioned characteristics. However, once they have graduated, it is essential for nurse practitioners to function within a supportive learning milieu that continues to encourage the synthesis of knowledge and critical thinking (Forbes et al., 2006; Heitz, Steiner, & Burman, 2004). Once in the new working environment, nurse practitioners can ensure a smooth transition by understanding the expectations associated with being a nurse practitioner (Stahl & Myers, 2002).

Not only do nurse practitioners need to understand the expectations of their role, but they also may need to overcome some barriers—such as a lack of knowledge about the nurse practitioner's scope of practice, lack of knowledge about the nurse practitioner's role, negative physician attitudes, lack of respect, poor communication, and patient and family reluctance to accept nurse practitioner care—if they want to facilitate a positive transition (Clarin, 2007). Fortunately, several useful strategies to overcome these barriers are easily implemented. For example, nurse practitioners can provide formal and informal education and orientation to physicians and medical students on nurse practitioners' scope of practice and roles (Clarin). In addition, they can develop and utilize integrated collaboration models when establishing a new nurse practitioner position within a particular organization or practice. Furthermore, nurse practitioners can attend interdisciplinary rounds to visibly show the patients and families their involvement with the medical management of care (Clarin). Moreover, nurse practitioners can advocate for medical students to be exposed to graduate nursing students early in their education as well as advocate for uniformity in nurse practitioner education and certification (Clarin). An essential part of overcoming these barriers and, therefore, of ensuring a successful transition is to demonstrate and showcase the positive outcomes that nurse practitioners can foster, such as decreased length of hospital stay, improved medical management resulting in decreased numbers of unnecessary office visits, more comprehensive patient education, improved health maintenance, and greater patient satisfaction (Clarin).

A smooth transition can also be fostered by novice nurse practitioners selecting preceptors who can help assure sufficient socialization and encourage the nurse practitioners' feelings of self-worth (Hayes, 1998). Mentors can certainly provide additional teaching of clinical skills if needed (Hayes). Moreover, they can help expose nurse practitioners to additional aspects of their role and boost their confidence in their capability to assume the role (Hayes). Novice nurse practitioners are more apt to assimilate other facets of the nurse practitioner role when they observe their preceptors in action (Hayes).

Finally, reflective journaling can be used as a strategy for promoting a successful transition. Reflective journaling can help novice nurse practitioners transition successfully into an expert role by keeping a written record in which they contemplate their professional experiences and learn from the process (Hamric & Taylor, 1989; Latham & Fahey, 2006). The method used can be as simple as daily written reflections on the following four questions: (1) What happened today? (2) What did I think about that? (3) How do I feel about it? (4) What did I learn? The very act of analyzing thoughts, ideas, and feelings helps to develop metacognitive skills by assisting nurse practitioners to self-evaluate and discern what they know versus what they have yet to learn. Such reflection, which addresses their cognitive, psychomotor, and emotional growth, will help nurse practitioners identify potential educational strategies to help them advance their professional development. The practice of analyzing the nurse practitioner's thoughts and feelings is especially useful for learning how to handle complicated situations that exceed a straightforward right or wrong response. A reflective journal can assist nurse practitioners in recognizing their capabilities, professional worth, and future educational needs critical to the development of their new nurse practitioner role (Latham & Fahey). Reflective journals can also be a positive way to map the nurse practitioner's growth and development (Latham & Fahey).

ENTERING THE JOB MARKET

To complete the transition from students to expert nurse practitioners working in the healthcare field, graduating nurse practitioner students will need to secure their first position. This section discusses some practical aspects to entering the job market, such as how to find open positions. In addition, it reviews the personal, marketplace, organization, and nurse practitioner–organization fit assessments that nurse practitioners should complete to prepare them for the job market. Furthermore, it presents practical ideas for developing a portfolio that can be shared with potential employers to highlight the possible benefits nurse practitioners can offer an organization. Additionally, specifics about applying for a job such as applications and interviews are reviewed.

Finding Nurse Practitioner Openings

A first step with regard to entering the job market is to locate nurse practitioner job openings. Nurse practitioners can find openings via print and online resources, professional memberships, and networking. These strategies are discussed next.

Print and Online Resources

Nurse practitioner job openings can be found via multiple media (Vilorio, 2011). The traditional way to find jobs has been in printed classified advertisements (Vilorio). Today, however, few practices or organizations post nurse practitioner job openings only in printed advertisements, if they publish them in printed form at all (Vilorio). Instead, most nurse practitioner job postings appear on the Internet (Vilorio). Job boards such as AdvancedPracticeJobs.com and nursepractitionerJobs.com may be of use (Vilorio). However, bear in mind that national job boards will attract larger numbers of job-seekers (Vilorio). As a result, the national job boards may not produce the results that nurse practitioners would like (Vilorio). Experts warn that it is difficult for nurse practitioners to differentiate themselves online; as such, it is more useful to follow leads through contacts and thorough research (Vilorio).

Professional Memberships

An initial step in nurse practitioners' job search should be to get involved in professional organizations such as the American Academy of Nurse Practitioners and the American College of Nurse Practitioners (Critchley, 2003; Hosking, 2010;

Mize, 2011a). Although paying dues may not be what a new practitioner wants to hear, it will be a key function in a successful job search as well as a successful career (Mize, 2011a). Actively participating on committees within their professional organizations will help develop nurse practitioners' knowledge about the national agenda and expose them to key issues and important individuals in the field (Critchley).

Networking

Referrals are one of the key ways of finding nurse practitioner employment opportunities, even for positions that are not being publicized (Hosking, 2010). In fact, research results indicate that approximately 70% of job postings are never advertised publicly (Owens & Young, 2008). In addition, referrals will help raise nurse practitioners' chances of having their curriculum vitae placed directly in front of the employer who is hiring (Hosking). Practices and organizations are apt to hire individuals with whom they are familiar and who are recommended by someone they trust (Vilorio, 2011). For this reason, it is suggested that nurse practitioners develop a network of professionals in the healthcare field (Hosking; Vilorio). A network involves cultivating relationships that are mutually beneficial (Owens & Young). Remember—it is not about who the nurse practitioner knows but who knows the nurse practitioner that will make a difference (Owens & Young).

When meeting individuals, it is imperative that nurse practitioners elicit feelings of liking, trusting, and knowing to establish a good rapport and relationship (Owens & Young, 2008). When nurse practitioners initially interact with individuals, they should ask these persons about themselves and their careers rather than immediately inquiring how they can get a job (Owens & Young). Having a personal contact may just get nurse practitioners the desired opportunity (Hosking, 2010; Vilorio, 2011). In addition to the professional healthcare network, nurse practitioners can utilize other contacts such as professors, alumni networks, former classmates, colleagues, family, friends, and employers both past and present (Mize, 2011a; Vilorio). Nurse practitioners should start developing their professional network while they are students (Vilorio). This can be done by becoming active in professional organizations, participating in professional conferences, attending continuing education programs, and partaking in volunteer work (Vilorio).

One of the benefits of networking is that it allows nurse practitioners the chance to create contacts with potential employers as well as to determine the work environment and employee morale in that organization or practice (Critchley, 2003; Vilorio). One word of caution is in order, however: Professional contacts will become leery if nurse practitioners talk about specific job opportunities before they have established a good rapport and trusted relationship (Vilorio). This kind of relationship can take some time to develop and foster (Vilorio). It is important to show genuine interest in each contact and learn about the individual and his or her job. For example, it is appropriate to ask what contacts' responsibilities are, what the most rewarding and challenging aspects of the role are, and what the work environment is like (Vilorio).

Nurse practitioners should take care to organize their networks (Owens & Young, 2008). One suggestion is to keep a file that lists all the contacts and identifies a little something of note about each person (Owens & Young). Then, when nurse practitioners review an article of interest or need a contact in a certain specialty, the network will be at their fingertips (Owens & Young). If the nurse practitioner's network list is short, then a simple tickler file based on a notebook, note cards, or business cards may be helpful (Owens & Young).

Nurse practitioners should make a conscious effort to stay in contact with the people in their network (Owens & Young, 2008). Although underutilized, "thank you" notes can help set nurse practitioners apart (Owens & Young). Techniques such as sending a note with a clipping from the paper or a journal relating to the individual's area of interest and sending a link to an appropriate online website are strategies to stay in contact (Owens & Young). Other strategies, such as arranging follow-up meetings over coffee, can also be helpful when trying to establish a mutually beneficial relationship.

Assessments to Prepare Nurse Practitioners for the Job Market

For nurse practitioners to promote their success in today's competitive job markets, they need to be prepared (Selph, 1998). Part of that preparation should involve an in-depth personal, marketplace, organizational, and nurse practitioner–organizational fit analysis.

Personal Assessment

Prior to engaging in pursuit for work, nurse practitioners should complete a comprehensive, honest, affirmative personal assessment (Shapiro & Rosenberg, 2002). This assessment should identify their strengths and weaknesses as well as their goals and objectives (Hosking, 2010; Shapiro & Rosenberg; Vilorio, 2011). Organizations and practices are seeking the most qualified nurse practitioners to fill their open positions (Mize, 2011a). If nurse practitioners want to stand out as the most qualified candidates to potential employers, then they will need to begin with an objective and constructive assessment of their strengths and weaknesses (Selph, 1998). Nurse practitioners should highlight the unique qualities that they offer and indicate how they complement the advanced practice nursing position (Mize, 2011a; Shapiro & Rosenberg). For example, nurse practitioners with the ability to speak more than one language may be an asset to the organization or practice (Shapiro & Rosenberg). In addition, nurse practitioners who have received special training, have expertise with central line placements, or have excellent suturing skills may be viewed as a benefit to particular institutions or practices (Shapiro & Rosenberg).

Likewise, deficiencies should be noted to provide a realistic description of the individual's performance as a nurse practitioner (Shapiro & Rosenberg, 2002). If nurse practitioners do not have the expertise that will help them stand apart, then they need to consider ways to make improvements to enhance their marketability (Hosking, 2010). In addition, nurse practitioners need to give some thought to their short- and long-term goals (Selph, 1998). Determining these goals will assist nurse practitioners in making appropriate decisions about their future employment (Mize, 2011a)

In addition to determining strengths, weaknesses, and goals, nurse practitioners should give thought to their personal financial and benefit needs (Selph, 1998). Assessing salary and benefit requirements will help nurse practitioners determine what their bottom line will be in the negotiations (Selph). Setting ranges prior to negotiations can help nurse practitioners balance or adjust certain elements to design the best possible benefits package (Selph). There are many factors to consider. Does the organization/practice include malpractice insurance in the benefits package? If this is not the case, nurse practitioners may wish to negotiate for an increased salary to cover this expense (Selph). Sometimes there are other benefits besides salary that nurse practitioners need to consider, such as work hours (on-call, required weekends), flexible scheduling, potential for growth, and vacation time (Selph).

Lastly, nurse practitioners' personal assessment should include an evaluation of the work location and setting as well as the professional environment requirements (Selph, 1998). Nurse practitioners will need to consider their constraints regarding the location. Are they willing to relocate? Do they want to stay in the same location? If they want to stay locally, then do they have limits on the distance they are willing to commute? In addition, in which specialty and setting do they wish to work? With which populations are they qualified to work and enjoy working? Once the location and setting have been determined, nurse practitioners need to assess the time commitments required by the position, the professional development requirements, and the anticipated work environment (Selph). Nurse practitioners must decide how many hours are needed for the role and identify any personal constraints such as the necessity to leave the site at a particular time (Selph). The professional development assessment includes an evaluation of the needs for mentoring and orientation, the amount of autonomy preferred, and continuing education required to maintain licensure, certification, and credentialing (Selph). Continuing education time and expenses as well as cost of journals, professional organization membership fees, and licensure and certification costs should all be assessed (Selph). Having this knowledge may assist nurse practitioners when it comes time to negotiate the benefits package for the position (Selph). With regard to the work environment, nurse practitioners will need to assess the specific environment such as office space, support staff, pagers, cell phones, and computer (Selph).

Once nurse practitioners have completed the personal assessment, they will need to prioritize these elements to determine which are absolutely essential versus which are more flexible (Selph, 1998). Oftentimes, nurse practitioners may need to make adjustments based on information obtained from the current marketplace and organizational assessments (Selph).

Marketplace Assessment

After the nurse practitioner completes the personal assessment, it is time to begin a marketplace assessment. This assessment comprises an evaluation of the regional and national marketplace and political atmosphere (Selph, 1998). When evaluating the regional and national marketplace, nurse practitioners need to take into account the state rules and regulations that guide advanced practice, the need for nurse practitioner roles, the number of qualified nurse practitioners, typical financial packages/salary, nurse practitioner scope of

practice, and chief surrounding competitors (Hupcey, 1993; Selph).

Organizational Assessment

Once the preceding information is obtained, nurse practitioners need to determine the specific practice or institution that they would like to pursue as an employer (Vilorio, 2011). Making that determination will require additional effort and research (Vilorio). It is important to find a practice or an organization that nurse practitioners admire and wish to work for (Vilorio). Nurse practitioners should pursue organizations and practices, not job openings (Vilorio).

Assessing the qualities of a particular practice or organization will require nurse practitioners to complete additional research. Some experts maintain that it is inexcusable for applicants not to know the fundamentals of an organization (or practice) (Vilorio, 2011). Thus nurse practitioners need to know which services their potential employer provides and how the organization compares to its competitors (Vilorio). Nurse practitioners should gather data about the organization's privileging and nurse practitioner scope of practice policies, recent political concerns, and the exposure the healthcare team has had to nurse practitioners (Selph, 1998). In addition, they should assess whether there are any competitors for the position or role they are seeking to fill (Selph). If they face competition, nurse practitioners will need to develop a strategy to advocate for their specific skills, expertise, and contributions (Selph). If possible, nurse practitioners will want to find out as many details as possible by looking for answers to the following questions (Brox, 2010; Selph; Shapiro & Rosenberg, 2002; Vilorio, 2011):

- Which population does the organization service?
- What are common diagnoses?
- What are the strengths and weaknesses of the organization/practice?

- What is the average daily census? What is the number of patient visits per day?

- How many outpatient and inpatient facilities does the organization have? Where are they located?

- Is the organization a teaching institution with medical teaching staff? What is the relationship between nurse practitioners and the medical teaching staff—that is, how is the work shared? Is there clear role delineation?

- What are the reporting mechanisms? Do nurse practitioners report to the nursing department? If so, are nurse practitioners expected to fulfill other obligations such as participating in annual educational in-service programs?

- Who will be completing the nurse practitioner's evaluation?

- How many nurse practitioners work in the institution/practice?

- How have they structured their practices and services? Are there specialty practices? Is the practice based primarily on consultation? Are there primary care providers?

- What is the reimbursement scheme and payer mix? Can revenue be generated from the services that the nurse practitioner can offer?

- What is the organizational structure?

- What is the organizational culture? Is the organization accepting of nurse practitioners? Are nurses empowered in the organization?

- What is the reputation of the organization in the community and among other professionals?

This information should be found through nurse practitioners' network contacts if possible; otherwise, jobseekers should seek it out through newspaper articles, healthcare publications, employer websites, employee blogs, and online discussions (Vilorio, 2011).

The preceding information will help nurse practitioners evaluate the specific practice char-

acteristics. This information, paired with the results of the personal assessment, will help nurse practitioners determine their fit with an organization. In addition, down the line it may help them negotiate for an established position or help to develop and design a new position (Selph, 1998).

Nurse Practitioner–Organizational Fit Assessment

At this point, it is time to see whether the personal assessment fits with the organizational assessment. This initial evaluation is intended to decide whether a good relationship between the nurse practitioner and the particular organization is viable. However, nurse practitioners cannot fully complete the fit assessment until they have had a chance to interview for the position and interact with the particular healthcare environment. In fact, nurse practitioners will not know for sure whether the fit is a good one until they are employed for some period of time. Nurse practitioner–organizational fit is essential for a good long-term relationship, as research studies have linked congruence between individual and organizational values (fit) with positive affect (Mount & Muchinsky, 1978; Spokane, 1985; Chatman, 1989) and a greater likelihood of staying with the organization (Chatman; Meir & Hasson, 1982), commitment, satisfaction, and performance (Chatman).

Causal mapping and storytelling are two strategies that, when combined, may be helpful in determining nurse practitioner–organizational fit (Billsberry, Ambrosini, Moss-Jones, & March, 2005). Causal mapping in this context entails reflecting on factors that have an effect on nurse practitioners' fit in an organization (Billsberry et al.). Nurse practitioners should contemplate which factors determine their fit in an organization (Billsberry et al.). Given that nurse practitioners begin this evaluation before they are actually working at the institution, they will want to draw upon their past experiences and determine which factors were most important to them. Through the reflections, nurse practitioners can begin to learn the particular individual factors that influence their sense of fit in an organization (Billsberry et al.). Causal mapping involves creating a graphic depiction of what affects the sense of fit. Nurse practitioners add to the picture by reflecting on what influences their sense of fit and then what happens to cause that effect. They continue to develop this map by reflecting on additional questions that help them get more specific about what causes the feelings. Nurse practitioners should continue to reflect until they are unable to come up with additional information. At that point, they should try to recall an individual work experience that influenced fit and tell a story about it. Some nurse practitioners may have difficulty determining what has influenced their fit in an organization and, therefore, will have trouble creating a map. In that instance, it will be useful to utilize the storytelling technique in which nurse practitioners recount stories from their work that illustrate how they felt about their employer. These two techniques help nurse practitioners to reflect on the underlying factors and provide an initial exploration of the nurse practitioner's sense of fit.

Portfolio Development

Nurse practitioners entering the job market need to be able to promote their positive personal and professional qualities to potential employers (Selph, 1998). Some organizations may not be familiar with the scope of practice and competencies of nurse practitioners (Selph). As a consequence, nurse practitioners will need to educate prospective employers as they concurrently negotiate for a position (Selph).

One strategy nurse practitioners can utilize to educate key individuals in an organization as well as to develop a strong base for negotiation is a well-prepared career portfolio (Selph). A good portfolio must be paired with an attitude of confidence and competence to ensure success (Selph). Nurse practitioners will want all

observers to see their positive attitude, which arises from their education, clinical knowledge and skills, adaptability, effective communication skills, and a strong conviction in the capability of the nurse practitioner to contribute to positive patient and financial outcomes (Selph). Successful negotiations begin with nurse practitioners' passionate belief in the worth and benefits of this advanced nursing practice role (Selph). If they lack the conviction that nurse practitioners offer a valuable service, candidates will run the risk of making compromises that will undermine their professional and personal goals (Selph). It is helpful to have data to support the notion that nurse practitioners can have a positive impact on practice (Selph).

Professional portfolios can be an effective means for conveying the significant worth of nurse practitioners (Selph, 1998). Portfolios can educate potential employers who are unacquainted with the role and scope of nurse practitioners as well as highlight the contributions that nurse practitioners can make in the practice setting (Selph). When possible, nurse practitioners should present data that support the value of the nurse practitioner role (Selph). Nurse practitioners can display evidence of professional knowledge, skills, expertise, work experiences, clinical experience, professional accomplishments, and scholarly work in the professional portfolio (Selph). Most of this information can be located in the nurse practitioner's personal and organization assessments (Selph). The most positive impact occurs when nurse practitioners present and organize this information in a professional manner while maintaining attention to detail to ensure a polished project.

The portfolio can contain the following components: curriculum vitae, professional development and continuing education activities, references, clinical experiences, legal regulations, standards and scope of practice, collaborative practice agreements, reimbursement guidelines, procedures, hospital privileging, job descriptions, scholarly work, protocols, advance practice documentation, and professional expenses (Shapiro & Rosenberg, 2002).

Curriculum Vitas

Some experts recommend that nurse practitioners include a curriculum vitae as opposed to a résumé (Hinck, 1997). Although the two documents are similar, there are some significant differences (Hinck). A résumé is typically a one- to two-page document that gives an overview of education, employment history, and achievements (Hinck). The curriculum vitae, by comparison, is typically longer and more detailed. Such profiles are typically used in academia, although medical and nursing professionals often use them as well.

The curriculum vitae is a practical tool that can highlight the nurse practitioner's abilities, skills, and accomplishments and promote his or her career (Hinck, 1997). It is a wonderful opportunity for nurse practitioners to make a positive impression. Of course, this document can quickly make a negative impression if it is poorly constructed or contains errors. Nurse practitioners should carefully proofread the curriculum vitae, as misspellings, typographical errors, and grammatical errors will likely give the impression that they lack attention to detail and professionalism (Hosking, 2010). In one recent study, more than 75% of organization leaders interviewed indicated that only one or two typographical errors in the curriculum vitae would eliminate the candidate from consideration for a position (Hosking).

The curriculum vitae should be printed on high-quality paper, on only one side (Hinck, 1997). Some experts suggest using a 10- to 14-point Times New Roman font as it is easy to read (Hinck). All information in the curriculum vitae must be honest and accurate (Hinck). Providing false information or embellishing one's accomplishments is not just unethical, but can also cause nurse practitioners great trouble when the information is verified (Hinck). Nurse

practitioners should modify their curriculum vitae at frequent intervals to ensure inclusion of all accomplishments (Hinck; Hosking, 2010; Selph, 1998).

When applying for a job, nurse practitioners should include a cover letter explaining how they could benefit the employer (Hinck; Hoskings). In addition, the content of the cover letter should express that they are familiar with the organization and explain how they can make an immediate contribution to its success (Hinck; Hosking)

The curriculum vitae can be organized in different ways depending on the nurse practitioner's preferences (Hinck, 1997). There are no strict rules that have to be applied (Hinck). Typically, this document contains the general categories reviewed in the following template in **Exhibit 29-1** (Critchley, 2003; Hinck; Selph, 1998).

Professional Development and Continuing Education Activities

Nurse practitioners may wish to include information in the portfolio about their professional development or continuing education activities. Doing so will help highlight the nurse practitioner's dedication to lifelong learning. In this section, nurse practitioners should outline any ongoing specialty training that was received (Hinck, 1997). The information can be displayed in a simple table that notes the date and title of the program as well as the organization that provided the education.

References

If nurse practitioners have letters of support or recommendation available, they can be included in this section of the portfolio. If such letters are not available, nurse practitioners can either note that references will be available upon request or list people who are willing to serve as references (Hinck, 1997). Nurse practitioners can ask current or former managers and colleagues if they would be willing to serve as a

EXHIBIT 29-1	Curriculum Vitae Template

Name, credentials

Home Address:

Work Address: (if desired)

Phone:

Email Address:

Education: (list highest degree first)
  Degree
  Graduation date
  University
  University's Address

Professional Employment: (list most recent nursing position first)
  Dates of employment
  Employer
  Position title: brief description of responsibilities and achievements

Licensure and Certifications:
  List licenses
  License number
  State(s) where qualified to practice
  List certifications
  Certification number
  Credentialing body
  Dates certification is valid

Professional Honors and Recognition: (list most recent first)
  Professional and community awards, scholarships, honorary degrees, fellowship and/or prizes
  Name of the award
  Presenting organization
  Date
  Reason for the award

Research/Grant History:
  Research fellowships
  Master's theses
  Doctoral dissertations
  Grants (do not list a project if funding was denied)

Lectures, Courses, and Presentations: (may include presentations given to colleagues, healthcare professionals, or the community)
  List of names of course/lecture/presentations
  Dates given

EXHIBIT 29-1 Curriculum Vitae Template *(continued)*

Professional Service:
 Peer review groups/grant study sections
 Journal service: (served as a reviewer for a journal)
  Dates of service
  Journal name
 Professional organizations:
  Names of organizations in which current membership is held
  Dates of membership
  Offices held
  Committees served in each organization
 Consultative service:
  Names of organizations where salaried consulting work was provided
  Address of the organization
  Type of consulting work
  Dates
 Organizational service:
  Dates
  Committees and task forces
  Role on the committee (i.e., member or chairperson)
  If appropriate, note any major accomplishment of the committee
 Hospital boards and committees

Public/Community Service:
 Community agency where volunteer work was completed
 Type of service (e.g., parish nursing, fundraising, educational sessions to non-nursing groups)
 Population served
 Date

Bibliography: (Use the American Psychological Association format for listing publications; list the publications in chronological order by year. Group types of publications separately, such as by the following groupings.)
 Peer-reviewed manuscripts
 Case reports, technical notes, letters
 Reviews, chapters, books
 Papers in press
 Peer reviews of presentations

(Note in the footer the date on which the curriculum vitae was last revised.)

reference for them as they enter the job market in the new role of a nurse practitioner (Hosking, 2010). Do not list people as references before obtaining their permission to do so, as that will increase the risk of the reference not being prepared for the call or giving a negative response to the caller (Hinck; Hosking). When listing references, nurse practitioners should include each reference's name, title, work address, and telephone number (Hinck).

Clinical Experience

Nurse practitioners should include a section in the career portfolio that underscores their clinical experience. To demonstrate their proficiency, a summary of the types of patients managed, age ranges, diagnoses, procedures performed, preceptor, and practice setting and location should be provided (Burgess & Misener, 1997; Selph, 1998). When possible, the nurse practitioner should try to obtain letters of reference to strengthen this section (Selph).

Legal Regulations

If the organization that nurse practitioners hope to enter has little or no experience with the advanced practice nurse role, then they will want to be sure to include a section on legal regulations in the portfolio (Selph, 1998). Nurse practitioners should begin by including a copy of the state's nurse practice act as well as regulations regarding advanced practice nursing (Selph). In addition, documentation should be provided that verifies nurse practitioners' prescriptive authority if appropriate. If nurse practitioners do not have prescriptive authority, then describe the process of how it is obtained (Selph, 1998). This information indicates that nurse practitioners are concerned with the legal aspects of their clinical practice while simultaneously educating the employer (Burgess & Misener, 1997; Hravnak & Magdic, 1997; Selph).

Standards and Scopes of Practice

The portfolio ought to include the *Standards of Clinical Practice and Scope of Practice for the Acute Care Nurse Practitioner,* as it provides the principles for competent care (Selph, 1998). In addition, this document serves as the basis for performance evaluation and a quality review program (Burgess & Misener, 1997; Selph).

Collaborative Practice Agreements

Sample collaborative practice agreements included in the portfolio can be useful for potential employers who are not familiar with this information and would like to review a copy (Shapiro & Rosenberg, 2002). Collaborative practice agreements are printed contracts among physicians and nurse practitioners that outline the scope of the collaborative practice (Shapiro & Rosenberg). The agreement should note how the two healthcare professional groups will organize and manage care, and the breadth or constraints of the APN practice (Shapiro & Rosenberg).

Reimbursement Guidelines

Including reimbursement guidelines in the portfolio will help educate employers regarding the types of payments that are available for nurse practitioner services (Burgess & Misener, 1997; Selph, 1998). Nurse practitioners should be sure to include current information regarding the guidelines or statutes concerning reimbursement, as these criteria change frequently (Selph). To do so, nurse practitioners should ascertain the practice payer mix and directly communicate with the payers to determine which nurse practitioner services they will reimburse for (Selph). Nurse practitioners can utilize the resources that are available such as the billing department or practice manager to help determine what is typically billed for by the practice and how often (what percentage) it uses each provider (Selph).

Scope of Practice: Procedures

A list of procedures that are typically performed by nurse practitioners in their state should be provided in the portfolio (Selph, 1998). The procedures that nurse practitioners can perform within their scope of practice are typically noted in the state's nurse practice act (Selph). In this section of the portfolio, nurse practitioners should list which procedures they have performed with supervision and which procedures they are prepared to learn (Selph). Nurse practitioners should highlight any special training received, the number of completed procedures, and outcomes (Selph). When possible, they should provide information regarding reimbursement for the procedure, which will help in the negotiation process (Selph).

Hospital Privileging

If nurse practitioners are hoping to gain employment in a hospital, they will need to be privileged based on the medical staff bylaws and policies for advanced practice nurses (Selph, 1998). Specific procedures must be followed and documentation must be submitted, which a committee will review and use as the basis for making a recommendation (Selph). If the institution has not utilized nurse practitioners in the past, procedures may not have been established to allow privileging of nurse practitioners. In this case, nurse practitioners will want to research best practices for privileging and provide this information in the portfolio. This effort will help prepare nurse practitioners to assist in developing a plan to implement a procedure (Selph).

Job Description

Depending on the individual nurse practitioner's situation, a job description may or may not be included in the portfolio. If nurse practitioners are well established in the potential employer's institution, then providing information about job descriptions may not be necessary. However, a sample job description can be a good tool for delineating particular instances in which nurse practitioners can use knowledge and skills to influence patient care (Selph, 1998). As such, nurse practitioners may wish to provide a sample job description that

highlights how their skills can positively influence the healthcare environment (Selph). The job description should be individualized for the setting in which the nurse practitioners will be working and include specific roles and responsibilities (Selph).

Scholarly Work

In this part of the portfolio, nurse practitioners can demonstrate their writing skills and showcase professional expertise by supplying a copy of publications, papers, or abstracts that are germane to the practice setting (Selph, 1998). These examples will illustrate nurse practitioners' capability for additional scholarly activities and lay the groundwork for negotiating time for such work and attendance at professional meetings (Selph).

Protocols

In many states, nurse practitioners utilize protocols and guidelines to inform their practice (Selph, 1998). In turn, they may wish to provide a sample protocol for the management of a clinical situation particular to the specialty of interest in their portfolio (Selph). Such protocols and guidelines are useful tools to demonstrate the responsibilities nurse practitioners will have with regard to diagnostic reasoning, treatments, and outcomes (Selph).

Advanced Practice Documentation

In this section of the portfolio, nurse practitioners can provide affirmation of advanced practice documentation ability by presenting examples of admission notes, history and physicals, orders, progress notes, and discharge summaries (Selph, 1998). Remember to remove all identifying patient information from these samples (Selph). If possible, the documents should be related to the population with whom the nurse practitioner intends to work (Selph). These examples can serve as a powerful testament of the nurse practitioner's clinical expertise and can show the distinct abilities that the nurse practitioner can provide within the practice, particularly in healthcare settings where the nurse practitioner is a new role (Selph).

Professional Expenses

This section of the portfolio includes a detailed inventory of the nurse practitioner's expected professional expenses (Selph, 1998). Nurse practitioners may choose to hold this information aside until it is time for negotiating a benefits package; nevertheless, it is important to be cognizant of the professional costs. When developing the record of expenses, nurse practitioners should think about all of their expenses, including one-time costs such as the initial application for a certification or for prescriptive authority as well as annual costs such as malpractice insurance and fees for license renewal (Selph). Other expenses that can be included are the cost of continuing specialty certifications, continuing education expenses, professional organization memberships, journals, and books (Selph). The more detailed the list, the more prepared the nurse practitioner will be to articulate his or her needs and expectations (Selph).

Applying for the Job

Once nurse practitioners have completed their personal, marketplace, organizational, and nurse practitioner–organizational fit assessments, they can present themselves to the employer, feeling empowered with the information provided in the career portfolio (Shapiro & Rosenberg, 2002). The next step in entering the job market is to place an application; this step is followed by the job interview.

Applications

An increasing number of employers are moving to an online application process (Vilorio, 2011). Of course, although an online process might be used, there is still a human being at the receiving end who will be doing the hiring (Vilorio). Nurse practitioners will increase their chances of being hired if they contact the hiring individual instead of relying solely on computer contact (Vilorio). Online processes have increased the number of applications an organization receives (Vilorio). As a result, many organizations utilize software that can somewhat automate the selection process by rejecting candidates based on minimum qualifications or keywords (Vilorio). For this reasons, nurse practitioners are advised to customize the cover letter, curriculum vitae, and application for each position that they apply to (Vilorio). To avoid being removed by the automatic culling software, they should be sure to include the words in the job posting and to emphasize the connection between their education and skills, and the duties necessary for the desired position (Vilorio).

Experts recommend that nurse practitioners use extreme caution when posting identifying personal data online, particularly on social media websites such as LinkedIn and Facebook (Hosking, 2010; Vilorio, 2011). Many organizations will conduct an online information check to evaluate potential hires (Hosking; Vilorio). Many social media programs have loose privacy settings, which make it easy for members of the public to access users' personal information (Hosking; Vilorio). One way to manage this access is to search one's own name online to see which information is available to the general public as well as to adjust privacy settings to protect personal information and photos, control what others share about the user, and reduce information that can compromise being hired (Hosking; Vilorio). All personal data should be kept private; however, nurse practitioners can certainly share professional accomplishments such as publications or awards or other information that presents a professional image (Hosking; Vilorio).

When possible, it is helpful for nurse practitioners to talk with the hiring manager, as this individual is responsible for choosing candidates and has a vested interest in finding a qualified nurse practitioner candidate who can meet the job responsibilities and fulfill the mission of the organization (Vilorio, 2011). If nurse practitioners have existing contacts within the organization, perhaps those individuals might be able to arrange an informational meeting with the hiring manager (Vilorio). Such a meeting will help nurse practitioners learn more about the job responsibilities and the institution while also giving them a chance to impress the individual responsible for hiring (Vilorio). During this meeting, nurse practitioners should be sure to demonstrate initiative while remaining polite and being mindful of the hiring channels (Vilorio).

After submitting an application and curriculum vitae, nurse practitioners should follow up with the hiring manager within 2 weeks of sending the application (Hosking, 2010). Experts recommend sending a brief email or calling the organization or practice after submitting the information to confirm the nurse practitioner's interest in the post and offer to respond to any questions the employer might have about the application (Hosking). This sort of professional attention to detail can set nurse practitioners apart in this process (Hosking).

Once nurse practitioners have submitted an application, they should be prepared to respond when the organization calls (Brox, 2010). The first impression begins with that call (Brox). Sometimes organizations use this initial phone conversation as a screening tool (Brox). As a result, nurse practitioners may wish to let the call go to voicemail so that they have time to adequately prepare and make a polished first impression (Brox).

Interviewing

Being brought in for an interview indicates that an organization is interested in the applicant's background (Brox, 2010). The interview is a critical time when nurse practitioners will have the opportunity to dazzle the employer and secure a position (Vilorio, 2011). According to experts, the main reason why people are not successful in interviews is a lack of preparation (Brox). Role-playing mock interviews with an individual who is knowledgeable about the process can help nurse practitioners develop and hone their interviewing skills (Brox). It may also help nurse practitioners to correct some potentially damaging behaviors (Brox). For example, many people are unaware that they use words and phrases such as "you know," "like," and "um" while speaking. Eliminating this habit can help nurse practitioners obtain a job (Brox). During the interview, nurse practitioners will want to attempt to work in all their career highlights (Brox). They should practice both delivering this information in a charming and natural fashion and telling engaging stories that help make what is listed on their curriculum vitae memorable (Brox).

Nurse practitioners should prepare for the interview by developing answers to questions that the employer might potentially ask (Brox, 2010). The employer will certainly ask questions to determine the applicant's knowledge, skills, and interests (Vilorio, 2011). Nurse practitioners should not be vague when responding to questions, but rather should provide the employer with specific details of how they solved problems and brought situations to a positive resolution (Brox). Potential employers will most likely ask nurse practitioners to respond to some behaviorally based questions that elicit how they would respond in specific situations (Brox; Vilorio). In addition, they may ask generic questions such as the following (Brox; Vilorio): What do you see yourself doing in 5 years? What are your strengths and weaknesses? Why would you like to be employed here? How do you handle conflict with peers? What do you consider to be your greatest accomplishment? What can you tell me about your reasons for leaving your last job? What was the most challenging issue you have encountered and how did you deal with it? Nurse practitioners should attempt to keep the responses positive even when discussing negative topics (Brox).

In addition, nurse practitioners should have a list of questions to ask the hiring manager (Vilorio, 2011). If they have not obtained details about the position and its associated responsibilities, then the interview is the time to ascertain this information (Shapiro & Rosenberg, 2002). Nurse practitioners should find out details about specific responsibilities such as completion of patient histories, physical examinations, and daily progress notes (Shapiro & Rosenberg). How many patients will the nurse practitioner be responsible for (Shapiro & Rosenberg)? Are nurse practitioners expected to respond to emergencies and if so, which backup systems are in place (Shapiro & Rosenberg)? Does the organization/practice utilize protocols? What are the steps in the credentialing and privileging process (Shapiro & Rosenberg)? Which kinds of orientation, support, and supervision will be offered (Shapiro & Rosenberg)?

A main purpose of the interview is to help nurse practitioners and the employer determine if the candidate is a good fit for the organization (Vilorio, 2011). Nurse practitioners should be positive and truthful about everything they say, but especially when discussing previous managers and colleagues (Brox, 2010; Vilorio). Nurse practitioners' interactions should be assertive and courteous while avoiding presumptions and aggression (Vilorio). For example, if nurse practitioners have information in their employment history that potentially might be perceived as negative, such as gaps in employment or frequent job changes, then they should succinctly acknowledge the situation and then redirect the discussion toward something positive, such as what has been learned from the experience and constructive actions that have been taken to prepare for the new position (Vilorio). Nurse practitioners need to sell themselves and be clear what they can bring to the organization (Mize, 2011b).

It might sound simple, but first impressions really do make a difference. The hiring individual wants to know that the candidate nurse practitioner will be a good representative on behalf of the organization or practice (Mize, 2011b). As such, nurse practitioners should show common sense and professionalism in all dealings with the possible new employer (Vilorio, 2011). At the very least, they should be on time, professionally dressed, and polite to all staff regardless of their position (Mize, 2011b; Vilorio). With any job, nurse practitioners need to bring a positive "can do and will do" attitude (Mize, 2011b). In particular, they should be prepared to respond to questions that require them to give examples of previous problem-solving and time-management scenarios (Mize, 2011b).

Nurse practitioners should thank the interviewer in person as well as in writing with a "thank you" letter (Vilorio, 2011). According to experts, it is most effective to hand-write the note, but an email "thank you" letter is also considered acceptable (Vilorio). The "thank you" note gives nurse practitioners one more opportunity to emphasize their positive qualifications and skills as well as confirm their interest in the position (Vilorio). The length of the hiring process can vary greatly between organizations. As such, nurse practitioners may wish to follow up with a phone call or email to reassert their interest in the position (Vilorio).

Salary Negotiation

Many organizations' human resources departments have guidelines and structures in place to help determine what the starting pay level will be (Mize, 2011b). As a result, nurse practitioners' negotiations may not yield the results they wished for. When assessing their compensation, however, nurse practitioners need to consider the entire benefits package, which includes such items as life insurance, health insurance, dental and vision care, vacation, and retirement/pension plans (Mize, 2011b). In addition, the nurse practitioner should consider whether the organization will provide compensation for professional memberships, continuing education opportunities, and travel expenses (Mize, 2011b). It is important to consider these factors in conjunction with the salary (Mize, 2011b).

FOSTERING DEVELOPMENT

Once nurse practitioners are in their new roles, they will need to continue their education and foster their growth and development. Nurse practitioners begin their first advanced practice positions as novices and will need to put structures and strategies in place to support their growth and development so that they can become expert nurse practitioners (Ackerman, Norsen, Martin, Wiedrich, & Kitzman, 1996; Doerksen, 2010). Continuing education and ongoing training are obvious ways to promote development. A few additional strategies are discussed in this section as well.

Formal and Informal Mentorship

Formal and informal mentorship has been noted in the literature as a method to address the professional development needs of nurse practitioners (Doerksen, 2010). Formal mentorship is often offered by an institution/practice with some prescribed components. Each organization goes about the process differently. Ideally, a needs assessment will be completed to develop an individualized program that meets the specific needs of the new nurse practitioner (Doerksen). In addition, novice nurse practitioners may be paired with experienced nurse practitioners who have agreed to serve in the mentor role (Doerksen). Once an agreement has been reached between the two parties, they will discuss the process to be used as well as goals and expectations. Ground rules and a contract should be established to facilitate a positive experience. Some organizations provide a welcoming package including a directory of potential mentors, which lists the areas of interest and strengths of the individuals (Doerksen). This tool can be very useful for beginning nurse practitioners who

would like to identify a colleague who can help them develop their professional interests.

Informal mentoring can also be a useful tool for fostering the development of novice nurse practitioners. Informal mentoring in this context refers to speaking with another professional who can offer assistance, provide encouragement, and stimulate growth. Being open and willing to learn and grow is the first step in developing informal mentoring relationships. Informal mentoring is less structured, with nurse practitioners scheduling their own time with the mentor perhaps meeting in the office or casually over coffee (Doerksen, 2010).

The ongoing professional development needs of nurse practitioners will most likely be met through multiple mentors, and these needs will likely change over time (Doerksen, 2010). Initially, nurse practitioners will need to learn about the daily ins and outs of their role (Doerksen). New nurse practitioners may need assistance with specific clinical activities as well as policies and procedures (Doerksen). With time, they will become more comfortable and confident with the daily functions, with their attention for mentoring focusing on additional growth in the role (Doerksen). The need for mentoring regarding research has been identified as a need that will increase for nurse practitioners over time (Doerksen). Onsite mentors for research can be a useful way to meet that need if the facility is lacking in such expertise (Doerksen). Visiting nurse practitioners from other institutions and practices can help both with conducting research and determining how this role can be implemented in a variety of ways (Doerksen). Physicians may be able to help nurse practitioners identify gaps in clinical knowledge and help by serving as mentors for research. However, nurse practitioners need to be cognizant of the professional obligation to further not just medical and healthcare research but nursing research as well.

Experiential Learning and Reflective Narratives

Nurse practitioners can foster their growth and development via experiential learning embedded in narratives (Cathcart, Greenspan, & Quin, 2010). In this context, experiential learning involves nurse practitioners actively reflecting on their work experiences with the assistance of written entries (Cathcart et al.). Nurse practitioners' work environments can provide an opportunity to acquire new skills and develop new knowledge if they are open to these events, have self-initiative, and are willing to self-evaluate. Making meaning from work experiences will require nurse practitioners to be attentive to pertinent occurrences, actively reflect on the situation by using analytical skills, consider alternative ways to handle the encounter, and develop new ideas from the experience (Cathcart et al.).

Written reflections can help nurse practitioners recognize the skilled knowledge and accomplishments they have achieved (Cathcart et al., 2010). Without contemplation, nurse practitioners' achievements or difficulties may be seen as merely isolated occurrences, possibly not remembered until the next time a similar event happens (Benner, 1984; Benner, Tanner, & Chesla, 2009; Benner, Sutphen, Leonard, & Day, 2010; Cathcart et al.). Writing about experiences at work will give nurse practitioners an opportunity to remember the event and start to understand the importance and implication of the incidents (Cathcart et al.). It will also help them appreciate why the specific incident was important and how their judgment and actions influenced the situation (Cathcart et al.). Written narratives reinforce the notion that nurse practitioners' professional development is a lifelong process based on constant exposure to a variety of experiences (Cathcart et al.).

Online Listservs

Online listservs are another practical strategy for fostering professional growth and develop-ment; they provide nurse practitioners with a network of support and informal knowledge sharing (Hew & Hara, 2008). In this context, listservs comprise an electronic mailing list management system that lets nurse practitioners subscribe to a mailing list of other nurse practitioners or healthcare professionals. Listservs can help nurse practitioners stay current with the latest changes in their area of expertise, which in turn may assist them in making informed decisions about clinical practice (Hew & Hara). Listservs provide nurse practitioners with a professional network to which they can pose questions or ideas to regarding clinical practice (Hew & Hara). Nurse practitioners will often gladly share their knowledge, as they feel a sense of obligation if they have been given assistance previously from others or if they hope to receive help in the future (Hew & Hara). Nurse practitioners tend to provide information to the listserv because they want to improve patient outcomes and assist their fellow nurse practitioners by imparting the needed information (Hew & Hara).

There are some downsides to listservs, however. Notably, the nurse practitioner should be certain to verify the information obtained via a listserv prior to using it in practice. In addition, although listservs can provide some pearls of wisdom, often the nurse practitioner will receive redundant messages that can overload their email in-boxes.

Grand Rounds

Grand rounds are a useful venue to promote and demonstrate nursing practice as well as foster growth and development (Furlong et al., 2007). If grand rounds are not available in the institution in which the nurse practitioner is practicing, then Benner's theoretical framework of skill acquisition can guide this process (Furlong et al.). Grand rounds are often held quarterly and are expected to connect evidence-based practice literature to practice (Furlong et al.). In this learning activity, healthcare professionals gather to hear about a clinical issue or particular patient case (Furlong et al.). For nurse practitioners, grand rounds serve as a means to improve nursing care by focusing on the educational needs of their clinical practice (Furlong et al.). In addition, they offer a way to recognize nurse practitioners for their clinical knowledge and skills, foster networking among nurse practitioners and other healthcare professionals, and provide recognition of the value of nursing's contribution to practice (Furlong et al.).

Recognition Programs

Recognition programs have been noted in the literature as a way to foster nurse practitioners' growth and development (Sullivan, Arlington, Madsen, & Guidry, 2006). Organizations develop and implement recognition programs as a way to publicly acknowledge contributions to meeting the goals and objectives of the institution. Typically, the goals and objectives in health care will involve obtaining positive patient, staff, institutional, and community outcomes. If the nurse practitioner's institution has not developed a recognition program, he or she might propose developing one to recognize the numerous contributions of the healthcare professionals in that institution, including advanced practice nurses (Sullivan et al.). Such a program can be utilized to acknowledge nurse practitioners' competency in the role, achievement of goals above and beyond their job expectations, and promotion of nursing practice (Sullivan et al.).

SUMMARY

Nurse practitioner educational programs are limited in their ability to fully assist students with the transformation that is necessary as they move from pupil, to novice, and eventually to expert nurse practitioner. This transition has been described in the recent literature as a process that involves three stages: identity loss, transitional role, and incorporation.

Nurse practitioner programs attempt to facilitate this transition by providing students with a framework that emphasizes evidence-based practice, research, collaboration, and consultation as a way to inform nursing practice (Spoelstra & Robbins, 2010). Although nurse practitioner programs may assist students with this process, other strategies to facilitate a positive transition can be implemented as well, such as understanding expectations and overcoming commonly encountered barriers such as a lack of knowledge about the nurse practitioner's scope of practice, lack of knowledge about the nurse practitioner role, poor physician attitudes, lack of respect, poor communication, and patient and family reluctance to accept nurse practitioner care (Clarin, 2007). Strategies to overcome these barriers include educating healthcare professionals about the nurse practitioner's scope of practice and roles, using integrated collaboration models, attending interdisciplinary rounds, advocating for medical students to be exposed to graduate nursing students early in their education, advocating for uniformity in nurse practitioner education and certification, and demonstrating positive outcomes fostered by the nurse practitioner role (Clarin). Other useful strategies include enlisting the help of mentors and reflective journaling.

The transition from student to expert nurse practitioner cannot be fully achieved until graduating students have secured their first position. As graduating students prepare for the job marketplace, they will need to locate job openings and conduct the following assessments: personal, marketplace, organization, and nurse practitioner–organization fit. In addition, a professional portfolio will be helpful to demonstrate the benefits that nurse practitioners can offer to an employer. Finally, nurse practitioners will need to present themselves favorably in the application and interview process.

Once nurse practitioners have begun a new position, it will be essential that they develop a lifelong learning plan that includes measures to foster their growth and development. Some suggested methods to promote development are formal and informal mentorships, experiential learning and reflective narratives, online listservs, grand rounds, and recognition programs.

DISCUSSION QUESTIONS

1. As you lay the foundation for professional advanced nursing practice, which concerns do you have regarding life after graduation?

2. Which strategies can the novice nurse practitioner employ to have a successful transition to the professional role?

3. Following a self-, marketplace, and organizational assessment, which factors are most important to consider when selecting an advanced practice position?

REFERENCES

Ackerman, M. H., Norsen, L., Martin, B., Wiedrich, J., & Kitzman, H. (1996). Development of a model of advanced practice. *American Journal of Critical Care, 5*, 68–73.

American Academy of Nurse Practitioners. (2010a). Annual report. Retrieved July 28, 2011, from http://www.aanp.org/NR/rdonlyres/97CD0283-59DF-4964-819B-61E58864B4F8/0/2010AANP_AnnualReport.pdf

American Academy of Nurse Practitioners. (2010b). *Nurse practitioner cost effectiveness.* Retrieved July 28, 2011, from http://www.aanp.org/NR/rdonlyres/197C9C42-4BC1-42A5-911E-85FA759B0308/0/CostEffectiveness4pages.pdf

American Academy of Nurse Practitioners. (2010c). Nurse practitioners in primary care. Retrieved July 28, 2011, from http://www.aanp.org/NR/rdonlyres/9AF1A29F-5C82-4151-98CB22D1F20A9BD9/0/NPsInPrimaryCare324.pdf

American Academy of Nurse Practitioners. (2007). The nurse practitioner: Your partner in health. Retrieved July 28, 2011, from http://www.aanp.org/NR/rdonlyres/E65B35D1-5810-4F38-8E45-DFFC999B6B4B/0/EnglishNPBrochure.pdf

Barton, T. D. (2007). Student nurse practitioners: A rite of passage? The universality of Van Gennep's model of social transition. *Nurse Education in Practice, 7*, 338–347.

Benner, P. (1984). *From novice to expert: excellence and power in clinical nursing practice.* Menlo Park, CA: Addison-Wesley.

Benner, P., Tanner, C., & Chesla, C. (2009). *Expertise in nursing practice,* 2nd ed. New York: Springer.

Benner, P., Sutphen, M., Leonard, V., & Day, L. (2010). *Educating nurses: A call for radical transformation.* San Francisco, CA: Jossey-Bass.

Billsberry, J., Ambrosini, V., Moss-Jones, J., & March, P. (2005). Some suggestions for mapping organizational members' sense of fit. *Journal of Business and Psychology, 19*(4), 555–570.

Brox, D. (2010). Mastering the interview. *PM Network,* 51–53.

Bryant-Lukosius, D., & DiCenso, A. (2004). A framework for the introduction and evaluation of advanced practice nursing roles. *Journal of Advanced Nursing, 48*(5), 530–540.

Burgess, S. E., & Misener, T. R. (1997). The professional portfolio: An advanced practice nurse job search marketing tool. *Clinical Excellence for Nurse Practitioners, 1*(7), 468–471.

Cathcart, E. B., Greenspan, M., & Quin, M. (2010). The making of a nurse manager: The role of experiential learning in leadership development. *Journal of Nursing Management, 18*, 440–447.

Chatman, J. A. (1989). Improving interactional organizational research: A model of person-organization fit. *Academy of Management Review, 14*(3), 333–349.

Clarin, O. A. (2007). Strategies to overcome barriers to effective nurse practitioner and physician collaboration. *Journal for Nurse Practitioners,* 538–548.

Cleary, M., Matheson, S., & Happell, B. (2009). Evaluation of a transition to practice programme for mental health nursing. *Journal of Advanced Nursing,* 844–850.

Critchley, D. (2003). Moving house or moving jobs: What's the difference? *Nursing Management, 10*(2), 12–14.

Doerksen, K. (2010). What are the professional development and mentorship needs of advanced practice nurses? *Journal of Professional Nursing, 26*(3), 141–151.

Forbes, A., While, A., Mathes, L., & Griffiths, P. (2006). Evaluating MS specialist nurse program. *International Journal of Nursing Studies, 43*, 985–1000.

Furlong, K. M., D'Luna-O'Grady, L., Macari-Hinson, M., O'Connel, K. B., & Pierson, G. S. (2007). Implementing nursing grand rounds in a community hospital. *Clinical Nurse Specialist, 21*(6), 287–291.

Hamric, A. B., & Taylor, J. W. (1989). Role development of CNS. In A. B. Hamric & J. Spross (Eds.), *The clinical nurse specialist in theory and practice* (2nd ed., pp. 41–82). Philadelphia: W. B. Saunders.

Hayes, E. (1998). Mentoring and nurse practitioner student self-efficacy. *Western Journal of Nursing Research, 20,* 521–525.

Heitz, L. J., Steiner, S. H., & Burman, M. E. (2004). RN to nurse practitioner: A qualitative study of role transition. *Journal of Nursing Education, 43,* 416–420.

Hew, K. H., & Hara, N. (2008). An online listserve for nurse practitioners: A viable venue for continuous nursing professional development? *Nurse Education Today, 28,* 450–457.

Hinck, S. (1997). A curriculum vitae that gives you a competitive edge. *Clinical Nurse Specialist, 11*(4), 174–177.

Hosking, R. (2010). Top 10 tips for job seekers. *OfficePro, 70*(2), 5.

Hravnak, M., & Magdic, K. (1997). Marketing the acute care nurse practitioner. *Clinical Excellence Nursing Practice , 1,* 9–13.

Hupcey, J. E. (1993). Factors and work settings that may influence nurse practitioner practice. *Nursing Outlook, 41,* 181–185.

Latham, C. L., & Fahey, L. J. (2006). Novice to expert advanced practice nurse role transition: Guided student self-reflection. *Journal of Nursing Education, 45*(1), 46–48.

Lindblad, E., Hallman, E. B., Gillsjo, C., Lindblad, U., & Foerstrom, L. (2010). Experiences of the new role of advanced practice nurses in Swedish primary health care: A qualitative study. *International Journal of Nursing Practice, 16,* 69–74.

Meir, E., & Hasson, R. (1982). Congruence between personality type and environment type as a predictor of stay in an environment. *Journal of Vocational Behavior, 21,* 309–317.

Mize, S. (2011a, March). Future leaders: Finding a job in a tight market. *Parks & Recreation,* 39–40.

Mize, S. (2011b, April). Future leaders: Your first job. *Parks & Recreation,* 41–41.

Mount, M., & Muchinksy, P. (1978). Person-environment congruence and employee job satisfaction: A test of Holland's theory. *Journal of Vocational Behavior, 13,* 84–100.

Owens, L. A., & Young, P. (2008). You're hired! The power of networking. *Journal of Vocational Rehabilitation, 29*(1), 23–28.

Pye, S. (2011). Professional development for an advance practice nursing team. *Journal of Continuing Education in Nursing, 40*(5), 217–222.

Selph, A. M. (1998). Negotiating an acute care nurse practitioner position. *AACN Clinical Issues, 9*(2), 269–276.

Shapiro, D., & Rosenberg, N. (2002). Acute care nurse practitioner collaborative practice negotiations. *AACN Clinical Issues, 12*(3), 470–478.

Spoelstra, S. L., & Robbins, L. B. (2010). A qualitative study of role transition from RN to APN. *International Journal of Nursing Education Scholarship, 7*(1), 1–14.

Spokane, A. (1985). A review of research on person-environment congruence in Holland's theory of career. *Journal of Vocational Behavior, 26,* 306–343.

Stahl, M. S., & Myers, J. (2002). The advanced practice nursing role with multiple responsibilities. *Critical Care Nursing Clinics of North America, 14,* 299–305.

Sullivan, T., Arlington, R., Madsen, V., & Guidry, V. (2006). Development and implementation of a recognition and development model for advanced practice nurses: An opportunity for professional growth. *Oncology Nursing Forum, 33*(2), 420.

U.S. Department of Health and Human Services Health Resources and Services Administration. (2010). The registered nurse population findings from the 2008 national sample survey of registered nurses. Retrieved July 28, 2011, from http://bhpr.hrsa.gov/healthworkforce/rnsurveys/rnsurveyfinal.pdf

Vilorio, D. (2011). Focused job seeking: A measure approach to looking for work. *Occupational Health Quarterly,* 2–11.

CHAPTER 30

Interprofessional Collaboration for Improving Patient and Population Health

Laurel Ash and Catherine Miller

CHAPTER OBJECTIVES

1. Identify workforce and regulatory issues that affect interprofessional collaboration in the clinical setting.

2. Discuss barriers to and drivers of effective collaboration among interprofessional healthcare teams.

3. Discuss stages of effective team development.

4. Analyze components of a work culture that supports collaboration.

5. Review leadership theories and consider the roles that leaders play in improving population health.

INTRODUCTION

The Consensus Model for APRN Regulation (2008)—prepared by the APRN Consensus Work Group and the National Council of State Boards of Nursing APRN Advisory Committee and endorsed by numerous nursing organizations—defines APRN practice as nurses practicing in one of four recognized roles: certified nurse practitioners, certified nurse-midwives, clinical nurse specialists, and certified registered nurse anesthetists. The primary focus of an APRN's practice includes provision of direct patient or population care. Conventionally, APRNs are prepared in accredited programs, sit for national certification, and meet regulatory requirements authorizing them (via license) to practice as an APRN. A number of nurses with advanced graduate preparation function in specialties that do not fall into these categories, yet advance the health of an organization, population, or aggregate or provide indirect patient care. Such roles may include administration, informatics, education, and public health. Discussions are ongoing as to how these specialty practices fit within the traditional definition of APRN practice and subsequently the doctor of nursing practice (DNP) role. This chapter uses the term *APRN* to reflect all advanced roles of nursing practice.

Numerous research studies have thoroughly documented the impact APRNs have on health outcomes, including the ability to deliver excellent quality, cost-effective care with high levels of patient satisfaction (Cunningham, 2004; Dailey, 2005; Horrocks, Anderson, & Salisbury, 2002; Ingersoll, McIntosh, & Williams, 2000; Lambing, Adams, Fox, & Divine, 2004; Laurant et al., 2004; Miller, Snyder, & Lindeke, 2005; Mundinger et al., 2000). The world is changing, and APRNs must position themselves to be at the table with other disciplines and professionals to emphasize the influence of nursing care on the health of an individual or population. The complexity of the current healthcare delivery system, trends in patient demographics, epidemiological changes of disease and chronic conditions, economic challenges, the need for improved patient safety, and the call for a redesign or reform of the healthcare delivery system will challenge all professionals to envision health care in new ways.

Healthcare reform is a prominent issue for health professionals, policymakers, and the public. During the 2008 presidential campaign, now-President Barack Obama announced a comprehensive healthcare reform proposal (Kaiser Family Foundation, 2008). This proposal outlines key points regarding restructuring our present system. As a foundation, all individuals and communities must be guaranteed a set of essential preventive care services. Reform must include measures to improve health outcomes and safeguard patients from

preventable medical error. President Obama's platform supports programs that use collaborative teams as a means to deliver comprehensive, cost-effective, and safe care to persons with chronic conditions (Kaiser Family Foundation, 2008). Access to safe, effective, and affordable health care is a concern shared by the American public and rated of significant importance in a national poll conducted by researchers from the Kaiser Family Foundation and the Harvard School of Public Health released in January 2009.

The professions of nursing and medicine agree on the need to create organizational environments that promote interprofessional collaboration. The American Nurses Association report *Nursing's Agenda for Health Care Reform* (2008) places particular emphasis on the role of collaboration in chronic disease management and patient safety. The American College of Physicians (ACP, 2009) also acknowledges that the future of healthcare delivery requires interprofessional teams who are prepared to meet the diverse, multifaceted health issues of the population. Providers, policy leaders, and health systems will need to shift their mind-set from traditional models of linear, disease-focused care to new delivery approaches. In the redesigned model, each discipline brings specialized skills and abilities, practices at the highest level of the individual provider's scope, assumes new roles, and participates in a collaborative manner with other professionals to provide high-quality, safe, cost-effective, patient-focused care. This call to action demands that APRNs perform at the highest level of clinical expertise, the doctor of nursing practice (DNP), and collaborate interprofessionally to improve patient and population health outcomes.

Merriam-Webster's Collegiate Dictionary (2005) defines *collaborate* as "to labor together, to work jointly with others" (p. 224). Leaders in the business world further describe collaboration as a concept involving "strategic alliances" or "interpersonal networks" in an effort to accomplish a project (Ring, 2005). As healthcare professionals, we can learn from successful business and management practices and use the collaboration processes of communicating, cooperating, transferring knowledge, coordinating, problem solving, and negotiating to more effectively reach a healthcare goal or outcome. The ACP (2009) suggests that collaboration involves mutual acknowledgment, understanding, and respect for the complementary roles, skills, and abilities of the interprofessional team. Effective collaborative partnerships promote quality and cost-effective care through an intentional process that allows members to exchange pertinent knowledge and ideas and subsequently engage in a practice of shared decision making. The purpose of this chapter is to generate a better understanding of interprofessional collaboration, distinguish the elements DNPs must possess to successfully collaborate with other professionals to improve the health status of persons or groups, and provide an overview of models of interprofessional collaboration in the real world.

IMPROVING HEALTH OUTCOMES

The Institute of Medicine's (IOM) 2001 report, *Crossing the Quality Chasm: A New Health System for the 21st Century,* identifies four key issues contributing to poor quality of care and undesirable health outcomes: the complexity of the knowledge, skills, interventions, and treatments required to deliver care; the increase in chronic conditions; inefficient, disorganized delivery systems; and challenges to greater implementation of information technology. The report goes on to outline 10 recommendations intended to improve health outcomes, one of which focuses on interprofessional collaboration. It emphasizes the need for providers and institutions to actively collaborate, exchange information, and make provisions for care coordination because the needs of any persons or population are beyond the expertise of any single health profession (IOM, 2001; Yeager,

2005). An earlier IOM report (1999), entitled *To Err Is Human: Building a Safer Health System,* addresses issues related to patient safety and errors in health care. This report articulates interprofessional communication and collaboration as primary measures to improve quality and reduce errors.

Accrediting and regulatory bodies such as the Joint Commission (2008) recognize interprofessional collaboration as an essential component of the prevention of medical error. This organization's mission is to continuously improve the safety and quality of care through the measure and evaluation of outcomes data. It has targeted improved communication and collaboration among providers, staff, and patients as a means to better protect patients from harm. Improved patient safety outcomes can also be facilitated through collaborative efforts such as development of interdisciplinary clinical guidelines and interprofessional curricula that incorporate proven strategies of team management and collaboration processes. Doctorally prepared APRNs are well positioned to participate and lead interprofessional collaborative teams in efforts to improve health outcomes of the individual patient or target population (American Association of Colleges of Nursing [AACN], 2006b).

INTERPROFESSIONAL COLLABORATION

The terms *interdisciplinary* and *interprofessional* are often used interchangeably in the literature about collaborative teams, but each has a slightly different connotation. Interprofessional collaboration describes the interactions among individual professionals who may represent a particular discipline or branch of knowledge, but who additionally bring their unique educational backgrounds, experiences, values, roles, and identities to the process. Each professional may possess some shared or overlapping knowledge, skills, abilities, and roles with other professionals with whom he or she collaborates.

Hence, the term "interprofessional" offers a broader definition than "interdisciplinary," which is more specific to the knowledge ascribed to a particular discipline. DNPs are well suited to serve as effective collaborative team leaders and participants not only because of the scientific knowledge, skills, and abilities related to their distinctive advanced nursing practice disciplines, but also because of their comprehension of organizational and systems improvements, outcome evaluation processes, healthcare policy, and leadership. This new skill set will be critical for DNPs leading teams in the complex and ever-changing health arena. The AACN's *Essentials of Doctoral Education for Advanced Nursing Practice* (2006b) adds that collaborative teams must remain "fluid depending upon the needs of the patient (population) . . . and [DNPs] must be prepared to play a central role in establishing interprofessional teams, participating in the work of the team and assuming leadership of the team when appropriate" (p. 14).

The concept of interprofessional collaborations to improve health outcomes is not new; it has been and continues to be the cornerstone of public health practice. Effective public health system collaborations are critical to protect populations from disease and injury and to promote health. Public health collaborations have involved not only vested professionals but also systems of communities, governmental agencies, nonprofit organizations, and private-sector groups to address a common goal or complex health outcome (Wilson & Bekemeir, 2004). DNPs can benefit from the experiences of public health colleagues and expand the definition of interprofessional panel collaboration. This is particularly relevant when considering potential stakeholders and in assembling the team. Successful implementation of a system or organizational improvement may require collaborations outside the typical healthcare team. The purpose or outcome of the project may dictate the need to include patient or family repre-

sentation in accordance with their ability and willingness to participate, as well as professionals from information and technology, health policy, administration, governing boards, and library science.

Interprofessional Healthcare Teams

Many healthcare practitioners indicate they practice within an interprofessional team. Often, this involves each professional addressing a particular portion of patient or population care, working independently and in parallel or in sequence to one another, with the physician frequently assuming the role of team leader (Robert Wood Johnson Foundation [RWJF], 2008). Drinka and Clark (2000) reinforce the need to function interdependently and engage in collaborative problem solving. All too often competition exists between roles, with each discipline holding to the belief that it is the most qualified to manage the patient or problem, thus negatively influencing the functioning of the team. In effective interprofessional teams, members recognize and value dissimilar professional perspectives and overlapping roles and share decision making and leadership to best meet the needs of the patient or problem at hand (Drinka & Clark, 2000).

To achieve optimal health outcomes, it is essential for DNPs and other health professionals to engage in true collaborative interprofessional practices. These types of collaborative practices will be most successful when (1) the complexity of the problem is high, (2) the team shares a common goal or vision for the outcome, (3) members have distinctive roles, (4) members recognize the value of one another's positions, and (5) each member offers unique contributions toward the improved patient or population outcome (ACP, 2009; Drinka & Clark, 2000; RWJF, 2008). This model for interprofessional healthcare teams will require DNPs to have a thorough understanding of effective collaboration, in addition to a firm grounding in effective communication, team processes, and leadership, to bring forth innovative strategies to improve health and health care.

Benefits of Collaboration

The literature of the past two decades well documents the numerous benefits of collaborative practices, including reduced error rates, decreased length of stays, improved health, better pain management, improved quality of life, and higher patient satisfaction (Brita-Rossi et al., 1996; Chung & Nguyen, 2005; Cowan et al., 2006; D'Amour & Oandasan, 2005; Drinka & Clark, 2000; Grady & Wojner, 1996; IOM, 1999; Joint Commission, 2008; Yeager, 2005). Nelson et al. (2002) and Sierchio (2003) note the additional benefits to healthcare systems of cost savings and healthy work environments. High-performing collaborative teams promote job satisfaction (D'Amour & Oandasan, 2005; Hall, Weaver, Gravelle, & Thibault, 2007; Sierchio, 2003), support a positive workplace atmosphere, and provide a sense of accomplishment while valuing the unique work and contributions of team members. These issues are particularly relevant to nursing practice. Addressing concerns of nursing shortages, improving working environments, and promoting measures to increase job satisfaction all have been found to correlate with lower rates of nurse burnout (Vahey, Aiken, Sloane, Clarke, & Vargas, 2004) and in turn indirectly influence nurse retention and recruitment.

The concept of "value added" has been discussed as an indirect benefit of effective collaboration (Dunevitz, 1997; Kleinpell et al., 2002). The term *value added* indicates the growth or improvement experienced in a group, project, or organization over a period, which yields an indirect "value" gained by a patient or population. Such value-added contributions may be the improvement to patient care delivery over time because of the rich professional interactions and exchanges that occur within an interprofessional team meeting. This enhanced communication would be more beneficial than the communication required from professionals working independently of one another. Value-added benefits may additionally be evident from the process itself, such as the creative problem solving that occurs during a brainstorming session designed to address a community health problem.

BARRIERS TO AND DRIVERS OF EFFECTIVE COLLABORATION IN INTERPROFESSIONAL HEALTHCARE TEAMS

Barriers

In spite of the mandates or recommendations by IOM, RWJF, the American Nurses Association (ANA), and the Joint Commission, effective interprofessional collaboration has yet to be adopted in any widespread form in the United States to improve patient or population outcomes. Literature from both Canada and Britain also makes recommendations for interprofessional collaboration to improve care (Oandasan et al., 2004), along with illuminating current thinking as to why healthcare systems have not adopted interprofessional healthcare teams. Some of the barriers to interprofessional collaboration include (1) gender, power, socialization, education, status, and cultural differences between professions (Hall, 2005; Whitehead, 2007); (2) lack of a payment system and structures that reward interprofessional collaboration; (3) misunderstanding of the scope and contribution of each profession; and (4) turf protection (Patterson, Grenny, McMillan, & Switzler, 2002). The DNP will need a comprehensive understanding of these barriers to provide fresh, creative thinking and leadership for the healthy development and sustainment of collaboration.

Nursing and medicine were and are often considered central players in healthcare teams; an examination of the issues related to these two professions is prudent. Nurse and physician role differences are easier to understand in light of the historical roles of gender. In the 19th century, nurses cared for patients in hospitals, while physicians cared for patients in their offices or patients' homes. According to Lynnaugh and Reverby's *Ordered to Care: The Dilemma of American Nursing 1850–1945* (1990), whereas physicians were "welcome visitors," hospitals were run by lay boards and often staffed by "live-in" nurses (p. 26). That situation changed when medicine became more science oriented and medical practitioners realized that hospitals were full of sick patients to whom they could apply their newly developed knowledge of science. Medicine soon controlled hospitals and defended this control with the argument that it owned the "special knowledge" needed to diagnose and treat disease. Physicians were able to convince the public that nurses were not trustworthy enough to manage medications or capable of obtaining the "special knowledge" that physicians had (often citing the menstrual cycle as the source of nurses' unreliability). Nurses soon became handmaidens to physicians; they needed to be "self-less, knowledgeless and virtuous" (Gordon, 2005, p. 63).

Nursing education in the 20th century was designed to provide cheap labor for hospitals while educating its new workforce. Nurses came to view themselves as working for doctors, not patients. Nurses were valued for their virtue, not for their knowledge (Buresh & Gordon, 2006). Most nurse leaders either accepted this subjugated role or were unable to change it. As nursing lost power, medicine increased its social status through the introduction of high-tech innovations in acute care (along with reimbursement for these advances). Healthcare delivery became fragmented based on physician specialty care for patients with acute care needs. Indeed, medicine dominated health care in the 20th century.

It can be argued that this physician-dominant, fragmented care has driven up healthcare costs, promoted polypharmacy, and encouraged "silo" practices. Wheatley (2005) compares organizations to the biological natural world. In the biological world, if a species becomes too dominant and loses its ability to work when the environment shifts, the entire system can collapse. According to *Healthy People 2010* (U.S. Department of Health and Human Services, 2000), the U.S. healthcare system will be challenged to provide effective chronic disease prevention and treatment. The current system, which is based on episodic care, will not serve the needs of the population. To meet the needs of the public in the early 21st century, DNPs will need to bring a full nursing perspective into the healthcare environment, along with the empowerment of other members of the team to improve the viability and strength of the healthcare system.

Physicians have also been closely aligned with the financial success of healthcare organizations (often hospitals) and, therefore, have often been designated leaders for any clinically based team. Even today, the American College of Physicians (2009) concludes that the "patient is best served by a multidisciplinary team where the clinical team is led by the physician" (p. 2). Although physicians may have the most training in diagnosis and treatment of disease, they may not always be the best choice to lead teams. Haas and Shaffir (1987) discuss the "cloak of competence" that is expected of physicians by society. Medical students eventually adopt this cloak to meet societal expectations, and may bring this "decisiveness" to the interprofessional arena. This perception may lead the physician to believe he or she must always make the final decision in the team, which may lead to a professional power imbalance whereby physicians have more power than other members of the team.

The issue of "disruptive behavior" in the workplace has been studied recently in light of the connection between poor communication and adverse events (Joint Commission, 2008). Rosenstein's (2002) qualitative study of physician–nurse relations found that almost all nurses in the study experienced some sort of "disruptive physician behavior," including verbal abuse. Rosenstein and O'Daniel (2008) repeated this work, expanded to include disruptive behavior by both nurses and physicians. This second report concluded that whereas "physician disruptive behavior is usually more direct and overt, nurse disruptive behaviors more frequently take the form of back-door undermining, clique formation, and other types of passive-aggressive behavior" (Rosenstein & O'Daniel, p. 467).

Drivers

In its *Essentials of Doctoral Education for Advanced Nursing Practice,* the AACN (2006b) discusses the need for interprofessional healthcare teams to function as high-performance teams. High-performance teams emphasize the skills, abilities, and unique perspective of each team member. If the nurses (or other team members) remain invisible, the overall effectiveness of the team will be impaired.

To work on interprofessional teams, nurses will need to articulate the role they play in improving patient care. The work that nurses perform is often not recognized by other healthcare professionals and reimbursement systems or found within the nomenclature of electronic health records. Many tasks that nurses perform are difficult to quantify, such as supporting a family through a crisis. A vital responsibility of the DNP (likely collaborating with other nursing PhD colleagues) is to articulate to the public, insurers, and policymakers the role that nurses play in promoting positive patient and family outcomes.

Another key factor in empowering nurses in interprofessional collaboration is the importance of role identification and clarity. In the United States, there is confusion about the education and titling of nurses. Although many states protect the title of "nurse," the public (including other healthcare professionals) continues to be confused about just who nurses are.

Nurses in administration may not identify themselves as nurses, whereas some medical assistants may call themselves "nurses." Although the work that medical assistants do with patients is valuable, it is not nursing. The first step to getting our voices heard is to identify who we are and call ourselves "nurses" at all levels. It is important that as nurses work to gain visibility and voice, they remain open to listening to other voices on the team.

SUCCESSFUL TEAM DEVELOPMENT

What are the stages of development that transform groups of disparate professionals into high-performance teams? Tuckman and Jensen (1977), and many others, believe that teams go through phases including forming, storming, norming, performing, and adjourning. Amos, Hu, and Herrick (2005) recommend that nurses understand these developmental stages to promote the development of a successful team.

Forming is the stage when the team first comes together to serve a specific purpose. Team members come into the group as individuals and get to know one another while determining the mission of the team along with their roles and responsibilities. The development of trust is key in this stage. Davoli and Fine (2004) suggest incorporating activities that are designed to show the human side of each team member, such as "icebreakers" or "member check-in" (p. 269).

An interdisciplinary team is likely to include members from diverse professions, all of whom have their own culture and language. An important first task of an interdisciplinary team is to discuss and understand the scope of each profession represented (Hall, 2005). It is likely there will be both overlap and diversity of function and skills among the professions. It is also important to develop a sense of shared language by reducing the use of professional jargon. Although it may be unintentional, jargon can prevent knowledge sharing, hinder communication, and promote power imbalances.

Standardized tools such as SBAR (situation, background, assessment, and recommendation), developed and used by Kaiser Permanente, can be used by interprofessional teams for discussion and problem solving regarding patient situations (Leonard, Graham, & Bonacum, 2004).

In the storming stage, team members have not fully developed trust, and conflict inevitably arises. Within interprofessional teams, members come from diverse disciplines and worldviews. It is highly likely that there will be a wide range of opinions and thoughts related to the issues and work of the team. It is important to face this conflict directly, however, so that the team can move on to the next stage. During the storming stage, it is vital that members learn to listen to one another with tolerance and patience (Lee, 2008). If the team does not go through this stage successfully, differences between individuals will not be brought into the team process and outcome. Conflict resolution is discussed at length later in this chapter.

Norming is the stage in which team members begin to develop a team identity. It is still important for the team to elicit differences of opinion to prevent "groupthink."

In the performing stage, team members work together to achieve team goals. Individual and professional turf needs will be set aside for the team to be effective in its mission. At this stage, the team members also learn to be flexible in tasks and roles to achieve the team's goals. Finally, the stage of adjourning concludes the formation of a team. The team evaluates its performance and progress by reviewing whether or not outcomes were met.

The following factors assist teams to progress through the stages of team development:

- Shared purpose, goal, and buy-in of members
- Reciprocal trust in team members
- Recognition and value of the unique role or skills each team member brings
- Functioning at the highest level of skill, ability, or practice

- Clear understanding of roles and the responsibilities of team members to meet goals
- Work culture and environment that embrace the collaborative process
- Collective cognitive responsibility and shared decision making

Shared Purpose

For a team to be effective, there must be a shared purpose or vision (Kouzes & Pozner, 2007). The purpose of the interprofessional healthcare team is based on improving some aspect of patient or population health outcomes. Competing needs of team members must be tabled in favor of the greater purpose. Turf wars and politicized thinking have no place in an effective interprofessional healthcare team. The leader must inspire this shared vision and elicit buy-in from each member. As Wheatley (2005) suggests, creativity is unleashed in people when they find "meaning" or purpose in "real" work. Meaningful teamwork can create synergistic solutions from members when the team has shared meaning or vision. Patterson et al. (2002) describe how free-flowing dialogue helps "fill the pool" of shared meaning. By allowing dialogue to be safe, more people can add their meaning to the "shared pool," giving the group a higher IQ. Learning to make dialogue safe is a skill that drives trust.

Team Members and Reciprocal Trust

An effective team must include the development of reciprocal trust between members. According to Kouzes and Pozner (2007), members of a high-trust team must continue to work to maintain interpersonal relationships with one another. In addition to the group mission and goals, the work of the group must include getting to know one another. The leader or facilitator who is willing to trust others in the group enough to show vulnerability and give up control often begins a culture of trust. The leader needs to be self-confident enough to be willing to be the first to be transparent;

because trust is contagious, others will likely follow suit. Team members and leaders need to listen intently and value the unique viewpoints of others in the group. If the group members fail to develop trust or to listen and value one another, it is likely that they will resist and sabotage the group's efforts (Wheatley, 2005). Many authors describe this aspect of team leadership as leading with the heart: looking at how the heart can help shape dialogue and goals (Kouzes & Pozner; Patterson et al., 2002).

Because of economic and time constraints, many teams meet in virtual formats. The question many have is, Are face-to-face encounters between team members vital to the development of trust building? Kouzes and Pozner (2007) propose that a group can become a team only when members have met face to face four to five times. These authors suggest that "virtual trust, like virtual reality, is one step removed from the real thing" (p. 241). Other sources discuss the very real possibility of developing trust via virtual means (Grabowski & Roberts, 1999; Greenberg, Greenberg, & Antonucci, 2007). Because of the lack of eye contact and body language in virtual interactions, communication patterns should be more deliberate.

Greenberg et al. propose that trust building in virtual teams intentionally includes activities that promote both cognitive and affective trust. Cognitive trust is implicated in the formation of "swift, but fragile trust" during the early development of the team (Greenberg et al., p. 325). For cognitive trust to develop, individual team members need to believe that group members have both ability (competence) and integrity. One action to promote a sense of competence in individual team members is to have the team leader introduce members, endorse their abilities, and explain why they were chosen for the team. Another important asset for building the sense of integrity is for team members to keep deadlines and stay engaged in the process (no freeloading). Affective trust is essential during later stages of the team's development and is vital to the functioning of team members to complete the task. Development of affective trust is based on benevolence and relies on team members seeing the humanity in one another, with development of true caring and concern.

G. Boelhower (personal communication, April 10, 2009) recommends that virtual teams begin their time with "check-in, story-telling, deep questioning and dialogue, and affirmation." He goes on to state that he "sees the level of trust develop regularly" in online groups when the human side of individuals is shared. As discussed earlier in this chapter, this type of sharing may be started with icebreakers, check-ins, and checkouts. DNPs will likely have experience with online relationship building during their education process and can continue to experiment with team building in face-to-face and virtual formats based on the current evidence.

Recognition and Value of Each Team Member

According to Burkhardt and Alvita (2008), "each person is a moral agent and must be recognized as worthy of dignity and respect" (p. 219). Without respect, the work of the group cannot move forward; dialogue is halted. Respect among team members is vital because, as Patterson et al. (2002) note, "Respect is like air. If it goes away, it is all people can think about" (p. 71). Each member's voice must be heard and respected whether he or she is the highest educated member or not. To do this, team members must recognize the moral agency of each member and his or her unique skills and abilities, often based on the individual's professional skill set.

Using structure in interprofessional team dialogue may be called for as a result of the entrenched perceived power and authority of individual members and the professions they represent. Such methods as the Indian talking stick and Johari window can be used proactively to be sure that all team members feel they have a voice, are understood, and are free to share their thoughts and feelings. The concept behind the talking stick is that only the person who is holding the stick may speak. When the person finishes speaking, the stick is passed to the next speaker. That next person may not argue or disagree with the former speaker, but is to restate what has been said. This process allows for all team members to be and feel understood (Covey, 2004).

The Johari window is a tool developed in 1955 by Joseph Luft and Harry Ingham (Chapman, 2008). It is used to help build trust among group members by encouraging appropriate self-disclosure. The Johari window has four quadrants: the open area, the blind area, the hidden area, and the unknown area. The goal is to increase the open area so that team members can be more productive because communication is not hampered by "distractions, mistrust, confusion, conflict and misunderstanding" (Chapman, p. 4.) One team member (the subject) is given a list of 55 adjectives and is told to pick 5 or 6 that describe himself or herself. A team member is given the same list and also picks out 5 or 6 words that describe the subject. The adjectives are then placed in the four quadrants:

1. Both team members know the open area.
2. Only the subject, not the other team member, knows the hidden area.
3. Only the team member, not the subject, knows the blind spot.
4. The unknown area include adjectives not picked by either subject nor team member and may or may not be applicable to the subject (Chapman, 2008).

The Johari tool can assist team members to learn about both themselves and one another. Appropriate and sensitive increases in the open area can be promoted by the use of team-building exercises and games, along with teams engaging in non-work-time activities.

Functioning at the Highest Level

American health care is expensive, but not always effective. There is pressure for innovative models of care that are cost-effective and improve outcomes for patients. Many clinical systems have begun to use episodic treatment groups (ETGs) to measure patient outcomes and provider performance (Fortham, Dove, & Wooster, 2000). Examples of ETGs are those for chronic diseases such as diabetes, asthma, depression, and hypertension. Guideline development by such groups as the Institute for Clinical Systems Integration (ICSI) can provide evidence-based pathways of care for the various ETGs.

In the past, physicians have felt the need to perform all the primary care tasks for patients. Given the current complexity and expense of health care, it is not possible for one group to do it all. This realization has led to the concept of having all healthcare providers work to the top of their licenses. This involves a shifting of tasks, often with each discipline giving up some tasks that can be done by another care provider more cost-effectively. An example of working to the top of one's license is for advanced practice nurses to take more responsibility for routine chronic and acute care and health maintenance, while physicians perform the diagnosing and treatment of more complex unstable patients, and RNs assume the role of care coordinator (including pre- and post-visit planning), coach, and educator. In this example, all disciplines may need to give up some tasks to be cost-effective. An exemplar of a program that utilizes healthcare providers at the top of their licenses is the DIAMOND (Depression Improvement Across Minnesota, Offering a New Direction) project (ICSI, 2007). At the center of the DIAMOND project is a case manager (typically an RN) who has 150 to 200 patients with depression in an outpatient setting. The case manager works with a consulting psychiatrist to review patients on a weekly basis (typically 2 hours per week). This has proven to be a cost-effective model that provides better depression outcomes than standard care. The challenge is to provide a payment structure that rewards this type of innovative care.

Clear Understanding of Roles and Responsibilities

During the forming stage of the team (and beyond), it is vital that each team member understand his or her role and responsibilities. Role uncertainty can lead to conflict among team members and decrease team functioning (Baker, Baker, & Campbell, 2003). The leader should be certain that each team member has a clear understanding of his or her role by having the members restate their roles to the team. This type of candid discussion can occur only if the team feels that open communication is safe. A clear understanding of each team member's role helps to prevent role overlap as well as tasks falling through the cracks (Lewis, 2007).

Work Culture That Embraces Collaboration

Components of a work culture that embraces collaboration include (1) a culture of psychological safety, (2) a flattened power differential (hierarchy), (3) administrative support and resultant resources allocated for collaboration (Kelly, 2008), and (4) physical space design that promotes collaboration, such as rooms for interdisciplinary interaction (Lindeke & Sieckert, 2005).

According to Edmonson (2006), organizations that support "upward voice" promote a culture of psychological safety. She goes on to state that "upward voice is communication directed to someone higher in the organizational hierarchy with perceived power or authority to take action on the problem or suggestion" (Edmonson, p. 1). Tangible evidence of this culture includes leaders who walk around the organization and initiate conversation, suggestion boxes placed around the organization, and an "open door" policy. Individuals must have the sense that they can readily ask questions, try out new ideas and innovations, and ask for support from others.

Another way to promote psychological safety within an organization is to enhance employee confidence that there will not be a penalty for admitting to mistakes. Safety culture research is shifting from focusing on only the role of individuals in errors to the role of systems in such mistakes. Healthcare leaders have had to explore other industry successes that promote safety, such as aviation, where the focus of safety improvement is on the systems in which individuals operate (Feldman, 2008). Authors such as Snijders, Kollen, Van Lingen, Fetter, and Molendijk (2009) recommend implementation of a nonpunitive incident reporting system to improve safety standards. A nonpunitive incident reporting system helps ensure that issues are brought to the forefront so that improvements can be made. The Agency for Healthcare Research and Quality (2009) has developed evaluation tools for primary care offices, nursing homes, and hospitals with questions related to psychological safety and communication. DNPs will be required to provide leadership and recommend resources to champion the culture of both psychological and systems safety within the organizations they serve.

Collective Cognitive Responsibility and Shared Decision Making

As fundamental as it is for each team member to have a clear understanding of individual roles and responsibilities, it is also essential for high-performance teams to have a culture of shared decision making or collective cognitive responsibility. Scardamalia (2002) describes collective cognitive responsibility in terms of team members having responsibility not only for the outcome of the group, but also for staying cognitively involved in the process as things unfold. She describes the functioning of a surgical team, in which members not only perform their assigned tasks but also keep involved in the entire process. The responsibility for the outcome lies not just with the leader of the surgical team, but with the entire team as a whole.

A key component of shared decision making is that it usually occurs at the point of service

(Golanowski, Beaudry, Kurz, Laffey, & Hook, 2007; Porter-O'Grady, 1997). Porter-O'Grady states that "the point of decision making in the clinical delivery system is the place where patients and providers meet" (p. 41), which has implications for including patients as collaborators on the interprofessional team.

Healthcare systems, as complex adaptive systems, require flexibility and continuous participation, learning, and sharing (Begun, Zimmerman, & Dooley, 2003). All of the interprofessional healthcare team members must stay engaged in the process at the point of service for the outcome of care to be successful.

STRONG LEADERSHIP

There is no dispute that redesigning health care will require strong leadership. As opposed to "management," which seeks to control and manage, leaders seek to create and inspire change (Kotter, 1990). Leadership theories generally fall under the classifications of behavioral, contingency, contemporary, and Wheatley's "new leadership" approaches (Kelly, 2008). Behavioral theories posit that leadership style or behavior is the most important factor in the outcome desired. Behavioral approaches include autocratic, democratic, and laissez-faire, based on the point at which the power or decision making occurs and the type of worker or task involved. Contingency theories recognize that there is more to leadership than the leader's behavior. One type of contingency theory is situational leadership, developed by Hershey and Blanchard, in which follower maturity is evaluated and determines the amount of direction, support, or delegation from the leader to the follower. Contemporary theories include transformational leadership, which IOM (2003) deemed vital to the achievement of the transformation of health care.

Transformational Leadership

The IOM (2003) report recommends transformational leadership as a means to make the necessary changes to improve patient safety. The theory of transformational leadership, developed first by Burns (1978), is based on the concept of empowering all team members (including the leader) to work together to achieve a shared goal. This fits with Covey's (2004) definition of leadership: "Leadership is communicating to people their worth and potential so clearly that they come to see it in themselves" (p. 98).

The transformational leader need not be in a formal position of administration, but can lead from any position within the organization and operates through an ethical and moral perspective. Transformational leaders lead with a clear vision and use coaching, inspiring, and mentoring to transform themselves, followers, and organizations (Burns, 1978; Kelly, 2008).

"New Leadership"

Wheatley (2005) describes a "new way" of leadership, which is contrary to the Western style of linear, hierarchical organizations. She bases her view of organizations on biology, which is self-organizing and complex. Instead of seeing change as negative, Wheatley views change as life itself. She states, "Nothing alive, including us, resists creative motions. However, all of life resists control. All of life reacts to any process that inhibits its freedom to create itself" (Wheatley, 2005, p. 28). She recommends that teams self-organize to build communities that are no longer ruled by "command and control" (Wheatley, p. 68). Instead of viewing organizations and workers as machines, Wheatley suggests that organizations model themselves after living systems, which are adaptive, creative, and depend on one another for growth and sustainability.

Leadership Versus Management

Whereas management is the coordination of resources to meet organizational goals, leadership is built on relationships. Kouzes and Pozner (2007), in their seminal book *The Leadership*

Challenge, examined leaders over 25 years and determined that leadership is a relationship in which leaders do five things:

1. *Model the way.* The leader must be aware of his or her own values and live a life that expresses those values.

2. *Inspire a shared vision.* The leader must be able to imagine the future and inspire others to share that vision.

3. *Challenge the process.* Leaders are engaged in the processes of the team and continually looking for innovations. They are willing to take risks and learn from experiences.

4. *Enable others to act.* Leaders help to build trust in relationships through collaboration and competence.

5. *Encourage the heart.* Leaders identify the contributions of each individual team member and encourage celebration when victories occur.

Anyone can be a leader; a formal title is not necessary.

EFFECTIVE COMMUNICATION

> Remember not only to say the right thing in the right place, but far more difficult still, to leave unsaid the wrong thing at the tempting moment.
>
> —*Benjamin Franklin*

All of the work of interprofessional collaborations involves communication. Success or failure of the team depends on the effectiveness of the communication processes. Communication is a complex process of transmitting a message between a sender and a receiver. The sender must effectively deliver the content, and the receiver must in turn correctly interpret or decipher the message. Many sources of error can occur within this exchange, and skilled communicators must make a concerted effort to deliver clear, consistent messages to prevent misinterpretation and loss of meaning.

Communication is more than the exchange of verbal information; in fact, the majority of communication is nonverbal. The DNP must be accomplished not only in the art of verbal and written communication but also in the interpretation and effective use of nonverbal communiqués such as silence, gestures, facial expressions, body language, tone of voice, and space (Sullivan, 2004).

In addition to sending congruent verbal and nonverbal messages, it is vital for DNPs to employ strategies that enhance communication within the interprofessional team setting. Determining the timing and best medium for what, how, and when to deliver a message is a necessary skill (Sullivan, 2004). Appropriate timing of key messages increases the likelihood that the message will have the desired impact on the recipient. The message may be phrased well but rejected if the intended audience is not receptive. Consider the availability and state of mind of the recipient. Is there adequate time for the discussion? Is the recipient distracted, emotionally or physically? Are other issues more pressing now? Such factors may contribute to misinterpretation or lack of objectivity regarding the communication. Reflect as to whether an alternative time, venue, or medium may provide a more appropriate means by which to deliver the message. For instance, if the message is of a sensitive, confidential matter, face-to-face communication would be preferable to an email, voicemail correspondence, or team discussion (Sullivan, 2004). In group settings, it is imperative to allow participants enough time to provide objective information and express thoughts, viewpoints, and opinions about the situation for meaningful collaboration to occur.

Buresh and Gordon, in their book *From Silence to Voice: What Nurses Know and Must Communicate to the Public* (2006), suggest use of the "voice of agency" when communicating the role of nursing to others. Within the collaborative team it is imperative that DNP members clearly communicate nursing's involvement in a patient care scenario or clinical project and, more importantly, articulate the level of clinical judgment and rationale required for such actions. It is important and necessary to embrace the opportunity to communicate to the team the role of the DNP in enhanced care delivery. This "voice of agency" is neither boastful nor an attempt to be superior, but rather an accurate acknowledgment of the unique contributions, value added, and improved patient outcomes resulting from expert nursing care. Conversely, it may reflect the negative consequences or potential for error averted as a result of the expertise, skills, and knowledge of doctorally prepared nurses. Davoli and Fine (2004) offer a similar perspective and note, "Collaboration gives providers an opportunity to be introspective and solidify their role through the contributions they make. A successful collaborative process will enhance one's professional identity" (p. 268). Draye, Acker, and Zimmer (2006), in their article on the practice doctorate in nursing, propose that the educational preparation of DNPs include opportunities for students to convene an interprofessional team. This experience allows students to incorporate strategies to promote effective team functioning while communicating the unique contributions of nursing required for the improved health outcome.

Buresh and Gordon (2006) go on to discuss the role self-presentation plays in communicating information regarding the competency and credibility of the DNP to team members, patients, or the public. Attire and manner of address influence the perceptions of others. What does dress communicate if Mary wears teddy bear scrubs rather than street clothes and a lab coat to a committee meeting? How might the DNP's role be valued if she were introduced as "Mary from Pediatrics" versus "Dr. Mary Jones, Pediatric Nurse Practitioner"? How are physician colleagues addressed in similar workplace encounters? Introductions using one's full name and credentials convey professionalism, respect, and credibility on par with other healthcare professional colleagues (Buresh & Gordon, 2006).

Ineffective communication is a major obstacle in interprofessional collaboration, is directly related to quality of patient care, and contributes to adverse health outcomes (Clarin, 2007; IOM, 1999). Some barriers that lead to communication breakdowns are specific to interactions between the sender and the receiver, whereas others relate to the organizational system. Defensiveness on the part of either participant can hamper communications (Sullivan, 2004). These behaviors may result from lack of self-confidence, a fear of rejection, or perceived threat to self-image or status. Defensiveness impedes communication by displacing anger via verbal aggression or conflict avoidance. Awareness of this mechanism and developing an approach to manage it in the context of the collaborative team are necessary attributes of an effective DNP leader.

As healthcare teams become more global and virtual, the potential for language and cultural communication barriers increases. Misreading body language or misinterpretation of the spoken or written message often results from a lack of understanding regarding language (especially in translation) and cultural differences (Sullivan, 2004). What one group finds acceptable, another may consider offensive, such as eye contact, physical touch, or the use of space. Room for misinterpretation exists in translation. Language used by Western cultures typically is direct and explicit, in which the background is not necessarily required to interpret the meaning of the message. This approach may differ from that employed in cultures using indirect communication, in which the intent of the message often relies upon the context in which it is used (Brett, Behfar, & Kern, 2006). DNPs and interprofessional colleagues have an obligation to increase their cultural competence and understanding of health issues and healthcare disparities to dispel any misconceptions, particularly if the team is composed of persons from diverse cultures.

Jargon is another "language" that can pose a barrier to understanding (Davoli & Fine, 2004;

Sullivan, 2004). Unfamiliar terms can lead to confusion and error and should be avoided to prevent unfavorable outcomes. Although professional jargon may serve as a type of verbal shorthand among some group members, it can also be a form of intimidation or exclusion and contribute to an imbalance of knowledge or power within the team (Davoli & Fine, 2004). Lindeke and Block (2001) stress that collaborative teams communicate with a shared, inclusive (i.e., "we," "our") language to prevent this imbalance and promote participation of all members. Effective communication involves the use of a common, shared language that is understood by all members of the team.

Preconceived assumptions and biases prevent the listener from tuning in and focusing on the content (Sullivan, 2004). This hinders the communication process because the receiver has formulated a predetermined judgment or drawn a conclusion before all the information is shared or facts validated. Effective communicators need to suspend judgments until all viewpoints are shared.

Gender differences in style and approach to communication can also pose obstacles (Sullivan, 2004). Subtle differences exist in how men and women perceive the same message. In collaborative teams, women may strive for consensus whereas men may place emphasis on hierarchy and "leading the team." Differences exist in the use of questions and interruptions in communications. An appreciation and understanding of these dissimilarities can prepare the DNP to function more effectively in teams of mixed gender.

Organizations and systems may pose additional obstacles to effective interprofessional communications. Outdated, limited, or unavailable technologies, such as video conferencing, messaging or paging systems, or lack of electronic health record interoperability between systems, can significantly impair the ability of members to communicate on a timely basis. This can be of vital importance to patient safety when attempting to communicate critical changes in patient status, medications, or lab values. The system further contributes to communication problems when the roles and responsibilities of team members are unclear. Participants may be hesitant or resistant to engage in exchanges or knowledge sharing. Clear designation of roles is of particular importance in virtual organizations and teams (i.e., electronically linked providers). In these collaborative environments, risks can be mitigated if members have a clear understanding of what is expected of each other and have a preestablished path of communication (Grabowski & Roberts, 1999) (see **Table 30-1**).

TABLE 30-1 Measures to Improve Communication

- Maintain eye contact: Convey interest, attentiveness (United States/Canada).
- Speak concisely: Avoid jargon.
- Use questions wisely: Clarify or elicit further information.
- Avoid qualifiers or tags (i.e., "sort of," "kind of," "I don't know if you would be interested"): These reduce the effectiveness of one's message.
- Be aware of gestures, facial expressions, posture: Send positive nonverbal signals (e.g., smiling conveys warmth, leaning forward indicates receptivity, and open-palm gestures suggest accessibility).
- Avoid defensiveness.
- Avoid responding emotionally: Never raise your voice, yell, or cry.

CONFLICT RESOLUTION

As both leaders and members of interprofessional teams, DNPs will need to develop and continue to refine skills related to conflict resolution. Conflicts are inevitable, and are even vital for interprofessional team effectiveness. Conflict is defined in many ways, but generally includes disagreement, interference, and negative emotion (Barki & Hartwick, 2001). If conflict is disruptive or dysfunctional, team efforts can decrease communication and, therefore, team functioning. Conversely, conflict that is constructive leads to superior results by including the "shared pool of meaning" of all team members. According to Patterson et al. (2002), the "larger the shared pool, the smarter the decisions" (p. 21).

As stated earlier, nurses over the last century have often used passive-aggressive methods to resolve conflict, such as avoidance, withholding, smoothing over, and compromising (Feldman, 2008). These methods do not promote dialogue, the most central means to attain the shared pool of meaning of the entire team. DNPs need to lead nurses and other professionals in using techniques that promote dialogue and, thereby, collaboration between professionals. The purpose of collaborative conflict management is to promote win–win versus win–lose solutions. The skills for conflict resolution and improving dialogue can be learned. According to Patterson et al. (2002) in their book *Crucial Conversations,* conflict resolution includes such methods as starting with the heart, making conversation safe, staying in dialogue when emotions are high, using persuasion, and promoting positive actions. Most of the skills related to collaborative conflict management are intertwined with effective communication skills and the development of emotional intelligence.

Chinn (2008) offers suggestions that are foundational for the transformation of conflict into solidarity and diversity. These recommendations begin before there is any conflict in a group or team and include rotating leadership, practicing critical reflection, and adopting customs to value diversity. By rotating leadership, the team members all have a stake in the outcome of the team goals and processes. When a conflict arises, involved parties can step back while other members rise up to help lead the team. Critical reflection can be accomplished by incorporating a closing time at which all team members can share their thoughts and feelings about the team process. By practicing ways to value diversity, such as developing team processes during meetings that show appreciation and value for each individual, conflict can move from violence to peaceful recognition of the diversity of alternative views.

EMOTIONAL INTELLIGENCE

Emotional intelligence (EI) is yet another valuable attribute of successful interprofessional leadership. EI is the awareness of the role emotion plays in personal relationships and the purposeful use of emotion to communicate, build rapport, and motivate self and others. These characteristics have been found to play a far greater role than cognitive abilities in the success or failure of a leader (Goleman, Boyzatsis, & McKee, 2002).

Goleman et al. outline five realms of EI: self-awareness, self-regulation, motivation, empathy, and social skills. Self-awareness involves recognizing your own emotions and the effect your mood and confidence level have on persons. Maintaining your composure in high-emotion meetings or challenging clinical situations is an example of effectual self-regulation. Conflict is a natural process of interprofessional teamwork, which can lead to positive or negative group functioning, depending on leadership style. Emotionally intelligent leaders have the ability to adapt, withhold judgment, and exhibit self-control in emotionally charged situations. An optimistic attitude, passion, and commitment to pursuing the goals of the group and desire for excellence help provide the motivation factor of EI. Leaders who are sensitive and empathetic to the needs and perspectives of others encourage the group to carry on and perform to its best ability.

Drinka and Clark (2000) talk about the role of "reflective practice" in interprofessional team practice. This concept builds on the self-awareness and empathy qualities of EI: the understanding of how our professional cultures, preparations, and experiences shape how we function in teams, as well as the ability to appreciate the similar and dissimilar perspectives of other interprofessional team members.

A fifth element is that of social skill: The ability to build rapport, network, communicate, and facilitate change. As an effective leader, it is imperative to foster a system of open, timely communication, whether by face-to-face communication, phone, or electronic means, to meet the desired outcomes for the project, patient, or population successfully. Regularly practicing calming relaxation techniques and rehearsing responses prior to anticipated stressful encounters allow one to manage reactions in an emotionally intelligent manner. DNPs can develop these skills with regular practice, self-reflection, coaching, and feedback from colleagues, and can use "EQ" (emotional intelligence quotient) as a tool to gauge their performance as leaders.

McCallin and Bamford (2007) suggest that EI is integral to effective interdisciplinary team functioning. Healthcare providers may be highly skilled in practicing emotionally intelligent interactions with their patients and families but may receive little preparation in promoting emotionally intelligent, healthy communication and functioning between professionals. Miller et al. (2008) specifically explored the role of EI in nursing practice as it relates to interprofessional team functioning. In this qualitative study, the ability of the nurse to effectively collaborate on interprofessional teams was influenced by his or her degree of EI. Nurses who engaged in esprit de corps (significant role embracing to the exclusion of other professionals) were considerably less able to function successfully on the team, less able to

have other members appreciate nursing's contribution to patient care, and generally less engaged in team processes. These researchers support the need to address not only the cognitive aspects of interprofessional teamwork but also the emotional aspects of optimal team functioning. DNP leaders versed in EI work are well suited to recognize individual and personality differences among team members and can build on them, mentor colleagues, and use EI to influence the effectiveness of the team and improve patient outcomes and satisfaction among interprofessional team members.

NECESSITIES FOR COLLABORATION

The objective of interprofessional collaboration is, of course, to generate a practice or systems enhancement to improve the health of an individual or population. Whether implementing an evidence-based practice effort or a quality improvement initiative, some sort of change is required. Even what many group members view as a desirable change will inevitably encounter some reluctance or resistance. The ability to facilitate change or serve as an agent of change is a key function required for successful collaboration. DNPs must be versed in one or more theories of change to effectively motivate and move the collaborative team to the optimal goal.

Change Agent: Lewin's Model

Lewin's force field analysis model (1951) is a classic framework for understanding the process of change within a group, system, or health initiative. Lewin's theory recognizes change as a constant factor of life ensuing from a dynamic balance of driving and opposing forces. The desired change results from the addition of driving forces or the diminishing of opposing forces and progresses over a series of three stages: unfreezing, moving, and refreezing. Unfreezing necessitates assessing the need and preparing members to move from the status quo to an improved level of practice, whereas the movement phase involves the addition of driving forces to motivate and empower members to adopt the improved perspective while simultaneously minimizing restraining forces that pose barriers to the desired change (Lewin, 1951; Miller, 2008). Driving forces must outweigh opposing forces to shift the equilibrium in the direction of the desired change. The improvements must then be secured, or allowed to refreeze, to maintain the desired change (Lewin, 1951; Miller, 2008).

Continuous Reflective Learning

The drivers of effective interprofessional teams discussed in this chapter will evolve in teams over time. Knowing the drivers is the first step in the development of both personal and team skills, but individual team members and the team as a whole will need continuous reflection. Each leader and follower should develop habits that build in time for personal reflection and growth. Many find that reading sacred texts or poetry, listening to music, practicing yoga, praying, meditating, exercising, connecting with spiritual leaders, or being in nature allow for deep reflective thinking and learning. Covey (1991) calls this "sharpening the saw" (p. 38), and recommends that people proactively plan for daily time to renew themselves. The wholeness of each team member is vital for the best functioning of the entire team.

Teams within healthcare organizations in the 21st century will need to practice continuous reflective learning (developed by Senge, 1990) to adapt to the rapid changes taking place. Interprofessional teams can utilize the vast organizational behavior research on the significance of continuous reflective learning. Edmonson (1999) defines team learning as "the activities carried out by team members through which a team obtains and processes data that allow it to adapt and change" (p. 352). Spending some time on reflection regarding team functioning will be vital to learning. Structural practices that foster team

learning include providing time during each meeting for reflection, leaving the worksite for retreats, conducting "critical incident" evaluations, discussing errors and failures, using patient satisfaction surveys and interviews, and celebrating successes.

The Patient and Family as Interprofessional Team Members

As health care reorganizes into interprofessional teams in which primary care is the hub of the system, central team members will be patients and their families. Patients and their families will need to be invited and supported into the interprofessional collaboration process through actions that promote meaningful dialogue, patient empowerment, self-efficacy, and activation (Hibbard, Stockard, Mahoney, & Tusler, 2004). Some tools the DNP may want to recommend include patient or family focus groups, satisfaction surveys, personal health records, decisional guides such as the *Ottawa Personal Decision Guide* (O'Connor, 2006), and advanced directives, along with ongoing patient education regarding the patients' and families' role in health care.

MODELS FOR IMPLEMENTATION: FROM PROJECT TO PRACTICE

Value of Incorporating Collaborative Work into Educational Preparation Curricula

Although there is a growing body of evidence regarding the benefits of collaboration between disciplines in the delivery of optimal patient care, few healthcare professionals have received any formal training in this concept during their educational preparation. Students in health professional programs often are taught in both the classroom and the clinical setting by faculty from the same professional background. They have little opportunity to learn about the work of other disciplines or participate in any shared learning experience. Brewer (2005) describes this pattern of education as "silo" preparation, in which each discipline believes it is best qualified to care for the patient. Without a formal structure and support for learning and practicing a team approach to care delivery in the educational setting, negative attitudes, prejudices, and misunderstanding of roles can occur. This contributes to an inability to collaborate effectively and consult with other providers as practicing professionals and may lead to discipline overlap and competition rather than collaboration for delivery of care.

A Cochrane systematic review of interprofessional education interventions (Reeves et al., 2008) examined six studies (four randomized control and two controlled before-and-after designs in a variety of settings). Interprofessional education was defined as any type of educational experience or learning opportunity in which interactive learning occurred between two or more health-related disciplines. Although a number of positive outcomes were noted, further rigorous studies are needed to draw conclusive evidence supporting core elements of interprofessional education and the subsequent impact of interprofessional collaborative education on health outcomes.

In an effort to increase the ability of health professional teams to deliver optimal patient care, RWJF funded educational programs (Partnerships for Quality Education [PQE]) designed to improve interprofessional collaboration, chronic disease management, systems-based care, and quality (RWJF, 2008). These initiatives were developed to provide nurse practitioners, physicians, and other allied healthcare providers with educational experiences, skills, and attitudes to deliver care that is of better quality than that which could be provided by any single discipline. One funded model was Collaborative Interprofessional Team Education (CITE); the objective of this program was to design collaborative clinical and educational interventions for health professional students from medicine, nursing, so-

cial work, and pharmacy (RWJF, 2008). The program did make some strides toward improvement in participants' understanding and attitudes toward other professions.

Whitehead (2007) offers some insight into the challenges of engaging medical students in interprofessional educational programs. Real and perceived power, high degree of status, professional socialization, and decision-making responsibility can limit the ability of physicians to collaborate with other members of the healthcare team unless efforts to change the culture, flatten hierarchy, and share responsibility are promoted. A number of additional obstacles prevented full implementation of the CITE initiative, including differing academic schedules and a lack of faculty practicing in teams to effectively mentor and model for students (RWJF, 2008).

The primary objective of Achieving Competence Today (ACT), another PQE initiative, was to promote interprofessional collaboration and quality improvement in the curriculum of healthcare professionals within two academic health centers (Ladden, Bednash, Stevens, & Moore, 2006; RWJF, 2008). Four disciplines worked jointly to plan and implement a quality improvement project. As a result, core competencies necessary for successful interprofessional teams were identified, and researchers suggested measures for incorporating these competencies into the educational preparation of future students as a means to improve quality and safety in health care.

DNP programs can build on concepts of interprofessional education by allowing and encouraging programs to use faculty from a variety of disciplines to prepare DNP students. Interprofessional faculty can add a depth and richness to the DNP curriculum by bringing and sharing skills, knowledge, and the highest level of expertise in areas of clinical practice—whether it be business and management, pharmacy, public policy, psychology, medicine, or informatics (AACN, 2006a). Educational experience related to interprofessional collaboration as a means to improve quality or promote safety should be highly visible within the scholarly DNP project.

Role of the Scholarly Project: Real Interdisciplinary Collaboration

The Essentials of Doctoral Education for Advanced Nursing Practice (AACN, 2006) refers to the final DNP scholarly project or capstone as a culminating, immersion experience that affords the opportunity to integrate and synthesize all elements of doctoral education competencies within an interprofessional work environment. DNP-led scholarly projects provide a venue for students to assume leadership roles for effective interprofessional collaboration to improve health care, patient outcomes, and healthcare systems.

The DNP project "Optimal Use of Individualized Asthma Action Plans in an Electronic Health Record" (Miller, 2008) involved a number of opportunities for interprofessional collaboration. This process improvement project involved a systems change designed to improve pediatric asthma care delivery in a regional health system. An asthma action plan tool built into the electronic health record of a multispecialty regional health system served as a vehicle for the delivery of evidence-based practice. Distinct DNP-led interprofessional teams collaborated during various stages of program planning, implementation, and evaluation. Collaboration with nursing professionals and professionals in the fields of informatics, information technology, statisticians, and management was active throughout the project, particularly during tool development and in the implementation phase. Key to ensuring effective communication within this group was the use of a common language and developing a clear understanding of one another's roles and contributions. A second opportunity for interprofessional collaboration occurred during the implementation phase. All of the members of the pediatric asthma team—the DNP, clinical nurse specialist, and physician—came to the project with their own agendas and perspectives. Frequent revisiting of desired project outcomes, goals, and objectives was necessary early on to develop a cohesive, unified collaboration.

A third DNP-led collaboration took place at the pilot project site, a regional primary care clinic. This collaboration, which initially presented many challenges, involved physicians, nursing, administrative management, and administrative support. This site had recently been acquired by the parent organization. Previous quality improvement initiatives had been attempted and, due to a variety of factors, were not successfully implemented. A number of barriers to collaboration were anticipated at this site, including a sense of mistrust and resistance to change. Building trusting, nonthreatening relationships with staff and providers was a much-needed starting point. Issues of power were foreseeable between the physicians and the project manager. Initially, this group expressed hesitancy with the concept of anyone other than the physician being responsible for the optimal delivery of pediatric asthma care. It is important to acknowledge that providers might experience competing loyalties as they struggle to prioritize and balance the additional time needed to implement a project along with time required to see other patients or perform other duties. Avoiding these barriers requires mutual respect for each other's role, purpose, and workload. It is vital to continually clarify and communicate the shared vision of the collaborative project—in this case, it was improved asthma care for children. Building relationships, seeking team member input, and developing a shared vision play a critical role in negotiating hurdles for interprofessional collaboration and for effective project implementation and evaluation.

In the DNP project "Developing a Population-Focused Student Health Service" (Ash, 2005), interprofessional collaboration morphed from providers within the student health services

(SHS) to a broad range of professionals. The ecologic approach (NASPA, 2004) was used in the final stages of the student DNP project, which broadened the base of stakeholders and thus the collaborating professionals. The ecologic perspective views the connections between health and learning within the campus setting (Sacher et al., 2005). The initial task force led by the DNP student included a project mentor who was an expert in group work as a result of his education and experience as a master of social work. His skills in the so-called softer side of team development molded the experience by bringing all the team members into the process. He was also continually willing to try new approaches and then evaluate the outcomes. The project mentor had direct access to the vice president of student affairs, who was also known to be innovative and skilled in human relationships due to his background in counseling.

Unlike with many healthcare-related projects, there were no physicians on the interprofessional team. This may have changed the leadership and political issues that have plagued nurse–physician relationships in the past. The DNP student may have struggled to lead a team that included a physician. If, however, a physician was part of the team, increased efforts could have been conducted to develop reciprocal trust and to recognize and value each profession. Having a physician from outside the college may have afforded an opportunity for increased networking of the interprofessional team within the community in which the college is situated.

Some of the drivers of interprofessional team functioning (such as trust, recognition and value of team members, and a shared purpose) were already present on this team at some level. Team members knew one another and had passion for the team purpose: developing a culture that embraces health and well-being. The team members work within a college that espouses "Benedictine values" (College of St.

Scholastica, 2009), which include community, hospitality, and stewardship. This emphasis on Benedictine values provided a work culture that embraced collaboration, which is a driver of interprofessional teams.

One of the barriers that plagued the team was the lack of clear understanding of roles and responsibilities. The team met and formed ideas that the team leader and mentor needed to follow through on. This team structure has changed since the end of the DNP project to four separate working groups focused on student health, faculty and staff health, marketing, and academic integration, respectively. The project, now entitled Well U, has been in full swing for over four years.

The use of Wheatley's "new leadership" approach helps account for the success of this project. The college campus, in relationship to health, could be seen as chaotic; once the relationships were formed between team members, however, information and ideas flowed. The team came to understand that all connections were vital to the development of a collegewide culture that embraced health and well-being. A long-term approach to building cultural change continues in this project. **Table 30-2** shows interprofessional team members in the DNP project.

SUMMARY

Given their advanced preparation, DNPs are well positioned to participate in and lead interprofessional teams. Recognizing obstacles and developing strategies to reduce such barriers are key functions of interprofessional team leadership. All members of the interprofessional team need to have preparation and opportunities to rehearse this new approach to patient care delivery. Incorporating shared interdisciplinary learning experiences in the educational preparation of healthcare professionals provides the foundation for forming partnerships rather than competition for patient care delivery. Further study is needed to demonstrate the

TABLE 30-2	Interprofessional Team Members
Initial Task Force	Final Multi-Interprofessional Team
DNP student	DNP student
MSW mentor	MSW mentor
RN from SHS	RN from SHS
Student	Student
	Director of Institutional Research and Assessment
	VP for Enrollment Management
	Registrar
	Manager, Wellness Center
	International student advisor
	Department chair, Physical Therapy

most effective educational interventions to prepare healthcare providers for successful collaborative work.

Workforce and regulatory issues may present both challenges and opportunities for interprofessional collaborations. Shortages of physician primary care providers, particularly in rural settings, are likely to influence both the configuration and function of the interprofessional team (ACP, 2009; Minnesota Department of Health [MDH], 2009). DNP-prepared primary care providers can help to fill this gap, but must be allowed (regulatory-wise) to practice at the top of their education and scope; this will necessitate that physician colleagues reexamine and relinquish some of the responsibilities and tasks traditionally "owned" by medicine. Nursing and medicine will need to work together to devise a vision for this new collaborative practice model to most efficiently and effectively address the needs of the population and improve the quality of care provided.

The American Academy of Pediatrics' concept of "medical home" suggests that all individuals, particularly those with complex or chronic health conditions, should receive a comprehensive, coordinated approach to health care and social services (MDH, 2009). The proposed Health Care Home initiatives expand the definition of primary care provider to include physicians, APRNs, and physician assistants (MDH, 2009). The primary care provider will lead and coordinate the efforts of the interprofessional team to best meet the needs of the patient. Nurse practice acts, regulations, and reimbursement issues must be reviewed and revised to support the ability of APRNs to assume this role and deliver comprehensive care. Continued research is needed to identify the full impact of workforce and regulatory issues on these collaborations as well as strategies to address these concerns. DNPs in both direct (CNP, CNS, CRNA, CNM) and indirect provider roles (health policymakers, administrators, informatics specialists, public health experts) must continue to effectively work with other members of the healthcare team to deliver comprehensive, patient-centered care. Interprofessional collaborations are an important facet of a reformed healthcare delivery system and a vital step toward improving health outcomes and reducing medical error.

DISCUSSION QUESTIONS ——————

1. What is the difference between shared decision making and collective cognitive responsibility?

2. How does leadership differ from management?

3. Consider a conflict in your clinical practice setting. As an advanced practice nurse, what is your role in assisting the team to resolve the issue(s)?

4. What is your vision of the ideal interdisciplinary team?

REFERENCES ——————

Agency for Healthcare Research and Quality. (2009). Patient safety culture surveys. Retrieved from http://www.ahrq.gov/qual/patientsafetyculture/

American Association of Colleges of Nursing. (2006a). DNP roadmap task force report, October 20, 2006. Retrieved from http://www.aacn.nche.edu/DNP/pdf/DNProadmapreport.pdf

American Association of Colleges of Nursing. (2006b). *The essentials of doctoral education for advanced nursing practice.* Washington, DC: Author.

American College of Physicians. (2009). *Nurse practitioners in primary care* [Policy monograph]. Philadelphia: Author.

American Nurses Association. (2008, February). *Nursing's agenda for health care reform.* Silver Spring, MD: Author. Retrieved from http://www.nursingworld.org/MainMenuCategories/HealthcareandPolicyIssues/HSR/ANAsHealthSystemReformAgenda.aspx

Amos, M., Hu, J., & Herrick, C. (2005). The impact of team building on communication and job satisfaction of nursing staff. *Journal for Nurses in Staff Development, 21*(1), 10–16.

APRN Consensus Work Group & National Council of State Boards of Nursing APRN Advisory Committee. (2008, July). Consensus model for APRN regulation: Licensure, accreditation, certification and education. Retrieved from http://www.nonpf.com/Joint%20Dialogue%20ReportFinal0708.pdf

Ash, L. (2005). *Developing a population-focused student health service* (Unpublished doctoral project). Rush University, Chicago, IL.

Baker, S., Baker, K., & Campbell, M. (2003). *Complete idiot's guide to project management.* Indianapolis, IN: Alpha.

Barki, H., & Hartwick, J. (2001). Interpersonal conflict and its management in information system development. *MIS Quarterly, 25*(2), 195–228.

Begun, J., Zimmerman, B., & Dooley, K. (2003). Health care organizations as complex adaptive systems. In S. M. Mick & M. Wyttenbach (Eds.), *Advances in health care organization theory* (pp. 253–288). San Francisco: Jossey-Bass. Retrieved from http://www.change-ability.ca/Complex_Adaptive.pdf

Brett, J., Behfar, K., & Kern, M. (2006, November). Managing multicultural teams. *Harvard Business Review, 84*(11), 84–91. Retrieved from Business Source Premier database.

Brewer, C. (2005). The health care workforce. In A. Kovner & J. Knickman (Eds.), *Health care delivery in the United States* (pp. 320–326). New York: Springer.

Brita-Rossi, P., Adduci, D., Kaufman, J., Lipson, S. J., Totte, C., & Wasserman, K. (1996). Improving the process of care: The cost-quality value of interdisciplinary collaboration. *Journal of Nursing Care Quality, 10*(2), 10–16.

Buresh, B., & Gordon, S. (2006). *From silence to voice: What nurses know and must communicate to the public.* Ithaca, NY: Cornell University Press.

Burkhardt, M., & Alvita, K. (2008). *Ethics and issues in contemporary nursing.* Clifton Park, NY: Thomson Delmar Learning.

Burns, J. (1978). *Leadership.* New York: Harper and Row.

Chapman, A. (2008). Johari window: Ingham and Luft's Johari window model diagrams and examples—for self-awareness, personal development, group development and understanding relationships. Retrieved from www.businessballs.com/johariwindowmodel.htm

Chinn, P. (2008). *Peace and power.* Sudbury, MA: Jones and Bartlett.

Chung, H., & Nguyen, P. H. (2005). Changing unit culture: An interdisciplinary commitment to improve pain outcomes. *Journal for Healthcare Quality: Official Publication of the National Association for Healthcare Quality, 27*(2), 12–19.

Clarin, O. A. (2007). Strategies to overcome barriers to effective nurse practitioner and physician collaboration. *Journal for Nurse Practitioners, 3*(8), 538–548.

College of St. Scholastica. (2009). Guiding documents. Retrieved from http://www.css.edu/About/Leadership/Guiding-Documents.html

Covey, S. (1991). *Principle-centered leadership.* New York: Summit Books.

Covey, S. (2004). *The eighth habit: From effectiveness to greatness.* New York: Free Press.

Cowan, M. J., Shapiro, M., Hays, R. D., Afifi, A., Vazirani, S., Ward, C. R., et al. (2006). The effect of a multidisciplinary hospitalist/physician and advanced practice nurse collaboration on hospital costs. *Journal of Nursing Administration, 36*(2), 79–85.

Cunningham, R. (2004, March). Advanced practice nursing outcomes: A review of selected empirical literature. *Oncology Nursing Forum, 31*(2), 219–232. Retrieved from CINAHL Plus with Full Text database.

Dailey, M. (2005, April). Interdisciplinary collaboration: Essential for improved wound care outcomes and wound prevention in home care. *Home Health Care Management & Practice, 17*(3), 213–221. Retrieved from CINAHL Plus with Full Text database.

D'Amour, D., & Oandasan, I. (2005). Interprofessionality as the field of interprofessional practice and interprofessional education: An emerging concept. *Journal of Interprofessional Care, 19,* 8–20.

Davoli, G. W., & Fine, L. J. (2004). Stacking the deck for success in interprofessional collaboration. *Health Promotion Practice, 5*(3), 266–270.

Draye, M. A., Acker, M., & Zimmer, P. A. (2006). The practice doctorate in nursing: Approaches to transform nurse practitioner education and practice. *Nursing Outlook, 54*(3), 123–129.

Drinka, T., & Clark, P. (2000). *Health care teamwork: Interdisciplinary practice and teaching.* Westport, CT: Auburn House.

Dunevitz, B. (1997). Perspectives in ambulatory care: Collaboration—in a variety of ways—creates health care value. *Nursing Economics, 15*(4), 218–219.

Edmonson, A. (1999). Psychological safety and learning behavior in work teams. *Administrative Science Quarterly, 44*(2), 350–383.

Edmonson, A. (2006). Do I dare say something? *Harvard Business School Working Knowledge.* Retrieved from https://www.iterasi.net/openviewer .aspx?sqrlitid=j0ercd12deaukxst2bsbta

Feldman, H. (2008). *Nursing leadership: A concise encyclopedia.* New York: Springer.

Fortham, M., Dove, H., & Wooster, L. (2000). Episodic treatment groups (ETGs): A patient classification system for measuring outcomes performance by episode of care. *Topics in Healthcare Information Management, 21*(2), 51–61. Retrieved from http://www.thedeltagroup.com/Corporate /Pubs/ETGs.pdf

Golanowski, M., Beaudry, D., Kurz, L., Laffey, W., & Hook, M. (2007). Interdisciplinary shared decision-making: Taking shared governance to the next level. *Nursing Administration Quarterly, 31*(4), 341–353.

Goleman, D., Boyzatsis, R., & McKee, A. (2002). *Primal leadership: Realizing the power of emotional intelligence.* Boston: Harvard Business School Press.

Gordon, S. (2005). *Nursing against the odds.* Ithaca, NY: Cornell University Press.

Grabowski, M., & Roberts, K. (1999, November). Risk mitigation in virtual organizations. *Organization Science, 10*(6), 704–721. Retrieved from Business Source Premier database.

Grady, G. F., & Wojner, A. W. (1996). Collaborative practice teams: The infrastructure of outcomes management. *AACN Clinical Issues: Advanced Practice in Acute & Critical Care, 7*(1), 153–158.

Greenberg, P., Greenberg, R., & Antonucci, Y. (2007). Creating and sustaining trust in virtual teams. *Business Horizons, 50*(4), 325–333.

Haas, J., & Shaffir, W. (1987). Taking on the role of doctor. In D. Coburn, C. D'Arcy, & G. M. Torrance (Eds.), *Health and Canadian society.* Markham, Ontario, Canada: Fitzhenry & Whiteside.

Hall, P. (2005). Interprofessional teamwork: Professional cultures as barriers. *Journal of Interprofessional Care, 19*(Suppl. 1), 188–196.

Hall, P., Weaver, L., Gravelle, D., & Thibault, H. (2007). Developing collaborative person-centered practice: A pilot project on a palliative care unit. *Journal of Interprofessional Care, 21*(1), 69–81.

Hibbard, J. H., Stockard, J., Mahoney, E. R., & Tusler, M. (2004). Development of the patient activation measure (PAM): Conceptualizing and measuring activation in patient and consumers. *Health Services Research, 39*(4), 1005–1026.

Horrocks, S., Anderson, E., & Salisbury, C. (2002, April 6). Systematic review of whether nurse practitioners working in primary care can provide equivalent care to doctors. *BMJ: British Medical Journal, 324*(7341), 819–823. Retrieved from CINAHL Plus with Full Text database.

Ingersoll, G. L., McIntosh, E., & Williams, M. (2000). Nurse sensitive outcomes of advanced practice. *Journal of Advanced Nursing, 32*(5), 1272–1281.

Institute for Clinical Systems Integration. (2007). DIAMOND initiative: Depression improvement across Minnesota: Offering a new direction. Retrieved from http://www.icsi.org/colloquium _2007/diamond_panel.html

Institute of Medicine. (1999). *To err is human: Building a safer health system.* Washington, DC: National Academies Press.

Institute of Medicine. (2001). *Crossing the quality chasm: A new health system for the 21st century.* Washington, DC: National Academies Press.

Institute of Medicine. (2003). *Health professions education: A bridge to quality.* Washington, DC: National Academies Press.

The Joint Commission. (2008). Accreditation program: Ambulatory health care national patient safety goals. Retrieved from http://www.joint commission.org/NR/rdonlyres/979098FA-74FD-4F25-AF41-EDD48FBD300E/0/AHC_NPSG.pdf

Kaiser Family Foundation. (2008). President-elect Barack Obama's health care reform proposal. Retrieved from http://www.kff.org/uninsured /upload/Obama_Health_Care_Reform_Proposal .pdf

Kaiser Family Foundation/Harvard School of Public Health Survey. (2009). The public's health care agenda for the new president and congress (Publication No. 7853). Retrieved from http://www .kff.org/kaiserpolls/upload/7853.pdf

Kelly, P. (2008). *Nursing leadership and management.* Clifton Park, NY: Delmar.

Kleinpell, R. M., Faut-Callahan, M. M., Lauer, K., Kremer, M. J., Murphy, M., & Sperhac, A. (2002). Collaborative practice in advanced practice nursing in acute care. *Critical Care Nursing Clinics of North America, 14*(3), 307–313.

Kotter, J. (1990). What leaders really do. *Harvard Business Review, 68,* 104.

Kouzes, J., & Pozner, B. (2007). *The leadership challenge.* San Francisco: Wiley.

Ladden, M., Bednash, G., Stevens, D., & Moore, G. (2006). Educating interprofessional learners for quality, safety and systems improvement. *Journal of Interprofessional Care, 20*(5), 497–509.

Lambing, A., Adams, D., Fox, D., & Divine, G. (2004, August). Nurse practitioners' and physicians' care activities and clinical outcomes with an inpatient geriatric population. *Journal of the American Academy of Nurse Practitioners, 16*(8), 343–352. Retrieved from CINAHL Plus with Full Text database.

Laurant, M., Reeves, D., Hermens, R., Braspenning, J., Grol, R., & Sibbald, B. (2004, December). Substitution of doctors by nurses in primary care. *Cochrane Database of Systematic Reviews.* Retrieved from CINAHL Plus with Full Text database.

Lee, S. (2008). The five stages of team development. Retrieved from http://ezinearticles.com/?The-Five-Stages-of-Team-Development&id=1254894

Leonard, M., Graham, S., & Bonacum, D. (2004). The human factor: The critical importance of effective teamwork and communication in providing safe care. *Quality and Safety in Health Care, 13*(Supp. 1), 85–90.

Lewin, K. (1951). Frontiers in group dynamics. In D. Cartwright (Ed.), *Field theory in social science* (pp. 188–237). New York: Harper.

Lewis, J. (2007). *Fundamentals of project management.* New York: AMACOM.

Lindeke, L. L., & Block, D. E. (2001). Interdisciplinary collaboration in the 21st century. *Minnesota Medicine, 84*(6), 42–45.

Lindeke, L. L., & Sieckert, A. M. (2005). Nurse-physician workplace collaboration. *Online Journal of Issues in Nursing, 10*(1). Retrieved from http ://www.nursingworld.org/MainMenuCategories /ANAMarketplace/ANAPeriodicals/OJIN/Tableof Contents/Volume102005/No1Jan05/tpc26_416011 .aspx

Lynnaugh, J., & Reverby, S. (1990). *Ordered to care: The dilemma of American nursing 1850–1945.* New York: Cambridge University Press.

McCallin, A., & Bamford, A. (2007). Interdisciplinary teamwork: Is the influence of emotional intelligence fully appreciated? *Journal of Nursing Management, 15*(4), 386–391.

Merriam-Webster's Collegiate Dictionary (11th ed.). (2005). Springfield, MA: Merriam-Webster.

Miller, C. (2008). *Optimal use of individualized asthma action plans in an electronic health record* (Unpublished doctoral project). University of Minnesota, Minneapolis, MN.

Miller, K.-L., Reeves, S., Zwarenstein, M., Beales, J. D., Kenaszchuk, C., & Gotlib Conn, L. (2008). Nursing emotion work and interprofessional collaboration in general medicine wards: A qualitative study. *Journal of Advanced Nursing, 64*(4), 332–343.

Miller, M., Snyder, M., & Lindeke, L. (2005, September). Forces of change. Nurse practitioners: current status and future challenges. *Clinical Excellence for Nurse Practitioners, 9*(3), 162–169. Retrieved from CINAHL Plus with Full Text database.

Minnesota Department of Health. (2009). *Health workforce shortage study report: Report to the Minnesota legislature 2009.* St. Paul, MN: Author.

Mundinger, M., Kane, R., Lenz, E., Totten, A., Tsai, W., Cleary, P., et al. (2000). Primary care outcomes in patients treated by nurse practitioners or physicians: A randomized trial. *Journal of the American Medical Association, 283*(1), 59-68. Retrieved from CINAHL Plus with Full Text database.

NASPA. (2004). Leadership for a healthy campus: An ecological approach for student success. Retrieved from www.longwood.edu/Health/. . ./leadership_for_a_healthy_campus.pdf

Nelson, E. C., Batalden, P. B., Huber, T. P., Mohr, J. J., Godfrey, M. M., Headrick, L. A., et al. (2002). Microsystems in health care: Part 1. Learning from high-performing front-line clinical units. *The Joint Commission Journal on Quality Improvement, 28*(9), 472–493.

Oandasan, I., D'Amour, D., Zwarenstein, M., Barker, K., Purden, M., Beaulieu, M.-D., et al. (2004). Interprofessional education for collaborative patient-centered practice: An evolving framework [Executive summary]. Retrieved from www.hc-sc.gc.ca/hcs-sss/hhr-rhs/strateg/interprof/summ-somm-eng.php

O'Connor, A. (2006). *Ottawa personal decision guide* [Pamphlet]. University of Ottawa: Ottawa Health Research Institute.

Patterson, K., Grenny, J., McMillan, R., & Switzler, A. (2002). *Crucial conversations: Tools for talking when stakes are high.* New York: McGraw Hill.

Porter-O'Grady, T. (1997). *Whole systems shared governance.* Gaithersburg, MD: Aspen.

Reeves, S., Zwarenstein, M., Goldman, J., Barr, H., Freeth, D., Hammick, M., et al. (2008). Interprofessional education: Effects on professional practice and health care outcomes [Review]. *Cochrane Database of Systematic Reviews, 1,* CD002213. doi:10.1002/14651858.CD002213.pub2

Ring, P. (2005, January). Collaboration. In *Blackwell encyclopedic dictionary of organizational behavior.* Retrieved from Blackwell Encyclopedia of Management Library database.

Robert Wood Johnson Foundation. (2008, April). Partnerships for quality education (Robert Wood Johnson Grant Results Reports). Retrieved from http://www.rwjf.org/reports/npreports/pqe.htm

Rosenstein, A. (2002). The impact of nurse–physician relationships on nurse satisfaction and retention. *American Journal of Nursing, 102*(6), 26–34.

Rosenstein, A., & O'Daniel, M. (2008). A survey of the impacts of disruptive behaviors and communication defects on public safety. *The Joint Commission Journal on Quality and Patient Safety, 34*(8), 464–471.

Sacher, L., Moses, K., Fabiano, P., Haubenreiser, J., Grizzel, J., & Mart, S. (2005). *College health: Stretch your definitions of the core concepts, assumptions and practices.* American College Health Association. PowerPoint presentation at NASPA (Student Affairs Administration in Higher Education) session, March 22, 2005, Washington, DC.

Scardamalia, M. (2002). Collective cognitive responsibility for the advancement of knowledge. In B. Smith (Ed.), *Liberal education in a knowledge society* (pp. 67–98). Chicago: Open Court.

Senge, P. (1990). *The art and discipline of the learning organization.* New York: Doubleday.

Sierchio, G. P. (2003). A multidisciplinary approach for improving outcomes. *Journal of Infusion Nursing, 26*(1), 34–43.

Snijders, C., Kollen, B., Van Lingen, R., Fetter, W., & Molendijk, H. (2009). Which aspects of safety culture predict incident reporting behavior in neonatal intensive care units? A multilevel analysis. *Critical Care Medicine, 37*(1), 61–67.

Sullivan, E. J. (2004). *Becoming influential: A guide for nurses.* Upper Saddle River, NJ: Pearson Prentice Hall.

Tuckman, B. W., & Jensen, M. A. C. (1977). Stages of small-group development revisited. *Group & Organization Management, 2*(4), 419–427. doi:10.1177/105960117700200404

U.S. Department of Health and Human Services. (2000). *Healthy People 2010.* Rockville, MD: Author. Retrieved from http://www.healthypeople.gov/

Vahey, D. C., Aiken, L. H., Sloane, D. M., Clarke, S. P., & Vargas, D. (2004). Nurse burnout and patient satisfaction. *Medical Care, 42*(Suppl. 2), 1157–1166.

Wheatley, M. (2005). *Finding our way: Leadership for an uncertain time.* San Francisco: Berrett-Koehler.

Whitehead, C. (2007). The doctor dilemma in interprofessional education and care: How and why will physicians collaborate? *Medical Education, 41*(10), 1010–1016.

Wilson, J., & Bekemeir, B. (2004). Public health. In *Encyclopedia of leadership* (Vol. 3, pp. 1271–1274). Thousand Oaks, CA: Sage.

Yeager, S. (2005). Interdisciplinary collaboration: The heart and soul of healthcare. *Critical Care Nursing Clinics of North America, 17*(2), 143–148.

Index

Exhibits, figures, and tables are indicated by exh, f, and t following the page number.